Mitochondria-Targeted Drug Delivery

Mitochondria-Targeted Drug Delivery

Editor

Joanna Kopecka

MDPI • Basel • Beijing • Wuhan • Barcelona • Belgrade • Manchester • Tokyo • Cluj • Tianjin

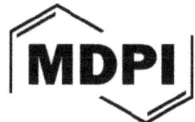

Editor
Joanna Kopecka
University of Turin
Italy

Editorial Office
MDPI
St. Alban-Anlage 66
4052 Basel, Switzerland

This is a reprint of articles from the Special Issue published online in the open access journal *Pharmaceutics* (ISSN 1999-4923) (available at: https://www.mdpi.com/journal/pharmaceutics/special_issues/mitochondria_targeted_delivery).

For citation purposes, cite each article independently as indicated on the article page online and as indicated below:

LastName, A.A.; LastName, B.B.; LastName, C.C. Article Title. *Journal Name* **Year**, *Volume Number*, Page Range.

ISBN 978-3-0365-4039-9 (Hbk)
ISBN 978-3-0365-4040-5 (PDF)

© 2022 by the authors. Articles in this book are Open Access and distributed under the Creative Commons Attribution (CC BY) license, which allows users to download, copy and build upon published articles, as long as the author and publisher are properly credited, which ensures maximum dissemination and a wider impact of our publications.

The book as a whole is distributed by MDPI under the terms and conditions of the Creative Commons license CC BY-NC-ND.

Contents

About the Editor ix

Joanna Kopecka
Mitochondria-Targeted Drug Delivery
Reprinted from: *Pharmaceutics* **2022**, *14*, 178, doi:10.3390/pharmaceutics14010178 1

Yoon-ha Jang, Sae Ryun Ahn, Ji-yeon Shim and Kwang-il Lim
Engineering Genetic Systems for Treating Mitochondrial Diseases
Reprinted from: *Pharmaceutics* **2021**, *13*, 810, doi:10.3390/pharmaceutics13060810 5

Emanuela Bottani, Costanza Lamperti, Alessandro Prigione, Valeria Tiranti, Nicola Persico and Dario Brunetti
Therapeutic Approaches to Treat Mitochondrial Diseases: "One-Size-Fits-All" and "Precision Medicine" Strategies
Reprinted from: *Pharmaceutics* **2020**, *12*, 1083, doi:10.3390/pharmaceutics12111083 25

Francesca Forini, Paola Canale, Giuseppina Nicolini and Giorgio Iervasi
Mitochondria-Targeted Drug Delivery in Cardiovascular Disease: A Long Road to Nano-Cardio Medicine
Reprinted from: *Pharmaceutics* **2020**, *12*, 1122, doi:10.3390/pharmaceutics12111122 89

Jeffrey Farooq, You Jeong Park, Justin Cho, Madeline Saft, Nadia Sadanandan, Blaise Cozene and Cesar V. Borlongan
Stem Cells as Drug-like Biologics for Mitochondrial Repair in Stroke
Reprinted from: *Pharmaceutics* **2020**, *12*, 615, doi:10.3390/pharmaceutics12070615 113

Ekaterina M. Fock and Rimma G. Parnova
Protective Effect of Mitochondria-Targeted Antioxidants against Inflammatory Response to Lipopolysaccharide Challenge: A Review
Reprinted from: *Pharmaceutics* **2021**, *13*, 144, doi:10.3390/pharmaceutics13020144 129

Martina Godel, Giacomo Ortone, Dario Pasquale Anobile, Martina Pasino, Giulio Randazzo, Chiara Riganti and Joanna Kopecka
Targeting Mitochondrial Oncometabolites: A New Approach to Overcome Drug Resistance in Cancer
Reprinted from: *Pharmaceutics* **2021**, *13*, 762, doi:10.3390/pharmaceutics13050762 153

Faustino Mollinedo and Consuelo Gajate
Mitochondrial Targeting Involving Cholesterol-Rich Lipid Rafts in the Mechanism of Action of the Antitumor Ether Lipid and Alkylphospholipid Analog Edelfosine
Reprinted from: *Pharmaceutics* **2021**, *13*, 763, doi:10.3390/pharmaceutics13050763 169

Jae-Seon Lee, Jiwon Choi, Seon-Hyeong Lee, Joon Hee Kang, Ji Sun Ha, Hee Yeon Kim, Hyonchol Jang, Jong In Yook and Soo-Youl Kim
Oxoglutarate Carrier Inhibition Reduced Melanoma Growth and Invasion by Reducing ATP Production
Reprinted from: *Pharmaceutics* **2020**, *12*, 1128, doi:10.3390/pharmaceutics12111128 197

Haoran Zhang, Aijun Zhang, Anisha A. Gupte and Dale J. Hamilton
Plumbagin Elicits Cell-Specific Cytotoxic Effects and Metabolic Responses in Melanoma Cells
Reprinted from: *Pharmaceutics* **2021**, *13*, 706, doi:10.3390/pharmaceutics13050706 211

Sergejs Zavadskis, Adelheid Weidinger, Dominik Hanetseder, Asmita Banerjee, Cornelia Schneider, Susanne Wolbank, Darja Marolt Presen and Andrey V. Kozlov
Effect of Diphenyleneiodonium Chloride on Intracellular Reactive Oxygen Species Metabolism with Emphasis on NADPH Oxidase and Mitochondria in Two Therapeutically Relevant Human Cell Types
Reprinted from: *Pharmaceutics* **2021**, *13*, 10, doi:10.3390/pharmaceutics13010010 . . . . **227**

Consuelo Ripoll, Pilar Herrero-Foncubierta, Virginia Puente-Muñoz,
M. Carmen Gonzalez-Garcia, Delia Miguel, Sandra Resa, Jose M. Paredes,
Maria J. Ruedas-Rama, Emilio Garcia-Fernandez, Mar Roldan, Susana Rocha,
Herlinde De Keersmaecker, Johan Hofkens, Miguel Martin, Juan M. Cuerva and Angel Orte
Chimeric Drug Design with a Noncharged Carrier for Mitochondrial Delivery
Reprinted from: *Pharmaceutics* **2021**, *13*, 254, doi:10.3390/pharmaceutics13020254 . . . . **247**

Michał Burdukiewicz, Katarzyna Sidorczuk, Dominik Rafacz, Filip Pietluch,
Mateusz Bakała, Jadwiga Słowik, Przemysław Gagat
CancerGram: An Effective Classifier for Differentiating Anticancer from Antimicrobial Peptides
Reprinted from: *Pharmaceutics* **2020**, *12*, 1045, doi:10.3390/pharmaceutics12111045 . . . . **265**

About the Editor

Joanna Kopecka received her PhD degree from the University of Turin, Italy in 2013. Her research focuses on the basis of chemoresistance and immunoresistance in cancer cells. In particular, she is interested in finding new therapeutic approaches through which resistant cancer cells can be targeted, using both pharmacological and molecular biology tools. She has coauthored more than 70 scientific papers, abstracts and reviews.

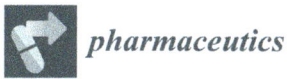

Editorial

Mitochondria-Targeted Drug Delivery

Joanna Kopecka

Department of Oncology, University of Torino, Via Santena 5/bis, 10126 Torino, Italy; joanna.kopecka@unito.it

Citation: Kopecka, J. Mitochondria-Targeted Drug Delivery. *Pharmaceutics* **2022**, *14*, 178. https://doi.org/10.3390/pharmaceutics14010178

Received: 6 January 2022
Accepted: 11 January 2022
Published: 13 January 2022

Publisher's Note: MDPI stays neutral with regard to jurisdictional claims in published maps and institutional affiliations.

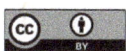

Copyright: © 2022 by the author. Licensee MDPI, Basel, Switzerland. This article is an open access article distributed under the terms and conditions of the Creative Commons Attribution (CC BY) license (https://creativecommons.org/licenses/by/4.0/).

Mitochondria, organelles surrounded by a double membrane and with their own small genome, are the cells' energy centres. Besides the production of ATP through cellular respiration, mitochondria play a pivotal role in other aspects of the life and death of a cell: heat production, programmed cell death, regulation of metabolic activity, immunity, and calcium homeostasis. A number of diseases are associated with mitochondrial dysfunction, including cardiovascular, neurological, inflammatory, metabolic disorders and cancer. Mitochondria therefore represent an important therapeutic target, and it is not surprising that a number of different treatment strategies have emerged. Approaches targeting mitochondria can be split into two opposite categories: drugs that restore mitochondrial function and drugs that trigger mitochondria-mediated cell death. Targeted drug delivery to obtain a selective accumulation of drug molecules in mitochondria is complex and involves methods such as direct drug modification or encapsulation into nanocarriers.

This Special Issue's goal is to present the current state of the art in the field. We invite reviews or original articles on mitochondria as a promising target for treating a wide range of human diseases and pathological conditions, as well as articles on recent approaches for mitochondria-targeted drug delivery.

In this Special Issue, 76 authors representing 71 affiliations from 7 countries over 3 continents have made 12 contributions, and it is my great privilege and pleasure to introduce this collective work which summarizes important insights in this field of research.

As mentioned above, mitochondria contain DNA and therefore are involved in genetic disorders reviewed in this Special Issue by Jang et al. Jang et al. showed relevant core genetic components involved in mitochondria linked diseases and recent genetic approaches to alleviate and/or reverse negative effects of the core component mutations on the physiology and functions of mitochondria [1]. In particular mutations in the mitochondrial genome or in the nuclear genes encoding for proteins involved in oxidative phosphorylation (OXPHOS) may cause primary mitochondrial diseases (PMD). A group of severe often inherited genetic disorders that now are under intensive investigation aimed to find the best experimental treatments. The therapeutic approaches to treat PDM was reviewed by Bottani et al. presenting both more general approaches and precision medicine strategies [2]. Besides, genetic disorders mitochondria play also a key role in cardiovascular disfunctions as nicely summed up by Forini et al. In this interesting review, authors discuss advance in nanotechnology research aimed to improve pharmacokinetic and biocompatibility in mitochondria-targeted drug delivery systems to contrast cardiovascular diseases [3]. In line with importance of mitochondria in cardiovascular pathologies, review of Farooq et al. describes tissue condition after the stroke where sufficient mitochondrial activity is necessary for cell survival. Lacking mitochondria in damaged tissues can be obtained from astrocytes in order to rescue them, however without the capacity to completely repair damaged tissues. Farooq et al. investigate current literature about mitochondrial transfer pathway as a target of future therapeutic strategies with an emphasis on stem cells as a source of healthy mitochondria [4]. Tissue damage and mitochondria in the contest of inflammation due to the response to lipopolysaccharide (LPS) present in outer membrane of Gram-negative bacteria is an object of Fock and Parnova's review. The authors describe the newest finding in the field of protection against LPS induced inflammatory response. LPS causes oxidative stress and mitochondrial dysfunction therefore application of different mitochondria-targeted antioxidants have beneficial influence on the cells and protects cells and tissues from damage [5]. Mitochondria are also important in cancer. Alternated tricarboxylic acid cycle leads to production of oncometabolites increasing cancer aggressiveness and drug resistance as reviewed by Godel et al. In addition to detailed description of oncometabolites role in response to anticancer therapy, authors of this review describe the state of the art in pharmacological strategies targeting oncometabolites production in order to improve the efficacy of cancer treatment [6]. Targeting mitochondria often aims to enhance apoptosis of cancer cells. For example, Mollinedo and Gajate reviewed the involvement of cholesterol transport and cholesterol-rich lipid rafts in the interactions between the organelles as well as in the role of mitochondria in the regulation of apoptosis in cancer cells and cancer therapy. In particular they concentrate their effort on the role of alkylphospholipid analogs such as ether lipid edelfosine that induces the redistribution of lipid rafts from the plasma membrane to the mitochondria, reorganization of raft-located mitochondrial proteins that critically modulate cell death or survival [7]. Targeting mitochondria often aims to inhibit cancer growth. Indeed, Lee et al. have showed that blocking of oxoglutarate carrier decreased transport of NADH from cytosol to mitochondria, resulting in efficient inhibition of melanoma growth in vitro and in vivo due to suppression of mitochondrial activity and reduction of ATP production [8]. Interestingly, efficacy of drugs targeting mitochondria depends on cell metabolism as demonstrated by Zhang et al. They showed that distinctive mitochondrial metabolism in melanoma cells characterized by different invasiveness influences cytotoxic effects of plumbagin (PLB). PLB anticancer effects are mediated partially by modulation of mitochondrial electron transport and induction of reactive oxygen species. Indeed, PLB displays stronger cytotoxic effects on A375 cells, which exhibit lower respiratory function than SK-MEL-28 cells with higher respiratory function. At contrary to SK-MEL-28, A375 cells after the treatment with PLB have decreased mitochondrial OXPHOS and ATP production with elevated mitochondrial membrane potential [9]. Similar results were obtained by Zavadskis et al. using human amniotic membrane mesenchymal stromal cells (hAMSCs), human bone marrow mesenchymal stromal cells (hBMSCs) and MG-63 cells. They have showed that cytotoxic effect of diphenyleneiodonium (DPI) depends on type of the metabolism used by the cells. Thus, in cell types prevalently using glycolysis, DPI predominantly interacts with nicotinamide adenine dinucleotide phosphate oxidase, while the mitochondria remain unaffected. In contrast, in cells with aerobic energy metabolism, the mitochondria become an additional target for DPI. As a result, cells relying more on aerobic metabolism such as MG-63 or osteoblast-like cells are more sensitive to the toxic effects of DPI, while cells predominantly living from glycolysis, such as hAMSCs, are more resistant to the toxic effects of DPI suggesting that undifferentiated cells rather than differentiated parenchymal cells should be considered as potential targets for DPI [10]. To effectively target mitochondria drugs need to be delivered specifically and although some drugs may accumulate prevalently in mitochondria due to their physicochemical nature, often a targeting vehicle is needed. Ripoll et al, have showed promising new carrier to target mitochondria based on nonprotonable, noncharged thiophene ring. Authors used this construction to prepare chimeric drug deliver using the carrier and pyruvate dehydrogenase kinase inhibitor dichloroacetate demonstrating utility of thiophene moiety as a noncharged carrier for targeting mitochondria with metabolism-targeting drugs [11]. Alternatively, the drugs maybe designed specifically. For instance, Burdukiewicz et al. have showed a robust computational tool, CancerGram helping researchers to find appropriate anticancer peptides to target mitochondria in the cancer cells [12].

In conclusion, this Special Issue underlines importance of mitochondria in pathophysiological situation such as: genetic disorders [1,2], cardiovascular diseases [3,4], inflammation [5] and cancer [6–10]. Indicates new tools to selective target mitochondria in order to: rescue aberrant cell phenotype, change cell metabolism or induces mitochondria dependent cell death [1–12].

Funding: This research received no external funding.

Conflicts of Interest: The author declares no conflict of interest.

References

1. Jang, Y.-h.; Ahn, S.R.; Shim, J.-y.; Lim, K.-i. Engineering Genetic Systems for Treating Mitochondrial Diseases. *Pharmaceutics* **2021**, *13*, 810. [CrossRef] [PubMed]
2. Bottani, E.; Lamperti, C.; Prigione, A.; Tiranti, V.; Persico, N.; Brunetti, D. Therapeutic Approaches to Treat Mitochondrial Diseases: "One-Size-Fits-All" and "Precision Medicine" Strategies. *Pharmaceutics* **2020**, *12*, 1083. [CrossRef] [PubMed]
3. Forini, F.; Canale, P.; Nicolini, G.; Iervasi, G. Mitochondria-Targeted Drug Delivery in Cardiovascular Disease: A Long Road to Nano-Cardio Medicine. *Pharmaceutics* **2020**, *12*, 1122. [CrossRef] [PubMed]
4. Farooq, J.; Park, Y.J.; Cho, J.; Saft, M.; Sadanandan, N.; Cozene, B.; Borlongan, C.V. Stem Cells as Drug-like Biologics for Mitochondrial Repair in Stroke. *Pharmaceutics* **2020**, *12*, 615. [CrossRef] [PubMed]
5. Fock, E.M.; Parnova, R.G. Protective Effect of Mitochondria-Targeted Antioxidants against Inflammatory Response to Lipopolysaccharide Challenge: A Review. *Pharmaceutics* **2021**, *13*, 144. [CrossRef] [PubMed]
6. Godel, M.; Ortone, G.; Anobile, D.P.; Pasino, M.; Randazzo, G.; Riganti, C.; Kopecka, J. Targeting Mitochondrial Oncometabolites: A New Approach to Overcome Drug Resistance in Cancer. *Pharmaceutics* **2021**, *13*, 762. [CrossRef] [PubMed]
7. Mollinedo, F.; Gajate, C. Mitochondrial Targeting Involving Cholesterol-Rich Lipid Rafts in the Mechanism of Action of the Antitumor Ether Lipid and Alkylphospholipid Analog Edelfosine. *Pharmaceutics* **2021**, *13*, 763. [CrossRef] [PubMed]
8. Lee, J.-S.; Choi, J.; Lee, S.-H.; Kang, J.H.; Ha, J.S.; Kim, H.Y.; Jang, H.; Yook, J.I.; Kim, S.-Y. Oxoglutarate Carrier Inhibition Reduced Melanoma Growth and Invasion by Reducing ATP Production. *Pharmaceutics* **2020**, *12*, 1128. [CrossRef] [PubMed]
9. Zhang, H.; Zhang, A.; Gupte, A.A.; Hamilton, D.J. Plumbagin Elicits Cell-Specific Cytotoxic Effects and Metabolic Responses in Melanoma Cells. *Pharmaceutics* **2021**, *13*, 706. [CrossRef] [PubMed]
10. Zavadskis, S.; Weidinger, A.; Hanetseder, D.; Banerjee, A.; Schneider, C.; Wolbank, S.; Marolt Presen, D.; Kozlov, A.V. Effect of Diphenyleneiodonium Chloride on Intracellular Reactive Oxygen Species Metabolism with Emphasis on NADPH Oxidase and Mitochondria in Two Therapeutically Relevant Human Cell Types. *Pharmaceutics* **2021**, *13*, 10. [CrossRef] [PubMed]
11. Ripoll, C.; Herrero-Foncubierta, P.; Puente-Muñoz, V.; Gonzalez-Garcia, M.C.; Miguel, D.; Resa, S.; Paredes, J.M.; Ruedas-Rama, M.J.; Garcia-Fernandez, E.; Roldan, M.; et al. Chimeric Drug Design with a Noncharged Carrier for Mitochondrial Delivery. *Pharmaceutics* **2021**, *13*, 254. [CrossRef] [PubMed]
12. Burdukiewicz, M.; Sidorczuk, K.; Rafacz, D.; Pietluch, F.; Bąkała, M.; Słowik, J.; Gagat, P. CancerGram: An Effective Classifier for Differentiating Anticancer from Antimicrobial Peptides. *Pharmaceutics* **2020**, *12*, 1045. [CrossRef] [PubMed]

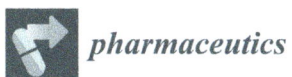

Review

Engineering Genetic Systems for Treating Mitochondrial Diseases

Yoon-ha Jang [1,†], Sae Ryun Ahn [2,†], Ji-yeon Shim [1] and Kwang-il Lim [1,2,*]

- [1] Department of Chemical and Biological Engineering, Sookmyung Women's University, Yongsan-gu, Seoul 04310, Korea; miin_yj@sookmyung.ac.kr (Y.-h.J.); 94sjy@naver.com (J.-y.S.)
- [2] Industry Collaboration Center, Industry-Academic Cooperation Foundation, Sookmyung Women's University, Yongsan-gu, Seoul 04310, Korea; saeryun@sookmyung.ac.kr
- * Correspondence: klim@sookmyung.ac.kr; Tel.: +82-2-710-7627
- † These authors contributed equally to this work.

Abstract: Mitochondria are intracellular energy generators involved in various cellular processes. Therefore, mitochondrial dysfunction often leads to multiple serious diseases, including neurodegenerative and cardiovascular diseases. A better understanding of the underlying mitochondrial dysfunctions of the molecular mechanism will provide important hints on how to mitigate the symptoms of mitochondrial diseases and eventually cure them. In this review, we first summarize the key parts of the genetic processes that control the physiology and functions of mitochondria and discuss how alterations of the processes cause mitochondrial diseases. We then list up the relevant core genetic components involved in these processes and explore the mutations of the components that link to the diseases. Lastly, we discuss recent attempts to apply multiple genetic methods to alleviate and further reverse the adverse effects of the core component mutations on the physiology and functions of mitochondria.

Keywords: mitochondrial disease; gene therapy; mitochondrial DNA; heteroplasmy; mitochondrial gene delivery

1. Introduction

Mitochondria are intracellular organelles that produce cellular energy in the form of adenosine triphosphate (ATP) through oxidative phosphorylation. Mitochondria have their own genomes as circular forms of DNA. Mitochondrial DNA (mtDNA) encodes 13 messenger RNAs (mRNAs), 2 ribosomal RNAs (rRNAs), and 22 transfer RNAs (tRNAs) required for the production of 13 protein subunits of the electron transport chain that performs oxidative phosphorylation [1]. Most cells have hundreds of mitochondria containing 2–10 copies of mtDNA [2]. More than one type of mtDNA molecule coexist in a cell. The resulting mitochondrial genome sequence heterogeneity represents a state of mitochondrial heteroplasmy [3].

Hundreds of mutations at different mtDNA sites have been reported to reduce the expression of the functional gene products required for oxidative phosphorylation [4]. When the portion of mtDNAs with such mutations out of the total mtDNAs in a cell exceeds a threshold, typically ranging from 0.6 to 0.8, the corresponding cell can be in a disease state [5]. For example, when the portion of mtDNA with the m.8993T > C mutation within the MT-ATP6 gene is higher than 0.7, neurogenic muscle weakness, ataxia, and retinitis pigmentosa (NARP) syndrome can develop. A proportion of the mutant mtDNA > 0.9 links to the development of Leigh syndrome [6].

Mutations in protein-coding mitochondrial genes can cause diseases, including Leber's hereditary optic neuropathy (LHON), mitochondrial encephalopathy, lactic acidosis, stroke-like episodes (MELAS) syndrome, and cardiomyopathy, by resulting in the production of non-functional proteins that cannot perform oxidative phosphorylation or interfere with the reaction [7–9]. Given the limited resources for transcription and translation in mitochondria, such mutations can also indirectly cause a reduction in the production of functional proteins involved in the phosphorylation reaction. In addition, mutations in the regulatory regions and the genes encoding rRNA and tRNA in the mtDNAs can also lead to diseases such as Alzheimer's disease (AD), tubulointerstitial kidney disease, ataxia, maternally inherited deafness or aminoglycoside-induced deafness (DEAF), and MELAS by altering the copy number of mtDNAs and the efficiencies of transcription and translation in mitochondria [10–13]. Various products of the genes encoded in the nuclear DNA (nDNA) also actively participate in maintaining the physiology and functions of mitochondria. Therefore, we can easily expect that mutations of such genes also cause a reduction in the rates of the oxidative phosphorylation reaction, eventually inducing the disease state of ATP deficiency [14,15].

To date, multiple attempts have been made to treat the mitochondrial disease states caused by DNA mutations [16–19]. These include targeted degradation of the mtDNA with pathogenic mutations and the introduction of a corrected version of genetic components into cells to increase the production of key parts involved in ATP production of mitochondria. In this review, we first describe the key genetic components and regulations that maintain the physiology and functions of mitochondria. Next, we list the pathogenic mutations in the genetic components and the resulting diseases. Lastly, we discuss recent therapeutic approaches to treat mitochondrial dysfunction caused by the mutations.

2. Regulations of Expression of Mitochondrial Genes

Replication of mtDNA is needed to maintain the copy number of the genetic materials in mitochondria. The replication also dynamically affects the heteroplasmic states of mtDNAs [20,21]. The genes in mitochondrial mtDNAs are expressed within the matrix space [22]. Mitochondrial genes are transcribed to produce long polycistronic transcripts. Through processing and maturation, the long transcripts become mRNAs, rRNAs, and tRNAs. These RNAs are involved in the translation of mitochondrial proteins [15,23]. The expression level of mitochondrial genes critically affects the organelle functions. Thus, sophisticated regulations of mitochondrial gene expression are important to maintaining cellular physiology [15,24]. Many factors encoded in nDNA are also transported to mitochondria and participate in mitochondrial gene regulations [25]. In this section, we describe how the regulations of mtDNA replication and transcription affect the mitochondrial gene expression levels. In addition, we discuss the known mutations in mtDNA and nDNA that cause disease by altering mitochondrial gene expression.

2.1. mtDNA Replication
2.1.1. Overview of mtDNA Replication

Mammalian mtDNA is a circular, double-stranded molecule composed of a heavy (H) and a light (L) strand [26]. Each strand has a replication origin and nuclear-encoded replication factors mediate the synthesis of new strands of mtDNA through interactions with regulatory elements in mitochondrial genomes [27]. Most regulatory elements are concentrated in the mtDNA control region. According to the strand displacement model for mtDNA replication, the synthesis of the H-strand DNA is initiated at the replication origin of the H-strand (O_H) [28,29]. RNA primers required for the initiation of DNA replication are transcribed from the L-strand and then processed by RNase mitochondrial RNA processing (MRP) complex [30]. A G-quadruplex structure between nascent RNA and non-template DNA forms at the guanine-rich conserved sequence block 2, which is located downstream of the L-strand promoter. The G-quadruplex promotes premature termination of transcription [31]. Next, RNase H1 processes the 3′end of the produced RNA, making it accessible to DNA polymerase gamma (POLγ) and function as a primer for DNA synthesis [32]. The POLγ synthesizes the H-strand DNA with the help of hexameric DNA helicase (TWINKLE) and tetrameric single-stranded DNA-binding protein (SSBP1) [33,34]. TWINKLE uncoils double-stranded DNA at the replication fork. SSBP1 prevents the formation of secondary structures of the uncoiled DNA, which is a required condition for sufficient processivity of POLγ [33,34]. The synthesis of the H-strand continues until the replication machinery reaches the O_L, which is located approximately 11 kbp downstream of O_H. Next, the H-strand at the origin folds into a stem–loop structure containing a poly-dT stretch. The stem–loop prevents SSBP1 from binding and mitochondrial RNA polymerase (POLRMT) synthesizes short RNA primers of around 25 nucleotides (nt) from the loop region. After the short RNA synthesis, POLRMT is replaced by POLγ, and L-strand DNA synthesis is initiated from the 3′end of the RNA primer [35]. Synthesis of both DNA strands continues until two new mtDNA molecules are formed [27,36]. The mtDNA replication machinery composed of the nuclear-encoded POLγ, TWINKLE, and SSBP1 proteins, is the main player in the mtDNA replication reactions.

2.1.2. Mutations of the Replication Regulatory Elements Encoded in mtDNA

Mutations in the control region of mtDNA broadly affect the mitochondrial genetic system and are associated with mitochondrial diseases such as AD, Huntington's disease, and melanoma [37–39]. For example, in brain samples of AD patients, multiple mutations were identified at different sites in the control region of mtDNA. The samples harbored mutations in the control region at frequencies 63% higher than the frequencies for the control case. The frequencies of mutations in the upstream portion (within the first 100 bases) of the control region of mtDNA (approximately 1100 bases) were not different between the AD patients and the control cases. In contrast, the frequency of mutations in the central portion (between bases 101 and 570), where the regulatory elements are enriched, was clearly higher for the AD patient cases [40]. Mutations at the conserved sequence block I (CSBI) and mitochondrial transcription factor A (TFAM) binding sites are also often found in AD patients. The m.414T > G, m.414T > C, and m.477T > C mutations are representative examples.

Similarly, several studies have found additional mutations in the mtDNA control region, which are associated with other diseases, by obtaining the corresponding DNA sequences for patients [38,41]. The mutations, m.16145G > A and m.16311T > C are associated with a higher risk of stroke [11]. It was speculated that the m.16,145G > A mutation perturbs the premature termination of H-strand elongation. This speculation was based on the fact that the mutation site is located near the termination-associated sequence responsible for DNA replication termination [42]. It was also predicted that the mutation m.16311T > C can reduce the stability of the secondary structure of the local DNA region containing base 16,311 [41]. The secondary structure of the mtDNA control region affects the binding of regulatory factors involved in mtDNA replication and transcription. Thus, mutations in this region can alter mitochondrial physiology and functions [43]. On the other hand, mutations in mtDNA that include m.72T > C, m.73A > G, and m.16356T > C may decrease the progression of myocardial infarction (MI) [41]. In addition, single nucleotide polymorphisms in the control regions of mtDNA can increase (m.16069C > T, m.16126T > C, m.16189T > C, m.16519T > C, and m.16223C > T) or decrease (m.16150C > T, m.16086T > C, and m.16195T > C) the risk of Huntington's disease [38]. Various pathogenic mutations in the control region of mtDNA are listed in the Human Mitochondrial Genome Database (MITOMAP) [44].

2.1.3. Mutations of the Nuclear Genes Involved in mtDNA Replication

Similar to the mutations in the control regions of mtDNA, those in the nuclear genes that encode the factors involved in mtDNA replication can affect the physiology and functions of mitochondria [14]. In many cases, pathogenic mutations in this group of nuclear genes lead to mitochondrial diseases by reducing mtDNA replication efficiency and causing mtDNA depletion and multiple rearrangements (mostly deletions and rarely duplications) (Table 1) [45,46]. For example, mutations in the POLG gene that encodes POLγ are linked to various diseases, including progressive external ophthalmoplegia (PEO), mitochondrial recessive ataxia syndrome (MIRAS), Parkinsonism, and Alpers–Huttenlocher syndrome [47].

To determine the mechanisms by which mutations in nuclear genes cause mitochondrial dysfunction, genetic analysis of a patient with late-onset autosomal recessive PEO (arPEO) was performed. The analysis revealed two pathogenic heterozygous missense mutations in the POLG gene: c.590T > C; Phe197Ser and c.2740A > C; Thr914Pro. The Phe197Ser mutation in the 3'-5' exonuclease domain of POLγ reduced the exonuclease and polymerase activities of the enzyme. This reduced polymerase activity can lead to a pause of mtDNA replication during L-strand synthesis, eventually resulting in multiple mtDNA deletions. The protein with the Thr914Pro mutation has no DNA-binding affinity and therefore cannot support DNA synthesis [48].

Table 1. Diseases caused by mutations of the proteins regulating mtDNA replication.

Gene	Function	Disease	References
POLG	POLγ catalytic subunit	MIRAS, Parkinsonism, AHS, MCHS, MEMSA, ANS, ad/ar PEO, male infertility, testicular cancer	[47,51]
POLG2	POLγ accessory subunit	adPEO	[52]
TWINKLE	mtDNA helicase	PEO, hepatopathy, spinocerebellar ataxia, epileptic encephalopathy	[49]
RNASE H1	Endoribonuclease of the RNA-DNA hybrid	CPEO, exercise intolerance	[53]
SSBP1	Subunit of ssDNA-binding complex	optic atrophy	[50]
MGME1	Metal dependent ssDNA exonuclease	recessive multi-systemic mitochondrial disorder	[54]
TOP3A	Topoisomerase	CPEO plus syndrome	[55]
TFAM	Transcription factor	neonatal failure	[56]

Abbreviations: MIRAS, Mitochondrial recessive ataxia syndrome; AHS, Alpers–Huttenlocher syndrome; MCHS, myocerebrohepatopathy spectrum; MEMSA, myopathy sensory ataxia; ANS, ataxia neuropathy spectrum; CPEO, chronic progressive external ophthalmoplegia.

Pathogenic missense mutations were also found within four functional domains of TWINKLE: mitochondrial targeting sequence, trimase-like domain, linker region, and helicase domain. Mutations in each domain resulted in the disruption of the corresponding function required for the full activity of TWINKLE. These severely decreased functions are the causes of mitochondrial diseases such as autosomal dominant PEO (adPEO), Perrault syndrome 5, mtDNA depletion syndrome 7, and mitochondrial hepatopathy [49]. Del Dotto et al. also identified five SSBP1 mutations associated with an optic atrophy spectrum disorder by whole-exome sequencing of five unrelated families and analyzed the effects of the mutations on mtDNA maintenance. These mutations were shown to alter the stability and multimer formation of SSBP1. The SSBP1 mutations decreased the mtDNA copy number in cells by reducing the mtDNA replication rate and resulted in mitochondrial diseases. The levels of mitochondrial dysfunction varied depending on the type of mutation of the SSBP1 gene [50].

2.2. Mitochondrial Transcription

2.2.1. Overview of mtDNA Transcription

Transcription of mtDNA is initiated by the action of three promoters in the control region: light strand promoter (LSP), heavy strand promoter 1 (HSP1), and HSP2. LSP and HSP2 are responsible for synthesizing near-genome-length transcripts that are polycistronic, containing a single mRNA and eight tRNAs, and twelve mRNAs, thirteen tRNAs, and two rRNAs, respectively. In contrast, HSP1-mediated transcription produces a relatively short transcript containing two tRNAs and two rRNAs [57]. POLRMT initiates transcription of mtDNA by interacting with the three promoters to form transcription initiation machinery with TFAM and mitochondrial transcription factor B2 (TFB2M). After binding of TFAM upstream of the transcriptional start site, TFAM anchors POLRMT to the sites upstream of LSP and HSP1 and then recruits TFB2M, which later melts the promoter DNA sequence [58]. Once the transcription is initiated, the mitochondrial transcription elongation factor (TEFM) increases the processivity of POLRMT, resulting in the production of near-genome-length transcripts [59]. The individual mRNAs and rRNAs in the polycistronic transcripts are mostly separated by tRNAs. RNase P and elaC ribonuclease Z 2 (ELAC2) mediate the endonucleolytic cleavage at the 5' and 3' ends of the tRNAs, respectively, and release mRNA and rRNA from the polycistronic precursor RNA [60]. The processed mRNA, tRNA, and rRNA go through their respective maturation processes [61]. The mature tRNAs and rRNAs participate in mRNA translation in mitochondria.

2.2.2. Mutations of mtDNA Transcription Regulatory Elements

Mutations in the DNA sequences related to the regulation of mitochondrial transcription can lead to mitochondrial diseases [57,62]. In Section 2.1.2, we reviewed the mutations that occur in the mtDNA control region [40]. Most of these mutations are located near the LSP, which mediates the synthesis of RNA primers used for H-strand synthesis and L-strand transcription [63]. A quantitative analysis of mtDNA copy number and mitochondrial mRNAs revealed that the local mutations resulted in a 50% reduction of the number of mtDNA and a 2-fold reduction in the number of ND6 mRNA encoded in the L-strand of mtDNA [40]. In addition, Connor et al. identified m.547A > T mutations located within the HSP of mtDNA from a large family with tubulointerstitial kidney disease [64]. The patient-derived cells showed a reduced HSP transcriptional activity. The expression levels of tRNA^{Phe} and tRNA^{Leu} encoded in the H-strand were reduced compared with the level of tRNA^{Gln} as a control [64]. Regarding the mitochondrial tRNA processing, Veronika and Rita listed disease-causing mtDNA mutations with the corresponding molecular effects and associated phenotypes [61]. More than half of all the pathogenic mutations in mtDNA are in the tRNA-coding genes [65,66]. These tRNA mutations generally have detrimental effects on tRNA biogenesis, stability, and function [61]. The best-known mutation is m.3243A > G. It is located in the MT-TL1 gene encoding tRNA$^{Leu\,(UUR)}$, which is linked MELAS, chronic PEO (CPEO), and maternally inherited diabetes and deafness.

2.2.3. Mutations of Nuclear Genes Involved in mtDNA Transcription

Approximately 250–300 nuclear-encoding proteins would affect mitochondrial gene expression [14,61]. A previous study reported a prevalence of nDNA mutations related to adult mitochondrial disease of 2.9 per 100,000 people in Northeast England [67]. As an example of clinical manifestations associated with defects in the nuclear genes involved in mitochondrial transcription, knockout mice with disruption of the *Polrmt*, a nuclear gene, in heart tissue developed cardiomyopathy [68]. In addition, knockout mice with disruption of the *Tefm*, another nuclear gene, showed a significantly increased heart weight [69]. Haack et al. discovered pathogenic mutations in the *Elac2* gene, which is involved in mitochondrial RNA processing, through exome sequencing of five patients with infantile hypertrophic cardiomyopathy, lactic acidosis, and isolated complex I deficiency in skeletal muscle [70]. In muscle and fibroblasts of the affected individuals, accumulation of 5'-end-unprocessed mitochondrial mRNA and rRNA precursors was observed for all the genes adjacent to mitochondrial tRNAs. Several nuclear-encoded pathogenic genes associated with the processing of precursor transcripts were also listed in another review paper [61].

In this section, we describe the details of mtDNA replication and transcription and introduced examples of mitochondrial diseases that can be caused by mutations of the genetic components involved in mtDNA expression. The genetic components are encoded by both mtDNA and nDNA.

3. Methods to Treat Non-Ideal Mitochondrial Gene Expression

Non-ideal profile of mitochondrial gene expression can be caused by mutations in mtDNA or nuclear genes. Untreated non-ideal mitochondrial gene expression profiles are associated with various mitochondrial diseases. Multiple studies have suggested two approaches to treat this pathogenic state: reduction of the portion of mtDNAs with pathogenic mutations in cells and introduction of corrected versions of the mutated mitochondrial genes into cells. In comparison, there have been few attempts to reverse the negative effects of mutations in the nuclear genes involved in mtDNA gene expression. Therefore, in this section, we focus on recent studies targeting the treatment of non-ideal mitochondrial gene expression, which is mainly linked to mutations in mtDNAs.

3.1. Reduction of mtDNAs Harboring Mutations

Increasing the proportion of functional mtDNAs in cells by selectively degrading the mutated mtDNAs is one way to treat the state of non-ideal mitochondrial gene expression. This approach mostly employs endonucleases that can cut the mutated mtDNA sequences in a sequence-specific manner (Figure 1A). When endonucleases targeting the mutated sequences are imported into the mitochondrial matrix where mtDNAs exist, those create double-strand breaks at the mutated sites of mtDNAs. Because mitochondria lack the ability to repair double-strand breaks in DNA, the linearized DNAs were eventually degraded [71]. For example, Pst I and Sma I endonucleases transferred into the mitochondria of rodent and human cells increased cellular respiration by decreasing the proportion of mutated mtDNAs [72,73]. This approach has produced multiple successful examples of correcting the portion of functional mtDNAs in cells. However, this approach has a critical limitation in that some mutated sequences cannot be targeted because of the lack of endonucleases with the corresponding sequence specificity [74].

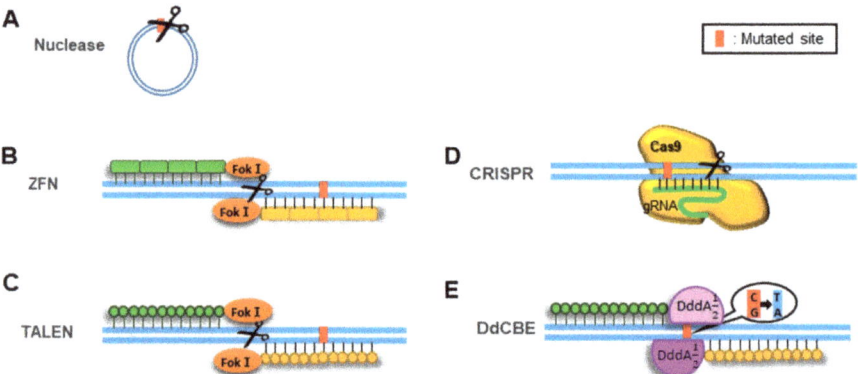

Figure 1. Methods of reducing mtDNAs harboring mutations to treat misregulation of mitochondrial gene expression. (**A**) Nuclease cleaves the target mutated sites. (**B**) ZFN: constructed by fusing the Fok I endonuclease with an array of zinc fingers, each having a recognition ability for a three-base DNA sequence. (**C**) TALEN: constructed by fusing Fok I with single base-recognizing domains, TALEs. (**D**) CRISPR: gRNA recognizes the mutation-including domain, and Cas9 cleaves mtDNA around the gRNA-bound site. (**E**) DdCBE: TALEs recognize the periphery of the mutation, and the two parts of DddA were fused to form the whole DddA toxin that can convert cytosine to thymidine.

3.1.1. Use of Zinc Fingers and Transcription Activator-Like Effectors (TALEs) as Sequence Targeting Modules

To overcome this limitation, sequence-specific DNA-binding protein domains have been fused to nucleases without sequence specificity. The first type of the domains is composed of an array of zinc fingers, each having a specificity for a three base pair DNA sequence. When multiple zinc fingers are combined, the complex can recognize longer DNA sequences (Figure 1B). The engineered mitochondria-targeted zinc-finger nuclease (mtZFN) contains a mitochondrial targeting sequence (MTS) and a synthetic endonuclease. The synthetic endonuclease was constructed by fusing the Fok I endonuclease with an array of zinc fingers [75]. This mtZFN could selectively eliminate the pathogenic mtDNAs with the m.8993T > G point mutation, which is associated with NARP and maternally inherited Leigh syndrome (MILS) [75].

Another type of DNA-binding domain is composed of an array of TALEs, each with specificity for a single DNA base. Multiple TALEs have been combined to target longer DNA sequences (Figure 1C). Mitochondria-targeted TALE nucleases (mtTALENs) have also been constructed by fusing Fok I with an array of TALEs and an MTS [76]. Two mtTALENs were used to cleave mtDNAs with the m.8344A > G mutation found in myoclonic epilepsy with ragged red fibers (MERRF) or m.13,513G > A mutation found in MELAS/Leigh [77,78].

The success of nuclease-based reduction of the portion of mutated mtDNAs highly depends on the delivery efficiency of sequence-specific nucleases into mitochondria. For enhanced delivery of nucleases viral vectors such as adeno-associated virus (AAV)-based ones have been applied. Newly expressed mtZFNs and mtTALENs after vector-mediated delivery of corresponding genes could eliminate the mutated mtDNAs and subsequently reduce the production of pathogenic factors [79–81]. This nuclease-based method decreases the number of mutated mtDNAs, resulting in an increase in the proportion of normal mtDNAs. The change in mtDNA heteroplasmy could persist because the long-term culture of cells expressing nucleases increases the proportion of normal mtDNAs [16,77]. To remove various mutated mtDNAs, more advanced methods for effectively constructing mtZFNs and mtTALENs are needed.

3.1.2. Use of CRISPR Cas9 to Target Mutated Sequences

A new technique based on clustered regularly interspaced short palindromic repeats (CRISPR) Cas9 has been widely used to cut the mutated sites of nDNAs. The key advantage of this technique is that it can target any sequence by only altering the guide RNA (gRNA) loaded inside the Cas9 enzyme (Figure 1D). However, the application of the technique to cleave the mutated mtDNAs can be more difficult than nDNA manipulation. The Cas9 enzyme is a very large protein. It can be difficult to deliver it into the mitochondria. In addition, for transfer into mitochondria, gRNAs should contain specific sequences that form certain stem–loop structures or MTS [82,83]. There is no effective way to deliver gRNAs into mitochondria. Moreover, it is difficult to experimentally confirm the translocation of gRNA into mitochondria. Even with these difficulties, some attempts based on Cas9 and gRNA targeting the mutated mtDNAs have been successful in reducing the proportion of mutated DNAs in cells [82,83].

A CRISPR-free mtDNA editing system based on the double-stranded deaminase A (DddA) toxin, which catalyzes the deamination of cytidines of dsDNA, has been recently developed [84]. This DddA-derived cytosine base editor (DdCBE) system was engineered to split DddA into two parts at G1333 or G1397, rendering it non-toxic and inactive before binding to the target DNA (Figure 1E). The split parts of DddA were fused to MTS-linked TALE proteins that bind two adjacent DNA sites within the mitochondrial ND6 gene. To increase DNA editing efficiency one uracil glycosylase inhibitor was appended to the C-terminus of each TALE-split DddA fusion. The resultant DdCBEs efficiently mediated base editing of the mitochondrial ND6 gene in HEK293T cells by converting cytosine to thymidine [84]. If mitochondrial targeting and editing accuracy are improved, more base editing tools can be applied to correct the pathogenic mutations in mtDNA.

3.2. Delivery of Genetic Components to Mitochondria

Mutations of mtDNA can disrupt the genetic components involved in maintaining the physiology and functions of mitochondria, and eventually induce serious illness. Direct correction of these mutations remains technically challenging. Instead of this difficult option, the introduction of corrected versions of genetic components into cells has been suggested for the treatment of mitochondrial diseases. In this section, we describe techniques used to introduce DNA or RNA components into mitochondria to mitigate the negative effects of mutated mtDNAs.

3.2.1. DNA Import into Mitochondria

Physical Methods

For nucleic acids to be delivered into mitochondria the genetic materials should pass through the plasma membrane, endosomes, and double layers of the mitochondrial membrane. Multiple physical methods have been applied to overcome these diffusion barriers [85]. One example of a physical method employed mechanical force to overcome the diffusion limitation. In one approach, a solution containing plasmid DNAs was injected into the skeletal muscle of rats using a hydrodynamic limb vein (HLV) injection system (Figure 2A). The introduced plasmid DNAs were successfully delivered into the nucleus and mitochondria without severe mitochondrial toxicity [86]. The HLV injection system promoted the flow of plasmid DNAs from vascular tissue into muscle tissue by the use of a sufficient amount of saline. The hydrodynamic forces reportedly induced temporary cell membrane openings [86]. This microinjection method is conceptually simple and direct, but its limitations include low efficiency and mechanical stress on cells [86]. In another approach, mitochondria were isolated from cells to directly introduce DNAs into them. Plasmids containing mtDNA sequences were successfully delivered into the mitochondria through electroporation that generated pores on mitochondrial membranes [87,88]. This electroporation-based method was only applied to isolated mitochondria. However, because outer mitochondria can be introduced into cells [89–91], one may treat cells that have defects in mtDNAs by isolating their mitochondria, transferring therapeutic DNAs into the mitochondria, and introducing the engineered mitochondria back into the cells.

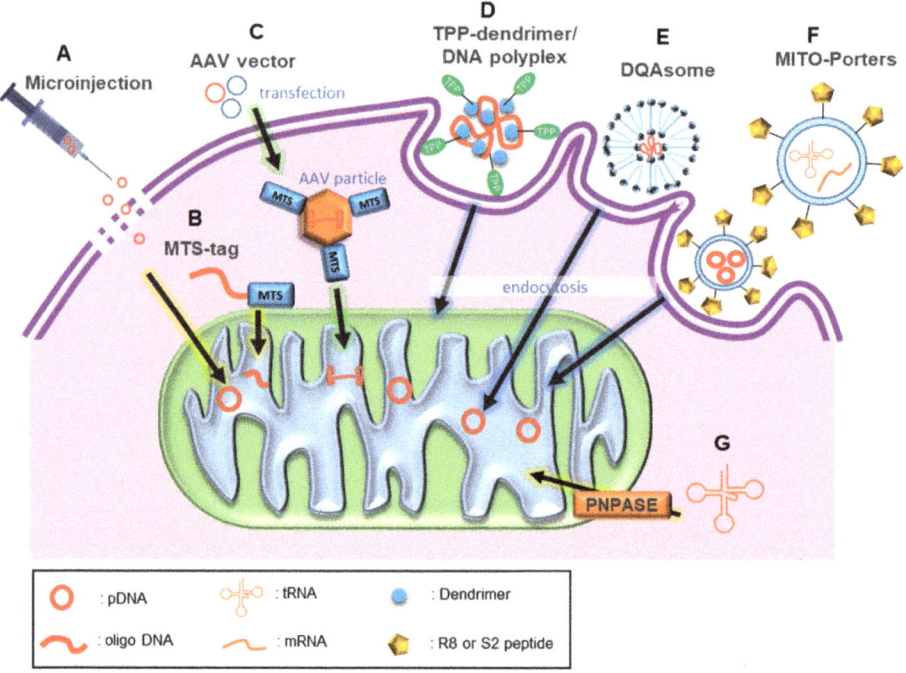

Figure 2. Methods for delivery of genetic components into mitochondria. (**A**) Microinjection is one of the physical methods. (**B**) MTS-mediated translocation can deliver DNAs into the mitochondrial matrix. (**C**) MTS-modified AAV particles can import target genes into mitochondria. (**D**) TPP-dendrimer/DNA polyplex is a dendrimer-based carrier that cannot import DNA into mitochondria but target mitochondria. Liposome-based carriers are DQAsome and MITO-Porter. (**E**) Mitochondrial expression of the gene transferred using DQAsome-mediated transfection system was confirmed. (**F**) MITO-Porters are surface-functionalized liposome-based carriers that increase transporting efficiency of target substances to mitochondria. (**G**) PNPASE can mediate the import of both small and large RNAs into mitochondria.

Biological and Chemical Methods

Thirteen mitochondrial proteins are encoded in the mitochondrial genome and the remaining proteins are encoded in the nuclear genome. The nuclear-encoded proteins are synthesized in the cytoplasm of cells and are transported into mitochondria via MTS-mediated translocation (Figure 2B). MTSs are 10–80 amino acids long. They are usually located at the N-terminus of mitochondrial proteins and often contain amphiphilic helices [92–94]. Mitochondrial import complexes comprising translocases of the outer membrane and inner membrane recognize the MTSs of nuclear-encoded proteins and translocate the proteins into the matrix space through mitochondrial membranes. MTSs are cleaved during translocation. The mitochondrial importing system and MTS tagging have also been utilized for the delivery of nucleic acids into mitochondria [95,96]. Short double-stranded linear DNAs (17 bp or 322 bp) were successfully transported into mitochondria by MTS tagging [97]. To conjugate cargo DNA and MTS peptide, a 39 nt oligodeoxynucleotide with an amino-modified deoxythymidine in the center of its palindromic sequence was designed. The oligodeoxynucleotides form a stable loop–stem structure composed of a reactive amino group at the loop region for coupling with a unique cysteine at the C-terminus of the peptide and sticky 5′-end for cargo DNA ligation [97]. Similarly, peptide nucleic acids (PNAs)—artificial nucleic acids with an aminoethyl (pseudopeptide) backbone—can be used as carriers for gene delivery because of their DNA or RNA binding capacity and resistance to nuclease or protease attack. Furthermore, PNAs can be readily internalized into various cell lines including human fibroblasts, HeLa cells, HepG2 cells, and SY5Y cells. For mitochondrial localization, PNAs were conjugated with MTS and the PNA-MTS conjugates were translocated into the mitochondrial matrix of cultured human myoblasts in a membrane potential-dependent manner [98]. In another study, PNA linked with yeast cytochrome oxidase (COX) IV mitochondrial targeting peptide successfully mediated the transport of oligonucleotides annealed to the PNA into the mitochondrial matrix of mouse myoblasts [99]. Transferred short oligo DNA can act as a selective inhibitor for mutated mtDNA replication or can mediate the repair of mtDNA with point mutations. Furthermore, MTS conjugation to various carriers applied for general gene therapy can be a strategy to introduce large nucleic acids, such as plasmid DNA, into the mitochondrial matrix.

AAV vectors have attracted much attention in the field of gene and cell therapy because they can transduce genes into many types of cells without severe adverse effects [100–102]. AAV is a parvovirus having a DNA genome of approximately 4.7 kb. Its single-stranded genome contains viral replicase (*rep*) and capsid (*cap*) genes between two inverted terminal repeats (ITRs) [102]. The *rep* gene encodes four enzymatic proteins (Rep78, Rep68, Rep52, and Rep40), and the *cap* gene encodes three capsid proteins (VP1, VP2, and VP3) [102]. For applications of AAV as gene delivery vectors, the AAV protein-coding sequences between the ITRs are substituted with therapeutic gene expression cassettes, and the *rep* and *cap* genes are provided *in trans* [103]. In this way, AAV vectors carrying the mitochondrial *ND4* gene expression cassette were generated [17]. The *ND4* gene can only be translated into mitochondria because the gene uses TGA, which is recognized as a tryptophan codon rather than as a stop codon in mitochondria. An MTS was inserted into the N-terminus of the capsid VP2 sequence to guide the AAV vectors to mitochondria (Figure 2C). The cytoplasmic hybrid (cybrid) cell lines containing mitochondria with the m.11778G > A mutation in the *ND4* gene were infected with the MTS-modified AAV vectors carrying a wild-type *ND4* gene. The delivered functional *ND4* gene was expressed in the cells and their defective respiratory function was rescued. In an in vivo study, AAV vectors that carry a functional *ND4* gene and MTS were injected into the eyes of mice. Two days later, AAV vectors carrying an *ND4* gene with a mutation of Arg340His, which is known to cause visual loss in rodents, were additionally injected into the eyes that were treated with the functional *ND4* gene. The introduced functional ND4 gene prevented visual impairment in the mice, and the therapeutic effects persisted for almost the entire life span of the mice [17]. In a subsequent study, the DNAs containing the *ND4* gene that were delivered by MTS-modified AAV vectors remained episomally in the mitochondrial matrix without integration into the mitochondrial genome [104]. These results suggest a possibility that viral vectors commonly used in gene therapy can be engineered to target mitochondria by tagging MTS to viral structural proteins.

Lipophilic cations such as ethidium, tetraphenylphosphonium (TPP), triphenylmethylphosphonium (TPMP), and tetraphenylarsonium (TPA) also have mitochondria-targeting capabilities. Lipophilic ions can permeate across biological membranes composed of phospholipid bilayers, and cationic molecules can accumulate in the negatively charged mitochondrial matrix as a result of the electrochemical equilibration of ions [105]. TPP has been applied to target various molecules to mitochondria by conjugation with the molecules directly or by carrier packaging of the molecules [106–109]. As an example of TPP-mediated DNA delivery, an 11-mer PNA conjugated with TPP was taken up by mitochondria within 143 B osteosarcoma cells [110]. The sequence of the PNA oligomer was designed to be complementary to the mtDNA containing the MERRF disease-causing m.8344A > G mutation to selectively inhibit the mutated mtDNA replication in cells. In another study, TPP was conjugated to polymer-based dendrimers that can condense genetic materials [111]. Plasmid DNAs containing the genes that encode enhanced green fluorescent protein or luciferase were incubated with TPP-conjugated dendrimers to generate TPP-dendrimer/DNA polyplexes (Figure 2D). The mitochondria-targeting ability of the polyplexes was experimentally demonstrated, but the mitochondrial import of the transferred DNA was not confirmed. The data collectively indicate that MTS actively transports cargo molecules into the mitochondrial matrix by passing through the channels on the mitochondrial membrane, while TPP passively diffuses depending on the mitochondrial membrane potential.

For the passage of negatively charged mitochondrial lipid bilayer membranes, liposome-based carriers have been used to encapsulate the DNA. The DQAsome is a liposome-like aggregate formed with dequalinium. Dequalinium can accumulate in mitochondria due to the delocalized cationic charge [112,113]. As DQAsomes can bind and condense plasmid DNA, DQAsome-DNA complexes (DQAplexes) were prepared by simply mixing the DNA with DQAsomes [114]. The applicability of DQAsomes as mitochondria-targeting carriers for DNA was investigated (Figure 2E). Fluorescence imaging of live BT20 cells exposed to DQAplexes revealed the endosomal escape of DQAplexes and the liberation of plasmid DNAs from DQAplexes at the site of mitochondria [114]. In addition, Weissig et al. provided evidence that DQAplexes release DNA upon contact with the mitochondrial membrane through experiments using cardiolipin-rich liposomes mimicking mitochondrial membranes and isolated mouse liver mitochondria [113,115]. DQAsomes were used to transfect plasmid DNA containing the GFP gene designed for mitochondrial expression (mtGFP) into several mammalian cell lines [116]. Mitochondrial expression of the mtGFP gene transferred by the DQAsome-mediated transfection system was experimentally confirmed. Although the expression level was low, the result was significant in that it is one of the few methods to date that has enabled mitochondrial expression of genes introduced into live cells. Another study showed that the mitochondria-targeting characteristics of DQAsomes can be enhanced by anchoring mitochondriotropic ligands such as TPP to the liposomal phospholipid bilayer [117].

Liposome-based carriers for mitochondrial gene delivery have been improved through surface modification and lipid composition optimization. MITO-Porters developed by Yamada et al. displayed octaarginine (R8) on the surface for cellular internalization of the liposome [118]. In addition, the original lipid component, egg yolk phosphatidylcholine, was substituted by 1,2-dioleoyl-sn-glycero-3-phosphatidylethanolamine (DOPE). This lipid composition increased the fusogenic activity of liposomes, consequently allowing endosome escape of the liposome-DNA complex and fusion between the liposomal membrane and mitochondrial membrane [118] (Figure 2F). In a subsequent study, dual-function MITO-Porter (DF-MITO-Porter) was generated to improve mitochondrial drug delivery efficiency [119]. The DF-MITO-Porter comprises a mitochondria-fusogenic inner lipid envelope and an endosome-fusogenic outer lipid envelope, whose surfaces are modified with R8. The penetration efficiency of this new liposome-based carrier for mitochondria was higher than that of conventional MITO-Porter (83.3% versus 25.0%) [119]. To evaluate the delivery of cargo molecules into the mitochondrial matrix, DNaseI protein was encapsulated in DF-MITO-Porter and mtDNA levels in the mitochondrial matrix were analyzed [119,120]. After DF-MITO-Porter-mediated mitochondrial delivery of DNase I, a substantial decrease in mtDNA levels was observed compared with the conventional MITO-Porter case [119,120]. Aside from the R8 peptide, five kinds of peptides with favorable properties for mitochondrial gene transfer were used as ligands for surface modification of MITO-Porters. MITO-Porter modified with S2 peptides (Dmt-$_D$-Arg-Phe-Lys-Dmt-$_D$-Arg-Phe-Lys, Dmt = 2, 6-dimethyltyrosine) showed a similar mitochondrial targeting activity, but lower cytotoxicity compared to those of the one modified with R8 [121]. Using the MITO-Porters, both short oligo DNAs and plasmid DNAs were successfully transferred into mitochondria in live HeLa cells [121–123]. Finally, mitochondrial localization of cy5-labeled oligo DNAs was observed using confocal laser scanning microscopy [121,122]. In another study, MITO-Porter modified with cell-penetrating KALA peptides delivered plasmid DNAs containing the gene that encodes luciferase using the mitochondrial codon system [123]. The potent CMV promoter derived from cytomegalovirus induced luciferase expression. This is one of the few examples of transgene expression in mitochondria.

3.2.2. RNA Import into Mitochondria

Efficient delivery of RNA into mitochondria can be an alternative to treat mitochondrial diseases caused by mutations in nDNAs or mtDNAs. Several methods to deliver RNA into mitochondria have utilized endogenous RNA import systems. Similar to mitochondrial proteins, some RNAs that function in the mitochondria are encoded and transcribed in the nucleus [124]. The pre-protein import apparatus mediates the mitochondrial uptake of cytosolic small RNAs depending on ATP. In mammals, three types of RNAs are imported into mitochondria: 5S rRNA, RNA component of RNase P (H1 RNA), and RNA component of RNase MRP (RMRP) [125]. These are all imported into mitochondria through the pre-protein import channel, and protein factors that direct the RNA translocation exist. For example, the mitochondrial ribosomal proteins MRP-L18 and rhodanese (thiosulfate sulfurtransferase) are protein factors involved in mitochondrial import of 5S rRNA [126,127]. MRP-L18 induces a conformational change of 5S rRNA by binding to the γ-domain and allows interaction between the rhodanese and the α-domain of 5S rRNA. Subsequently, the RNA-protein complex is imported into mitochondria [124].

In addition, polynucleotide phosphorylase (PNPASE) is a well-known protein that mediates the import of nuclear-encoded RNAs, including 5S rRNA, H1 RNA, and RMRP, into the mitochondrial matrix [128]. Mammalian PNPASE has an MTS at its N-terminus and recognizes a 20 nt stem–loop structure in H1 RNA. In similar, PNPASE interacts with a different 20 nt sequence forming a stem–loop structure in RMRP [129]. In a study, fusion of one of the stem–loop sequences to the 5'-end of the glyceraldehyde 3-phosphate dehydrogenase (GAPDH) RNA allowed the import of the RNA into isolated yeast mitochondria [128] (Figure 2G). The sequence forming a stem–loop structure also enabled the translocation of human mitochondrial tRNA^{trp} into isolated mouse liver mitochondria [128]. In the following study, this approach was also applied to transfer nuclear-encoded tRNAs into mitochondria to mitigate the disease state of MERRF caused by the m.8344A > G mutation in the mitochondrial tRNA^{Lys} and MELAS caused by the m.3243A > G mutation in the mitochondrial tRNA^{Leu} [130]. In addition to appending the RNA import sequence of H1 RNA to the tRNA precursor sequences, two more strategies were applied. First, the aminoacyl stems of the mitochondrial tRNA^{Lys} and tRNA^{Leu} precursors were extended by changing several unpaired ribonucleotides adjacent to the stem region to be paired to prevent cleavage of the H1 RNA import sequence from the tRNA precursors. Second, for RNA localization to the mitochondrial outer membrane, the 3'-untranslated region (UTR) of transcript for mitochondrial ribosomal protein S12 (*MRPS12*) was additionally appended to the 3′-end of the extended tRNA precursors with the H1 RNA import sequence. As a result, in MERRF and MELAS cybrid cells expressing the rationally engineered mitochondrial tRNA precursors, defects in mtRNA translation and cellular respiration were rescued. Furthermore, using the interaction between PNPASE and the H1 RNA import sequence, the import of relatively large mRNAs as well as tRNA precursors into the mitochondrial matrix was also confirmed. A mitochondrial-encoded mouse *COX2* gene was linked with the H1 RNA import sequence. The resultant DNA construct was introduced into HeLa cells via transient transfection. RT-PCR was used to examine the import of RNA transcribed from the introduced DNA. Only the genes fused to the H1 RNA import sequences were imported into the mitochondrial matrix [130]. PNPASE, which guides cytosolic small RNAs into mitochondria in cells, can mediate the import of both small and large RNAs. As this approach takes advantage of the proteins originally existing in mammalian cells, it is expected to have lower cytotoxicity than other approaches using artificial carriers.

Currently, it is known that tRNA^{Gln} is the only tRNA that translocates from the cytosol to mitochondria in mammalian cells [131]. In contrast, in yeast more types of tRNA can be imported into mitochondria. Therefore, there have been attempts to treat human mitochondrial dysfunction caused by mutations in tRNAs with yeast tRNAs. In a study, it was experimentally confirmed that several yeast tRNA^{Lys} derivatives can be internalized into isolated human mitochondria through the protein import channels [125]. In addition, mammalian cytosolic aminoacyl-tRNA synthetase mediated aminoacylation of the yeast tRNA^{Lys} efficiently as yeast aminoacyl-tRNA synthetase did [125]. Based on this result, Kolesnikova et al. suggested a therapeutic strategy to treat MERRF syndrome caused by mutations in mtDNA encoding the tRNA^{Lys} [18]. Plasmid DNA containing the yeast tRNA$^{Lys\ (CUU)}$ sequence was introduced into cybrid cells carrying the m.8344A > G mutation in mtDNA and MERRF patient-derived fibroblasts via transient transfection. Expression of the yeast tRNA^{Lys} partially rescued defects in mitochondrial functions such as mitochondrial translation, cellular respiration, and membrane potential generation [18]. This method is based on allotropic expression, in which DNAs encoding mitochondrial genes are transferred to the nucleus and the resultant gene products in the cytoplasm are re-localized to mitochondria.

In contrast, mtRNAs could be directly delivered to mitochondria by using the aforementioned liposome-based MITO-Porter [132]. Wild-type mitochondrial tRNA^{Phe} precursors produced via an in vitro transcription system with T7 RNA polymerase were complexed with protamine and encapsulated by MITO-Porter for mitochondrial localization. The resulting MITO-Porter complexes were introduced into fibroblasts derived from a patient carrying the m.625G > A mutation in the mitochondrial gene encoding tRNA^{Phe}. To confirm the effects of MITO-Porter-mediated RNA delivery, the fractions of mutant tRNA^{Phe} in the mitochondria of the control and treated cells were evaluated. The fraction of the mutant tRNA^{Phe} in the mitochondria of the untreated control cells was around 0.8. After transfection of MITO-Porter encapsulating wild-type tRNA^{Phe} that was modified with tRK1 sequence having the mitochondrial import activity, the fraction of the mutant was decreased to around 0.2. In another attempt, MITO-Porter was used to deliver an antisense RNA oligonucleotide (ASO) of 46 nt targeting the *COX2* gene [133]. The 5′-end of the ASO was modified with a Darm sequence that binds to the RNA import complex protein for mitochondrial targeting activity. Darm-ASOs were complexed with polyethyleneimine (PEI) polycation, and the complexes were encapsulated in MITO-Porter. The MITO-Porter enabled the RNA/PEI complex to reach the intermembrane space of mitochondria in HeLa cells, and the ASOs were imported into the mitochondrial matrix via the Darm import machinery. In cells transfected with Darm-modified ASOs, the expression level of COX2 protein was decreased, inhibiting ATP production, whereas ASOs without the Darm sequence did not affect the COX2 level [133]. This finding suggests that the expression of specific mitochondrial genes can be regulated through gene silencing by mitochondrial delivery of ASOs.

MITO-Porter can also mediate the delivery of relatively large mRNA [19]. The synthesis of ND3 mRNA was achieved by T7 promoter-driven in vitro transcription. ND3 mRNA formed a complex with positively charged protamine for encapsulation into MITO-Porter nanoparticles. MITO-Porters carrying normal ND3 mRNAs were introduced into fibroblasts from a Leigh syndrome patient harboring the m.10158T > C mutation in the *ND3* gene. To confirm the mitochondrial delivery of ND3, the proportion of mutant ND3 mRNA in the mitochondria of fibroblasts, which were obtained from a patient with Leigh syndrome caused by the m.10158T > C mutation in mtDNA, and the oxygen consumption rate indicating the mitochondrial respiratory activities were both evaluated. Compared with non-treated cells showing the mutant proportion of approximately 0.8, the mutant proportion of the treated cells was significantly decreased to 0.1 in a dose-dependent manner. In addition, the maximal oxygen consumption rate of the cells treated with the MITO-Porter carrying normal ND3 mRNAs was about 1.46-fold higher than that of the untreated cells. These data indicate that mitochondrial respiration activity can be improved by the introduction of normal mRNAs into mitochondria [19]. The use of MITO-Porters can be a potential therapeutic strategy for mitochondrial diseases caused by mutations in mtDNA because of their ability to encapsulate various forms of nucleic acids and pass through biological membranes, if the basal cytotoxicity of the liposome-based carriers can be overcome.

4. Concluding Remarks

Mutations in mitochondrial genomes can cause diseases involving malfunction of various organs, including the brain, nerves, eyes, and heart, due to impaired energy production. Correction of the mutations or introduction of functional genetic components into mitochondria can be a reasonable strategy to cure mitochondrial diseases. However, two separate lipid membranes of mitochondria do not allow easy access of therapeutic genetic components to the matrix space where the mitochondrial genetic system mainly operates. The mixed and heterogeneous nature of mitochondrial DNAs in a cell complicates the design and applications of the gene therapy strategy. In this review, we introduced multiple aspects of basic regulations of mitochondrial DNA replication and transcription. Mutations of the genetic components that affect the physiology and functions of mitochondria and linkages between the mutations and diseases have been also discussed. Various studies targeted to reduce the number of mutated DNAs in mitochondria and enhance the delivery system for the introduction of therapeutic genetic components into mitochondria. To reach the goal of treating and eventually curing mitochondrial diseases, various approaches, employing physical forces, newly constructed chemical complexes, and recombinant proteins, have been applied. Partial success in the studies encourages future ambitious attempts to effectively cure mitochondrial disease. A better understanding of molecular and genetic mechanisms involved in mitochondrial diseases and the fusion of multidisciplinary approaches will further fuel the advances in mitochondrial gene therapy.

Funding: This work was supported by grants from the National Research Foundation of Korea (NRF) (Grant numbers: 2016M3A9B6947831 and 2020R1A2C2005893). This work was also supported by Korea Institute of Planning and Evaluation for Technology in Food, Agriculture and Forestry (IPET) through Animal Disease Management Technology Development Program, funded by Ministry of Agriculture, Food and Rural Affairs (MAFRA) (Grant number: 118094-03), and Technology Development Program (Grant number: S2938432) funded by the Ministry of SMEs and Startups (MSS, Korea).

Conflicts of Interest: The authors declare no conflict of interest.

Abbreviation

ATP	adenosine triphosphate
AAV	adeno-associated virus
AD	Alzheimer's disease

adPEO	autosomal dominant PEO
AHS	Alpers–Huttenlocher syndrome
ANS	ataxia neuropathy spectrum
arPEO	autosomal recessive PEO
ASO	antisense RNA oligonucleotide
cap	capsid
COX	cytochrome oxidase
CPEO	chronic PEO
CPEO	chronic progressive external ophthalmoplegia
CRISPR	clustered regularly interspaced short palindromic repeats
CSBI	conserved sequence block I
DdCBE	DddA-derived cytosine base editor
DddA	double-stranded deaminase A
DEAF	deafness or aminoglycoside-induced deafness
DF-MITO-Porter	dual function MITO-Porter
DOPE	1,2-dioleoyl-sn-glycero-3-phosphatidylethanolamine
DQAplexes	DQAsome-DNA complexes
ELAC2	elaC ribonuclease Z 2
GAPDH	glyceraldehyde 3-phosphate dehydrogenase
gRNA	guide RNA
HLV	hydrodynamic limb vein
HSP1	heavy strand promoter 1
ITRs	inverted terminal repeats
LHON	Leber's hereditary optic neuropathy
LSP	light strand promoter
MCHS	myocerebrohepatopathy spectrum
MELAS	mitochondrial encephalopathy, lactic acidosis, stroke-like episodes
MEMSA	myopathy sensory ataxia
MERRF	myoclonic epilepsy with ragged red fibers
MI	myocardial infarction
MILS	maternally inherited Leigh syndrome
MIRAS	Mitochondrial recessive ataxia syndrome
MIRAS	mitochondrial recessive ataxia syndrome
mRNAs	messenger RNAs
MRP	mitochondrial RNA processing
MRPS12	mitochondrial ribosomal protein S12
mtDNA	mitochondrial DNA
MTS	mitochondrial targeting sequence (
mtTALENs	mitochondria-targeted TALE nucleases
mtZFN	mitochondria-targeted zinc-finger nuclease
NARP	neurogenic muscle weakness, ataxia, and retinitis pigmentosa
nDNA	nuclear DNA
nt	nucleotides
O_H	origin of the H-strand
PEI	polyethyleneimine
PEO	progressive external ophthalmoplegia
PNAs	peptide nucleic acids
PNPASE	polynucleotide phosphorylase
POLRMT	mitochondrial RNA polymerase
POLγ	DNA polymerase gamma
rep	replicase
RMRP	RNase MRP
rRNAs	ribosomal RNAs
SSBP1	single-stranded DNA-binding protein

TALEs	transcription activator-like effectors
TEFM	mitochondrial transcription elongation factor
TFAM	mitochondrial transcription factor A
TFB2M	mitochondrial transcription factor B2
TPA	tetraphenylarsonium
TPMP	triphenylmethylphosphonium
TPP	tetraphenylphosphonium
tRNAs	transfer RNAs
UTR	untranslated region

References

1. Chinnery, P.F.; Hudson, G. Mitochondrial genetics. *Brit. Med. Bull.* **2013**, *106*, 135–159. [CrossRef] [PubMed]
2. Fazzini, F.; Schöpf, B.; Blatzer, M.; Coassin, S.; Hicks, A.A.; Kronenberg, F.; Fendt, L. Plasmid-normalized quantification of relative mitochondrial DNA copy number. *Sci. Rep.* **2018**, *8*, 1–11. [CrossRef]
3. Lightowlers, R.N.; Chinnery, P.F.; Turnbull, D.M.; Howell, N. Mammalian mitochondrial genetics: Heredity, heteroplasmy and disease. *Trends Genet.* **1997**, *13*, 450–455. [CrossRef]
4. Tuppen, H.A.; Blakely, E.L.; Turnbull, D.M.; Taylor, R.W. Mitochondrial DNA mutations and human disease. *Biochim. Biophys. Acta Bioenerg.* **2010**, *1797*, 113–128. [CrossRef] [PubMed]
5. Stewart, J.B.; Chinnery, P.F. The dynamics of mitochondrial DNA heteroplasmy: Implications for human health and disease. *Nat. Rev. Genet.* **2015**, *16*, 530–542. [CrossRef]
6. Maeda, R.; Kami, D.; Maeda, H.; Shikuma, A.; Gojo, S. High throughput single cell analysis of mitochondrial heteroplasmy in mitochondrial diseases. *Sci. Rep.* **2020**, *10*, 1–10. [CrossRef]
7. Brown, M.D.; Trounce, I.A.; Jun, A.S.; Allen, J.C.; Wallace, D.C. Functional analysis of lymphoblast and cybrid mitochondria containing the 3460, 11778, or 14484 Leber's hereditary optic neuropathy mitochondrial DNA mutation. *J. Biol. Chem.* **2000**, *275*, 39831–39836. [CrossRef]
8. Mattiazzi, M.; Vijayvergiya, C.; Gajewski, C.D.; DeVivo, D.C.; Lenaz, G.; Wiedmann, M.; Manfredi, G. The mtDNA T8993G (NARP) mutation results in an impairment of oxidative phosphorylation that can be improved by antioxidants. *Hum. Molecul. Genet.* **2004**, *13*, 869–879. [CrossRef] [PubMed]
9. Wong, L.J.C. Pathogenic mitochondrial DNA mutations in protein-coding genes. *Muscle Nerve* **2007**, *36*, 279–293. [CrossRef]
10. Barthélémy, C.; de Baulny, H.; Lombès, A. D-loop mutations in mitochondrial DNA: Link with mitochondrial DNA depletion? *Hum. Genet.* **2002**, *110*, 479–487. [PubMed]
11. Smith, P.M.; Elson, J.L.; Greaves, L.C.; Wortmann, S.B.; Rodenburg, R.J.T.; Lightowlers, R.N.; Chrzanowska-Lightowlers, Z.M.A.; Taylor, R.W.; Vila-Sanjurjo, A. The role of the mitochondrial ribosome in human disease: Searching for mutations in 12S mitochondrial rRNA with high disruptive potential. *Hum. Molecul. Genet.* **2014**, *23*, 949–967. [CrossRef]
12. Ding, Y.; Ye, Y.; Li, M.; Xia, B.; Leng, J. Mitochondrial tRNAAla 5601C> T variant may affect the clinical expression of the LHON-related ND4 11778G> A mutation in a family. *Molecul. Med. Rep.* **2020**, *21*, 201–208. [CrossRef]
13. Ikeda, T.; Osaka, H.; Shimbo, H.; Tajika, M.; Yamazaki, M.; Ueda, A.; Murayama, K.; Yamagata, T. Mitochondrial DNA 3243A> T mutation in a patient with MELAS syndrome. *Hum. Genome Variat* **2018**, *5*, 1–4. [CrossRef] [PubMed]
14. Rusecka, J.; Kaliszewska, M.; Bartnik, E.; Tońska, K. Nuclear genes involved in mitochondrial diseases caused by instability of mitochondrial DNA. *J. Appl. Genet.* **2018**, *59*, 43–57. [CrossRef] [PubMed]
15. Pearce, S.F.; Rebelo-Guiomar, P.; D'Souza, A.R.; Powell, C.A.; Van Haute, L.; Minczuk, M. Regulation of mammalian mitochondrial gene expression: Recent advances. *Trends Bioc. Sci.* **2017**, *42*, 625–639. [CrossRef]
16. Yahata, N.; Matsumoto, Y.; Omi, M.; Yamamoto, N.; Hata, R. TALEN-mediated shift of mitochondrial DNA heteroplasmy in MELAS-iPSCs with m. 13513G> A mutation. *Sci. Rep.* **2017**, *7*, 1–11. [CrossRef]
17. Yu, H.; Koilkonda, R.D.; Chou, T.; Porciatti, V.; Ozdemir, S.S.; Chiodo, V.; Boye, S.L.; Boye, S.E.; Hauswirth, W.W.; Lewin, A.S. Gene delivery to mitochondria by targeting modified adenoassociated virus suppresses Leber's hereditary optic neuropathy in a mouse model. *Proc. Natl. Acad. Sci. USA* **2012**, *109*, E1238–E1247. [CrossRef] [PubMed]
18. Kolesnikova, O.A.; Entelis, N.S.; Jacquin-Becker, C.; Goltzene, F.; Chrzanowska-Lightowlers, Z.M.; Lightowlers, R.N.; Martin, R.P.; Tarassov, I. Nuclear DNA-encoded tRNAs targeted into mitochondria can rescue a mitochondrial DNA mutation associated with the MERRF syndrome in cultured human cells. *Hum. Molecul. Genet.* **2004**, *13*, 2519–2534. [CrossRef] [PubMed]
19. Yamada, Y.; Somiya, K.; Miyauchi, A.; Osaka, H.; Harashima, H. Validation of a mitochondrial RnA therapeutic strategy using fibroblasts from a Leigh syndrome patient with a mutation in the mitochondrial ND3 gene. *Sci. Rep.* **2020**, *10*, 1–13. [CrossRef]
20. Tyynismaa, H.; Sembongi, H.; Bokori-Brown, M.; Granycome, C.; Ashley, N.; Poulton, J.; Jalanko, A.; Spelbrink, J.N.; Holt, I.J.; Suomalainen, A. Twinkle helicase is essential for mtDNA maintenance and regulates mtDNA copy number. *Hum. Molecul. Genet.* **2004**, *13*, 3219–3227. [CrossRef]
21. Jackson, C.B.; Turnbull, D.M.; Minczuk, M.; Gammage, P.A. Therapeutic manipulation of mtDNA heteroplasmy: A shifting perspective. *Trends Molecul. Med.* **2020**, *26*, 698–709. [CrossRef]
22. Crimi, M.; Rigolio, R. The mitochondrial genome, a growing interest inside an organelle. *Internat. J. Nanomed.* **2008**, *3*, 51–57.

23. Garone, C.; Minczuk, M.; D'Souza, A.R. Mitochondrial transcription and translation: Overview. *Essays Biochem.* **2018**, *62*, 309–320. [CrossRef]
24. Garone, C.; Minczuk, M.; Boczonadi, V.; Ricci, G.; Horvath, R. Mitochondrial DNA transcription and translation: Clinical syndromes. *Essays Biochem* **2018**, *62*, 321–340. [CrossRef] [PubMed]
25. Ali, A.T.; Boehme, L.; Carbajosa, G.; Seitan, V.C.; Small, K.S.; Hodgkinson, A. Nuclear genetic regulation of the human mitochondrial transcriptome. *Elife* **2019**, *8*, e41927. [CrossRef]
26. Taanman, J.-W. The mitochondrial genome: Structure, transcription, translation and replication. *Biochim. Biophys. Acta Bioenerget.* **1999**, *1410*, 103–123. [CrossRef]
27. Garone, C.; Minczuk, M.; Falkenberg, M. Mitochondrial DNA replication in mammalian cells: Overview of the pathway. *Essays Biochem.* **2018**, *62*, 287–296. [CrossRef]
28. Bogenhagen, D.F.; Clayton, D.A. The mitochondrial DNA replication bubble has not burst. *Trends Biochem. Sci.* **2003**, *28*, 357–360. [CrossRef]
29. Hsieh, C.-L. Novel lines of evidence for the asymmetric strand displacement model of mitochondrial DNA replication. *Molecul. Cell. Biol.* **2019**, *39*, e00406–e00418. [CrossRef]
30. Moraes, C.T. What regulates mitochondrial DNA copy number in animal cells? *Trends Genet.* **2001**, *17*, 199–205. [CrossRef]
31. Wanrooij, P.H.; Hodgkinson, A.P.; Simonsson, T.; Falkenberg, M.; Gustafsson, C.M. G-quadruplex structures in RNA stimulate mitochondrial transcription termination and primer formation. *Proc. Natl. Acad. Sci. USA* **2010**, *107*, 16072–16077. [CrossRef]
32. Posse, V.; Al-Behadili, A.; Uhler, J.P.; Clausen, A.R.; Reyes, A.; Zeviani, M.; Falkenberg, M.; Gustafsson, C.M. RNase H1 directs origin-specific initiation of DNA replication in human mitochondria. *PLoS Genet.* **2019**, *15*, e1007781. [CrossRef]
33. Milenkovic, D.; Matic, S.; Kühl, I.; Ruzzenente, B.; Freyer, C.; Jemt, E.; Park, C.B.; Falkenberg, M.; Larsson, N. TWINKLE is an essential mitochondrial helicase required for synthesis of nascent D-loop strands and complete mtDNA replication. *Hum. Molecul. Genet.* **2013**, *22*, 1983–1993. [CrossRef]
34. Ciesielski, G.L.; Bermek, O.; Rosado-Ruiz, F.A.; Hovde, S.L.; Neitzke, O.J.; Griffith, J.D.; Kaguni, L.S. Mitochondrial single-stranded DNA-binding proteins stimulate the activity of DNA polymerase γ by organization of the template DNA. *J. Biol. Chem.* **2015**, *290*, 28697–28707. [CrossRef] [PubMed]
35. Fusté, J.M.; Wanrooij, S.; Jemt, E.; Granycome, C.E.; Cluett, T.J.; Shi, Y.; Atanassova, N.; Holt, I.J.; Gustafsson, C.M.; Falkenberg, M. Mitochondrial RNA polymerase is needed for activation of the origin of light-strand DNA replication. *Molecul. Cell.* **2010**, *37*, 67–78. [CrossRef]
36. Falkenberg, M.; Gustafsson, C.M. Mammalian mitochondrial DNA replication and mechanisms of deletion formation. *Crit. Rev. Biochem. Molecul. Biol.* **2020**, *55*, 509–524. [CrossRef]
37. Tanaka, N.; Goto, Y.; Akanuma, J.; Kato, M.; Kinoshita, T.; Yamashita, F.; Tanaka, M.; Asada, T. Mitochondrial DNA variants in a Japanese population of patients with Alzheimer's disease. *Mitochondrion* **2010**, *10*, 32–37. [CrossRef] [PubMed]
38. Mousavizadeh, K.; Rajabi, P.; Alaee, M.; Dadgar, S.; Houshmand, M. Usage of mitochondrial D-loop variation to predict risk for Huntington disease. *Mitochondrial DNA* **2015**, *26*, 579–582. [CrossRef]
39. Ebner, S.; Lang, R.; Mueller, E.E.; Eder, W.; Oeller, M.; Moser, A.; Koller, J.; Paulweber, B.; Mayr, J.A.; Sperl, W. Mitochondrial haplogroups, control region polymorphisms and malignant melanoma: A study in middle European Caucasians. *PLoS ONE* **2011**, *6*, e27192.
40. Coskun, P.E.; Beal, M.F.; Wallace, D.C. Alzheimer's brains harbor somatic mtDNA control-region mutations that suppress mitochondrial transcription and replication. *Proc. Natl. Acad. Sci. USA* **2004**, *101*, 10726–10731. [CrossRef]
41. Umbria, M.; Ramos, A.; Aluja, M.P.; Santos, C. The role of control region mitochondrial DNA mutations in cardiovascular disease: Stroke and myocardial infarction. *Sci. Rep.* **2020**, *10*, 1–10.
42. Jemt, E.; Persson, Ö.; Shi, Y.; Mehmedovic, M.; Uhler, J.P.; Dávila López, M.; Freyer, C.; Gustafsson, C.M.; Samuelsson, T.; Falkenberg, M. Regulation of DNA replication at the end of the mitochondrial D-loop involves the helicase TWINKLE and a conserved sequence element. *Nucl. Acids Res.* **2015**, *43*, 9262–9275. [CrossRef]
43. Pereira, F.; Soares, P.; Carneiro, J.; Pereira, L.; Richards, M.B.; Samuels, D.C.; Amorim, A. Evidence for variable selective pressures at a large secondary structure of the human mitochondrial DNA control region. *Molecul. Biol. Evol.* **2008**, *25*, 2759–2770. [CrossRef] [PubMed]
44. Ruiz-Pesini, E.; Lott, M.T.; Procaccio, V.; Poole, J.C.; Brandon, M.C.; Mishmar, D.; Yi, C.; Kreuziger, J.; Baldi, P.; Wallace, D.C. An enhanced MITOMAP with a global mtDNA mutational phylogeny. *Nucl. Acids Res.* **2007**, *35*, D823–D828. [CrossRef] [PubMed]
45. Tang, Y.; Schon, E.A.; Wilichowski, E.; Vazquez-Memije, M.E.; Davidson, E.; King, M.P. Rearrangements of human mitochondrial DNA (mtDNA): New insights into the regulation of mtDNA copy number and gene expression. *Molecul. Biol. Cell.* **2000**, *11*, 1471–1485. [CrossRef] [PubMed]
46. Chapman, J.; Ng, Y.S.; Nicholls, T.J. The maintenance of mitochondrial DNA integrity and dynamics by mitochondrial membranes. *Life* **2020**, *10*, 164. [CrossRef]
47. Hudson, G.; Chinnery, P.F. Mitochondrial DNA polymerase-γ and human disease. *Hum. Mol. Genet.* **2006**, *15*, R244–R252. [CrossRef]
48. Hedberg-Oldfors, C.; Macao, B.; Basu, S.; Lindberg, C.; Peter, B.; Erdinc, D.; Uhler, J.P.; Larsson, E.; Falkenberg, M.; Oldfors, A. Deep sequencing of mitochondrial DNA and characterization of a novel POLG mutation in a patient with arPEO. *Neurol. Genet.* **2020**, *6*, e391. [CrossRef]

49. Peter, B.; Falkenberg, M. TWINKLE and other human mitochondrial DNA helicases: Structure, function and disease. *Genes* **2020**, *11*, 408. [CrossRef]
50. Del Dotto, V.; Ullah, F.; Di Meo, I.; Magini, P.; Gusic, M.; Maresca, A.; Caporali, L.; Palombo, F.; Tagliavini, F.; Baugh, E.H. SSBP1 mutations cause mtDNA depletion underlying a complex optic atrophy disorder. *J. Clin. Invest.* **2020**, *130*, 108–125. [CrossRef]
51. Young, M.J.; Copeland, W.C. Human mitochondrial DNA replication machinery and disease. *Curr. Opin. Genet. Dev.* **2016**, *38*, 52–62. [CrossRef] [PubMed]
52. Longley, M.J.; Clark, S.; Man, C.Y.W.; Hudson, G.; Durham, S.E.; Taylor, R.W.; Nightingale, S.; Turnbull, D.M.; Copeland, W.C.; Chinnery, P.F. Mutant POLG2 disrupts DNA polymerase γ subunits and causes progressive external ophthalmoplegia. *Am. J. Hum. Genet.* **2006**, *78*, 1026–1034. [CrossRef] [PubMed]
53. Carreño-Gago, L.; Blázquez-Bermejo, C.; Díaz-Manera, J.; Cámara, Y.; Gallardo, E.; Martí, R.; Torres-Torronteras, J.; García-Arumí, E. Identification and characterization of new RNASEH1 mutations associated with PEO syndrome and multiple mitochondrial DNA deletions. *Front. Genet.* **2019**, *10*, 576. [CrossRef]
54. Kornblum, C.; Nicholls, T.J.; Haack, T.B.; Schöler, S.; Peeva, V.; Danhauser, K.; Hallmann, K.; Zsurka, G.; Rorbach, J.; Iuso, A. Loss-of-function mutations in MGME1 impair mtDNA replication and cause multisystemic mitochondrial disease. *Nat. Genet.* **2013**, *45*, 214. [CrossRef]
55. Nicholls, T.J.; Nadalutti, C.A.; Motori, E.; Sommerville, E.W.; Gorman, G.S.; Basu, S.; Hoberg, E.; Turnbull, D.M.; Chinnery, P.F.; Larsson, N.-G. Topoisomerase 3α is required for decatenation and segregation of human mtDNA. *Molecul. Cell.* **2018**, *69*, 9–23.e6. [CrossRef]
56. Stiles, A.R.; Simon, M.T.; Stover, A.; Eftekharian, S.; Khanlou, N.; Wang, H.L.; Magaki, S.; Lee, H.; Partynski, K.; Dorrani, N. Mutations in TFAM, encoding mitochondrial transcription factor A, cause neonatal liver failure associated with mtDNA depletion. *Mol. Genet. Metab.* **2016**, *119*, 91–99. [CrossRef]
57. Barshad, G.; Marom, S.; Cohen, T.; Mishmar, D. Mitochondrial DNA transcription and its regulation: An evolutionary perspective. *Trends Genet.* **2018**, *34*, 682–692. [CrossRef]
58. Bonawitz, N.D.; Clayton, D.A.; Shadel, G.S. Initiation and beyond: Multiple functions of the human mitochondrial transcription machinery. *Molecul. Cell.* **2006**, *24*, 813–825. [CrossRef] [PubMed]
59. Posse, V.; Shahzad, S.; Falkenberg, M.; Hällberg, B.M.; Gustafsson, C.M. TEFM is a potent stimulator of mitochondrial transcription elongation in vitro. *Nucl. Acids Res.* **2015**, *43*, 2615–2624. [CrossRef]
60. Lopez Sanchez, M.I.; Mercer, T.R.; Davies, S.M.; Shearwood, A.-M.J.; Nygård, K.K.; Richman, T.R.; Mattick, J.S.; Rackham, O.; Filipovska, A. RNA processing in human mitochondria. *Cell Cycle* **2011**, *10*, 2904–2916. [CrossRef]
61. Van Haute, L.; Pearce, S.F.; Powell, C.A.; D'Souza, A.R.; Nicholls, T.J.; Minczuk, M. Mitochondrial transcript maturation and its disorders. *J. Inherit. Metabol. Dis.* **2015**, *38*, 655–680. [CrossRef]
62. Powell, C.A.; Nicholls, T.J.; Minczuk, M. Nuclear-encoded factors involved in post-transcriptional processing and modification of mitochondrial tRNAs in human disease. *Front. Genet.* **2015**, *6*, 79. [CrossRef]
63. Clayton, D.A. Transcription and replication of mitochondrial DNA. *Hum. Reprod.* **2000**, *15*, 11–17. [CrossRef] [PubMed]
64. Connor, T.M.; Hoer, S.; Mallett, A.; Gale, D.P.; Gomez-Duran, A.; Posse, V.; Antrobus, R.; Moreno, P.; Sciacovelli, M.; Frezza, C. Mutations in mitochondrial DNA causing tubulointerstitial kidney disease. *PLoS Genet.* **2017**, *13*, e1006620. [CrossRef]
65. Florentz, C.; Sohm, B.; Tryoen-Toth, P.; Pütz, J.; Sissler, M. Human mitochondrial tRNAs in health and disease. *Cell. Molecul. Life Sci.* **2003**, *60*, 1356–1375. [CrossRef]
66. Yarham, J.W.; Elson, J.L.; Blakely, E.L.; McFarland, R.; Taylor, R.W. Mitochondrial tRNA mutations and disease. *Wiley Interdisc. Rev. RNA* **2010**, *1*, 304–324. [CrossRef]
67. Gorman, G.S.; Schaefer, A.M.; Ng, Y.; Gomez, N.; Blakely, E.L.; Alston, C.L.; Feeney, C.; Horvath, R.; Yu-Wai-Man, P.; Chinnery, P.F. Prevalence of nuclear and mitochondrial DNA mutations related to adult mitochondrial disease. *Annal. Neurol.* **2015**, *77*, 753–759. [CrossRef] [PubMed]
68. Kühl, I.; Miranda, M.; Posse, V.; Milenkovic, D.; Mourier, A.; Siira, S.J.; Bonekamp, N.A.; Neumann, U.; Filipovska, A.; Polosa, P.L. POLRMT regulates the switch between replication primer formation and gene expression of mammalian mtDNA. *Sci. Adv.* **2016**, *2*, e1600963. [CrossRef] [PubMed]
69. Jiang, S.; Koolmeister, C.; Misic, J.; Siira, S.; Kühl, I.; Silva Ramos, E.; Miranda, M.; Jiang, M.; Posse, V.; Lytovchenko, O. TEFM regulates both transcription elongation and RNA processing in mitochondria. *EMBO Rep.* **2019**, *20*, e48101. [CrossRef] [PubMed]
70. Haack, T.B.; Kopajtich, R.; Freisinger, P.; Wieland, T.; Rorbach, J.; Nicholls, T.J.; Baruffini, E.; Walther, A.; Danhauser, K.; Zimmermann, F.A. ELAC2 mutations cause a mitochondrial RNA processing defect associated with hypertrophic cardiomyopathy. *Am. J. Hum. Genet.* **2013**, *93*, 211–223. [CrossRef]
71. Peeva, V.; Blei, D.; Trombly, G.; Corsi, S.; Szukszto, M.J.; Rebelo-Guiomar, P.; Gammage, P.A.; Kudin, A.P.; Becker, C.; Altmüller, J. Linear mitochondrial DNA is rapidly degraded by components of the replication machinery. *Nat. Commun.* **2018**, *9*, 1–11. [CrossRef] [PubMed]
72. Srivastava, S.; Moraes, C.T. Manipulating mitochondrial DNA heteroplasmy by a mitochondrially targeted restriction endonuclease. *Hum. Molecul. Genet.* **2001**, *10*, 3093–3099. [CrossRef]
73. Tanaka, M.; Borgeld, H.-J.; Zhang, J.; Muramatsu, S.-i.; Gong, J.-S.; Yoneda, M.; Maruyama, W.; Naoi, M.; Ibi, T.; Sahashi, K. Gene therapy for mitochondrial disease by delivering restriction endonucleaseSmaI into mitochondria. *J. Biomed. Sci.* **2002**, *9*, 534–541. [CrossRef]

74. Reddy, P.; Ocampo, A.; Suzuki, K.; Luo, J.; Bacman, S.R.; Williams, S.L.; Sugawara, A.; Okamura, D.; Tsunekawa, Y.; Wu, J. Selective elimination of mitochondrial mutations in the germline by genome editing. *Cell* **2015**, *161*, 459–469. [CrossRef] [PubMed]
75. Gammage, P.A.; Rorbach, J.; Vincent, A.I.; Rebar, E.J.; Minczuk, M. Mitochondrially targeted ZFN s for selective degradation of pathogenic mitochondrial genomes bearing large-scale deletions or point mutations. *EMBO Molecul. Med.* **2014**, *6*, 458–466. [CrossRef]
76. Sun, N.; Zhao, H. Transcription activator-like effector nucleases (TALENs): A highly efficient and versatile tool for genome editing. *Biotechnol. Bioeng.* **2013**, *110*, 1811–1821. [CrossRef] [PubMed]
77. Hashimoto, M.; Bacman, S.R.; Peralta, S.; Falk, M.J.; Chomyn, A.; Chan, D.C.; Williams, S.L.; Moraes, C.T. MitoTALEN: A general approach to reduce mutant mtDNA loads and restore oxidative phosphorylation function in mitochondrial diseases. *Molecul. Ther.* **2015**, *23*, 1592–1599. [CrossRef]
78. Bacman, S.R.; Williams, S.L.; Pinto, M.; Peralta, S.; Moraes, C.T. Specific elimination of mutant mitochondrial genomes in patient-derived cells by mitoTALENs. *Nat. Med.* **2013**, *19*, 1111–1113. [CrossRef] [PubMed]
79. Gammage, P.A.; Viscomi, C.; Simard, M.-L.; Costa, A.S.; Gaude, E.; Powell, C.A.; Van Haute, L.; McCann, B.J.; Rebelo-Guiomar, P.; Cerutti, R. Genome editing in mitochondria corrects a pathogenic mtDNA mutation in vivo. *Nat. Med.* **2018**, *24*, 1691–1695. [CrossRef]
80. Bacman, S.R.; Kauppila, J.H.; Pereira, C.V.; Nissanka, N.; Miranda, M.; Pinto, M.; Williams, S.L.; Larsson, N.-G.; Stewart, J.B.; Moraes, C.T. MitoTALEN reduces mutant mtDNA load and restores tRNA Ala levels in a mouse model of heteroplasmic mtDNA mutation. *Nat. Med.* **2018**, *24*, 1696–1700. [CrossRef] [PubMed]
81. Minczuk, M.; Kolasinska-Zwierz, P.; Murphy, M.P.; Papworth, M.A. Construction and testing of engineered zinc-finger proteins for sequence-specific modification of mtDNA. *Nat. Prot.* **2010**, *5*, 342. [CrossRef] [PubMed]
82. Hussain, S.-R.A.; Yalvac, M.E.; Khoo, B.; Eckardt, S.; McLaughlin, K.J. Adapting CRISPR/Cas9 system for targeting mitochondrial genome. *bioRxiv* **2020**. [CrossRef]
83. Jo, A.; Ham, S.; Lee, G.H.; Lee, Y.-I.; Kim, S.; Lee, Y.-S.; Shin, J.-H.; Lee, Y. Efficient mitochondrial genome editing by CRISPR/Cas9. *BioMed Res. Internat* **2015**, *2015*. [CrossRef]
84. Mok, B.Y.; de Moraes, M.H.; Zeng, J.; Bosch, D.E.; Kotrys, A.V.; Raguram, A.; Hsu, F.; Radey, M.C.; Peterson, S.B.; Mootha, V.K. A bacterial cytidine deaminase toxin enables CRISPR-free mitochondrial base editing. *Nature* **2020**, *583*, 631–637. [CrossRef] [PubMed]
85. Jang, Y.-h.; Lim, K.-i. Recent advances in mitochondria-targeted gene delivery. *Molecules* **2018**, *23*, 2316. [CrossRef]
86. Yasuzaki, Y.; Yamada, Y.; Kanefuji, T.; Harashima, H. Localization of exogenous DNA to mitochondria in skeletal muscle following hydrodynamic limb vein injection. *J. Control. Rel.* **2013**, *172*, 805–811. [CrossRef] [PubMed]
87. Collombet, J.-M.; Wheeler, V.C.; Vogel, F.; Coutelle, C. Introduction of plasmid DNA into isolated mitochondria by electroporation: A novel approach toward gene correction for mitochondrial disorders. *J. Biol. Chem.* **1997**, *272*, 5342–5347. [CrossRef]
88. Yoon, Y.G.; Koob, M.D. Efficient cloning and engineering of entire mitochondrial genomes in Escherichia coli and transfer into transcriptionally active mitochondria. *Nucl. Acids Res.* **2003**, *31*, 1407–1415. [CrossRef] [PubMed]
89. Patananan, A.N.; Wu, T.-H.; Chiou, P.-Y.; Teitell, M.A. Modifying the mitochondrial genome. *Cell Metabol.* **2016**, *23*, 785796. [CrossRef] [PubMed]
90. Kitani, T.; Kami, D.; Matoba, S.; Gojo, S. Internalization of isolated functional mitochondria: Involvement of macropinocytosis. *J. Cell. Molecul. Med.* **2014**, *18*, 1694–1703. [CrossRef] [PubMed]
91. Kitani, T.; Kami, D.; Kawasaki, T.; Nakata, M.; Matoba, S.; Gojo, S. Direct human mitochondrial transfer: A novel concept based on the endosymbiotic theory. *Transplant. Proc.* **2014**. [CrossRef]
92. Von Heijne, G. Mitochondrial targeting sequences may form amphiphilic helices. *EMBO J.* **1986**, *5*, 1335–1342. [CrossRef]
93. Mukhopadhyay, A.; Heard, T.S.; Wen, X.; Hammen, P.K.; Weiner, H. Location of the actual signal in the negatively charged leader sequence involved in the import into the mitochondrial matrix space. *J. Biol. Chem.* **2003**, *278*, 13712–13718. [CrossRef] [PubMed]
94. Yoon, Y.G.; Koob, M.D.; Yoo, Y.H. Re-engineering the mitochondrial genomes in mammalian cells. *Anat. Cell. Biol.* **2010**, *43*, 97–109. [CrossRef]
95. Vestweber, D.; Schatz, G. DNA-protein conjugates can enter mitochondria via the protein import pathway. *Nature* **1989**, *338*, 170–172. [CrossRef] [PubMed]
96. Lu, Y.; Beavis, A.D. Effect of leader peptides on the permeability of mitochondria. *J. Biol. Chem.* **1997**, *272*, 13555–13561. [CrossRef]
97. Seibel, P.; Trappe, J.; Villani, G.; Klopstock, T.; Papa, S.; Reichmann, H. Transfection of mitochondria: Strategy towards a gene therapy of mitochondrial DNA diseases. *Nucleic Acids Res.* **1995**, *23*, 10–17. [CrossRef]
98. Chinnery, P.; Taylor, R.; Diekert, K.; Lill, R.; Turnbull, D.; Lightowlers, R. Peptide nucleic acid delivery to human mitochondria. *Gene Ther.* **1999**, *6*, 1919–1928. [CrossRef] [PubMed]
99. Flierl, A.; Jackson, C.; Cottrell, B.; Murdock, D.; Seibel, P.; Wallace, D. Targeted delivery of DNA to the mitochondrial compartment via import sequence-conjugated peptide nucleic acid. *Mol. Ther.* **2003**, *7*, 550–557. [CrossRef]
100. Naso, M.F.; Tomkowicz, B.; Perry, W.L.; Strohl, W.R. Adeno-associated virus (AAV) as a vector for gene therapy. *BioDrugs* **2017**, *31*, 317–334. [CrossRef]
101. Wang, D.; Tai, P.W.; Gao, G. Adeno-associated virus vector as a platform for gene therapy delivery. *Nat. Rev. Drug Discov.* **2019**, *18*, 358–378. [CrossRef] [PubMed]

102. Li, C.; Samulski, R.J. Engineering adeno-associated virus vectors for gene therapy. *Nat. Rev. Genet.* **2020**, *21*, 255–272. [CrossRef] [PubMed]
103. Kimura, T.; Ferran, B.; Tsukahara, Y.; Shang, Q.; Desai, S.; Fedoce, A.; Pimentel, D.R.; Luptak, I.; Adachi, T.; Ido, Y. Production of adeno-associated virus vectors for in vitro and in vivo applications. *Sci. Rep.* **2019**, *9*, 1–13. [CrossRef]
104. Yu, H.; Mehta, A.; Wang, G.; Hauswirth, W.W.; Chiodo, V.; Boye, S.L.; Guy, J. Next-generation sequencing of mitochondrial targeted AAV transfer of human ND4 in mice. *Mol. Vis.* **2013**, *19*, 1482.
105. Rottenberg, H. Membrane potential and surface potential in mitochondria: Uptake and binding of lipophilic cations. *J. Membr. Biol.* **1984**, *81*, 127–138. [CrossRef] [PubMed]
106. Yuan, P.; Mao, X.; Wu, X.; Liew, S.S.; Li, L.; Yao, S.Q. Mitochondria-targeting, intracellular delivery of native proteins using biodegradable silica nanoparticles. *Angewandte Chemie* **2019**, *131*, 7739–7743. [CrossRef]
107. Marrache, S.; Dhar, S. Engineering of blended nanoparticle platform for delivery of mitochondria-acting therapeutics. *Proc. Natl. Acad. Sci. USA* **2012**, *109*, 16288–16293. [CrossRef]
108. Biswas, S.; Dodwadkar, N.S.; Piroyan, A.; Torchilin, V.P. Surface conjugation of triphenylphosphonium to target poly (amidoamine) dendrimers to mitochondria. *Biomaterials* **2012**, *33*, 4773–4782. [CrossRef]
109. Smith, R.A.; Porteous, C.M.; Gane, A.M.; Murphy, M.P. Delivery of bioactive molecules to mitochondria in vivo. *Proc. Natl. Acad. Sci. USA* **2003**, *100*, 5407–5412. [CrossRef]
110. Muratovska, A.; Lightowlers, R.N.; Taylor, R.W.; Turnbull, D.M.; Smith, R.A.; Wilce, J.A.; Martin, S.W.; Murphy, M.P. Targeting peptide nucleic acid (PNA) oligomers to mitochondria within cells by conjugation to lipophilic cations: Implications for mitochondrial DNA replication, expression and disease. *Nucl. Acids Res.* **2001**, *29*, 1852–1863. [CrossRef]
111. Wang, X.; Shao, N.; Zhang, Q.; Cheng, Y. Mitochondrial targeting dendrimer allows efficient and safe gene delivery. *J. Mat. Chem. B.* **2014**, *2*, 2546–2553. [CrossRef]
112. Weissig, V.; Lasch, J.; Erdos, G.; Meyer, H.W.; Rowe, T.C.; Hughes, J. DQAsomes: A novel potential drug and gene delivery system made from dequalinium™. *Pharmaceut. Res.* **1998**, *15*, 334–337. [CrossRef] [PubMed]
113. Weissig, V.; Lizano, C.; Torchilin, V.P. Selective DNA release from DQAsome/DNA complexes at mitochondria-like membranes. *Drug Del.* **2000**, *7*, 1–5. [CrossRef] [PubMed]
114. D'Souza, G.G.; Rammohan, R.; Cheng, S.-M.; Torchilin, V.P.; Weissig, V. DQAsome-mediated delivery of plasmid DNA toward mitochondria in living cells. *J. Control. Rel.* **2003**, *92*, 189–197. [CrossRef]
115. Weissig, V.; D'Souza, G.; Torchilin, V.P. DQAsome/DNA complexes release DNA upon contact with isolated mouse liver mitochondria. *J. Control. Rel.* **2001**, *75*, 401–408. [CrossRef]
116. Lyrawati, D.; Trounson, A.; Cram, D. Expression of GFP in the mitochondrial compartment using DQAsome-mediated delivery of an artificial mini-mitochondrial genome. *Pharmaceut. Res.* **2011**, *28*, 2848–2862. [CrossRef] [PubMed]
117. Boddapati, S.V.; D'Souza, G.G.; Erdogan, S.; Torchilin, V.P.; Weissig, V. Organelle-targeted nanocarriers: Specific delivery of liposomal ceramide to mitochondria enhances its cytotoxicity in vitro and in vivo. *Nano Lett.* **2008**, *8*, 2559–2563. [CrossRef] [PubMed]
118. Yamada, Y.; Akita, H.; Kamiya, H.; Kogure, K.; Yamamoto, T.; Shinohara, Y.; Yamashita, K.; Kobayashi, H.; Kikuchi, H.; Harashima, H. MITO-Porter: A liposome-based carrier system for delivery of macromolecules into mitochondria via membrane fusion. *Biochim. Biophys. Acta Biomem.* **2008**, *1778*, 423–432. [CrossRef]
119. Yamada, Y.; Furukawa, R.; Yasuzaki, Y.; Harashima, H. Dual function MITO-Porter, a nano carrier integrating both efficient cytoplasmic delivery and mitochondrial macromolecule delivery. *Molecul. Ther.* **2011**, *19*, 1449–1456. [CrossRef]
120. Yamada, Y.; Harashima, H. Delivery of bioactive molecules to the mitochondrial genome using a membrane-fusing, liposome-based carrier, DF-MITO-Porter. *Biomaterials* **2012**, *33*, 1589–1595. [CrossRef] [PubMed]
121. Kawamura, E.; Yamada, Y.; Harashima, H. Mitochondrial targeting functional peptides as potential devices for the mitochondrial delivery of a DF-MITO-Porter. *Mitochondrion* **2013**, *13*, 610–614. [CrossRef]
122. Yamada, Y.; Kawamura, E.; Harashima, H. Mitochondrial-targeted DNA delivery using a DF-MITO-Porter, an innovative nano carrier with cytoplasmic and mitochondrial fusogenic envelopes. *J. Nanopart. Res.* **2012**, *14*, 1013. [CrossRef]
123. Yamada, Y.; Ishikawa, T.; Harashima, H. Validation of the use of an artificial mitochondrial reporter DNA vector containing a Cytomegalovirus promoter for mitochondrial transgene expression. *Biomaterials* **2017**, *136*, 56–66. [CrossRef]
124. Jeandard, D.; Smirnova, A.; Tarassov, I.; Barrey, E.; Smirnov, A.; Entelis, N. Import of non-coding RNAs into human mitochondria: A critical review and emerging approaches. *Cells* **2019**, *8*, 286. [CrossRef] [PubMed]
125. Entelis, N.S.; Kolesnikova, O.A.; Dogan, S.; Martin, R.P.; Tarassov, I.A. 5 S rRNA and tRNA import into human mitochondria: Comparison of in vitro requirements. *J. Biol. Chem.* **2001**, *276*, 45642–45653. [CrossRef]
126. Smirnov, A.; Comte, C.; Mager-Heckel, A.-M.; Addis, V.; Krasheninnikov, I.A.; Martin, R.P.; Entelis, N.; Tarassov, I. Mitochondrial enzyme rhodanese is essential for 5 S ribosomal RNA import into human mitochondria. *J. Biol. Chem.* **2010**, *285*, 30792–30803. [CrossRef]
127. Smirnov, A.; Entelis, N.; Martin, R.P.; Tarassov, I. Biological significance of 5S rRNA import into human mitochondria: Role of ribosomal protein MRP-L18. *Genes. Develop.* **2011**, *25*, 1289–1305. [CrossRef] [PubMed]
128. Wang, G.; Chen, H.-W.; Oktay, Y.; Zhang, J.; Allen, E.L.; Smith, G.M.; Fan, K.C.; Hong, J.S.; French, S.W.; McCaffery, J.M. PNPASE regulates RNA import into mitochondria. *Cell* **2010**, *142*, 456–467. [CrossRef]

129. Wang, G.; Shimada, E.; Koehler, C.M.; Teitell, M.A. PNPASE and RNA trafficking into mitochondria. *Biochim. Biophys. Acta Gene Regulat. Mechan.* **2012**, *1819*, 998–1007. [CrossRef] [PubMed]
130. Wang, G.; Shimada, E.; Zhang, J.; Hong, J.S.; Smith, G.M.; Teitell, M.A.; Koehler, C.M. Correcting human mitochondrial mutations with targeted RNA import. *Proc. Natl. Acad. Sci. USA* **2012**, *109*, 4840–4845. [CrossRef]
131. Rubio, M.A.T.; Rinehart, J.J.; Krett, B.; Duvezin-Caubet, S.; Reichert, A.S.; Söll, D.; Alfonzo, J.D. Mammalian mitochondria have the innate ability to import tRNAs by a mechanism distinct from protein import. *Proc. Natl. Acad. Sci. USA* **2008**, *105*, 9186–9191. [CrossRef] [PubMed]
132. Kawamura, E.; Maruyama, M.; Abe, J.; Sudo, A.; Takeda, A.; Takada, S.; Yokota, T.; Kinugawa, S.; Harashima, H.; Yamada, Y. Validation of gene therapy for mutant mitochondria by delivering mitochondrial RNA using a MITO-Porter, a liposome-based nano device. *Molecul. Ther. Nucl. Acids* **2020**, *20*, 687–698. [CrossRef] [PubMed]
133. Kawamura, E.; Hibino, M.; Harashima, H.; Yamada, Y. Targeted mitochondrial delivery of antisense RNA-containing nanoparticles by a MITO-Porter for safe and efficient mitochondrial gene silencing. *Mitochondrion* **2019**, *49*, 178–188. [CrossRef] [PubMed]

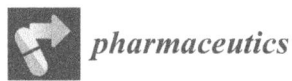

Review

Therapeutic Approaches to Treat Mitochondrial Diseases: "One-Size-Fits-All" and "Precision Medicine" Strategies

Emanuela Bottani [1,*], Costanza Lamperti [2], Alessandro Prigione [3], Valeria Tiranti [2], Nicola Persico [4,5] and Dario Brunetti [2,6,*]

1. Department of Diagnostics and Public Health, Section of Pharmacology, University of Verona, 37134 Verona, Italy
2. Medical Genetics and Neurogenetics Unit, Fondazione IRCCS Istituto Neurologico C. Besta, 20126 Milan, Italy; costanza.lamperti@istituto-besta.it (C.L.); valeria.tiranti@istituto-besta.it (V.T.)
3. Department of General Pediatrics, Neonatology, and Pediatric Cardiology, University Clinic Düsseldorf (UKD), Heinrich Heine University (HHU), 40225 Dusseldorf, Germany; Alessandro.Prigione@med.uni-duesseldorf.de
4. Department of Clinical Science and Community Health, University of Milan, 20122 Milan, Italy; nicola.persico@unimi.it
5. Fetal Medicine and Surgery Service, Fondazione IRCCS Ca' Granda, Ospedale Maggiore Policlinico, 20122 Milan, Italy
6. Department of Medical Biotechnology and Translational Medicine, University of Milan, 20129 Milan, Italy
* Correspondence: emanuela.bottani@univr.it (E.B.); dario.brunetti@unimi.it (D.B.)

Received: 9 October 2020; Accepted: 9 November 2020; Published: 11 November 2020

Abstract: Primary mitochondrial diseases (PMD) refer to a group of severe, often inherited genetic conditions due to mutations in the mitochondrial genome or in the nuclear genes encoding for proteins involved in oxidative phosphorylation (OXPHOS). The mutations hamper the last step of aerobic metabolism, affecting the primary source of cellular ATP synthesis. Mitochondrial diseases are characterized by extremely heterogeneous symptoms, ranging from organ-specific to multisystemic dysfunction with different clinical courses. The limited information of the natural history, the limitations of currently available preclinical models, coupled with the large variability of phenotypical presentations of PMD patients, have strongly penalized the development of effective therapies. However, new therapeutic strategies have been emerging, often with promising preclinical and clinical results. Here we review the state of the art on experimental treatments for mitochondrial diseases, presenting "one-size-fits-all" approaches and precision medicine strategies. Finally, we propose novel perspective therapeutic plans, either based on preclinical studies or currently used for other genetic or metabolic diseases that could be transferred to PMD.

Keywords: mitochondria; mitochondrial DNA; mitochondrial disorders; pharmacological therapy; gene therapy; precision medicine

1. Genetics of Mitochondrial Diseases

Primary mitochondrial disorders (PMD) are a group of rare diseases affecting approximately 1 in 4300 live birth and causing progressive, incurable defects often resulting in premature death. PMD are characterized by a high genetic, biochemical, and clinical complexity that arise from the dysfunction of the oxidative phosphorylation (OXPHOS), the essential, final pathway for aerobic metabolism [1]. Such impairment is caused by mutations in genes encoding for proteins involved in mitochondrial respiratory chain (MRC) biogenesis, (i.e., subunits of MRC complexes, assembly factors, or post-assembly quality controllers), or by mutations in genes involved in other mitochondrial functions, including fission and fusion machinery, mitochondrial DNA (mtDNA) maintenance, heme biosynthesis, and iron/sulfur metabolism, among others [2].

Each mitochondrion contains several mitochondrial DNA (mtDNA) molecules, the abundance of which spans from hundreds to thousands of copies per cell, depending on the tissue type. For years, it was trusted that in physiological conditions, all mtDNA molecules have the same sequence, a condition known as homoplasmy. When mutations in mtDNA occur, wild type and mutant molecules coexist in the same cell/organ, a condition known as heteroplasmy. However, recent deep resequencing analysis has shown that low-level mtDNA heteroplasmy is extremely common in humans, and, at very low levels (0.5–1%), heteroplasmy seems to be a universal finding [3].

MtDNA mutations could affect any gene encoding the 13 core subunits of the MRC complexes, the 22 mitochondrial tRNAs, or the two rRNAs. They can include point mutations, either homo- or heteroplasmic, and (invariably heteroplasmic) large-scale rearrangements. Heteroplasmic mutations lead to different clinical phenotypes, such as Leigh syndrome (LS) [4], myoclonic epilepsy with ragged red fibers (MERRF) [5], mitochondrial encephalomyopathy with lactic acidosis and stroke-like episodes (MELAS) [6], and neurogenic weakness, ataxia, and retinitis pigmentosa (NARP) [7]. The central disease entity associated with homoplasmic mtDNA mutations is Leber's hereditary optic neuropathy (LHON) [8]. Mutations in the same gene can lead to different clinical presentation; for instance, mitochondrial phenotypes described in patients with MT-ATP6 mutations span from maternally inherited Leigh syndrome and neurogenic muscle weakness, ataxia, and retinitis pigmentosa (NARP)[9], to Charcot–Marie–Tooth disease [10], late-onset hereditary spastic paraplegia-like disorder [11], and MERRF-like phenotype [12]. Rearrangements (single deletions or duplications) of mtDNA are responsible for sporadic progressive external ophthalmoplegia (PEO), Kearns–Sayre syndrome (KSS) [13], and Pearson's syndrome [14,15].

There are approximately 1500 predicted mitochondrial genes, that if mutated could lead to mitochondrial dysfunction [16], and so far, more than 300 have been linked to mitochondrial disorders [17,18]. Advanced diagnostic technologies, like next-generation sequencing, are leading to a rapid escalation in the discoveries of novel disease-causing genes. Therefore, a further, widely accepted, genetic classification of PMD is based on the function of the protein products encoded by the mutated genes and includes (i) structural subunits of complexes I-IV, and ATP synthase complex F_0F_1; (ii) assembly factors of complexes I-IV, and ATP synthase complex F_0F_1; (iii) factors performing or regulating replication, expression, and stability of mtDNA; (iv) proteins related to mitochondrial biogenesis or indirectly associated to OXPHOS; (v) proteins of the execution pathways, such as fission/fusion and apoptosis; (vi) proteins involved in the biosynthesis and metabolism of cofactors; or (vii) proteins involved in the biosynthesis and metabolism of mitochondrial membrane lipids.

The mitochondrial membrane potential ($\Delta\Psi m$) generated by proton-pumping Complexes I, III, and IV, is essential not only for the energy storage but also for the elimination of disabled mitochondria [19]. Genetic defects affecting these respiratory complexes often lead to dysfunctional $\Delta\Psi m$ with significant consequences to the viability of the cells. However, a comprehensive description of clinical features and genetic causes of PMD is beyond the scope of this manuscript; please refer to [20,21] for an exhaustive list.

Despite significant advances in understanding the pathophysiology, the extremely varied phenotype–genotype relationship of PMD [1] (Figure 1) has strongly limited the development of effective therapies. Currently, no approved cure exists for most of them, and existing treatments are focused on relieving complications. However, in recent decades, significant signs of progress have been reported. In this manuscript, we will review the most substantial advances in the treatment of PMD and discuss future therapeutic perspectives.

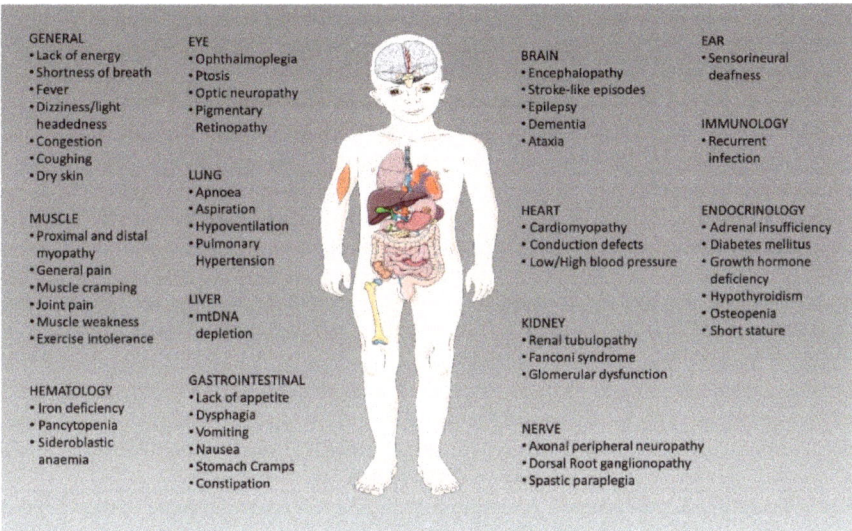

Figure 1. Clinical features of mitochondrial disorder: PMD arise from the dysfunction of the oxidative phosphorylation (OXPHOS) and are characterized by a high genetic, biochemical, and clinical complexity that hinder the prediction of disease progression and the development of therapeutic strategies.

2. Therapeutic Approaches to Treat Mitochondrial Disorders

In this manuscript, we choose to classify the current treatments as (i) "one-size-fits-all" strategies, which could, in principle, be used to treat different PMD, regardless the underlying genetic mutation; and (ii) "precision medicine" approaches, aimed at treating a specific PMD with a specific mutation or a peculiar metabolic hallmark. The reader should note, however, that such categorization does not act as unconditional rule, since some exceptions are indeed possible.

The 'one-size-fits-all' strategies include symptomatic interventions, mainly diet, exercise, exposure to hypoxia, and pharmacological therapy, which is based on drugs aiming at (i) inducing mitochondrial biogenesis; (ii) stimulating the pathway of nitric oxide synthase; (iii) increasing ATP synthesis; (iv) improving antioxidant defense; (v) enhancing the mitochondrial quality control pathway by stimulating dynamics (fission/fusion events) and degradation of damaged mitochondria (autophagy); (vi) targeting cardiolipin. Recent advances in understanding the underlying pathophysiology of several PMD have made possible the development of a 'precision medicine' approach in some cases. Specialized therapies include: (i) supplementation of nucleotides; (ii) replacing defective mtDNA in the oocyte; (iii) supplementation of exogenous mitochondria; (iv) gene- and cell-replacement therapies; (v) scavenging of poisoning metabolites; (vi) organ transplantation; (vii) mtDNA editing. Appendix A Table A1 summarizes the most relevant discussed approaches, distinguishing those that are currently only at preclinical level from therapies advanced in clinical trials or exploited in compassionate use.

3. "One-Size-Fits-All" Approaches

3.1. Physical Exercise

Although mitochondrial patients' clinical features are highly variable, neurological involvement is often present, best described as neuromuscular defect, including muscle weakness, exercise intolerance, and fatigue. The molecular defect in patients with mitochondrial myopathies (MM) commonly involves the mitochondrial genome, with either single, large-scale deletions, or point mutations, resulting in mosaicism of MRC-competent and MRC-affected muscle fibers [22]. Given the well-established positive effects of physical exercise on healthy subjects, exercise training has been suggested as an approach to improve physical capacity and quality of life. The rationale of endurance training is based on three fundamental aspects: (i) to counteract adverse physiological effects of deconditioning caused by habitual avoidance of activities, provoking the symptoms of fatigue; (ii) to ameliorate the disease process by increasing mitochondrial biogenesis and MRC activity in skeletal muscle; and, in case of mtDNA mutations/deletions; (iii) to stimulate the induction of muscle satellite cells, which have low or undetectable levels of mtDNA mutations, shifting the wild-type mtDNA templates to mature muscle.

Endurance exercise is a potent inducer of mitochondrial biogenesis [23], not only in skeletal muscle but also in the brain [24]. Exercise triggers mitochondrial proliferation through inducing the peroxisome proliferator-activated receptor-γ (PPAR-γ) coactivator 1α (PGC-1α), which is the master transcriptional regulator modulating mitochondrial biogenesis [25]. Endurance training also activates PGC-1β, AMP-dependent kinase (*AMPK*), p38γ MAPK, and hypoxia-inducible factors (HIFs) [26], contributing to the extensive metabolic and molecular remodeling that leads to the preservation of aerobic fitness and muscle strength. Also, physical activity upregulates endothelial nitric oxide synthase (eNOS) gene expression with the consequent increase of nitric oxide (NO) production, which in turn induces mitochondrial biogenesis and cell glucose uptake in skeletal and cardiac muscle [27,28]. Please refer to Section 3.6 for an extensive description of the molecular mechanisms.

Muscle satellite cells are dormant, committed myogenic cells reactivated as needed for muscle growth and repair. Since mutant mtDNA molecules are often undetectable in satellite cells cultured from affected muscles of MM patients [29,30], the stimulations of the proliferation and incorporation of satellite cells into existing myofibers through exercise training have been proposed as a method for normalizing the skeletal muscle mtDNA genotype in MM patients, with encouraging results [31,32]. Favorable effects of physical exercise have been demonstrated in preclinical models of PMD. Prolonged endurance exercise conferred muscular protection and prevented early mortality in the transgenic *PolG* mouse model, harboring a defect in the proofreading-exonuclease activity of mitochondrial polymerase gamma [33]. Significantly, such effects were not limited to skeletal muscle but also involved other organs, including brain, blood, and heart. Exercise training significantly improved aerobic fitness, OXPHOS activity, and muscle strength in the *Harlequin* mutant mouse, a model of complex I (CI) deficiency due to a proviral insertion in the apoptosis-inducing factor (*Aif*) gene. Significant activation of the mTORC1-mediated anabolic pathway in skeletal muscle was reported upon training [34]. Exercise training also remodeled MRC complexes organizations in skeletal muscle of healthy humans, increasing the amount of MRC complexes organized into supercomplexes (SC) and promoting the redistribution of CI from SC I+III$_2$ to SC I+III$_2$+IV$_n$ and of complex III (CIII) and complex IV (CIV) from free forms or SC I+III$_2$ into more functional SC species, such as the fully assembled SC I+III$_2$+IV$_n$ [35].

These and other findings [36,37] supported endurance training as a therapeutic strategy for patients affected by MM, and beneficial effects have been reported in open-label clinical studies. Twelve-week supervised rehabilitation endurance training increased maximal oxygen uptake, work output, minute ventilation, endurance performance, walking distance in shuttle walking test, peripheral muscle strength, and improved clinical symptoms in patients with MM [38]. Prolonged physical exercise increased VO$_{2MAX}$, citrate synthase activity, and mtDNA quantity in muscle biopsies of MM patients; these beneficial effects partially reverted after deconditioning [39]. Taivassalo and co-workers obtained similar training and detraining results, but they did not see an effect on mtDNA amount [40]. Endurance training also promoted heteroplasmic shifting, reducing the relative proportion of mutant to wild-type mtDNA in patients with heteroplasmic mtDNA deletions and point mutations [41,42]. However, other studies reported a trend toward the preferential proliferation of mutant genomes in MM patients with heteroplasmic mtDNA mutations following prolonged aerobic training, despite enhanced muscle OXPHOS, raising some concern proposing endurance training as a treatment option [43]. Finally, other studies suggested that muscle from MM patients may be exposed to greater levels of oxidative stress during the training, given to the reduced expression of DNA repair machinery, and reduced aconitase activity, despite the induction of the antioxidant enzyme Mn-superoxide dismutase (MnSOD) [44].

Therefore, physical exercise could ameliorate clinical conditions and OXPHOS activity in MM patients; however, further studies are needed to investigate whether a link between heteroplasmic shift towards mutant mtDNA and the level of physical activity may exist.

3.2. Dietary Approaches

Epilepsy is a common feature of PMD. The ketogenic diet (KD) is a high-fat (≈90%), low-carbohydrate diet that allows the generation of ketone bodies (KB) in the liver through mitochondrial β-oxidation of fatty acids. KB are then metabolized to acetyl-CoA, which feeds the tricarboxylic acid (TCA) cycle, thus serving as an alternative energy source for brain, heart, and skeletal muscle. KD can control seizures with an unclear mechanism [45], and for this reason, it has been proposed for PMD patients who have epilepsy. A comparative study reported that 7 out of 14 children with intractable epilepsy and various MRC complex defects treated with KD became seizure-free, while others had important seizure reduction, spanning 50% and 90% [46]. In another study, KD produced clinical progress, including seizure reduction and global functional improvement in 75% of the treated patients [47]. No severe side effects were reported in both studies.

Besides the curative effects on seizure, KD has also been proposed in patients suffering from inborn errors of pyruvate dehydrogenase complex (PDC) [48], given the alternative production of acetyl-CoA from KB rather than pyruvate. Patients treated with KD showed increased longevity and improved mental development [48]. KD was also proposed to treat CI defects, as it could promote the mitochondrial respiration through complex II (CII) activity and the oxidation of $FADH_2$, therefore bypassing the inactive CI [49,50].

KB also increased OXPHOS genes expression through a starvation-like response, resulting in the activation of many transcription factors and cofactors (including AMPK, SIRT1, and PGC-1α), with consequent increase of mitochondrial biogenesis [51]. Additional exciting observations have been reported in cellular models of PMD: KB alleviated mitochondrial dysfunction by restoring CI assembly in cybrid model of MELAS [52], and reduced the mutation load of a heteroplasmic mtDNA deletion in a cybrid cell line from a Kearns–Sayre syndrome patient [53], although the mechanisms of such improvements still need to be deciphered. Similarly, a high-fat diet (HFD) protected fibroblasts with CI deficiency and delayed the neurological phenotype of the *Harlequin* mouse [54]. A preclinical trial in the *Deletor* mouse, overexpressing a mutant replicative helicase Twinkle, revealed slowing of mitochondrial myopathy progression in mice treated with the KD [55]. *BCS1L*-mutated mice with CIII deficiency and progressive hepatopathy fed with KD significantly attenuated liver disease [56]. However, other studies reported that KD could worsen the mitochondrial defect in the *Mpv17* knockout (ko) mouse, characterized by profound mtDNA depletion in the liver [57], in the *Pank2* ko mouse model [58] or in the astrocyte-specific ko mouse of the replicative mtDNA helicase *Twinkle* ($TwKO^{astro}$), a model of spongiotic mitochondrial encephalopathy with mtDNA depletion [59].

A modified ketogenic Atkins diet (mAD) was recently tested in patients with MM and progressive external ophthalmoplegia with single or multiple deletions [60]. All patients developed progressive muscle pain and rhabdomyolysis within two weeks; muscle ultrastructure analysis revealed selective fiber damage [60]. These adverse events determined the interruption of the trial. Incredibly, a two-year follow-up showed an increase in muscle strength, suggesting that, following the acute damage, an injury-induced muscle repair by satellite cells—which do not carry deleted mtDNA molecules—was stimulated. [60].

Other dietary approaches include the use of anaplerotic compounds to treat mitochondrial fat oxidation disorders. An example is the odd-chain fatty acid *triheptanoin*, an anaplerotic compound inducing a rapid increase of plasmatic C4- and C5-ketone bodies, the latter being a precursor of propionyl-CoA, which is then converted into succinyl-CoA. Treatment with *triheptanoin* permanently abolished chronic cardiomyopathy, rhabdomyolysis, and muscle weakness in patients with very-long-chain acyl-CoA dehydrogenase (VLCAD) deficiency [61].

In conclusion, in vitro and in vivo shreds of evidence suggest that dietary manipulation promotes different responses in different tissues and cell types, highlighting the need for disease-specific treatments based on their molecular pathophysiology knowledge.

3.3. Exposure to Hypoxia

Hypoxia response, a mechanism that helps cells adapting when oxygen is limited, was identified in 2016 as a potent suppressor of mitochondrial dysfunction, and therefore proposed as a therapeutic approach for mitochondrial diseases [62]. The authors identified the inhibition of the Von Hippel-Lindau (VHL) factor as the most effective suppressor of the mitochondrial dysfunction. VHL factor is a critical protein in cellular responses to oxygen availability, being required for the oxygen-dependent proteolysis of α subunits of hypoxia-inducible factor-1 (HIF). VHL factor negatively regulates HIFs, so downregulation of VHL activates the HIF transcriptional response, which induced the partial shift of cellular bioenergetic reliance on mitochondrial OXPHOS [62]. Genetic or pharmacological activation of the HIF pathway in cellular and zebrafish models, as well as chronic normobaric hypoxic treatment in the murine *Ndufs4* ko model of Leigh syndrome, prevented the development of the disease. Hypoxia markedly improved lifespan (from 58 to 270 days), body weight, body temperature, behavior, neuropathology, and disease biomarkers in *Ndufs4* ko mouse, a model of severe infantile Leigh syndrome; on the contrary, hyperoxia (55% O_2) worsened all the parameters analyzed [62]. Alternate hypoxia/normoxia and moderate hypoxic conditions (17% O_2) failed to improve the clinical phenotype in *Ndufs4* ko mice [63]. Confirmation of hypoxia's therapeutic effects in additional models of PMD and an in-depth explanation of the still unclear mechanistic details would open the possibility of pharmacological treatment.

3.4. Strategies to Increase ATP Levels

The observation that combined oral administration of febuxostat—an inhibitor of xanthine oxidoreductase (XOR) used to treat gout and hyperuricemia—and inosine elevated both hypoxanthine and ATP levels in peripheral blood of healthy subjects [64], let Kamatani and colleagues hypothesize that PMD patients may potentially benefit from such treatment.

Purine nucleoside phosphorylase catalyzes the conversion of inosine to hypoxanthine, that is further processed to urate by XOR. The concomitant administration of febuxostat and inosine caused a significant increase of the serum hypoxanthine levels. Hypoxanthine is then converted to IMP, while elevated levels of ATP were observed [64,65]. Two PMD patients—one with homoplasmic mutation (m.12192G>A) in the tRNA histidine (*MT-TH*) and mitochondrial cardiomyopathy, and the other one with mitochondrial diabetes, carrying a heteroplasmic mutation in tRNA leucine 1 (*MT-TL1*)—received concurrent administrations of inosine and febuxostat. In the first case, the specific marker of heart failure brain natriuretic peptide (BNP), was decreased by 31%, and in the second case, the insulinogenic index increased 3.1 times, suggesting a favorable action of the treatment [65]. However, further studies are needed to confirm these findings.

3.5. Pharmacological Stimulation of Mitochondrial Biogenesis

Standard features of OXPHOS-related PMD include reduced ATP production and subsequent energy failure. It has been well established that the onset of the clinical phenotype may appear once the residual mitochondrial activity drops below a critical threshold [66]. In this context, the activation of mitochondrial biogenesis could favor the cells residing in affected tissues to improve the 'mitochondrial energy units' and ameliorate their energy metabolism. However, debates exist regarding potential harmful consequences of increasing a mitochondrial mass composed mainly of damaged mitochondria, variably characterized by enhanced ROS production and mtDNA damage [67].

Nevertheless, several molecules pharmacologically targeting the mitochondrial biogenesis pathway have been tested in the last decades.

The mitochondrial biogenesis is regulated by a complex signaling cascade requiring coordinated transcription of several proteins encoded by the nuclear and mitochondrial genome. The mitochondrial biogenesis pathway has been extensively investigated in brown adipose tissue and skeletal muscle. The so-called master gene of mitochondrial biogenesis is the Peroxisome proliferator-activated receptor gamma coactivator 1-alpha (*PGC-1α*). This transcriptional coactivator physiologically acts as a sensor of various external and internal stimuli (i.e., cold, exercise, nutritional status) to modulate the mitochondrial mass to meet the energy requirements of the cells.

PGC-1α is a transcriptional coactivator of many transcription factors, including the nuclear respiratory factors (NRF1 and NRF2) that control the transcript levels of OXPHOS-related genes [68], the peroxisomal proliferator activator receptors (PPARs) that modulate fatty acid oxidation, as well as estrogen-related receptor α (ERRα) [69], thyroid hormone receptor [70], that modulate thermogenesis but also mitochondrial respiration [71]; transcription factor Yin-Yang 1 (YY1) implicated in respiratory chain expression [72].

Genetic manipulations of preclinical models have confirmed the beneficial effects of the activation of mitochondrial biogenesis pathway in MM. Transgenic mice overexpressing *PGC-1α* in skeletal muscle had enhanced endurance performance and a fiber type conversion from type II to type I, with concurrent activation of genes related to mitochondrial oxidative metabolism [73]. When *PGC-1α* is overexpressed in the skeletal muscle of *Surf1* ko [74] and other OXPHOS-deficient mice, including *Acta-Cox15* ko and *Sco2* knockin-knockout (kiko) mice, a significant amelioration of the phenotypic and molecular aspects of MM occurs (Bottani E, personal observations). On the contrary, selective depletion of *PGC-1α* leads to a blunting of exercise-induced increase of MRC proteins in muscle [75,76].

PGC-1α gene expression is modulated by many stimuli, which share some common molecular pathways despite the proven tissue-specificity of these mechanisms. Some of them include the PKA/CREB pathway, the calmodulin-dependent protein kinase IV (CaMKIV) and calcineurin A (CnA) pathway, and the NOS/cGMP/PGK pathway (for an extensive review, see [25]). Post-translational modifications modulate PGC-1α activity; in particular, it is activated by phosphorylation triggered by AMPK [77] or by deacetylation operated by the nuclear deacetylase Sirtuin 1 (SIRT1) [78]. The pharmacological modulation of both AMPK and SIRT1 activities is possible, and it has been exploited to activate PGC-1α [25]. AMPK is a highly conserved sensor of intracellular adenosine nucleotide levels activated when even modest decreases in ATP production result in relative increases in AMP or ADP. In response, AMPK promotes catabolic pathways to generate more ATP and inhibits anabolic pathways [79]. SIRT1 is an NAD^+-dependent deacetylase that acts on various substrates and is involved in an extensive assortment of physiological functions, comprising control of gene expression, metabolism, and aging [80].

In the last decade, the PGC-1α signaling cascade has become an attractive therapeutic target to manipulate mitochondrial function, and several drugs acting on the PGC-1α pathway have been tested in preclinical models of PMD [74,81]. A schematic representation of PGC-1α pathway and modulating factors are exemplified in Figure 2.

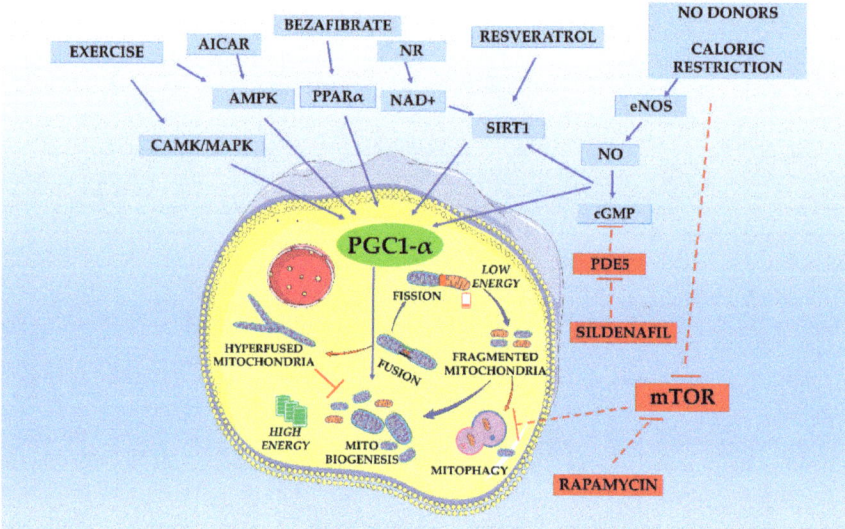

Figure 2. Schematic representation of the pathways regulating mitochondrial biogenesis, dynamics, and mitophagy. External factors (exercise, caloric restriction, or drugs such as bezafibrate, 5-aminoimidazole-4-carboxamide ribonucleoside (AICAR), resveratrol, or nicotinamide riboside (NR) upregulate the expression of *PGC-1α*, which in turn activates essential mitochondrial genes. Other drugs can act on NO pathway (PDE5 inhibitors as Sildenafil) or mitochondrial autophagy (Rapamycin). Blue arrows and squares indicate positive regulations, while red arrows and squares indicate negative regulations.

3.5.1. 5-Aminoimidazole-4-Carboxamide Ribonucleoside (AICAR)

The AMP analogue 5-aminoimidazole-4-carboxamide ribonucleoside (AICAR) has been used to induce PGC-1α-dependent mitochondriogenesis via the activation of the AMPK. We reported a robust induction of OXPHOS-related gene transcription with consequent increase of MRC complex activities in three preclinical models of COX deficiency, a *Surf1* ko mouse, a *Sco2* kiko mouse, and a muscle-specific Cox15 ko mouse [74]. The increase in the MRC activities was paralleled by a significant improvement in the kiko mouse's motor performance, which has a mild MM, but not in *Acta-Cox15* models. This difference is likely due to the severity of the *Acta-Cox15* ko mouse model's clinical phenotype, which could not be corrected despite a clear, although incomplete, rescue of the CIV activity. We also generated an *Acta-Cox15* ko mouse model overexpressing PGC-1α in the skeletal muscle. This mouse (*Acta-Cox15ko–PGC-1α*) also showed improved motor performance compared to naive *Acta-Cox15* ko littermates, but this effect was transient, and, at six months of age, both *Acta-Cox15* ko and *Acta-Cox15ko–PGC-1α* displayed comparable motor performance, suggesting that the overexpression of *PGC-1α* in the skeletal muscle delayed, but did not arrest, the clinical course of the disease. Intriguingly, chronic (three months) AICAR administration improved CIV activity, rescued the motor phenotype, and delayed the onset of the myopathy in a mouse model of slowly progressing MM (*Cox10-Mef2c-Cre*), either in pre-symptomatic or post-symptomatic administration protocol [82]. However, the authors attributed the effects of AICAR in promoting the regeneration of muscle fibers rather than activation of mitochondrial biogenesis [82]. Interestingly, Golubitzky and co-workers identified AICAR as the most effective compound able to induce mitochondrial biogenesis without altering mitochondrial membrane potential ($\Delta\psi$). AICAR also improved growth and ATP content while decreasing ROS production in CI deficient cells [83].

Nevertheless, the use of AICAR to treat CNS disease is limited by its low blood–brain barrier penetrance. Conversely, peripheral stimulation of AMPK and mitochondrial biogenesis may have some beneficial effects on MM.

3.5.2. Bezafibrate and Other PPAR Agonists

Bezafibrate is a fibrate drug, pan-agonist of the isoform alpha of the peroxisome proliferator-activated receptor (PPARα), displaying anti-lipidemic activity. The mechanism of action of fibric acid derivatives was elucidated in the 1990s, after identifying PPARs as targets of these drugs. Upon activation, PPARs bind as obligate heterodimers with the retinoid X receptor (RXR) to specific recognition sequences, called PPAR-response elements (PPRE), in the regulatory region of target genes, leading to cis-activation of gene transcription. There are three isoforms of *PPARs* (α, β/δ, and γ) characterized by different physiological functions and tissue specificity with high expression in liver, heart, and skeletal muscle, where they promote upregulation of genes encoding enzymes of the oxidation pathway [84,85] and fatty acid catabolism [86]. Initial experiments performed by Bastin et al. revealed that bezafibrate administration exerted positive effects on MRC activities. In particular, both control and MRC-deficient patients' fibroblasts with some residual respiratory chain function level upregulated the expression of several nuclear genes encoding subunits of CI, CIII, or CIV and augmented the enzymatic activities of MRC complexes [87]. These effects were accompanied by the increased expression of PGC-1α, NRF1/2, and Transcription Factor A, Mitochondrial (TFAM), the latter controlling the transcription and replication of the mitochondrial genome. Encouraging results were also obtained in *SCO2* mutant fibroblasts, in which bezafibrate rescued the cytochrome c oxidase (COX) defect [88]. Bezafibrate was also tested in fibroblasts of patients with a de novo heterozygous c.1084G>A (p.G362S) *DNM1L* mutation [89]. In this case, Bezafibrate effectively normalized growth on glucose-free medium, ATP production and oxygen consumption, and improved mitochondrial morphology, although it caused a mild increase in ROS production at the same time [89].

However, controversial preclinical results in the activation of PGC-1α were obtained by using bezafibrate [74,90]. Bezafibrate failed to induce mitochondrial biogenesis in vivo in two different mouse models of COX deficiency [74]. Bezafibrate administration significantly delayed the accumulation of COX-negative fibers and multiple mtDNA deletions in the *Deletor* mouse without inducing mitochondrial biogenesis. On the contrary, mtDNA copy number, transcript, and MRC protein amounts decreased in both *Deletor* and wild-type mice. Furthermore, bezafibrate induced severe lipid oxidation effects, with hepatomegaly and loss of adipose tissue, through a mechanism involving lipid mobilization by high hepatic expression of fibroblast growth factor 21 (FGF21) cytokine [90]. An 8-month bezafibrate treatment of the *Mutator* mouse—a premature aging model that harbors a proofreading-deficient mtDNA polymerase γ—delayed hair loss and improved skin and spleen aging-like phenotypes, without a generalized increase in mitochondrial markers, or improvements in muscle function or lifespan [91].

Recently, the results of an open-label observational experimental medicine study of six patients with MM caused by the m.3243A>G *MTTL1* mutation were published [92]. The aim of this study was to establish preliminary safety and efficacy evidence of bezafibrate on mitochondrial metabolism. No clinically adverse events were reported after the administration of 600–1200 mg bezafibrate daily for 12 weeks to the enrolled patients [92]. A reduction in the number of COX-immunodeficient muscle fibers and improved cardiac function were observed in treated patients. Curiously, some biomarkers, comprising the level of m.3243A>G heteroplasmy in urinary sediments or the exercise physiology, were extremely erratic, explaining why these do not always correlate with clinical severity. Moreover, the known serological biomarkers for PMD, FGF-21, and growth and differentiation factor 15 (GDF-15), were significantly elevated and paralleled by a strong imbalance in amino acid and fatty acid metabolism [92]. This alteration of mitochondrial disease patients' metabolomic signature following bezafibrate administration suggests being cautious with eventually possible adverse events in long-term treatment.

Thiazolidinediones are a class of heterocyclic compounds used to treat type 2 diabetes mellitus that display a high affinity for the PPARγ receptor. Once activated, the PPARγ binds to DNA in conjunction with the RXR receptor, and this heterodimer interacts with transcriptional coactivators, including PGC-1α [93]. Several lines of evidence support the mitochondriogenic effects of thiazolidinediones compounds, both in in vitro and in vivo models [94–96]. Interestingly, *Rosiglitazone* (a member of this family) simulated mitochondrial biogenesis in mouse brain through an apolipoprotein (Apo) E isozyme-independent manner. Rosiglitazone induced both mtDNA and estrogen-stimulated related receptor alpha (ESRRA) mRNA, a key regulator of mitochondrial biogenesis. PPARγ agonism induced neuronal mitochondrial biogenesis and glucose utilization, leading to progressed cellular function [97]. However, studies on preclinical models of PMD are lacking.

3.5.3. Modulating NAD$^+$ Pool

Another strategy to stimulate mitochondrial biogenesis is based on pharmacological activation of SIRT1, a nuclear deacetylase that utilizes the NAD$^+$ moiety to deacetylate acetyl-lysine residues of proteins. Downstream targets of SIRT1 are the Forkhead box O (FOXO), PGC-1α, the myocyte-specific enhancer factor 2 (MEF2), and the tumor suppressor p53 [98], which are involved in the transcriptional regulation of mitochondrial function. As SIRT1 activity is directly regulated by NAD$^+$ availability, NAD$^+$'s intracellular regulation may represent a strategy to promote SIRT1 activity and its downstream cascade. Various approaches can increase intracellular NAD$^+$ concentrations, including (I) supplementation with NAD$^+$ precursor [99,100]; (II) pharmacological inhibition of poly (ADP) ribosyl polymerase 1 (Parp1), an NAD$^+$ consumer, and SIRT1 competitor [101,102]; or (III) by inhibition of aminocarboxymuconate semialdehyde decarboxylase [103], which results in increased de novo synthesis of NAD$^+$ from tryptophan.

Vitamin B3 is a NAD$^+$ precursor and exists in several forms: nicotinic acid (niacin), nicotinamide (NAM), and nicotinamide riboside (NR) [100,104,105]. Supplementation with NR and reduction of NAD$^+$ consumption by inhibiting the Parp enzymes were tested in *Sco2* kiko mice leading to activation of SIRT1, and induction of OXPHOS genes via the PGC-1α axis, resulting in clinical improvement of the motor performance of treated mice up to normal values [81]. Similarly, NR's administration activated mitochondrial biogenesis, improved mitochondrial ultrastructure, prevented the generation of multiple mtDNA rearrangements, and delayed the MM in the *Deletor* mouse model [106]. It was also reported that NR administration improved mitochondrial function in iPSC-derived neurons from Parkinson's Disease (PD) patients and rescued neuronal loss and motor deficits in *GBA-PD Drosophila melanogaster* [107]. Nicotinamide mononucleotide (NMN), another NAD$^+$ precursor, significantly extended the lifespan of the *Ndufs4* ko mice by approximately 2-fold [108]. NMN also attenuated NAD$^+$ redox imbalance, protein hyperacetylation, and suppressed lactate levels in the skeletal muscle, while brain was not responsive [108].

A recent paper from Katsyuba and co-workers demonstrated that cellular NAD$^+$ levels are also controlled by α-amino-β-carboxymuconate-ε-semialdehyde decarboxylase (ACMSD), the enzyme that limits the proportion of ACMS able to undergo spontaneous cyclization in the de novo NAD$^+$ synthesis pathway, through a conserved evolutionary mechanism from *C. elegans* to the mouse [103]. RNAi of ACMDS led to increasing mitochondrial mass and respiration, and ultimately lifespan of worms through the activation of the mitochondrial stress response. Moreover, ACMSD inhibitors effectively modulate NAD$^+$ levels and mitochondrial function in vitro and in vivo, particularly in mouse models of liver and kidney injury [103].

A systemic NAD$^+$ deficiency has recently been reported in patients with an adult-onset type of MM. An elevated dose of niacin (to 750–1000 mg/day) was administered in 416 patients and their matched controls, for 10 or 4 months, respectively (ClinicalTrials.gov identifier NCT03973203). Blood NAD$^+$ grew to 8-fold in all participants, and the patients' muscular NAD$^+$ achieved the control level. Mitochondrial mass and muscle strength increased in all patients; furthermore, muscle metabolism normalized, and liver fat dropped by as much as 50% in patients. Lessened concentration of hemoglobin and erythrocytes and increased muscle glycogen have been identified as potential adverse reactions which need focus and follow-up. Similar increases in circulating NAD$^+$ were reported with NR treatment in healthy subjects [109]. These data point to a possible interference of NAD$^+$ precursors with erythropoiesis and/or iron metabolism, which require an appropriate supervising in the context of B3 supplementation [105]. However, these data suggest niacin as a good candidate to treat MM with NAD$^+$ deficiency, whereas possible curative effects on other PMD are still unclear.

3.5.4. I-BET 525762A

Through a high-throughput chemical screen, Barrow and co-workers identified I-BET 525762A, a bromodomain inhibitor, as a top hit that augments COX5a protein levels in CI-mutant cybrid cells. In parallel, bromodomain-containing protein 4 (BRD4), a target of I-BET 525762A, was identified using a genome-wide CRISPR screening to search for genes whose loss of function rescues the death of CI-impaired cybrids. Furthermore, I-BET525762A administration, or loss-of-Brd4, remodeled the mitochondrial proteome and increased the levels and activity of OXPHOS protein complexes, rescuing the CI defects and cell death [110]. BRD4 is a chromatin-bound transcriptional regulator linked to the expression of genes associated with different biological processes, including tumor progression or inflammation [111]. These findings suggest that these programs integrate with mitochondrial energetics and metabolic control, although the precise mechanism(s) needs still to be deciphered.

3.5.5. Polyphenols and Other Pharmacognostic Products

Resveratrol (2,3,4'-trihydroxystilbene) is a polyphenol that received attention for a range of potentially beneficial effects, including mitochondrial function improvement, anti-inflammatory properties, and protection against metabolic diseases and neuronal dysfunction. In 2003, resveratrol (RSV) was identified as the most potent SIRT1 activator molecule in a drug screening [112]. Since then, many studies have pointed to the ability of RSV to upregulate the Sirt1-mediated mitochondrial biogenesis and the functions of other key players as AMPK and PGC-1α. Although the effects of RSV in inducing mitochondrial biogenesis are well established and reproducible [113,114], concerns exist on the molecular mechanism(s) of action. Some authors reported that RSV acts primarily on AMPK activation [115,116], and that the activation of SIRT1 by RSV is an artifact [117–119]. In line with this hypothesis, Jee-Hyun Um et al. showed that RSV was unable to exert its pharmacological effects in AMPK deficient mice, proving that AMPK is a crucial target of RSV [120]. Other authors instead reported that RSV might first activate SIRT1 in vivo, leading to AMPK activation [121,122], and deacetylation of PGC-1α [114]. However, different RSV dosages preferentially activate SIRT1 or AMPK in vivo, further increasing the complexity of these pathways [113]. Besides the molecular mechanisms, studies based on preclinical neurodegenerative disease models reported positive effects of RSV in improving mitochondrial function and neurological symptoms [123,124]. More recently, the effects of RSV administration on mitochondrial respiration of skin fibroblasts from PMD-patients have been reviewed [125]. It appeared clear that responses to RSV are not uniform but highly patient- or mutation-dependent. Further studies on proper cellular models are needed to evaluate the effects of RSV on PMD.

Quercetin is a potent antioxidant flavonoid, more specifically a flavonol, with a reported ability to activate SIRT1 and PGC-1α and increases mtDNA and cytochrome c content in skeletal muscle and brain [126,127]. The use of quercetin for the treatment of neurodegenerative disorders with mitochondrial involvement has been exploited in preclinical models of Alzheimer's Disease [128] and Parkinson's disease [129].

Hydroxytyrosol (HT) is a polyphenol which activated PGC-1α through SIRT1 de-acetylation and induced mitochondrial biogenesis in vitro [130] and in skeletal muscle in vivo [131]. Furthermore, HT exerted dose-dependent effects on SC assembly in exercised animals through enhancing mitochondrial function [132]. Prolonged HT administration significantly activated AMPK, SIRT1, and PGC-1α, and increased the MRC complexes' levels in the brain of db/db mice. Likewise, targets of the antioxidative transcription factor nuclear factor erythroid 2 related factor 2 (NRF2), including p62 (sequestosome-1), heme oxygenase 1 (HO-1), and superoxide dismutase 1 and 2 increased, and protein oxidation significantly decreased upon treatment [133]. Recently, by using three different *C. elegans* models of PD, it was shown that HT enhanced locomotion in worms suffering from α-synuclein-expression in muscles or rotenone exposure, reduced α-synuclein accumulation in muscle cells, and prevent neurodegeneration in α-synuclein-containing dopaminergic neurons [134].

Curcumin—a dietary polyphenol derived from turmeric—also stimulated different mitochondrial biogenesis markers in vivo when administered to the senescence-accelerated mouse-prone 8 (SAMP8) strain. In particular, curcumin upregulated PGC-1α protein expression in the brain, improving MMP and ATP levels and restoring mitochondrial fusion [135]. In another study, curcumin dietary supplementation increased the expression of TFAM and PGC-1α, and ATP levels in mouse brains [136]. Curcumin also showed antioxidant effects in patients affected by β-Thalassemia [137,138]. Therefore, curcumin was proposed to treat LHON patients in phase 3 clinical trial (ClinicalTrials.gov identifier NCT00528151). Seventy patients with 11,778 LHON mutation were randomly treated with oral curcumin (500 mg/day) or placebo for one year. The visual acuity, computerized visual field, electrophysiologic parameters, and oxidative stress enzymes in plasma were compared before and after treatment at 3-, 6-, and 12-month intervals. Although the study was completed in 2007, results have not been published to date.

Despite the wide choice of molecules with a potential effect on mitochondrial biogenesis, more effort is needed to clarify which drug is most effective in patients affected by PMD. Bezafibrate gave highly variable results; AICAR presents several limitations for chronic use [139,140]; furthermore, the potential mutagenic effects of PARP inhibitors are still to be thoroughly evaluated, although data collected in patients treated with Olaparib (AZD-2281) suggest low mutational toxicity [141]. On the contrary, the possibility of translating into clinical practice supplementation with NAD^+ precursors seems to be more realistic, based on the high tolerability and substantial lack of adverse effects [142–144].

3.6. Pharmacological Modulation of the NO/cGMP/PKG Pathway

Nitric oxide (NO) is an intra- and extra-cellular gaseous second messenger that acts on various signaling pathways in target cells and orchestrates a plethora of physiological processes, including neuronal signaling, modulation of ion channels, immune response, inflammation, and cardiovascular homeostasis, among others. NO is catalytically produced from L-arginine and L-citrulline—the latter is converted to L-arginine via argininosuccinate synthase and argininosuccinate lyase—by the three isoforms of the enzyme nitric oxide synthase (NOS): the neuronal NOS (nNOS, or NOS1), inducible NOS (iNOS or NOS2), and endothelial NOS (eNOS or NOS3). Since mitochondria also produce NO, the existence of a putative mitochondrial NOS (mtNOS) is feasible, yet still controversial [145–147]. The enzymatic reaction generating NO involves the transfer of electrons from NADPH, via the flavins in the C-terminal reductase domain, to the heme in the N-terminal oxidase domain of NOS, where the substrate L-arginine is oxidized to L-citrulline and NO [148]. Stimulation of NOS leads to the generation and release of NO, which causes the activation of soluble guanylate cyclase (sGC) and cGMP production. The biological effects of cGMP are mediated by three major groups of cellular targets: cGMP-dependent protein kinases (PKGs), cGMP-gated ion channels, and phosphodiesterases (PDEs) [149]. Once activated by cGMP, PKGs initiates a cascade of phosphorylation events on various target proteins, resulting in modification of physiological processes, including calcium homeostasis, smooth muscle contraction, and cardiac function [149]. cGMP-gated channels are non-selective ion channels that function in response to cGMP binding and have important signal transduction roles in retinal photoreceptors and olfactory receptor neurons [150]. However, it should be noted that, other than cGMP-gated channels, many other ion channels are indirectly regulated by cGMP through PKG-consensus motifs on their sequence [151,152]. Lastly, the cGMP level is determined by the balance between sGC and PDEs activities, the latter breaking down cGMP molecules [149]. Notably, it has been reported that the NOS/NO/sGC/cGMP signaling upregulates

PGC-1α [153] in diverse cell types, including neurons [154,155]. The mechanisms by which cGMP activate PGC-1α may involve the PKG-driven modulation of the CREB signaling pathway, which has been recently reviewed elsewhere [156].

NO deficiency occurs in PMD and may be due to multiple factors, although not fully elucidated. The first hypothesis points to a generalized impairment of endothelial function, as observed in PMD [157]. Flow-mediated vasodilation (FMD), which is a function of NO synthesized by endothelial cells in response to reperfusion, is impaired in individuals with MM, MELAS, MERRF, MIDD (maternally inherited diabetes and deafness), and CPEO [158]. As often reported, abnormal mitochondrial proliferation may cause NO sequestration by CI and CIV binding [159]. Finally, reduced levels of NO precursors [160–162] and of sarcoplasmic NOS activity in COX-negative fibers from patients with PEO, MM, and MELAS syndrome were reported [163]. Beyond the cause(s), NO depletion may play a significant role in the onset of several observed complications, including stroke-like episodes, myopathy, diabetes, and lactic acidosis [164]. Subjects with MELAS syndrome have lower concentrations of NO metabolites (nitrite and nitrate) during stroke-like episodes [165] and low L-citrulline levels, suggesting that MELAS strokes may be caused by unstable NO homeostasis that leads to vascular endothelial dysfunction [161].

3.6.1. L-Arginine and L-Citrulline

As L-arginine and L-citrulline are NO precursors, their supplementation was proposed to treat NO deficiency-related manifestations of PMD [161,166,167]. L-Arginine supplementation increased the NO production rate [164] and improved FMD in MELAS patients [162]. An open-label trial showed that intravenous L-arginine administration to MELAS patients during stroke-like episodes led to an improvement in the clinical symptoms associated with these episodes, and oral L-arginine supplementation at the interictal phase decreased their frequency and severity [165]. A series of open-label studies confirmed these findings in MELAS patients with the common m.3243A>G mutation [162,168]. Interestingly, the NO synthesis rate effectively increased upon L-citrulline supplementation, rather than L-arginine, indicating that L-citrulline is a more powerful NO precursor than L-arginine [164,169]. Moreover, L-arginine and L-citrulline administration reduced plasmatic alanine and lactate concentrations, suggesting that such supplementation may improve lactic acidemia in MELAS syndrome by improving NO-mediated perfusion and oxygen delivery in all microvasculature compartment [167]. So, the L-citrulline and L-arginine supplementation may also be extended to treat other clinical features of PMD, e.g., lactic acidosis, muscle weakness, exercise intolerance, and diabetes. As such, a randomized crossover study (ClinicalTrials.gov identifier NCT02809170 was performed to evaluate the impact of L-citrulline and L-arginine supplementation on endothelial dysfunction in pediatric PMD patients. The primary outcomes were the changes in reactive hyperemic index, which reflects endothelial function, but results are not yet available. Currently, a Phase-1 clinical trial is recruiting patients to establish dose and safety of L-citrulline treatment of NO deficiency in MELAS (ClinicalTrials.gov identifier NCT03952234). Placebo-controlled randomized clinical trials are necessary before L-arginine and L-citrulline can be definitively recommended to ameliorate or treat stroke-like episodes in MELAS and other PMD.

3.6.2. Natriuretic Peptides and Cyclic Guanosine Monophosphate

Natriuretic peptides (NPs) induce natriuresis (i.e., the excretion of sodium by the kidney). NPs regulate vascular tone via GC, cGMP, and PKG [170]. The polypeptide hormones Atrial natriuretic peptide (ANP) and brain natriuretic peptide (BNP) regulate the vascular tone and natriuresis. ANP and BNP stimulate the production of cGMP via a selective binding to their receptors, the natriuretic peptide receptors A and B (NPRA/GC-A and NPRB/GC-B, respectively) which so activate their intracellular guanylate cyclase domains [170]. Transgenic mice overexpressing BNP or PKG increased the mitochondrial muscle content and fat oxidation through upregulation of PGC-1α and PPARδ, preventing obesity and glucose intolerance; moreover, treatment of myotubes with ANP and BNP stimulates mitochondrial biogenesis and mitochondrial respiration [171]. Exercise induced expression of NPRA/GC-A and was correlated with the expression of PGC-1α-dependent genes in muscle [172]. Whitaker et al. showed that phosphodiesterase type-3 (PDE3) inhibitors cilostamide and trequinsin increased PGC-1α levels, mRNA expression of mitochondrial genes, and mtDNA copy number both in renal proximal tubular cells and in the renal cortex [173]. However, these compounds have not been tested on PMD models yet, and therefore, future studies are necessary to exploit their potential therapeutic effects.

3.6.3. PDE5 Inhibitors

Sildenafil is the first specific phosphodiesterase type-5 (PDE5) inhibitor (PDE5i) marketed to treat erectile dysfunction. PDE5 is expressed in many tissues where it hydrolyzes intracellular cGMP; thus, PDE5i potentiates the endogenous increase of cGMP by inhibiting its breakdown [174]. Sildenafil restored mitochondrial biogenesis and favored renal recovery in mice after folic acid-induced acute kidney injury [173]. A recent study showed that sildenafil treatment induced mitochondrial biogenesis, increased UCP-1 expression, and promoted subcutaneous white adipose tissue browning in healthy mice [175]. Moreover, PDE5is have emerged from drug screening on MILS-neuronal progenitor cells (NPCs) as the most effective drug to ameliorate mitochondrial function. NPCs derived from patients carrying a deleterious homoplasmic mutation (m.9185T>C) in the mitochondrial gene *MT-ATP6* showed defective ATP production and abnormally high mitochondrial membrane potential (MMP), with altered calcium homeostasis [176].

Avanafil, a PDE5i, rescued the calcium defect in patient NPCs and differentiated neurons [176]. However, the NO pathway was not evaluated in this study; instead, a possible link with the activation of Ca^{2+}-activated potassium channels mediated by cGMP was speculated [176]. Nevertheless, the beneficial effects of PDE5i to treat PMD are still poorly understood, since preclinical studies [177,178] and case reports [179] gave controversial results; further investigations on the mechanisms need to be implemented.

3.7. Antioxidants

Reactive oxygen species (ROS) are unstable molecules containing oxygen that can quickly react with other molecules within cells. They are generated primarily as by-products of the enzymatic activities of the mitochondrial electron transport chain. ROS molecules comprise superoxide, hydrogen peroxide, hydroxyl radical, and hydroxyl ion. Hydrogen peroxide is not as reactive as the hydroxyl radical, yet the latter is readily generated by the former in the presence of Fe^{3+}, through the so-called Fenton reaction. Mitochondria are the primary site of ROS production within the cell. In physiological conditions, ROS act as signaling molecules through a tightly regulated process in cell proliferation [180], development, immunity, apoptosis, among others [181], while are scavenged by different antioxidant enzymes that include various isoforms of glutathione peroxidase (GP), superoxide dismutase (SOD), and peroxiredoxin (Prx) [182]. In pathological conditions due to mutations in genes involved in the OXPHOS system, the inefficient transfer of electrons among the four respiratory chain complexes causes an accumulation of electrons that react with molecular oxygen to form superoxide anions (O_2^-) [183], superoxide dismutase enzymes then convert that to H_2O_2, which can be further reduced to hydroxyl radical (OH^-), the most potent oxidizing agent among the ROS [183]. Therefore, ROS generation is enhanced, leading to ROS-mediated, irreversible cellular damage, including lipid peroxidation, DNA modifications, and cell death [182]. Moreover, ROS further damage MRC complexes, including NADH dehydrogenase, cytochrome c oxidase, and ATP synthase, and alter mitochondrial membrane permeability and structure, resulting in a complete shutdown of mitochondrial energy production (for a detailed review, see Guo et al. [184]).

Therefore, using antioxidant drugs in mitochondrial disease treatment is mainly related to the mitigation of such toxic effects. Antioxidant drugs do not target any specific biochemical pathways directly but help improve cellular energy metabolism regulation. Due to their non-specific mechanism, these drugs can be used in various PMD with an accumulation of mitochondrial ROS. Several antioxidant drugs have variable degrees of efficacy in terms of longevity and mitigation of oxidative stress in preclinical models of CI defects, pointing at the importance of such treatments in the therapy of PMD [185]. The currently used antioxidant drugs, their clinical uses in MRC diseases, and clinical trials results are discussed below.

3.7.1. Glutathione

Glutathione (GSH; γ-glutamyl-cysteinyl-glycine) is a tripeptide that contains an unusual γ-amide bond; it is a critical intracellular antioxidant agent that is the substrate of several peroxidases, helping to destroy peroxides generated by oxidases. Reduced blood GSH and redox imbalance have been reported in various PMD-patients [186,187]; therefore, supplementation of glutathione precursors may counteract ROS-driven damage. Cysteine donors have received increasing attention as cysteine is the rate-limiting substrate for glutathione biogenesis. However, a 30-day, double-blind, cross-over study providing an oral supplement with a glutathione precursor significantly reduced the oxidative stress biomarkers yet did not modify lactate concentration, clinical scale, or quality of life of the individuals [188]. Beyond its role of GSH precursor, cysteine is required for the 2-thiomodification of mitochondrial tRNAs, which is therefore useful for treating mtDNA mutations affecting mitochondrial transfer tRNA. Supplementation with cysteine, but not N-acetyl-cysteine, partially rescued the mitochondrial translation defect in fibroblasts of patients carrying the m.3243A>G and m.8344A>G mutations, suggesting a possible benefit in a subgroup of patients with impaired mitochondrial translation [189].

3.7.2. Cysteamine

Cysteamine is an amino thiol that is synthesized in mammals, including humans, through the breakdown of Coenzyme A. Cysteamine is an FDA-approved drug for the treatment of cystinosis. This lysosomal storage disease results from defects in the lysosomal cystine transporter (cystinosis), leading to a pathological accumulation of cystine-crystals in lysosomes [190]. Cysteamine exerts its function by entering into the lysosomes where it converts cystine into cysteine and cysteine-cysteamine disulfide, both of which can exit the lysosome [191]. Therefore, cysteamine increases the glutathione precursor cysteine availability, raising the possibility of its repositioning as a drug for PMD. A recent study evaluated cysteamine bitartrate's therapeutic potential in three different models of mitochondrial disorders: *C. elegans* model of CI defect, *FBXL4* mutant human fibroblast, and zebrafish models of pharmacologically-induced CI and CIV defects [192]. Although a therapeutic potential has been observed, no evident modulation of total glutathione levels was reported, raising concerns about its application in MRC diseases [192].

The microsphere formulation of Cysteamine bitartrate delayed-release (RP103) [193] has been used in a clinical trial. An open-label, dose-escalating study assessing safety, tolerability, efficacy, pharmacokinetics, and pharmacodynamics of RP103 in children affected by inherited PMD was completed in November 2017. RP103 was administered up to 1.3 g/m^2/day in two divided doses, every 12 h, for up to 6 months. The primary outcome measured focused on changes from baseline in Newcastle Paediatric Mitochondrial Disease Scale Score (NPMDS). Secondary outcomes focused on the measurement of glutathione, lactate, glutathione disulfide, lactate, and evaluation of myopathy by 6 Minute Walk Test. The data analysis is ongoing (ClinicalTrials.gov Identifier NCT02023866).

3.7.3. N-Acetylcysteine

N-acetylcysteine (NAC) also increases glutathione synthesis by increasing cysteine availability, which is, as mentioned above, a rate-limiting substrate for GSH biosynthesis [194]. NAC has been successfully used in a mouse model of ethylmalonic encephalopathy [195]. Ethylmalonic encephalopathy is a severe, fatal disorder caused by mutations in the *ETHE1* gene which encodes a mitochondrial sulfur dioxygenase necessary for the detoxification of sulfide [196]; therefore, mutations in *ETHE1* gene lead to the accumulation of hydrogen sulfide, that is a potent inhibitor of cytochrome c oxidase [197]. Since the supplementation of NAC replenishes the intracellular pool of reduced glutathione, the sulfide is effectively buffered. NAC supplementation is currently used in patients with ethylmalonic encephalopathy [198–200], with encouraging results.

3.7.4. Lipoic Acid

Lipoic acid (also called α-lipoic acid) is an essential cofactor covalently bound to several mitochondrial multi-enzymatic complexes, including the ketoglutarate dehydrogenase and pyruvate dehydrogenase [201], involved in energy metabolism. Lipoic acid is also a potent ROS scavenger [202] and antioxidant regenerator in vitro (mainly of CoQ_{10}, vitamin C, and glutathione) [203]. However, any increase in radical scavenging activity in vivo is unlikely to be sustained [204], due to the rapid elimination of its free form from cells. Nevertheless, lipoic acid is often administered with other antioxidants to PMD patients [205]. A randomized, double-blind, placebo-controlled, crossover study with 16 patients with mitochondrial diseases demonstrated that the supplementation of lipoic acid combined with creatine monohydrate and CoQ_{10} was able to decrease the levels of oxidative stress markers measured in urine, with parallel amelioration of clinical symptoms [206].

3.7.5. Vitamin C

Limited cases are documenting some improvements with Vitamin C administration, alone or in combination with other drugs. Progressive spasticity in a patient with familial spastic paraparesis and multiple MRC defects was arrested by combined treatment with CoQ_{10}, carnitine, vitamin C, and K [207]. Other patients with CIII defect showed mild recovery of some clinical symptoms by combining vitamin C and vitamin K administration [208,209]. However, other patients failed to respond to similar treatment [210].

3.7.6. Vitamin E

The vitamin E-derivative Trolox has been successfully used as ROS scavenger in fibroblasts from patients with CI defect, ameliorating the enzymatic activity's deficit, supporting evidence that CI expression may be controlled by the cell's oxidative balance [211]. Moreover, chronic Trolox administration in patients' fibroblasts with CI defects did restore mitochondrial membrane potential and normalized ER Ca^{2+} uptake without affecting control cell lines [212].

3.7.7. Coenzyme Q_{10}

Coenzyme Q_{10} (CoQ_{10}, or ubiquinone) is an endogenous, small lipophilic redox-active benzoquinone derivative with an isoprenoid side chain synthesized in every cell apart of erythrocytes. CoQ_{10} is an essential mobile electron carrier, which transfers electrons to mitochondrial respiratory chain CIII from CI and II and the oxidation of fatty acids and branched-chain amino acids. Moreover, CoQ_{10}, in its reduced form (ubiquinol), is an effective lipophilic antioxidant that protects cellular membranes from ROS-mediated oxidation and maintains the vitamin E and vitamin C in their reduced form [213]. CoQ_{10} supplementation may be expected to benefit patients with disorders of the mitochondrial respiratory chain by several mechanisms that are not mutually exclusive. First, it would be useful in patients affected by primary or secondary CoQ_{10} deficiencies, in which there is a pathological reduction of CoQ_{10} due to mutations in genes directly or indirectly involved in the CoQ_{10} biosynthetic pathway, that are, therefore, clinically heterogeneous [214,215]. Second, for the electron carrier properties mentioned above, CoQ_{10} could facilitate electron transport by circumventing a block in the electron transport chain, similar to what has been demonstrated for CIII defect treated with high doses of vitamin C and vitamin K3 [216]. Third, because of its antioxidant properties, CoQ_{10} may accept electrons from disrupted electron transport and reduce ROS formation risk that might cause various cellular damage [217,218]. This is the most general mechanism, potentially applicable to any defect of electron transport [219]. CoQ_{10} is the most common supplement used in PMD patients because it is well tolerated and lacks any chronic side effects. Recent work also provided evidence that CoQ_{10} may act as an enhancer of Parkin-mediated mitophagy flux in trans-mitochondrial cybrids, fibroblasts, and mutant-induced neurons derived from a MERRF patient, with partial improvement of the cellular bioenergetics and pathophysiology [220].

The first paper reporting beneficial effects of CoQ_{10} administration in vivo was published in 1986 and described the effects in five patients with Kearns–Sayre syndrome (KSS). The administration of CoQ_{10} as monotherapy improved abnormal metabolism of pyruvate, as seen by pyruvate/lactate ratio in the cerebrospinal fluid, and NADH oxidation in skeletal muscle, with concomitant amelioration of neurologic symptoms [221]. Since then, many studies have assessed the therapeutic potential of CoQ_{10} administration in patients with mitochondrial respiratory chain disorders. One-year treatment with 120 mg/day of CoQ_{10} in seven patients with KSS and other mitochondrial myopathies with CPEO demonstrated a progressive reduction of serum lactate and pyruvate levels following standard muscle exercise and generally improved neurological functions. Consistent findings on the normalization of pyruvate and lactate levels after exercise have been reported in many clinical studies [222–224]. A patient with mitochondrial encephalomyopathy with COX deficiency was treated for two years with a high dose of CoQ_{10} with beneficial effects on pyruvate metabolism and neurological function [225]. Another chronic, 2-year treatment with CoQ_{10} in oral doses of 150–100 mg/day in a patient with KSS syndrome and significantly reduced levels of CoQ_{10} in serum and skeletal muscle biopsy resulted in a marked physical and behavioral improvement. Tremor and ataxia disappeared, but external ophthalmoplegia, retinal degeneration, and cardiac function were unchanged [226]. Treatment with CoQ_{10} improves mitochondrial respiration in skeletal muscle and brain. One study reported that 6 months of treatment with CoQ_{10} (150 mg/day) in 10 patients with mitochondrial cytopathies remarkably improved all brain MRS-measurable variables and muscle rate mitochondrial respiration in all subjects [227]. Supplementation of CoQ_{10} and succinate resulted in clinical improvement of the respiratory function of a patient with Kearns-Sayre and chronic external ophthalmoplegia plus (KS/CEOP). In this case, the patient had virtually no CI activity as a consequence of 4.9 kDa mtDNA deletion; thus, the rationale of the combined treatment was a bypass of the CI defect by feeding the electron transport chain with succinate, plus the electron shuttle CoQ_{10}. A direct association between treatment regime and improved clinical status of the patient was documented [228].

In contrast, other studies failed to demonstrate any significant, reproducible, objective clinical improvement following CoQ_{10} administration in a variety of PMD patients [229]. However, the authors reported only a short treatment (2 months). CoQ_{10} treatment also failed to improve ptosis and CPEO [230]. Clinical trials also reported little if no benefit in patients with PMD: a study that enrolled 12 patients with different OXPHOS defects failed to demonstrate any clinical improvement upon CoQ_{10} treatment, regardless of its ability to promote ATP synthetic capacity in peripheral lymphocytes [231]. A randomized, double-blind, cross-over trial was performed in 30 patients with mitochondrial disorders, who received 1200 mg/day CoQ_{10} for 60 days. Although the treatment benefited from aerobic capacity and post-exercise lactate, it did not affect other clinically relevant variables [232]. In a multicenter study, eight patients with different PMD and documented CoQ_{10} defect received 300 mg/day of ubiquinone for 12 months; only subjective improvements on exercise intolerance, fatigue, and stiffness were reported, without any other significant amelioration of other clinical signs [233]. In the same study, CoQ_{10} was also administered to 15 patients with myopathy and normal CoQ_{10} levels in muscle. Only one patient, presenting with encephalomyopathy and an unknown genetic defect, reported subjective improvement of fatigue [233]. A phase 3 trial of CoQ_{10} (ClinicalTrials.gov identifier: NCT00432744) in children with PMD has been designed and implemented; the future outcomes will highlight any therapeutic effects [234].

3.7.8. Idebenone

Since the CoQ_{10} is lipophilic, water insoluble, and poorly absorbed in the gut, novel formulations with improved bioavailability have been developed. Idebenone is an organic molecule of the quinone family, with hydrophilic and redox-active properties, that increases the ATP production, reduces free radicals, inhibits lipid peroxidation, and consequently protects the lipid membranes and mitochondria from oxidative damage [235]. Its pharmacokinetic profile is more favorable than that of its analogue CoQ_{10} [236]. In rats and dogs, the idebenone plasma plateau is reached after 15 min from the administration, with a variable decline of half-life; moreover, idebenone is quickly and homogeneously distributed in the body, but the brain tends to lose its drug content very rapidly [235].

Idebenone is the only EU approved drug for the treatment of LHON. Treatment of fibroblasts from LHON patients with idebenone gave rise to increased CI activity, but yielded contradictory results on mitochondrial respiration, leading to impairment in some cases and stimulation in others [237]. Another study on LHON fibroblasts displayed metabolic alterations that were reversed by idebenone treatments, together with a significant rescue of CI activity [238]. The pharmacological effects of idebenone in retinal ganglion cells (RGC, which are inactive but viable in LHON patients) and in a mouse model of LHON were protective on retinal toxicity and visual impairment induced by CI dysfunction [239]. The first complete randomized, placebo-controlled, double-blind clinical trial in LHON (Rescue of Hereditary Optic Disease Outpatient Study "RHODOS", ClinicalTrials.gov identifier: NCT00747487) was conducted in 85 LHON patients with m.3460G>A, m.11778G>A, and m.14484T>C mutations. This study demonstrated the safety and well tolerability of idebenone (900 mg/day for 24 weeks) and reported amelioration of the visual outcome in a subgroup of patients [240]. Another randomized, double-blind placebo-controlled intervention study investigated the red–green (protan) and blue–yellow (tritan) color contrast sensitivity in 39 LHON patients, demonstrating significant protection from loss of color vision in subjects receiving idebenone for 6 months [241]. A clinical trial consisting of a single visit follow-up observational study in a subset of patients enrolled in the RHODOS study (RHODOS-OFU, ClinicalTrials.gov identifier: NCT01421381) demonstrated that the beneficial effect of idebenone treatment persisted despite discontinuation of therapy [242]. Additional studies are required to confirm these initial observations.

While use for LHON patients is well described, the exact mechanism is still undeciphered. However, beneficial effect of idebenone administration was described in an old adolescent patient suffering from an infantile-onset neurodegenerative disorder with severe cerebellar atrophy, epilepsy, dystonia, optic atrophy, and peripheral neuropathy, diagnosed with an homozygous stop mutation in Thioredoxin 2 (*TXN2*). TXN2 is a small mitochondrial redox protein essential for controlling the homeostasis of mitochondrial reactive oxygen species; based on the established defect in ROS regulation, TXN2 patient was treated with Idebenone (900 mg/day) in a compassionate use. During the 4 months follow-up period the, patient showed an improvement of feeding behavior (less tube feeding required), a considerable weight gain and increased physical capacity [243].

Idebenone has also been used to treat *OPA1*-dependent Dominant Optic Atrophy. Dominant optic atrophy (DOA) arises from heterozygous mutations in the *OPA1* gene that promotes fusion of the inner mitochondrial membrane and plays a role in maintaining ATP levels. Patients display optic disc pallor, RGC loss, and bilaterally reduced vision [244]. A randomized, placebo-controlled trial of idebenone at 2000 mg/kg/day in *Opa1* mutant mice with visual loss revealed limited therapeutic effects on RGC dendropathy and visual functions and showed a detrimental effect of idebenone in wild-type mice [245]. Nevertheless, patients' results are more encouraging: a pilot study on seven DOA patients documented encouraging results after 1-year of idebenone administration, with some improvement of visual function [246]. A recent retrospective cohort study investigated the effect of off-label idebenone administration on visual outcome in a DOA group of 87 patients, demonstrating that the treatment was significantly associated with stabilization/recovery of visual acuity [247].

3.7.9. MitoQ

MitoQ is a CoQ_{10} analogue that contains the antioxidant quinone moiety covalently attached to a lipophilic triphenylphosphonium cation (TPP^+), specifically designed to be accumulated by mitochondria in vivo, driven by the plasma- and mitochondrial-membrane potential [248]. To enter mitochondria, alkyl triphenylphosphonium cations first bind to the inner membrane's outer surface, then permeate the phospholipid bilayer's hydrophobic potential energy barrier, before binding to the inner surface of the membrane [249]. Once imported into mitochondria, nearly all the molecule is adsorbed into the IMM matrix surface, where it is continuously recycled to the antioxidant quinol form by the succinate-CoQ reductase [249,250]. However, MitoQ does not work as an electron carrier because it is a poor substrate for CI, CIII, and electron-transferring flavoprotein (ETF): quinone oxidoreductase (ETF-QOR) [250]. The selective accumulation of MitoQ prevents mitochondrial oxidative damage far more efficiently than untargeted antioxidants, although an intact mitochondrial membrane potential is required for its efficacy [251]. In vivo studies assessed that MitoQ can be safely administered for long term treatments [252,253]. Therefore, it has been developed as a pharmaceutical compound by Antipodean Pharmaceuticals Inc. and tested in few clinical trials to evaluate the beneficial effect of its antioxidant properties. The PROTECT study (ClinicalTrials.gov identifier: NCT00329056) evaluated the effect of MitoQ administration on the progression of Parkinson's Disease, which showed no significant improvement compared to the placebo group [254]. Some encouraging results have instead been obtained in age-related vascular dysfunction [255]. Although MitoQ is the most extensively studied mitochondria-targeted antioxidant in several disease contexts ranging from diabetes [256] to ageing [257] and heart failure [258] among others, MitoQ efficacy has never been evaluated in patients with PMD.

3.8. Redox-Active Molecules

3.8.1. EPI-Molecules

Modifications of the redox head and lipid tail of the CoQ_{10} molecule accomplished by Enns and co-workers [259] led to new experimental, redox-active molecules. Such new drugs, including the EPI-743, EPI-A0001, EPI-589 work as pro-oxidant, electron shuttles, and also display antioxidant properties. Importantly, the chemical modifications of the quinone ring, i.e., the substitution of the two methoxy groups with two methyl groups, significantly increased the redox properties of EPI-743, which undergo oxidation-reduction at a redox potential offset by −75 mV compared to CoQ_{10} and idebenone [259]. The changes at the isoprene tail significantly reduce these three molecules' lipophilicity, thus raising their bioavailability.

EPI-743 (Vatiquinone) is a drug belonging to the class of para-benzoquinones, a group of potent cellular oxidative stress protectants. EPI-743 targets the enzyme NADPH quinone oxidoreductase 1 (NQO1), increasing the biosynthesis of glutathione and modulating the redox control of metabolism [259]. It is an orally bioavailable molecule that can efficiently cross the blood–brain barrier [259]. The first clinical trial in 2011 enrolled 14 participants, who were selected based on two criteria: (I) genetically confirmed mitochondrial disease; and (II) possibility of end-of-life care starting within 90 days. All but one patient had an encephalomyopathy phenotype. Subjects were treated with EPI-743 orally or via gastrostomy tube for 12 weeks in a subject controlled, open-label study. Two patients died; the twelve survivors showed a modified disease progression, with a significant improvement of quality of life, brain imaging parameters, and clinical in >90% of the cases [259]. A prospective single-arm subject-controlled trial of EPI-743 was conducted in 2012 in children with genetically confirmed Leigh syndrome, at least moderately severe disease and MRI confirmation of necrotizing encephalopathy [260]. Subjects were treated for six months, with 100 mg of EPI-743 three times daily orally or via a gastrostomy tube. The clinical outcome showed that all children demonstrated arrested of the disease progression and/or reversal [260]. Analysis of blood samples in other children with mitochondrial encephalopathy showed EPI-743 administration's ability to restore reduced glutathione pools [261]. A recent case report documented the visible improvement of a pediatric patient with Leigh syndrome due to a mutation in the mitochondrially encoded ND3 gene treated with EPI-743. She was the only child surviving after four years of age, suggesting that EPI-743 could modify the natural course of the syndrome and contribute to the patient's long-term survival [262]. In a small open-label trial, EPI-743 arrested disease progression and reversed vision loss in most treated patients with LHON, suggesting that the previously described irreversible priming to retinal ganglion cell loss may be reversed by EPI-743 administration [263]. Other clinical trials evaluating the efficacy of EPI-743 in mitochondrial disease are still ongoing: one study has recruited 31 patients with Leigh syndrome to evaluate the long-term safety and neurodevelopmental effects of EPI-743 administration the dose of 15 mg/kg, up to a total 200 mg three times daily. The estimated primary completion date is December 2021 (ClinicalTrials.gov Identifier: NCT02352896). Another non-randomized, double-blind, placebo-controlled, cross-over study has finished recruiting children aged 2–11 with PMD in 2019. The primary outcome measures the effects of EPI-743 on quality of life. Secondary outcome measures include various biochemical, imaging, and clinical abnormalities (ClinicalTrials.gov Identifier: NCT01642056). Other molecules of the EPI series could be applied in the treatment of PMD due to OXPHOS defect, such as EPI-A0001 and EPI-589 although they have not been tested yet. EPI-A0001 (α-tocopheryl quinone) is a potent antioxidant, that has been tested for the treatment of Friedreich ataxia [264]. Only one double-blind, randomized, placebo-controlled, 28-days trial of two doses of EPI-A0001 in 31 patients reported encouraging results in terms of improvement of neurological function (ClinicalTrials.gov Identifier: NCT01035671). However, no other further studies have been reported. EPI-589, also known as (R)-troloxamide quinone, is expected to increase the reserves of antioxidant molecules, but to date, there are no published data regarding its mechanism of action. It is currently used for the treatment of ALS and in a clinical trial for Parkinson's Disease.

3.8.2. JP4-039

The affinity of the antibiotic Gramicidin S for the bacterial membrane has inspired the chemical structure of the JP4-039 molecule, a new, mitochondrial-targeted antioxidant drug [265]. JP4-039 displayed electron scavenger properties in animal models and in several tumor cell lines, as well as to improve mitochondrial respiration and scavenge ROS in *ACAD9*- [266] and in Very Long-Chain Acyl-CoA Dehydrogenase (*VLCAD*)- mutant fibroblasts [267]. Similar results have been reported in *ETHE1* and *MOCS1* mutant cell lines, in which JP4-039 treatment did increase the oxygen consumption rate, ATP production, and decrease superoxide levels. Preliminary pharmacokinetics after intravenous administration suggested fair tissue distribution, including in the brain, opening future perspectives for mitochondrial neurological disease therapies.

3.8.3. KH176

The ROS-Redox modulator KH176 was developed by the optimization of the Trolox-derivatives molecules [268]. KH176 has a dual effect: (I) it successfully reduces cellular ROS levels, and (II) it protects against redox perturbation by targeting the thioredoxin/peroxiredoxin system. The mechanism of action of KH176 requires its conversion into the quinone metabolite KH176m [268]. KH176 could counteract the ROS production and mitigate the altered cellular redox state in cellular models of CI defects [268]. The therapeutic efficacy of KH176 was tested in preclinical models of PMD. Long-term KH176 treatment ameliorated the clinical phenotype and the brain microstructural coherence of the CI-deficient *Ndufs4* ko mouse model [269,270]; however, no further improvement was observed with combined treatment with the PPAR agonist clofibrate [270]. A Phase 1 clinical trial in healthy adult male volunteers deemed that KH176 is well tolerated up to single doses of 800 mg and multiple doses of 400 mg b.i.d. and has a pharmacokinetic profile supportive for a twice-daily dose (ClinicalTrials.gov Identifier NCT02544217) [271]. Phase 2, double-blind, randomized, placebo-controlled, single-center, two-way cross-over trial has also been performed [272] (The KHENERGY STUDY - ClinicalTrials.gov Identifier NCT02909400). This study recruited patients with m.3242A>G mutation and aimed to explore the effects of treatment with KH176 for 4 weeks on clinical signs and symptoms and biomarkers of PMD and evaluate the KH176-related safety and pharmacokinetics. Results confirmed that KH176 was well tolerated and appeared safe at the 100-mg twice a day dose regimen; a significant improvement of the patients' overall mental health status was also documented [272]. Recently, KH176 (*Sonlicromanol*, developed by the biopharmaceutical company Khondrion, The Netherlands), received a rare pediatric disease (RPD) designation from the United States Food and Drug Administration (FDA), for the treatment of patients with MELAS syndrome [273]. Sonlicromanol is currently in Phase IIb clinical development (The KHENERGYZE Study, ClinicalTrials.gov Identifier: NCT04165239).

3.8.4. SKQ1

The mitochondria-targeted antioxidant 10-(6′-plastoquinonyl)-decyl-triphenyl-phosphonium (SKQ1) is a cationic plastoquinone derivative containing a positively charged phosphonium connected to plastoquinone by a decane linker. The antioxidant activities of mitochondria-targeted cationic plastoquinone derivatives (SKQs) are accomplished in two different ways: (I) by preventing peroxidation of cardiolipin [274] (mediated by quinol moieties) and (II) by fatty acid cycling, resulting in mild uncoupling that inhibits the formation of ROS in mitochondrial State IV (mediated by cation moieties) [275]. SKQ1 can effectively mitigate the oxidation induced either by hydrogen peroxide or by organic hydroperoxide in vitro [276]. SKQ1 has mainly been tested in several pathological cellular and pre-clinical models in which ROS-mediated mitochondrial dysfunction and cell death play a crucial role, such as Alzheimer's Disease [277,278], multiple sclerosis [279], and Parkinson's Disease [280]. In contrast, only one work tested its efficacy in a PMD model [281]. Shabalina and co-workers reported that chronic administration of SKQ1 to the *Mutator* mouse ameliorated mitochondrial ultrastructure in several tissues and significantly improved age-related phenotypic features, including the occurrence of hair loss, kyphosis, loss of estrus cycle, body weight loss, reduced lipid stores, hypothermia, immobility, and torpor-like states. Most importantly, SKQ1 administration significantly increased the lifespan of the *Mutator* mice [281]. However, increased oxidative damage has not been observed in the mtDNA *Mutator* mice (as reviewed by Edgar and Trifunovic [282]).

3.9. Pharmacological Modulation of Mitochondrial Dynamics

Mitochondria are highly dynamic organelles that undergo coordinated cycles of fission and fusion, referred to as "mitochondrial dynamics", to maintain their shape, distribution, and size [283]. Mitochondrial shape and mass are finely tuned by the activity of the pro-fusion proteins Mitofusin 1 (MFN1) and Mitofusin 2 (MFN2)—acting on the outer mitochondrial membrane (OMM)—and optic atrophy protein 1 (OPA1)—acting on the inner mitochondrial membrane (IMM)—plus the antagonist action of pro-fission proteins, such as dynamin-related protein 1 (DRP1) and mitochondrial fission 1 protein (FIS1) [284]. OPA1 is a multitasking GTPase with a total of eight long and short isoforms, which are involved in two independent mechanisms: (I) tighten of mitochondrial cristae of the IMM [285], that favors MRC supercomplexes assembly and optimizes mitochondrial respiration [286] (II) elongation of the mitochondrial network, promoting mitochondrial fusion [287]. Modifying these processes may benefit different PMD [98].

Genetic disorders of mitochondrial dynamics comprise defects of mitochondrial fusion triggered by mutations in *MFN2* or *OPA1*, exhibiting as Charcot–Marie–Tooth type 2A and autosomal dominant optic atrophy, respectively [288–290], and impaired mitochondrial fission caused by mutations in *DRP1* [291] and *MFF* [292]. The observation that the overexpression of OPA1 increased respiratory efficiency by stabilizing the respiratory chain SC [287] suggested that moderate overexpression of OPA1 could be beneficial in MRC defects models. Significant amelioration of mitochondrial encephalopathy and myopathy was obtained in a mouse model of COX defect crossed with a transgenic *Opa1* mouse model [293]. Furthermore, *Opa1* overexpression also prevented kidney focal glomerulosclerosis in the *Mpv17* ko mouse [294]. The recent discovery of chemical modulators of mitochondrial fusion (M-hydrazone) and fission (MDIVI-1 and P110) may represent a therapeutic option for OXPHOS defect [295–297].

Mitochondrial dynamics could be indirectly modulated, targeting the cytoskeleton organization, which has a significant role in supporting the mitochondrial network [298]. Recently, the *Escherichia coli* protein toxin called Cytotoxic Necrotizing Factor 1 (CNF1), which acts on the Rho GTPases regulators of the actin cytoskeleton [299], was tested in OXPHOS deficient patients' cells [300]. CNF1 effectively induced mitochondrial elongation, rescuing the wild-type-like mitochondrial morphology and increasing the ATP content in fibroblasts derived from a MERRF patient with m.8344A>G mutation [300]. Further studies are needed to assess the potential use of these drugs on preclinical models of PMDs.

3.10. Pharmacological Protection of Cardiolipin

Among experimentally new drugs for PMD, there is Elamipretide (also known as MTP-131, SS-31, and Bendavia), a small aromatic-cationic tetrapeptide (D-Arg-dimethylTyr-Lys-Phe-NH$_2$) that readily penetrates cell membranes in a non-energy requiring and non-saturable manner, and transiently localizes to the IMM, where reversibly binds to cardiolipin [301]. Cardiolipin is a unique phospholipid that is only located on the IMM and plays essential structural roles in modulating the IMM curvature leading to cristae formation and organizing the electron transport chain complexes into SC to facilitate optimal electron transfer and energy production. Cardiolipin also plays a role in anchoring cytochrome c to the inner membrane facilitating electron transfer from CIII to CIV [302]. When oxidized, cardiolipin participates in cell death. It is highly vulnerable to oxidative damage because it contains many unsaturated fatty acids and is located close to reactive oxygen species' production site. Oxidation of cardiolipin leads to the disruption of intimal microregions and the loss of membrane curvature and cristae [303]. Elamipretide binds selectively to cardiolipin via electrostatic and hydrophobic interactions and protects it from oxidation, keeping mitochondrial cristae, promoting oxidative phosphorylation, and inhibiting mitochondrial permeability transition pore opening [205]. The idea is that elamipretide restores energy production, reduces the production of reactive oxygen species, and ultimately increases the energy supply to affected cells and organs. It has been shown that elamipretide consistently improves mitochondrial, cellular, and organ function in both in vitro and in vivo disease models for which mitochondrial dysfunction is understood to be an essential component, including cardiovascular, renal, metabolic, skeletal muscle, neurodegenerative, and mitochondrial genetic disease [304–308].

Elamipretide is metabolized via sequential C-terminal degradation to the tripeptide M1 and the dipeptide M2. The apparent plasma half-life ($t_{\frac{1}{2}}$) of M1 was comparable to that of elamipretide, whereas $t_{\frac{1}{2}}$ of M2 was longer than that of elamipretide. elamipretide and its metabolites are excreted primarily through the kidneys. Elamipretide was initially used in preclinical models to treat ischemia/reperfusion injury, a common complication of interventional procedures for acute myocardial infarction and coronary bypass surgery [309].

As of November 2017, the U.S. FDA Office of Orphan Products Development has granted Orphan Drug Designation to Stealth's investigational drug candidate, elamipretide, to treat patients with primary mitochondrial myopathy (MM). SPIMM-301 was a Phase 3, multicentered, double-blind, parallel-group, placebo-controlled trial followed by an open-label treatment extension (ClinicalTrials.gov Identifier: NCT03323749). It evaluated the efficacy and safety of elamipretide over 32 weeks in 218 patients, ages 16 to 80, with MM. Enrolled subjects received in Part 1 single daily 40 mg/mL subcutaneous injections of fixed doses of elamipretide/placebo for up to 24 weeks; in Part 2 received single daily 40 mg/mL subcutaneous injections of fixed doses of elamipretide for up to 144 weeks. The trial was conducted at 28 clinical sites across North America, Europe, and Australia. The primary endpoints assessed efficacies were the 6-min walk test (6MWT) and the Primary Mitochondrial Myopathy Symptom Assessment (PMMSA) Total Fatigue Score. The 6MWT measures the distance an individual can walk over a total of 6 min on a hard, flat surface. PMMSA is a patient-reported outcome tool developed by Stealth in which individuals with PMM report their fatigue, muscle weakness, and other symptoms on a scale from 1 (least severe) to 4 (most severe). Safety results showed that treatment with elamipretide was well-tolerated with most adverse events mild to moderate in severity, but it did not produce significant improvements in 6MWT and PMMSA assessments [310].

Elamipretide is now in late-stage clinical studies in other three PMD: Barth syndrome (ClinicalTrials.gov Identifier: NCT03098797), Leber's hereditary optic neuropathy (ClinicalTrials.gov

Identifier: NCT02693119), as well as a clinical study in dry age-related macular degeneration (AMD) with non-central geographic atrophy (ClinicalTrials.gov Identifier: NCT03891875).

3.11. Pharmacological Modulation of Autophagy

Autophagy is an evolutionarily conserved process that degrades cargoes-like aggregate-prone proteins, pathogens, damaged organelles, and macromolecules via delivery to lysosomes, to warrant cellular quality control. Targets for degradation are first encircled into specific, double-membrane structures termed autophagosomes, whose formation (phagophore), elongation, and closure are controlled by autophagy-related (ATG) proteins [311]. Autophagosomes are fused with lysosomes to generate autophagolysosomes that carry out the degradation of the substrates. Stimulation of autophagy has been proposed as a therapeutic approach to target and eliminate dysfunctional mitochondria. The most widely used inhibitor of (macro) autophagy is rapamycin, which acts by blocking the target of rapamycin (mTOR) complex 1 (mTORC1) [312]. Johnson and co-workers first published the results of a chronic treatment of a PMD mouse model with the mTOR inhibitor Rapamycin in 2013. The authors reported a significant delay in the disease progression and fatal outcome of the *Ndufs4* ko mouse [313]. These results were further confirmed in other preclinical models of OXPHOS, including (I) a muscle-specific *Cox15* ko mouse [314], (II) an *ND2*-deficient *Drosophila* model of LS [315], (III) iPSCs-derived neurons carrying a mutation in the *MT-ATP6* gene [316], and (IV) the gas-1 (fc21) nematodes [317]. These encouraging results led to developing a clinical study (ClinicalTrials.gov Identifier: NCT03747328) in four MELAS patients treated with *Everolimus*, a rapamycin analogue. Patients' derived primary fibroblasts showed improvement of mitochondrial morphology, membrane potential, and replicative capacity [318]. Recently, *Everolimus* was used to treat two children affected by Leigh disease or MELAS. The latter failed to respond and died of progressive disease 10 months after starting the treatment [319], whereas the child with Leigh syndrome improved health status. Brain MRI reduced the bilateral signal hyperintensity in thalami and brainstem after 6 months of treatment. Further improvements were documented after 19 months of treatment, being the patient able to walk independently with a slightly ataxic gait, and with no longer required of tracheostomy and gastrostomy. However, although these data support the idea that rapamycin may be useful in several PMD, others recently reported that rapamycin treatment exacerbated the disease progression in mice with CoQ_{10} deficiency [320] and failed to rescue the cerebral pathological features of TwKO^{astro} mice [59], indicating that not all metabolic defects may benefit from rapamycin therapy. Moreover, mTORC1 inhibitors are linked to immunosuppressive outcomes [321], and it is currently unknown whether this effect could be detrimental for PMD patients in the long-term.

3.12. Bypassing cI-cIII-cIV Defects with Alternative Enzymes

A recent therapeutic strategy concerns the possibility to by-pass OXPHOS defects by using the alternative enzymes NADH dehydrogenase/CoQ_{10} reductase (NDI1), plant alternative NADH dehydrogenases (NDH-2), and CoQ_{10}/O_2 alternative oxidase (AOX). AOX and NDI1 are single-peptide enzymes present in yeast, plants, and lower eukaryotes where they act as alternative components of the respiratory chain. NDI1 substitutes CI in yeast, where it transfers electrons to CoQ_{10} and regenerates the NAD^+ pool, while AOX bypasses CIII and CIV by accepting electrons from CoQ_{10}. In contrast to *Saccharomyces Cerevisiae* NDI1, which enzymatically competes with endogenous CI [322], plant alternative NDH-2 naturally coexists with endogenous CI and supports the oxidation of NADH only in specific physiological conditions [323], e.g., when CI is metabolically inactive, or the concentration of matrix NADH exceeds a certain threshold. It should be noted that such alternatives electron transfer activities are not linked to a proton pumping across the inner mitochondrial membrane. Expression of these enzymes has been used to bypass CI deficiency in *Drosophila melanogaster* [324], combined CI-III-IV deficiencies in ρ^0 mouse cells [325], CIII-IV deficiencies in human cells [326] and *Drosophila melanogaster* [327], raising the possibility to use these genes to treat OXPHOS-related disorders. Adeno-associated virus (AAV) expressing *NDI1* (AAV-NDI1) was shown to protect retinal ganglion cells (RGCs) in a rotenone-induced murine model of LHON, significantly reducing RGC death by 1.5-fold and optic nerve atrophy by 1.4-fold and considerably preserving retinal function [328]. Recently, the effects of the expression of NDI1 in vivo have been tested in a mouse model of Leigh syndrome due to the lack of the 18-KDa complex I subunit Ndufs4 [329]. McElroy and co-workers generated a mouse that conditionally expressed the yeast *NDI1*, while the *Ndufs4* was lost, specifically in the brain. NDI1 expression was sufficient to dramatically prolong lifespan without significantly ameliorate the ataxic phenotype [329].

Interestingly, the authors demonstrated that mitochondrial CI activity in the brain supports organismal survival through its NAD^+ regeneration capacity, while optimal motor control requires the bioenergetic function of mitochondrial CI [329]. When transgenic *Ciona intestinalis AOX* mice were crossed with CIII-deficient $Bcs1l^{p.S78G}$ knock-in mice—a model of GRACILE syndrome (growth retardation, aminoaciduria, cholestasis, iron overload, lactic acidosis, and early death) [330,331], with multiple visceral manifestations and premature death—AOX expression was able to increase lifespan, prevent lethal cardiomyopathy, and ameliorate renal and cerebral manifestations. On the contrary, when the transgenic *AOX* mouse was crossed with the *Acta-Cox15* ko model, the double ko-*AOX* mutants showed a decreased lifespan and a substantial worsening of the myopathy compared to the ko alone. Decreased ROS production in ko-*AOX* versus ko mice led to impaired AMPK/PGC-1α signaling and PAX7/MYOD-dependent muscle regeneration, blunting compensatory responses [332].

Recently, the two different mitochondrially-targeted *NDH-2* (AtNDA2 and AtNDB4) from *Arabidopsis thaliana* (At) were used to bypass the OXPHOS defect in human CI deficient fibroblasts and reduce oxidative stress [333]. However, a competition between AtNDA2 and endogenous CI for NADH oxidation was reported in control cell lines [333], raising some concern about its potential therapeutic application for human PMD.

4. Precision Medicine Approaches for PMD Caused by mtDNA Defects

4.1. Pre-Implantation Therapies to Prevent the Transmission of mtDNA Mutations

Each mammalian cell contains numerous copies of mtDNA. The coexistence of mutated and wild-type mtDNA molecules is called heteroplasmy, the percentage of which can range from negligible values to 100%. Heteroplasmy allows detrimental mutations to persist, and most importantly, to be transferred to the next generation. MtDNA molecules segregate unequally during primordial germline development. Upon oocyte maturation, such segregated pools of mtDNA expand within each egg cell. In the case of an asymptomatic mother carrying heteroplasmic mutations in her germline, the heterogeneous population of oocytes could develop offspring with vastly varying levels of heteroplasmy [334]. Therefore, pathogenic mutations of mtDNA are maternally transmitted [335] although a rare, paternal inheritance was debated in the last years, and recently reviewed by Wei and Chinnery [336]. Heteroplasmy is well tolerated until the percentage of the mutation (i.e., mutational load) exceeds a certain threshold, often greater than 60% mutated mtDNA, beyond which bioenergetic defect manifests, mainly in high energy demanding tissues. No effective therapies for mtDNA-linked disease exist, and several techniques can prevent the transmission of pathogenic mutations.

4.1.1. Pre-Implantation Genetic Diagnosis

Pre-implantation genetic diagnosis is a preventive approach that still represents families' best option with a known story of mtDNA mutations [337]. Pre-implantation diagnosis is an in vitro fertilization (IVF)-based approach in which the fertilized egg harboring the pathogenic mtDNA mutation is cultured until the stage of 6–8 cells [338] or blastocyst [339] and then biopsied for genetic analysis before implantation. However, the pre-implantation diagnosis has some limitations: (I) it will only benefit women who have low levels of mtDNA mutations in oocytes [340] and, (II) it assumes that the diagnosed heteroplasmy level is representative of that of the entire embryo and would not change over time.

4.1.2. Mitochondrial Donation: Maternal Spindle Transfer

Recently, mitochondrial replacement or mitochondrial donation (MD) has been proposed as a potential method for preventing transmission of mutated mtDNA from the mother to the offspring, by replacing the mitochondria in the oocytes of carrier women. The most recently exploited MD reproductive technologies include maternal spindle transfer (MST) [341] and pronuclear transfer (PNT) [342]. This technology is legally approved for use in the U.K., but the governments of Australia and Singapore are in the process of formal discussions aimed at MD legalization. However, the current state of MD-relevant activity and regulation remains largely elusive in many countries; please refer to [343] for a detailed overview. MST is a complex technique that involves the transfer of nuclear genetic material between a patient's egg with mutated mtDNA to an enucleated donor's unfertilized metaphase II oocyte with healthy mitochondria. MST generates an oocyte with a patient's nuclear DNA devoid of mutated mtDNA. MST is then followed by intracytoplasmic sperm injection (ICSI) and in vitro embryo culture (Figure 3A). A proof-of-principle use of MST to prevent the transmission of mutated mtDNA molecules was first reported in rhesus macaques by the group of Mitalipov in 2009 [344]. In that case, MST and subsequent ICSI resulted in the birth of healthy offspring (named Mito and Tracker) with undetectable levels of spindle donor's associated mtDNA [344]. The same group then translated this technique to human oocytes, and similar fertilization and blastulation rates between MST and control groups were observed, suggesting that embryo development was not compromised [345]. MtDNA analysis revealed that all examined spindle transfer zygotes and cleaving embryos contained more than 99% donor mtDNA. Similar outcomes were observed in 87% of embryonic stem (ES) cell lines established from spindle transfer blastocysts, regardless of donor mtDNA. However, a reversal of mtDNA haplogroup from donor to maternal mtDNA in a limited number of ES clones was reported, for which a mechanistic explanation based on replicative advantages conferred by some D-loops polymorphisms were proposed [345]. It should be noted that a further mtDNA analysis on those and others ES cell lines [346] raised some concerns about the evidence provided by Kang and co-workers [345]. At the American Society for Reproductive Medicine (ASRM) annual meeting 2016, Dr. John Zhang, New Hope Fertility Center of New York City reported the outcome of the use of MST in a woman carrying mtDNA mutation of Leigh syndrome (8993 T>G), which resulted in the birth of an healthy baby with less than 10% mutated mtDNA in tissues tested 2 days after the birth [347]. A case report was published in 2017 [348].

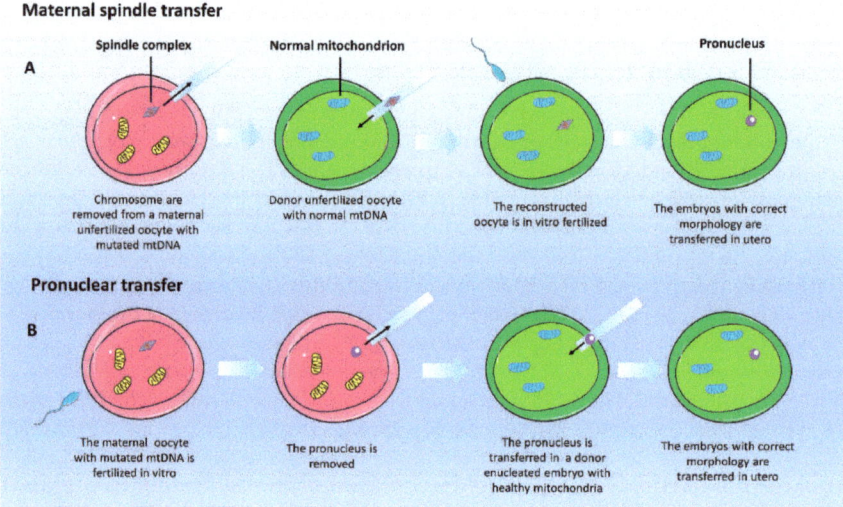

Figure 3. Mitochondrial donation (MD). (**A**) Maternal spindle transfer (MST) and (**B**) pronuclear transfer (PNT) represent the two principal strategies to prevent transmission of mtDNA disease. The techniques forecast the removal of nuclear genetic material from patient and maternal oocytes pre- or post-fertilization. The maternal genetic material is then transferred to enucleated oocyte or zygote from the donor, thereby generating an embryo characterized by the parental nuclear genetic material and by healthy mitochondria from the donor.

4.1.3. Mitochondrial Donation: Pronuclear Transfer

The pronuclear transfer (PNT) involves a first step of in vitro fertilization of the patient's oocyte, followed by the removal of the diploid nucleus, which is then transferred into a donor's enucleated zygote with healthy mitochondria (Figure 3B) [340]. PNT was proposed in 2005 to prevent transmission of mtDNA disease in the mito-mouse, a model that accumulates large-scale mtDNA deletions [349]. In this elegant paper, second polar bodies were used as biopsy samples to diagnose mtDNA genotypes of mito-mouse zygotes. Nuclear transplantation was carried out from mito-mouse zygotes to enucleated normal zygotes and was shown to rescue all of the F(0) progeny from the expression of respiration defects throughout their lives [349]. In a second report published in 2010, abnormally fertilized human zygotes were used, and reconstructed embryos developed following PNT showed the capacity to reach the blastocyst stage [340]. In 2016, the first preclinical evaluation of PNT using normally fertilized human embryos was reported [350]. Since the techniques used these studies [340] were not tolerated by normally fertilized zygotes, an alternative approach was developed, that significantly improved the efficient development to the blastocyst stage. This was based on performing the pronuclear transplantation immediately after completing meiosis rather than before the first mitotic division. Following this optimization, mtDNA carryover was reduced to less than 2% in the majority (79%) of PNT blastocysts. The study reported low levels of mtDNA carryover in PNT embryos and observed a reversion to the maternal haplogroup in a limited number of hESC clones derived from PNT inner cell mass embryos [350]. In conclusion, although PNT can reduce the risk of mtDNA disease, it may not guarantee prevention [350].

4.2. Personalized Therapies for mtDNA Disorders

4.2.1. Delivery of Nucleic Acids to the Mitochondria

Mutations in mitochondrial genes or mitochondrial tRNAs are associated with a variety of maternally inherited neuromyopathies. An effective therapy would imply delivery therapeutic genes or tRNAs to the mitochondrial matrix, where mtDNA resides.

Nucleic acid delivery into the mitochondrion has been attempted using liposome-based nanocarriers such as Mito-Porter [351,352] and dequalinium-based liposome-like vesicles (DQAsomes)-transfection system [353], or by RNA Import Complex [354]. Mito-Porter is a liposome-based carrier that introduces macromolecular cargos into mitochondria via membrane fusion. The authors provided evidence of nucleic acid delivery into the mitochondrial matrix either in isolated rat liver mitochondria and in living, intact cells [351]. As proof of principle, this method was further exploited to deliver wild-type mitochondrial pre-tRNA^{Phe} to decrease the mutation rate of tRNA^{Phe} in mitochondria of the patient's cell with a G625A heteroplasmic mutation in the tRNA^{Phe} of mtDNA, with a significant correction of the mutation rate [355]. Similarly, a therapeutic correction of ND3 mutant fibroblasts' mitochondrial respiration was obtained by reintroducing the wt mRNA of ND3 via Mito-Porter [356].

DQAsomes are the prototype for all mitochondria-targeted vesicular pharmaceutical nanocarrier systems. First described in 1998, they have been successfully explored to deliver DNA and low-molecular-weight molecules to mitochondria within living mammalian cells [357].

The RNA Import Complex (RIC) is a multi-subunit protein complex from the mitochondria of the Kinetoplastid protozoon *Leishmania tropica* that induces the transport of tRNA across natural and artificial membranes [358]. Observing that Kinetoplastid protozoa have evolved specialized systems for importing nucleus-encoded tRNAs into mitochondria, the RIC was used to import endogenous cytosolic tRNAs, including tRNA^{Lys}, and restored mitochondrial function in wild-type, MERFF, and KSS cybrids [354].

However, no effective treatment was translated into animal models despite this evidence of delivering the exogenous nucleic acids into the cellular mitochondria.

4.2.2. Heteroplasmic Shift

A second strategy to correct mtDNA mutations is based on the disruption of mutant molecules using selective nucleases to shift the heteroplasmy level below the critical, pathological threshold. To this aim, several approaches based on the following tools have been developed in the past years and are discussed below: (I) restriction enzymes; (II) antisense oligonucleotides; (III) molecular scissors; (IV) DddA.

The very first work carried out by Tanaka and co-workers in 2002 [359] implied the delivery of the restriction endonuclease SmaI into the mitochondria of cybrids to specifically degrade mtDNA in which the pathogenic 8993T>G mutation was present, creating a specific SmaI-restriction site [359]. SmaI specifically degraded mutant mtDNA, with consequent repopulation of mitochondrial genome by wild-type molecules, and subsequent restoration of intracellular ATP level and mitochondrial membrane potential [359].

Heteroplasmy shifting has also been achieved using antisense oligonucleotides in cybrids containing a heteroplasmic mtDNA deletion [360]. In this case, anti-replicative RNA molecules were designed and transfected into a cybrid cell line derived by a KSS patient's fibroblasts carrying an mtDNA deletion involving 65% of the mtDNA molecules. The anti-replicative effect of the RNA oligoribonucleotides complementary to the mutant mtDNA region specifically reduced the proportion of pathological mtDNA population, shifting the heteroplasmy level from 65% to 50% [360].

The Clustered Regularly Interspaced Short Palindromic Repeats (CRISPR)/Cas9 technology has been largely used for nuclear gene editing; however its application for the editing of the mitochondrial genome appears highly challenging mainly due to sub-efficient delivery of guide RNA and Cas9 enzyme complexes into mitochondria. However, in 2015, Jo and colleagues successfully manipulated the mtDNA with the CRISPR/Cas9 technology [361]. Despite the lack of MTS peptides, the authors showed that the flagged Cas9 localized into the mitochondria, while the gRNAs allowed specific depletion of targeted portions of mtDNA but not degradation of the entire molecule. This point was difficult to reconcile with the fact that mtDNA behaves as a unit [362].

A recent preprint study reported the editing of the *MT-ND4* gene accomplished by targeting the guide RNA to an RNA transport derived stem loop element (RP-loop), while expressing the Cas9 enzyme with a mitochondrial localization sequence [363]. However, due to the controversial nature of mammalian mitochondrial RNA import [364], the use of the CRISPR/Cas9 application for mtDNA editing is still debated.

Very recently, adeno-associated viral vectors (AAVs) were used to deliver molecular scissors (i.e., ZFNs, mitochondrial-targeted (mt) TALENs and mtZFNs) in vivo, to destroy mutated mtDNA selectively. Using the first available mouse model of heteroplasmic mitochondrial disease, bearing the point mutation m.5024C>T in mitochondrial tRNA^{ALA} (mt-tRNA^{ALA}) [365], both TALENs and mtZFNs were able to reduce the mtDNA heteroplasmy with the concomitant rescue of molecular and biochemical phenotypes [366,367].

However, the approaches described so far cannot introduce specific nucleotide changes in mtDNA and cannot be applied to homoplasmic mtDNA mutations because they would destroy all mtDNA copies. To overcome those issues, Mok et al. has recently set up a precision genome editing strategy. They obtained outbreaking results using the interbacterial toxin "double-stranded DNA deaminase toxin A", or DddA, encoded by *Burkholderia cenocepacia*, which catalyzes the deamination of cytidines within dsDNA [368]. Engineered split-DddA halves are inactive until simultaneously carried on the target DNA by adjacently bound programmable DNA-binding proteins. The fusions of the split-DddA halves, transcription activator-like effector (TALE) array proteins, and an uracil glycosylase inhibitor generated the RNA-free DddA-derived cytosine base editors (DdCBEs), which allows guided CG-to-TA changes in mtDNA without the need of double-strand breaks. This technique can potentially correct pathogenic mutations on mtDNA with high levels of purity and specificity [368]. Despite these findings looking extremely innovative, additional research aimed to improve the delivery of DdCBEs in vitro and in vivo is essential for exploring their therapeutic potential.

4.2.3. Allotopic Gene Expression

Allotopic gene expression is a method to overcome the mtDNA mutations by re-expressing the missing mtDNA-encoded protein from the nucleus. In this case, an engineered nuclear version of a mitochondrial gene encodes a protein that can be imported into the mitochondria due to an MTS presence. This approach was used to deliver the protein product of the MT-ATP6 gene to the mitochondria in cybrids containing the m.8993T>G mutation [369]. Such allotopic expression significantly improved the cell growth in selective medium and the ATP synthesis [369]. Similarly, allotopic expression of the MT-ND4 gene effectively prevented blindness in a rat model of LHON [370]. Consequently, a human clinical trial of gene therapy to treat LHON has been carried out. Although there was weak evidence of allotopic expression, Guy et al. reported the amelioration of visual acuity in the injected eyes [371]. Another clinical trial (ClinicalTrials.gov identifier NTC01267422) in which nine patients affected by LHON carrying the G11778A mutation were treated with a single dose (5×10^9 vg/0.05 mL) of rAAV2-*ND4* reported no adverse effects. In six out of nine patients, the injected eyes' visual acuity improved by at least 0.3 log MAR after nine months of follow-up. The visual field was enlarged, but the retinal nerve fiber layer remained relatively stable. The visual acuity improved, and the visual field was enlarged nine months after treatment, while other parameters were unchanged [372]. A third open-label phase I/II clinical trial (ClinicalTrials.gov identifier NCT02064569) investigated both safety and preliminary efficacy of a rAAV2/2-*ND4* in four dose-escalation cohorts. The treatment resulted in safe with mild adverse effects. Six out of 14 patients manifested a clinically relevant improvement in the best-corrected visual acuity. Taken together, these results suggest the possible use of gene therapy for LHON.

4.2.4. Mitochondrial Augmentation Therapy

Recently, Minovia Therapeutics developed a novel form of cellular therapy called Mitochondrial Augmentation Therapy (MAT). Its rationale is based on the capability of exogenous mitochondria to enter cells in culture [373,374], bringing their own genetic material, augmenting endogenous mitochondrial function, and content and fusing with the endogenous mitochondrial network. The mitochondrial uptake process was termed mitochondrial augmentation and is currently proposed for Kearns–Sayre syndrome (KSS) and Pearson Syndrome. KSS is a progressive retinitis pigmentosa and external ophthalmoplegia occurring at childhood due to de-novo mtDNA deletions [13]. Other systems may be involved over time, including hearing, heart, skeletal muscles, central nervous system, endocrine glands, and kidneys [13]. Pearson Syndrome is a rare disorder affecting the bone marrow and exocrine pancreas [14], also characterized by de-novo mtDNA deletion [15]. MAT approach enriches hematopoietic stem cells (HSCs) with healthy mitochondria before transplantation in patients. MAT involves a series of complex steps: first, mitochondria are extracted from white blood cells derived from the patient's mother (confirmed non-deleted); in turn, stem cells are collected from the patient, who receives treatment with *Neupogen* (filgrastim, by Amgen) to boost the production of white blood cells in the bone marrow, and with *Mozobil* (plerixafor, by Sanofi-Aventis) to mobilize the hematopoietic stem cells containing the CD34 protein marker into the bloodstream. The healthy mitochondria are then introduced into patient-derived stem cells and given back to the patient by intravenous infusion. A first human study was performed on three children with Pearson syndrome under a compassionate use program. Results were reported at the "Targeting Mitochondria Conference 2019" and at "Mitochondrial Medicine 2019 Meeting". Mitochondrial augmentation therapy improved the in vitro PS-derived HSC function, the metabolic determinants, the aerobic capacity, and the quality of life of the treated patients. The same company also promoted an open-label study (ClinicalTrials.gov identifier NCT03384420) to assess the MAT's safety and therapeutic effects. Recruitment of seven children is now in progress to analyze any treatment-related adverse events at one year, and any improvement in the quality of life, as assessed by the International Pediatric Mitochondrial Disease Scale.

Moreover, promising results of the first MAT treatment on a KSS patient were recently reported. The 14-year-old patient underwent leukapheresis, and positively selected CD34$^+$ cells were augmented with maternal mitochondria before infusion (2×10^6 cells/kg). Then, the patient was followed for clinical and metabolic parameters. Before MAT, she weighed only 19 kg, she could not sit, walk, express words, and experienced 1 or 2 seizures a week. Seven months after treatment, she gained weight, she could reach objects, sit independently, walk with assistance, and express herself in short sentences. Seizures were resolved 4 months after treatment. Her normalized functional score on the International Pediatric Mitochondrial Disease Score improved from 91% to 57%. Also, the ATP content of the peripheral blood lymphocytes was increased. Those impressive improvements of her physiological and metabolic status make MAT a potential therapy for KSS [375].

5. Precision Medicine Approaches for PMD Caused by Nuclear Defects

5.1. Gene Therapy Approaches

Gene therapy is the most straightforward option for treating disease caused by a single recessive genetic defect. Re-expressing the wild-type form of a mutated gene, or other therapeutic genes, using appropriate viral vectors is an attractive strategy, currently exploited for disorders affecting a single organ. In fact, while the expression of an ectopic gene in the whole body is still unfeasible, specific critical cells or tissue can be targeted with currently available technologies. AAVs are emerging as a suitable delivery method because they are not associated with any disease in humans or animals and remain episomic in the cells for a prolonged time, thus reducing the risk of insertional mutagenesis [376].

Moreover, the availability of several serotypes allows tissue-specific targeting [377]. Potential pitfalls concern the limited cloning capacity, the difficulty in achieving therapeutic expression levels in several tissues—especially skeletal muscle, due to is abundance and distribution- and the brain, due to the low blood–brain-barrier (BBB) penetrance. One of the first preclinical gene therapy studies applied to a mitochondrial myopathy was performed using the AAV2 carrying the *ANT1* cDNA in the *ANT1* ko mouse model. *ANT1* encodes the mitochondrial adenine nucleotide translocator, an integral IMM protein that forms homodimers or tetramers [378], acting as electrogenic pumps that export ATP out across the IMM in exchange for cytosolic ADP [379]. Mutations in *ANT1* lead to MM with progressive external ophthalmoplegia (PEO), caused by paralysis of the extraocular eye muscles [380]. AAV-*ANT1* transduction resulted in long-term stable expression in muscle precursor cells and differentiated muscle fibers. The transgenic ANT1 protein was targeted into the IMM, formed a functional ADP/ATP carrier, increased the mitochondrial export of ATP, and reversed the histopathological changes associated with the MM [381]. Furthermore, the efficacy of AAV-mediated gene therapy has been confirmed in several mouse models of mitochondrial disorders, including the models for hepato-cerebral forms of severe mtDNA depletion syndrome [57] and Leigh syndrome [382].

5.2. Liver Transplantation

Liver transplantation (LT) is a feasible approach to treat PMD, mainly affecting the single organ [383]. LT has been performed in individuals with hepatocerebral forms of mtDNA depletion syndromes, which frequently progress to liver failure, as those due to mutations in *MPV17* gene [384]. However, LT outcome has not been satisfactory, since almost fifty percent of the transplanted patients died in the post-transplantation period due to multiorgan failure. For this and other reasons, LT in mitochondrial hepatopathies remains controversial. LT is not recommended in patients with disorders characterized by a rapid progression of neurological manifestations, such as Alpers–Huttenlocher syndrome, but it may be beneficial in patients with an acceptable quality of life. LT may also differentially affect survival, e.g., patients with mtDNA depletion syndromes caused by mutations in *DGUOK* gene—encoding the mitochondrial deoxyguanosine kinase, which phosphorylates purines to the corresponding nucleotides in the mitochondrial nucleotides salvage pathway—show lower survival than those of patients with other PMD. Although a recent retrospective study on 12 PMD patients receiving LT confirmed these findings [385], others suggest that, even in the presence of neurological MRI findings, but in the absence of significant neurological symptoms, LT represents a viable option in DGUOK-deficient patients [386].

5.3. PMD Characterised by Systemic Accumulation of Toxic Compounds

5.3.1. Application of Gene Therapy Protocol

AAV therapy has been successfully achieved by targeting the missing gene to the liver when the underlying disease mechanism is linked to toxic compounds' systemic accumulation. This is the case of the ethylmalonic encephalopathy caused by mutations in the *ETHE1* gene encoding for a mitochondrial sulfur dioxygenase involved in the detoxification pathway of hydrogen sulfide (H_2S) [387]. Mutations in *ETHE1* lead to systemic accumulation of H_2S, which acts as a potent inhibitor of complex IV [197], leading to the onset of the phenotype (for a detailed description of the H_2S pathway, see Viscomi, Bottani et al., 2015 [388]). The re-expression of the *ETHE1* gene by a hepatotropic AAV2/8 serotype restored the missing enzymatic activity in the liver, with a significant clearance of H_2S from the bloodstream, a major amelioration of the phenotype and prolonged lifespan of the *Ethe1* ko mice [389]. Similarly, systemic accumulations of thymidine and deoxy uridine, which interfere with mtDNA replication and lead to mitochondrial dysfunction were corrected by hepatotropic AAV2/8 vector carrying the human *TYMP* in a mouse model of MNGIE [390]. The nucleoside reduction achieved by this treatment prevented deoxycytidine triphosphate (dCTP) depletion, which is the limiting factor affecting mtDNA replication in this disease [390].

AAV treatment may be useful also in mitochondrial neurodegenerative disorders: it was reported that the administration of AAV9 carrying the human *NDUFS4* partially rescued the phenotype of Ndufs4 ko mice only when simultaneously administered systemically and intracranially. AAV9 serotype did not efficiently cross the BBB, and mainly targeted glial cells when injected intracranially in new-borns. Interestingly, newly engineered serotypes AAV-PHP.eB and AAV-PHP.S showed great promises in their efficiency to transduce the central and peripheral nervous systems, crossing the BBB [391].

5.3.2. Application of Liver Transplantation Protocol

Like the gene therapy approach, the liver is an attractive target for pathologies triggered by systemic accumulation of toxic compounds. LT is proposed as an alternative approach to treat mitochondrial neurogastrointestinal encephalopathy (MNGIE) disease. MNGIE is caused by a deficiency of thymidine phosphorylase (TP) due to mutations in the nuclear gene *TYMP* [392]. TP is a cytosolic enzyme catalyzing the first step of thymidine (dThd) and deoxy uridine (dUrd) catabolism. Mutations in TYMP lead to the accumulation of dThd and dUrd systemically, which induce an imbalance of the cytosolic nucleotide pool. Because the mitochondrial nucleotide pool relies, in part, on nucleotides imported from the cytosol, an imbalanced cytosolic nucleotide pool lead to an imbalanced mitochondrial nucleotide pool, which ultimately has mutagenic effects on mtDNA, resulting in depletion, multiple deletions, and point mutations causing progressive mitochondrial deficiency and organ failure [392–394]. LT rapidly normalized serum levels of toxic nucleosides in a 25-year-old MNGIE patient, and his conditions were stable after 400 days of follow-up [395]. LT also resulted in an effective option to treat ethylmalonic encephalopathy due to mutation in *ETHE1* gene [396,397], since the replaced organ can substitute the deficient ETHE1 enzyme and clear the toxic H_2S that accumulate in this disorder, constituting a feasible therapeutic option in patients. Patients showed progressive improvement of the neurological functions and normalization or amelioration of the biochemical abnormalities [396,397]. However, the decision to perform LT remains difficult because neurological manifestations may worsen despite their absence before the transplant [398].

5.3.3. Cell Replacement

Cell therapy consists of using cells or cell-based products to replace dead or defective cells to restore the function of the affected tissue(s) [399]. Again, this approach has been proposed to treat MNGIE. While TP is not expressed in all tissues, cellular and plasmatic dThd and dUrd levels are in equilibrium among all body compartments. Therefore, replacing the lost enzyme in a circulating form—i.e., in the blood cells—should favor the catabolism of the toxic metabolites in plasma, thus clearing these freely diffusible substrates from the tissue compartments, normalizing the cellular nucleotide pools, and preventing further mtDNA damage.

Cell replacement therapies may offer a permanent cure to MNGIE. They comprise (I) Allogeneic Hematopoietic Stem Cell Transplantation (AHSCT) and (II) erythrocyte-encapsulated thymidine phosphorylase (EE-TP). Clinical and biochemical improvements following AHSCT have been reported in MNGIE patients [400,401]. Although AHSCT corrects biochemical abnormalities and improves gastrointestinal symptoms, the procedure is risky for subjects in poor medical conditions, as many MNGIE patients are. Since transplant-related morbidity and mortality increases with the progression of the disease and the number of comorbidities, MNGIE patients should be submitted to AHSCT when they are still relatively healthy, to minimize the complications of the procedure [401].

EE-TP consists of the ex-vivo encapsulation of *Escherichia coli* TP within the patient's autologous erythrocytes using a reversible hypo-osmotic dialysis process. Once inside the erythrocyte, the encapsulated enzyme catalyzes the deoxyribonucleosides' metabolism to the specific products thymine and uracil, which then exit the erythrocyte and flow into their physiological metabolic pathways. Recently, three adult MNGIE patients received escalating intravenous doses of EE-TP. EE-TP was well tolerated, and reductions in the disease-associated plasma metabolites, thymidine, and deoxy uridine were observed. Clinical ameliorations, including weight gain and improved disease scores, were observed in two patients, suggesting that EE-TP can reverse some aspects of the disease [401]. Advantages of the EE-TP are the prolonged circulatory half-life of the enzyme and the minimization of the immunogenic reactions compared to those frequently observed in enzyme replacement therapies administered by the conventional route [401].

5.4. Molecular Bypass Therapy in Disorders of mtDNA Instability

Syndromes characterized by mtDNA instability are usually due to mutations in nuclear genes involved either in the mtDNA replication machinery or deoxynucleotide triphosphate (dNTP) metabolism consequently affecting OXPHOS activities.

From the clinical perspective, these diseases are characterized by disorders that range from severe infantile hepatocerebral encephalopathy to childhood-onset myopathy or adult-onset PEO [402]. The TK2 gene provides an example. The protein product of this gene is a deoxyribonucleoside kinase with mitochondrial localization that specifically phosphorylates thymidine, deoxycytidine, and deoxyuridine. This enzyme is required for mtDNA synthesis. Recessive mutations in the human TK2 gene are responsible for the myopathic form of the mitochondrial depletion/multiple deletions syndrome [403]. Mitochondrial dNTPs pools are supplied either by *de novo* synthesis and import from the cytosol or by the mitochondrial deoxyribonucleoside salvage pathway [404]. Supplementation of the missing or insufficient dNTP may bypass the block restoring the deoxynucleotides triphosphate (dNTP) pools. Molecular bypass therapy (MBP) with deoxypyrimidine monophosphates (dCMP and dTMP) or substrate enhancement therapy with deoxypyrimidine nucleosides (dC and dT) were tested on the Tk2 knock-in (ki) mouse model in the early pre-symptomatic, but biochemically affected, stage [405]. Treatment with dCMP and dTMP raised dTTP concentrations, increase levels of mtDNA, ameliorated the defects of MRC enzymes, and significantly prolonged the lifespan (from 13 to 34 days) in a dose-dependent manner [406,407]. Late treatment of 29-day-old mice was ineffective.

Similar strategies were then extended in different models of PMD. The mtDNA depletion in human fibroblasts mutated in the DGUOK gene was ameliorated by the supplementation of deoxyguanosine [404], and similarly, pyrimidine and purine nucleoside administration, but not the corresponding monophosphate nucleotides, adjusted the mtDNA depletion induced by ethidium bromide in human RRM2B-mutant cells [408]. Similarly, deoxycytidine and tetrahydro uridine were also able to prevent mtDNA depletion in a cell model of the same syndrome [408]. Recently a mutant *dguok* zebrafish line was developed using CRISPR/Cas9 mediated mutagenesis; $dguok^{-/-}$ fishes have significantly reduced mtDNA levels compared to the wild-type counterpart. In contrast with previous cell culture studies, when supplemented with only one purine nucleoside (dGuo), mtDNA copy number in both mutant and wt juvenile animals was significantly reduced, possibly because of nucleotide pool imbalance. However, a significant increase in liver mtDNA was documented in adult $dguok^{-/-}$ zebrafish when supplemented with both purine nucleosides. [409].

Recently, an open-label study showed the results of deoxynucleoside monophosphates and deoxynucleoside administration under a compassionate program to 16 early-onset TK2-patients. Prolonged survival and improvement of motor abilities compared to untreated patients were recorded. Four of 5 patients who required enteric nutrition were able to discontinue using the feeding tube; and 1 of 9 patients who required mechanical ventilation became able to breathe independently. Out of 8, 3 non-ambulatory patients recovered the ability to walk. Out of 5, 4 patients with enteric nutrition discontinued the use of the feeding tube. Out of 9, 1 patient who required mechanical ventilation became able to breathe independently. Although diarrhea was the most common side effect manifested, discontinuation of the therapy was not necessary. Among 12 other TK2 patients treated with deoxynucleoside, two adults developed elevated liver enzymes normalized following discontinuation of therapy [410].

6. Future Perspectives

6.1. Fetal Gene Therapy

Current prenatal genetic technology can diagnose rare genetic diseases as early as the 12th week of pregnancy by chorionic villous sampling or from the 16th week by amniocentesis. Advances in fetal imaging and minimally invasive surgical equipment have also led to the development of interventional techniques for prenatal treatment of several fetal structural defects, such as congenital diaphragmatic hernia, myelomeningocele, pulmonary sequestration, hydrothorax, urinary tract obstruction, fetal tumours and others [411]. Also, intrauterine access to the fetal circulation through the umbilical vein is a well-described procedure, used to perform ultrasound-guided fetal blood or platelet transfusions, which are currently the standard of care in cases of fetal anemia and thrombocytopenia [412]. The option of fetal intervention is offered in specialized centers to reduce infant mortality and/or morbidity compared to postnatal treatment and, for each type of procedure, parents are extensively informed about the potential benefits balanced against the risks, which are mainly fetal death, miscarriage or preterm delivery.

For inherited genetic diseases, In-Utero Gene Therapy (IUGT) offers the potential of prophylaxis against early, irreversible, and lethal pathological change [413]. From a technical perspective, potential genetic therapeutic agents can be delivered to the fetus through infusion into the umbilical vein or via direct injection into the fetal organs. The rationale for IUGT is essentially based on the hypothesis that anticipating the treatment during fetal life could prevent or mitigate irreversible pathological changes associated with rare genetic disorders and improve clinical outcomes compared to postnatal therapy. Possible advantages of IUGT that may overcome some of the limitations encountered in postnatal gene therapy include: (i) the small fetal size (i.e., smaller area to be treated), (ii) the tolerogenic fetal immune system, (iii) the presence of highly proliferative and accessible stem/progenitor cells in multiple organs and, (iv) the ability to treat diseases in which irreversible pathological molecular and metabolic changes begin before birth [414].

Fetal therapeutic interventions could be especially useful for early-onset PMD in which mitochondrial dysfunction begins before birth, as the GRACILE syndrome. GRACILE syndrome initially develops with intrauterine growth retardation. A fatal lactic acidosis arises in the new-borns, often accompanied by nonspecific aminoaciduria, cholestasis, iron overload, and liver dysfunction [415].

Similarly, mitochondrial dysfunction likely starts before birth in SURF1-associated Leigh syndrome. Shreds of evidence suggest that *SURF1* mutations lead to metabolic impairments in neural progenitor cells (NPCs), which cannot switch from glycolytic to OXPHOS metabolism, with subsequent aberrant proliferation and insufficient support for neuronal morphogenesis [416]. A similar neuronal impairment was reported in a *SURF1* ko pig model [417]. Cerebral organoids from LS patients carrying *MT-ATP6* mutations also showed defective corticogenesis and suggest pre-natal impairment [418]. These findings suggest that OXPHOS defect could impair the NSC cellular metabolism in the early phase of the development leading to the onset of the neurological phenotypes; so prenatal intervention for pediatric PMD may be crucial for amelioration of the clinical course of the disease.

Fetal gene therapy may provide an alternative therapeutic approach for inherited diseases leading to early death or lifelong irreversible damage. Due to the lack of PMD-specific, fetal therapeutic approaches, curative strategies proposed for other genetic diseases should be considered. A recent study investigated the efficacy of human survival motor neuron (hSMN) gene expression after IU delivery in SMA mouse embryos. In the first part of the research report, authors showed that IU-intracerebroventricular injection of adeno-associated virus serotype-9 (AAV9)-EGFP led to an extensive expression of EGFP protein in different parts of the CNS with a significant number of transduced NSCs. SMA mouse fetuses receiving a single i.c.v. injection of a single-stranded or self-complementary AAV9-SMN vector extended their lifespan of 93 (median of 63) or 171 (median 105) days. Both muscle pathology and motor neuron survival improved upon treatments, with slightly better results from scAAV administration [413].

Additional evidence on the safety and efficacy of IUGT in a mouse model of neuronopathic Gaucher's disease were recently provided [419]. Fetal intracranial injection of an AAV9 carrying the curative gene improved neuronal inflammation and spectacularly increased the mice's overall survival. Of note, neonatal treatment did not achieve the same results of fetal therapy.

Maternal safety is a critical consideration in any fetal therapy. Possible maternal exposure to the viral vectors infused into the fetus should be considered in IUGT. Contact with the viral particles may result in maternal immune responses to the capsid protein or the recombinant protein, although the latter is unlikely, as the mother should already be producing—and therefore be tolerant to—the protein missing in the fetus.

Therapeutic viruses, including the AAV vectors, may undergo random integration in fetuses after IUGT; however, do evidences of germline integration have been reported. New technologies with more specific gene editing will possibly minimize off-target events of IUGT in future.

Despite promising preliminary results of IUGT, more experimental evidence on animal models is needed to demonstrate a significant improvement in the pathological hallmarks and the clinical course of the disease. Clinical trials involving human pregnancies would subsequently need to be setup, ensuring accurate monitoring of adverse events and long-term postnatal clinical follow-up. Randomized controlled trials on IUGT versus postnatal treatment may not be realistic due to the rarity of the investigated diseases and ethical concerns that may arise from offering randomization for conditions associated with a very severe if not lethal outcome. Also, rare genetic disorders currently lack any recommended screening policy in the general low-risk population. Therefore, most of the patients currently receiving a prenatal diagnosis of PMD have experienced a previously affected child's birth. In these cases, prenatal treatment parents could be offered within an experimental trial, after extensive counselling on the uncertainties regarding the clinical results and after discussion of other management options, which would be termination of pregnancy or postnatal therapy. It could be anticipated that the recruitment rate in such a context is likely to be extremely low. However, multicenter collaborative efforts may allow to collect and analyze a meaningful number of cases using a pre-defined shared protocol, to provide reliable information on the effects of IUGT on long-term postnatal development of infants affected by rare genetic disorders.

Ethical issues of fetal gene therapy have been reviewed by MacKenzie and collaborators [420]. Fetal treatment pivots on the concept of non-directive advising, in which the choices of no treatment and exploratory therapy—with all the conceivable risks and benefits—are rationalized without the physician's individual inclination. Rigorous preclinical trials and multidisciplinary debates will continue to advance the frontiers of fetal therapy, while these and other concerns deserve a continuous discussion [420].

6.2. Metabolic Rewiring

Pharmacological modulations of neuronal morphogenesis and neuronal maturation of the immature precursors, the neural stem cells (NSCs) have been proposed as an attractive therapeutic opportunity to treat several neurological diseases. NSCs require a metabolic shift towards oxidative phosphorylation during the process of neuronal differentiation [421]. Therefore, OXPHOS defects may inhibit this shift impairing neuronal differentiation and driving neural stem cells (NSCs) to a proliferative and less differentiated state [416]. We recently tested inductors of oxidative metabolism (developed and patented by Professional Dietetics, IT) composed of TCA cycle intermediates, specific amino acids, and co-factors that helped enhance mitochondrial function in different in vitro and in vivo models. Supplementing wild-type NSC-culture medium with these compounds during the differentiation phase enhanced the metabolic shift towards OXPHOS and mitochondrial function of mouse and human NSCs, improving their full differentiation capacity [422]. Neurons derived from treated-NSC changed the fission–fusion processing resulting in a mitochondrial elongated phenotype; moreover, the activation of the mTORC1 pathway with subsequent significant increase of ATP production was reported. Also, the antioxidant defense system was also triggered by the increase of the

NRF2 gene expression [422]. We observed similar metabolic and molecular changes in vivo, where they counteracted the pathological mitochondrial dysfunction occurring during the aging process. Three-month oral administration of metabolic inductor PD-0E7 (Professional Dietetics, IT) to the Senescence Accelerated Mouse-Prone 8 (SAMP8) mice significantly improved the sarcopenia and cognitive decline, enhancing oxidative metabolism by inducing mitochondrial biogenesis and increasing respiratory efficiency [423]. In particular, we documented a strong shift toward oxidative, COX-positive fibers and a general increase of the MRC enzymatic activities in the skeletal muscle of the 12-month-old PD-0E7-supplemented mice, which may explain the preserved physical endurance of the treated SAMP8 mice [423]. Also, the Opa1 isoforms were significantly increased in the skeletal muscle, as shown by western blot analysis, and this might support the improved stabilization of the CIII holocomplex into SCs that was detected by blue native gel electrophoresis (BNGE) analysis [423]. To note, the preserved cognitive function observed in the treated mice correlate with enhancement of the hippocampal mitochondrial proteostasis and with the upregulation of PITRM1, a mitochondrial matrix enzyme that digests the mitochondrial targeting sequences (MTS) and the mitochondrial fraction of amyloid beta [424,425].

Although the molecular mechanisms at the basis of the improvement of mitochondrial functions by such metabolic modulators were not fully elucidated, it is plausible that supplementation of TCA cycle intermediates and amino acids would feed the anaplerotic flux sustaining mitochondrial energy production. In support of this, it has recently been demonstrated that anaplerosis is protective in OXPHOS-deficient neurons with disruption of the *MFN2* gene, and that genetic blockage of the anaplerotic pathway further exacerbated the neuronal degeneration [426]. To date, triheptanoin is the only reported example of anaplerotic treatment in patients with very-long-chain acyl-CoA dehydrogenase (VLCAD) deficiency [61]. Studies of the effects of anaplerotic substrates in PMD should be encouraged.

7. Conclusions

The extreme clinical, genetic, and biochemical variability of PMD coupled with the low number of patients and the frequent lack of adequate preclinical models have limited identifying useful clinical outcomes and the development of effective therapy.

The enhancement of mitochondrial function and ATP production through the pharmacological stimulation of mitochondrial biogenesis, mitophagy, dynamics, and ROS detoxification using antioxidants may represent a general strategy to alleviate or at least partially corrected different clinical outcomes. Although these strategies do not solve the problem at the root, these are, in principle, adaptable to a large group of mitochondrial diseases and could help improve patients' everyday quality of life.

Conclusive cure for mitochondrial disease could be achieved by a precision medicine strategy that considers individual variability in genes, age, sex, stage of the disease, and tissues compromised for each patient (Figure 4). Although organ transplantation was already used successfully, cell replacement and gene therapy are still far to become routine for mitochondrial disease due to technical and regulatory reasons. However, given the recent exciting progress in gene editing and fetal surgery, we expect steps forward in the coming decades.

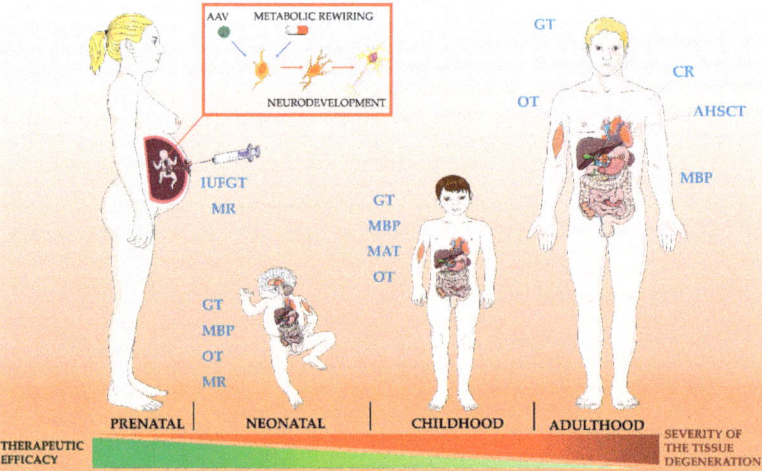

Figure 4. Severity of the tissue degeneration increases with age, impacting the efficacy of therapeutic interventions. IUFGT: In utero fetal gene therapy; MR: metabolic rewiring; MBP: Molecular Bypass Therapy; MAT: Mitochondrial Augmentation Therapy; GT: Gene Therapy; OT: Organ Transplantation; CR: Cell Replacement; AHSCT: Allogeneic Hematopoietic Stem Cell Transplantation.

Author Contributions: Conceptualization, E.B. and D.B.; methodology, D.B., E.B., C.L., N.P., A.P., and V.T. writing—original draft preparation, D.B., E.B., C.L., N.P., A.P., and V.T.; writing—review and editing, D.B. and E.B.; visualization, C.L., N.P., A.P., and V.T.; supervision D.B. and E.B.; funding acquisition, D.B. and C.L. All authors have read and agreed to the published version of the manuscript.

Funding: This study was supported by the Italian Ministry of Health (grants RF-2016-02361495, and "Ricerca Corrente").

Acknowledgments: D.B. acknowledge University of Milan, Grant number: BIOMETRA PSR2019-BRUNETTI; C.L. is members of the European Reference Network for Rare Neuromuscular Diseases (ERN EURO-NMD). This project was carried out in the Center for the Study of Mitochondrial Pediatric Diseases (http://www.mitopedia.org) funded by the Mariani Foundation.

Conflicts of Interest: The authors declare no conflict of interest.

Appendix A

Table A1. Summary of the therapeutic approaches discussed in this manuscript, with a distinction between those that have been tested in pre-clinical models and those that have already been used in clinical practice. This table is restricted to therapies used to treat PMD and does not include others that, although cited in the text, have not been tested in PMD models/patients.

Therapy	Model	Study	Ref.
	Strategies to increase ATP levels		
Febuxostat plus inosine	patients with homoplasmic mtDNA mutation	clinical	[65]
	patient with mitochondrial diabetes with heteroplasmic mutation in tRNA leucine 1	clinical	[65]
	Pharmacological stimulation of mitochondrial biogenesis		
AICAR	mouse models of COX defects	pre-clinical	[74]
	mouse model Cox10-Mef2c-Cre	pre-clinical	[82]
	CI deficient cells (NDUFS2, NDUFS4, NDUFAF4, C20ORF7, FOXRED1, NDUFA12L)	pre-clinical	[83]

Table A1. Cont.

Therapy	Model	Study	Ref.
Bezafibrate and other PPAR agonists	MRC-deficient patients' fibroblasts	pre-clinical	[87]
	SCO2 mutant fibroblasts	pre-clinical	[88]
	DNM1L mutant cells	pre-clinical	[89]
	mouse models of COX defects	pre-clinical	[74]
	Deletor mouse	pre-clinical	[90]
	Mutator mouse	pre-clinical	[91]
	patients with MM	clinical	[92]
NAD$^+$ precursors	*Sco2* ko mouse	pre-clinical	[81]
	Deletor mouse	pre-clinical	[106]
	GBA-PD *Drosophila melanogaster*	pre-clinical	[107]
	Ndufs4 ko mice	pre-clinical	[108]
Niacin	patients with MM	clinical (NCT03973203)	[109]
I-BET 525762A	cybrids carrying 3796A>G mutation	pre-clinical	[110]
Polyphenols and other Pharmacognostic Products			
Resveratrol	fibroblasts from MT-TL1, MT-TK, MT-ATP6-patients	pre-clinical	[125]
Curcumin	LHON patients	clinical (NCT00528151)	unpublished
Pharmacological modulation of the NO/cGMP/PKG pathway			
L-arginine and L-citrulline	MELAS patients	clinical (open-label trial)	[162,164,168]
	MELAS patients	clinical (open-label trial)	[165]
	various PMD patients	clinical (NCT02809170)	unpublished
	MELAS patients	Phase-1 clinical trial NCT03952234	unpublished
PDE5 inhibitors	NPCs with homoplasmic mutation in MT-ATP6	pre-clinical	[176]
	LHON	clinical (case report)	[179]
Antioxidant			
Glutathione	MM patients	clinical (double-blind cross-over study)	[188]
	fibroblasts of patients carrying the m.3243A>G and m.8344A>G mutations	pre-clinical	[189]
Cysteamine	*C. elegans* model of CI defect, FBXL4 mutant human fibroblast, and zebrafish models of pharmacologically induced CI and CIV defects	pre-clinical	[192]
Cysteamine bitartrate delayed-release (RP103)	PMD paediatric patients	clinical (NCT02023866)	unpublished
N-acetylcysteine	*Ethe1* mouse model	pre-clinical	[195]
	ETHE1 patients	clinical (compassionate use)	[198–200]
Lipoic acid and CoQ10	PMD patients	clinical (randomized, double-blind, placebo-controlled, crossover study)	[206]
Vitamin C and K	PMD patients	Clinical	[208–210]
Vitamin E	fibroblasts from patients with CI defect	pre-clinical	[211,212]

Table A1. *Cont.*

Therapy	Model	Study	Ref.
Coenzyme Q$_{10}$	MERRF cells	pre-clinical	[220]
	KSS patients	clinical	[221]
	KSS patents and other MM with CPEO	clinical	[222–224,226, 228,230]
	patient with mitochondrial encephalomyopathy with COX deficiency	clinical	[225]
	patients with mitochondrial cytopathies	clinical	[227]
	PMD patients	clinical	[229]
	patients with different OXPHOS defects	clinical	[231]
	PMD patients	randomized, double-blind, cross-over trial	[232]
	patients with different PMD; 15 patients with MM	clinical (multicenter study)	[233]
	PMD paediatric patients	clinical (NCT00432744)	[234]
Idebenone	fibroblasts from LHON patients	pre-clinical	[237,238]
	mouse model of LHON	pre-clinical	[239]
	85 LHON patients with to m.3460G>A, m.11778G>A, and m.14484T>C mutations	clinical ("RHODOS" study, NCT00747487)	[241]
	subset of LHON patients from RHODOS study	clinical (RHODOS-OFU, NCT01421381)	[242]
	patient with TXN2 mutation		[243]
	Opa1 mutant mice	pre-clinical	[245]
	seven DOA patients	clinial	[246]
	87 DOA patients	clinical (retrospective cohort study)	[247]
Redox-Active Molecules			
EPI-743	PMD patients	clinical	[259]
	patients with Leigh syndrome	clinical (prospective single-arm subject-controlled trial)	[260]
	children with mitochondrial encephalopathy	Clinical	[261]
	one patient with Leigh syndrome due to ND3 mutation	Clinical	[262]
	patients with LHON	clinical (open-label trial)	[263]
	patients with Leigh syndrome	clinical (NCT02352896)	unpublished
	PMD paediatric patients	clinical (NCT01642056)	unpublished
JP4-039	ACAD9- VLCAD-, ETHE1 and MOCS1 mutant fibroblasts	pre-clinical	[266,267]
KH176	cellular models of CI defects	pre-clinical	[268]
	Ndufs4 ko mouse model	pre-clinical	[269,270]
	patients with m.3242A>G mutation	clinical (KHENERGY STUDY, NCT02909400)	[272]
	patients with MELAS	clinical (KHENERGYZE Study, NCT04165239)	[273]
SKQ1	*Mutator* mouse	pre-clinical	[281]
Pharmacological modulation of mitochondrial dynamics			
Cytotoxic Necrotizing Factor 1 (CNF1)	MERRF fibroblasts	pre-clinical	[300]

Table A1. Cont.

Therapy	Model	Study	Ref.
Pharmacological protection of cardiolipin			
Elamipretide	patients with primary mitochondrial myopathy (MM)	clinical (NCT03323749)	[310]
	Barth syndrome	clinical (NCT03098797)	unpublished
	LHON patients	clinical (NCT02693119)	unpublished
	age-related macular degeneration (AMD) with non-central geographic atrophy	clinical (NCT03891875)	unpublished
Pharmacological modulation of autophagy			
Rapamycin	*Ndufs4* ko mouse	pre-clinical	[313]
	muscle-specific *Cox15* ko mouse	pre-clinical	[314]
	ND2-deficient Drosophila model of LS	pre-clinical	[315]
	MT-ATP6-mutant, iPSCs-derived neurons	pre-clinical	[316]
	gas-1 (fc21) nematodes	pre-clinical	[317]
	mice with CoQ_{10} deficiency	pre-clinical	[320]
	TwKO^{astro} mice	pre-clinical	[59]
Everolimus (rapamycin analogue)	MELAS patients	clinical (NCT03747328)	[318]
	children affected by Leigh disease or MELAS	Clinical	[319]
Bypassing cI-cIII-cIV defects with alternative enzymes			
NDI1	CI deficiency in *Drosophila melanogaster*	pre-clinical	[324]
	mouse model of LHON	pre-clinical	[238]
	mouse model of Leigh syndrome	pre-clinical	[239]
AOX, NDI1	ρ^0 mouse cells	pre-clinical	[325]
AOX	CIII-IV deficiencies in human cells	pre-clinical	[326]
	CIV deficient *Drosophila melanogaster*	pre-clinical	[327]
	Bcs1l$^{p.S78G}$ knock-in mice	pre-clinical	[330,331]
	Acta-Cox15 ko model	pre-clinical	[332]
NDH-2	human CI deficient fibroblasts	pre-clinical	[333]
Personalized therapies for mtDNA disorders			
Mitochondrial donation: maternal spindle transfer	legally approved for use in the U.K	clinical	[343]
	rhesus macaques	pre-clinical	[344]
	woman carrying mtDNA mutation of Leigh syndrome (8993 T>G)	clinical	[347,348]
Mitochondrial donation: pronuclear transfer	*mito*-mouse	pre-clinical	[349]
Delivery of nucleic acids to the mitochondria	patient's cell with a G625A heteroplasmic mutation in the tRNA^{Phe}	pre-clinical	[355]
	ND3 mutant fibroblasts	pre-clinical	[356]
	MERFF and KSS cybrids	pre-clinical	[354]
Heteroplasmic shift	various cells with heteroplasmic mutation	pre-clinical	[359–361]
	mouse model of heteroplasmic PMD	pre-clinical	[366,367]
Allotopic gene expression	cybrids with m.8993T>G mutation	pre-clinical	[369]
	rat model of LHON	pre-clinical	[370]
	LHON patients	clinical (NTC01267422; NCT02064569)	[371,372]
Mitochondrial augmentation therapy	children with Pearson syndrome	clinical	Unpublished
	children with KSS or Pearson Syndrome	clinical (NCT03384420)	unpublished
	KSS patient	clinical	[375]

Table A1. Cont.

Therapy	Model	Study	Ref.
Precision medicine approaches for PMD caused by nuclear defects			
Gene therapy approaches	*Ant1* ko mouse model	pre-clinical	[381]
	Tymp ko mouse model	pre-clinical	[390]
	Ethe1 ko mouse model	pre-clinical	[389]
	Ndufs4 mouse model	pre-clinical	[391]
	Mpv17 ko mouse model	pre-clinical	[58]
	mouse model of Leigh syndrome	pre-clinical	[382]
Liver transplantation	PMD patients	clinical	[385]
	DGUOK-deficient patients	clinical	[386]
	25-year-old MNGIE patient	clinical	[395]
	ETHE1 patients	clinical	[396,397]
Cell replacement	MNGIE patients	clinical	[400,401]
Molecular bypass therapy in disorders of mtDNA instability	*Tk2* mouse model	pre-clinical	[405–407]
	DGUOK mutant fibroblasts	pre-clinical	[404]
	RRM2B mutant fibroblasts	pre-clinical	[408]
	dguok$^{-/-}$ zebrafish	pre-clinical	[409]
	early-onset TK2-patients	clinical (open-label study)	[410]

References

1. Gorman, G.S.; Chinnery, P.F.; DiMauro, S.; Hirano, M.; Koga, Y.; McFarland, R.; Suomalainen, A.; Thorburn, D.R.; Zeviani, M.; Turnbull, D.M. Mitochondrial diseases. *Nat. Rev. Dis. Primers* **2016**, *2*, 16080. [CrossRef]
2. Wallace, D.C. A Mitochondrial Paradigm of Metabolic and Degenerative Diseases, Aging, and Cancer: A Dawn for Evolutionary Medicine. *Annu. Rev. Genet.* **2005**, *39*, 359–407. [CrossRef] [PubMed]
3. Stewart, J.B.; Chinnery, P.F. Extreme heterogeneity of human mitochondrial DNA from organelles to populations. *Nat. Rev. Genet.* **2020**, 1–13. [CrossRef] [PubMed]
4. Rahman, S.; Blok, R.B.; Dahl, H.-H.M.; Danks, D.M.; Kirby, D.M.; Chow, C.W.; Christodoulou, J.; Thorburn, D.R. Leigh syndrome: Clinical features and biochemical and DNA abnormalities. *Ann. Neurol.* **1996**, *39*, 343–351. [CrossRef] [PubMed]
5. Shoffner, J.M.; Lott, M.T.; Lezza, A.M.; Seibel, P.; Ballinger, S.W.; Wallace, D.C. Myoclonic epilepsy and ragged-red fiber disease (MERRF) is associated with a mitochondrial DNA tRNALys mutation. *Cell* **1990**, *61*, 931–937. [CrossRef]
6. Goto, Y.-I.; Nonaka, I.; Horai, S. A mutation in the tRNALeu(UUR) gene associated with the MELAS subgroup of mitochondrial encephalomyopathies. *Nat. Cell Biol.* **1990**, *348*, 651–653. [CrossRef]
7. Holt, I.J.; Harding, A.E.; Petty, R.K.; Morgan-Hughes, J.A. A new mitochondrial disease associated with mitochondrial DNA heteroplasmy. *Am. J. Hum. Genet.* **1990**, *46*, 428–433.
8. Wallace, D.C.; Singh, G.; Lott, M.T.; Hodge, J.A.; Schurr, T.G.; Lezza, A.M.; Elsas, L.J.; Nikoskelainen, E.K. Mitochondrial DNA mutation associated with Leber's hereditary optic neuropathy. *Science* **1988**, *242*, 1427–1430. [CrossRef]
9. Lopez-Gallardo, E.; Solano, A.; Herrero-Martin, M.D.; Martinez-Romero, I.; Castano-Perez, M.D.; Andreu, A.L.; Herrera, A.; Lopez-Perez, M.J.; Ruiz-Pesini, E.; Montoya, J. NARP syndrome in a patient harbouring an insertion in the MT-ATP6 gene that results in a truncated protein. *J. Med. Genet.* **2008**, *46*, 64–67. [CrossRef]
10. Pitceathly, R.D.; Murphy, S.M.; Cottenie, E.; Chalasani, A.; Sweeney, M.G.; Woodward, C.; Mudanohwo, E.E.; Hargreaves, I.; Heales, S.; Land, J.; et al. Genetic dysfunction of MT-ATP6 causes axonal Charcot-Marie-Tooth disease. *Neurology* **2012**, *79*, 1145–1154. [CrossRef]

11. Verny, C.; Guegen, N.; Desquiret-Dumas, V.; Chevrollier, A.; Prundean, A.; Dubas, F.; Cassereau, J.; Ferre, M.; Amati-Bonneau, P.; Bonneau, D.; et al. Hereditary spastic paraplegia-like disorder due to a mitochondrial ATP6 gene point mutation. *Mitochondrion* **2011**, *11*, 70–75. [CrossRef] [PubMed]
12. Bugiardini, E.; Bottani, E.; Marchet, S.; Poole, O.V.; Benincá, C.; Horga, A.; Woodward, C.; Lam, A.; Hargreaves, I.; Chalasani, A.; et al. Expanding the molecular and phenotypic spectrum of truncating MT-ATP6 mutations. *Neurol. Genet.* **2020**, *6*, e381. [CrossRef] [PubMed]
13. Moraes, C.T.; DiMauro, S.; Zeviani, M.; Lombes, A.; Shanske, S.; Miranda, A.F.; Nakase, H.; Bonilla, E.; Werneck, L.C.; Servidei, S.; et al. Mitochondrial DNA Deletions in Progressive External Ophthalmoplegia and Kearns-Sayre Syndrome. *N. Engl. J. Med.* **1989**, *320*, 1293–1299. [CrossRef] [PubMed]
14. Pearson, H.A.; Lobel, J.S.; Kocoshis, S.A.; Naiman, J.L.; Windmiller, J.; Lammi, A.T.; Hoffman, R.; Marsh, J.C. A new syndrome of refractory sideroblastic anemia with vacuolization of marrow precursors and exocrine pancreatic dysfunction. *J. Pediatr.* **1979**, *95*, 976–984. [CrossRef]
15. Baerlocher, K.E.; Feldges, A.; Weissert, M.; Simonsz, H.J.; Rötig, A. Mitochondrial DNA deletion in an 8-year-old boy with pearson syndrome. *J. Inherit. Metab. Dis.* **1992**, *15*, 327–330. [CrossRef] [PubMed]
16. Calvo, S.; Jain, M.; Xie, X.; Sheth, S.A.; Chang, B.; Goldberger, O.A.; Spinazzola, A.; Zeviani, M.; Carr, S.A.; Mootha, V.K. Systematic identification of human mitochondrial disease genes through integrative genomics. *Nat. Genet.* **2006**, *38*, 576–582. [CrossRef]
17. Vafai, S.B.; Mootha, V.K. Mitochondrial disorders as windows into an ancient organelle. *Nat. Cell Biol.* **2012**, *491*, 374–383. [CrossRef]
18. Stenton, S.L.; Prokisch, H. Genetics of mitochondrial diseases: Identifying mutations to help diagnosis. *EBioMedicine* **2020**, *56*, 102784. [CrossRef]
19. Zorova, L.D.; Popkov, V.A.; Plotnikov, E.Y.; Silachev, D.N.; Pevzner, I.B.; Jankauskas, S.S.; Babenko, V.A.; Zorov, S.D.; Balakireva, A.V.; Juhaszova, M.; et al. Mitochondrial membrane potential. *Anal. Biochem.* **2018**, *552*, 50–59. [CrossRef]
20. La Morgia, C.; Maresca, A.; Caporali, L.; Valentino, M.; Carelli, V. Mitochondrial diseases in adults. *J. Intern. Med.* **2020**, *287*, 592–608. [CrossRef]
21. Ghezzi, D.; Zeviani, M. Human diseases associated with defects in assembly of OXPHOS complexes. *Essays Biochem.* **2018**, *62*, 271–286. [CrossRef] [PubMed]
22. Taylor, R.W.; Turnbull, D.M. Mitochondrial DNA mutations in human disease. *Nat. Rev. Genet.* **2005**, *6*, 389–402. [CrossRef] [PubMed]
23. Freyssenet, D.; Berthon, P.; Denis, C. Mitochondrial Biogenesis in Skeletal Muscle in Response to Endurance Exercises. *Arch. Physiol. Biochem.* **1996**, *104*, 129–141. [CrossRef] [PubMed]
24. Steiner, J.L.; Murphy, E.A.; McClellan, J.L.; Carmichael, M.D.; Davis, J.M. Exercise training increases mitochondrial biogenesis in the brain. *J. Appl. Physiol.* **2011**, *111*, 1066–1071. [CrossRef]
25. Fernandez-Marcos, P.J.; Auwerx, J. Regulation of PGC-1α, a nodal regulator of mitochondrial biogenesis. *Am. J. Clin. Nutr.* **2011**, *93*, 884S–890S. [CrossRef] [PubMed]
26. Egan, B.; Zierath, J.R. Exercise Metabolism and the Molecular Regulation of Skeletal Muscle Adaptation. *Cell Metab.* **2013**, *17*, 162–184. [CrossRef]
27. Vettor, R.; Valerio, A.; Ragni, M.; Trevellin, E.; Granzotto, M.; Olivieri, M.; Tedesco, L.; Ruocco, C.; Fossati, A.; Fabris, R.; et al. Exercise training boosts eNOS-dependent mitochondrial biogenesis in mouse heart: Role in adaptation of glucose metabolism. *Am. J. Physiol. Metab.* **2014**, *306*, E519–E528. [CrossRef]
28. Miller, M.W.; Knaub, L.A.; Olivera-Fragoso, L.F.; Keller, A.C.; Balasubramaniam, V.; Watson, P.A.; Reusch, J.E. Nitric oxide regulates vascular adaptive mitochondrial dynamics. *Am. J. Physiol. Circ. Physiol.* **2013**, *304*, H1624–H1633. [CrossRef]
29. Weber, K.; Wilson, J.N.; Taylor, L.; Brierley, E.; Johnson, M.A.; Turnbull, D.M.; Bindoff, L.A. A new mtDNA mutation showing accumulation with time and restriction to skeletal muscle. *Am. J. Hum. Genet.* **1997**, *60*, 373–380.
30. Fu, K.; Hartlen, R.; Johns, T.; Genge, A.; Karpati, G.; Shoubridge, E.A. A novel heteroplasmic tRNAleu(CUN) mtDNA point mutation in a sporadic patient with mitochondrial encephalomyopathy segregates rapidly in skeletal muscle and suggests an approach to therapy. *Hum. Mol. Genet.* **1996**, *5*, 1835–1840. [CrossRef]
31. Clark, K.M.; Bindoff, L.A.; Chrzanowska-Lightowlers, Z.; Andrews, R.M.; Griffiths, P.G.; Johnson, M.A.; Brierley, E.J.; Turnbull, D.M. Reversal of a mitochondrial DNA defect in human skeletal muscle. *Nat. Genet.* **1997**, *16*, 222–224. [CrossRef] [PubMed]

32. Shoubridge, E.A.; Johns, T.; Karpati, G. Complete restoration of a wild-type mtDNA genotype in regenerating muscle fibres in a patient with a tRNA point mutation and mitochondrial encephalomyopathy. *Hum. Mol. Genet.* **1997**, *6*, 2239–2242. [CrossRef] [PubMed]
33. Safdar, A.; Bourgeois, J.M.; Ogborn, D.I.; Little, J.P.; Hettinga, B.P.; Akhtar, M.; Thompson, J.E.; Melov, S.; Mocellin, N.J.; Kujoth, G.C.; et al. Endurance exercise rescues progeroid aging and induces systemic mitochondrial rejuvenation in mtDNA mutator mice. *Proc. Natl. Acad. Sci. USA* **2011**, *108*, 4135–4140. [CrossRef] [PubMed]
34. Fiuza-Luces, C.; Valenzuela, P.L.; Laine-Menéndez, S.; La Torre, M.F.-D.; Bermejo-Gómez, V.; Rufián-Vázquez, L.; Arenas, J.; Martín, M.A.; Lucia, A.; Moran, M. Physical Exercise and Mitochondrial Disease: Insights from a Mouse Model. *Front. Neurol.* **2019**, *10*. [CrossRef] [PubMed]
35. Greggio, C.; Jha, P.; Kulkarni, S.S.; Lagarrigue, S.; Broskey, N.T.; Boutant, M.; Wang, X.; Alonso, S.C.; Ofori, E.; Auwerx, J.; et al. Enhanced Respiratory Chain Supercomplex Formation in Response to Exercise in Human Skeletal Muscle. *Cell Metab.* **2017**, *25*, 301–311. [CrossRef] [PubMed]
36. Voet, N.; Van Der Kooi, E.L.; Van Engelen, B.G.M.; Geurts, A.C.H. Strength training and aerobic exercise training for muscle disease. *Cochrane Database Syst. Rev.* **2013**, *2013*, CD003907. [CrossRef]
37. Tarnopolsky, M. Exercise as a Therapeutic Strategy for Primary Mitochondrial Cytopathies. *J. Child Neurol.* **2014**, *29*, 1225–1234. [CrossRef]
38. Cejudo, P.; Bautista, J.; Montemayor, T.; Villagómez, R.; Jiménez, L.; Ortega, F.; Campos, Y.; Sánchez, H.; Arenas, J. Exercise training in mitochondrial myopathy: A randomized controlled trial. *Muscle Nerve* **2005**, *32*, 342–350. [CrossRef]
39. Jeppesen, T.D.; Schwartz, M.; Olsen, D.B.; Wibrand, F.; Krag, T.; Duno, M.; Hauerslev, S.; Vissing, J. Aerobic training is safe and improves exercise capacity in patients with mitochondrial myopathy. *Brain* **2006**, *129*, 3402–3412. [CrossRef]
40. Taivassalo, T.; Gardner, J.L.; Taylor, R.W.; Schaefer, A.M.; Newman, J.; Barron, M.J.; Haller, R.G.; Turnbull, D.M. Endurance training and detraining in mitochondrial myopathies due to single large-scale mtDNA deletions. *Brain* **2006**, *129*, 3391–3401. [CrossRef]
41. Taivassalo, T.; Fu, K.; Johns, T.; Arnold, D.; Karpati, G.; Shoubridge, E.A. Gene shifting: A novel therapy for mitochondrial myopathy. *Hum. Mol. Genet.* **1999**, *8*, 1047–1052. [CrossRef] [PubMed]
42. Murphy, J.L.; Blakely, E.L.; Schaefer, A.M.; He, L.; Wyrick, P.; Haller, R.G.; Taylor, R.W.; Turnbull, U.M.; Taivassalo, T. Resistance training in patients with single, large-scale deletions of mitochondrial DNA. *Brain* **2008**, *131*, 2832–2840. [CrossRef] [PubMed]
43. Taivassalo, T.; Shoubridge, E.A.; Chen, J.; Kennaway, N.G.; DiMauro, S.; Arnold, U.L.; Ørngreen, M.C. Aerobic conditioning in patients with mitochondrial myopathies: Physiological, biochemical, and genetic effects. *Ann. Neurol.* **2001**, *50*, 133–141. [CrossRef] [PubMed]
44. Adhihetty, P.J.; Taivassalo, T.; Haller, R.G.; Walkinshaw, D.R.; Hood, D.A. The effect of training on the expression of mitochondrial biogenesis- and apoptosis-related proteins in skeletal muscle of patients with mtDNA defects. *Am. J. Physiol. Metab.* **2007**, *293*, E672–E680. [CrossRef]
45. Kossoff, E.; Wang, H.-S.; Eh, K.; Wang, H.-S. Dietary Therapies for Epilepsy. *Biomed. J.* **2013**, *36*, 2. [CrossRef]
46. Kang, H.-C.; Lee, Y.M.; Kim, H.D.; Lee, J.S.; Slama, A. Safe and Effective Use of the Ketogenic Diet in Children with Epilepsy and Mitochondrial Respiratory Chain Complex Defects. *Epilepsia* **2007**, *48*, 82–88. [CrossRef]
47. Lee, Y.M.; Kang, H.-C.; Lee, J.S.; Kim, S.H.; Kim, E.Y.; Lee, S.-K.; Slama, A.; Kim, H.D. Mitochondrial respiratory chain defects: Underlying etiology in various epileptic conditions. *Epilepsia* **2008**, *49*, 685–690. [CrossRef]
48. Wexler, I.D.; Hemalatha, S.G.; McConnell, J.; Buist, N.; Dahl, H.-H.M.; Berry, S.A.; Cederbaum, S.D.; Patel, M.S.; Kerr, D.S. Outcome of pyruvate dehydrogenase deficiency treated with ketogenic diets: Studies in patients with identical mutations. *Neurology* **1997**, *49*, 1655–1661. [CrossRef]
49. Rahman, S. Mitochondrial disease and epilepsy. *Dev. Med. Child Neurol.* **2012**, *54*, 397–406. [CrossRef]
50. Steriade, C.; Andrade, D.M.; Faghfoury, H.; Tarnopolsky, M.A.; Tai, P. Mitochondrial Encephalopathy with Lactic Acidosis and Stroke-like Episodes (MELAS) May Respond to Adjunctive Ketogenic Diet. *Pediatr. Neurol.* **2014**, *50*, 498–502. [CrossRef]
51. Nunnari, J.; Suomalainen, A. Mitochondria: In Sickness and in Health. *Cell* **2012**, *148*, 1145–1159. [CrossRef] [PubMed]

52. Frey, S.; Geffroy, G.; Desquiret-Dumas, V.; Gueguen, N.; Bris, C.; Belal, S.; Amati-Bonneau, P.; Chevrollier, A.; Barth, M.; Henrion, D.; et al. The addition of ketone bodies alleviates mitochondrial dysfunction by restoring complex I assembly in a MELAS cellular model. *Biochim. Biophys. Acta (BBA) Mol. Basis Dis.* **2017**, *1863*, 284–291. [CrossRef] [PubMed]
53. Santra, S.; Gilkerson, R.W.; Davidson, M.; Schon, E.A. Ketogenic treatment reduces deleted mitochondrial DNAs in cultured human cells. *Ann. Neurol.* **2004**, *56*, 662–669. [CrossRef] [PubMed]
54. Schiff, M.; Bénit, P.; El-Khoury, R.; Schlemmer, D.; Benoist, J.-F.; Rustin, P. Mouse Studies to Shape Clinical Trials for Mitochondrial Diseases: High Fat Diet in Harlequin Mice. *PLoS ONE* **2011**, *6*, e28823. [CrossRef] [PubMed]
55. Ahola-Erkkilä, S.; Carroll, C.J.; Peltola-Mjösund, K.; Tulkki, V.; Mattila, I.; Seppänen-Laakso, T.; Orešič, M.; Tyynismaa, H.; Suomalainen, A. Ketogenic diet slows down mitochondrial myopathy progression in mice. *Hum. Mol. Genet.* **2010**, *19*, 1974–1984. [CrossRef] [PubMed]
56. Purhonen, J.; Rajendran, J.; Mörgelin, M.; Uusi-Rauva, K.; Katayama, S.; Krjutskov, K.; Einarsdottir, E.; Velagapudi, V.; Kere, J.; Jauhiainen, M.; et al. Ketogenic diet attenuates hepatopathy in mouse model of respiratory chain complex III deficiency caused by a Bcs1l mutation. *Sci. Rep.* **2017**, *7*, 1–16. [CrossRef]
57. Bottani, E.; Giordano, C.; Civiletto, G.; Di Meo, I.; Auricchio, A.; Ciusani, E.; Marchet, S.; Lamperti, C.; D'Amati, G.; Viscomi, C.; et al. AAV-mediated Liver-specific MPV17 Expression Restores mtDNA Levels and Prevents Diet-induced Liver Failure. *Mol. Ther.* **2014**, *22*, 10–17. [CrossRef]
58. Brunetti, D.; Dusi, S.; Giordano, C.; Lamperti, C.; Morbin, M.; Fugnanesi, V.; Marchet, S.; Fagiolari, G.; Sibon, O.; Moggio, M.; et al. Pantethine treatment is effective in recovering the disease phenotype induced by ketogenic diet in a pantothenate kinase-associated neurodegeneration mouse model. *Brain* **2014**, *137*, 57–68. [CrossRef]
59. Ignatenko, O.; Nikkanen, J.; Kononov, A.; Zamboni, N.; Ince-Dunn, G.; Suomalainen, A. Mitochondrial spongiotic brain disease: Astrocytic stress and harmful rapamycin and ketosis effect. *Life Sci. Alliance* **2020**, *3*, e202000797. [CrossRef]
60. Ahola, S.; Auranen, M.; Isohanni, P.; Niemisalo, S.; Urho, N.; Buzkova, J.; Velagapudi, V.; Lundbom, N.; Hakkarainen, A.; Muurinen, T.; et al. Modified Atkins diet induces subacute selective ragged-red-fiber lysis in mitochondrial myopathy patients. *EMBO Mol. Med.* **2016**, *8*, 1234–1247. [CrossRef]
61. Roe, C.R.; Sweetman, L.; Roe, D.S.; David, F.; Brunengraber, H. Treatment of cardiomyopathy and rhabdomyolysis in long-chain fat oxidation disorders using an anaplerotic odd-chain triglyceride. *J. Clin. Investig.* **2002**, *110*, 259–269. [CrossRef] [PubMed]
62. Jain, I.H.; Zazzeron, L.; Goli, R.; Alexa, K.; Schatzman-Bone, S.; Dhillon, H.; Goldberger, O.; Peng, J.; Shalem, O.; Sanjana, N.E.; et al. Hypoxia as a therapy for mitochondrial disease. *Science* **2016**, *352*, 54–61. [CrossRef] [PubMed]
63. Ferrari, M.; Jain, I.H.; Goldberger, O.; Rezoagli, E.; Thoonen, R.; Cheng, K.-H.; Sosnovik, D.E.; Scherrer-Crosbie, M.; Mootha, V.K.; Zapol, W.M. Hypoxia treatment reverses neurodegenerative disease in a mouse model of Leigh syndrome. *Proc. Natl. Acad. Sci. USA* **2017**, *114*, E4241–E4250. [CrossRef] [PubMed]
64. Kamatani, N.; Hashimoto, M.; Sakurai, K.; Gokita, K.; Yoshihara, J.; Sekine, M.; Mochii, M.-A.; Fukuuchi, T.; Yamaoka, N.; Kaneko, K. Clinical studies on changes in purine compounds in blood and urine by the simultaneous administration of febuxostat and inosine, or by single administration of each. *Gout Nucleic Acid Metab.* **2017**, *41*, 171–181. [CrossRef]
65. Kamatani, N.; Kushiyama, A.; Toyo-Oka, L.; Toyo-Oka, T. Treatment of two mitochondrial disease patients with a combination of febuxostat and inosine that enhances cellular ATP. *J. Hum. Genet.* **2019**, *64*, 351–353. [CrossRef]
66. Rossignol, R.; Faustin, B.; Rocher, C.; Malgat, M.; Mazat, J.-P.; Letellier, T. Mitochondrial threshold effects. *Biochem. J.* **2003**, *370*, 751–762. [CrossRef]
67. Lee, H.-C.; Wei, Y.-H. Mitochondrial biogenesis and mitochondrial DNA maintenance of mammalian cells under oxidative stress. *Int. J. Biochem. Cell Biol.* **2005**, *37*, 822–834. [CrossRef]
68. Gleyzer, N.; Vercauteren, K.; Scarpulla, R.C. Control of Mitochondrial Transcription Specificity Factors (TFB1M and TFB2M) by Nuclear Respiratory Factors (NRF-1 and NRF-2) and PGC-1 Family Coactivators. *Mol. Cell. Biol.* **2005**, *25*, 1354–1366. [CrossRef]

69. Schreiber, S.N.; Emter, R.; Hock, M.B.; Knutti, D.; Cardenas, J.; Podvinec, M.; Oakeley, E.J.; Kralli, A. The estrogen-related receptor (ERR) functions in PPAR coactivator 1 (PGC-1)-induced mitochondrial biogenesis. *Proc. Natl. Acad. Sci. USA* **2004**, *101*, 6472–6477. [CrossRef]
70. Wu, Z.; Puigserver, P.; Andersson, U.; Zhang, C.; Adelmant, G.; Mootha, V.; Troy, A.; Cinti, S.; Lowell, B.; Scarpulla, R.C.; et al. Mechanisms Controlling Mitochondrial Biogenesis and Respiration through the Thermogenic Coactivator PGC-1. *Cell* **1999**, *98*, 115–124. [CrossRef]
71. Mullur, R.; Liu, Y.-Y.; Brent, G.A. Thyroid Hormone Regulation of Metabolism. *Physiol. Rev.* **2014**, *94*, 355–382. [CrossRef] [PubMed]
72. Scarpulla, R.C.; Vega, R.B.; Kelly, D.P. Transcriptional integration of mitochondrial biogenesis. *Trends Endocrinol. Metab.* **2012**, *23*, 459–466. [CrossRef] [PubMed]
73. Lin, J.; Wu, H.; Tarr, P.T.; Zhang, C.-Y.; Wu, Z.; Boss, O.; Michael, L.F.; Puigserver, P.; Isotani, E.; Olson, E.N.; et al. Transcriptional co-activator PGC-1α drives the formation of slow-twitch muscle fibres. *Nat. Cell Biol.* **2002**, *418*, 797–801. [CrossRef] [PubMed]
74. Viscomi, C.; Bottani, E.; Civiletto, G.; Cerutti, R.; Moggio, M.; Fagiolari, G.; Schon, E.A.; Lamperti, C.; Zeviani, M. In Vivo Correction of COX Deficiency by Activation of the AMPK/PGC-1α Axis. *Cell Metab.* **2011**, *14*, 80–90. [CrossRef] [PubMed]
75. Puigserver, P.; Wu, Z.; Park, C.W.; Graves, R.; Wright, M.; Spiegelman, B.M. A Cold-Inducible Coactivator of Nuclear Receptors Linked to Adaptive Thermogenesis. *Cell* **1998**, *92*, 829–839. [CrossRef]
76. Geng, T.; Li, P.; Okutsu, M.; Yin, X.; Kwek, J.; Zhang, M.; Yan, Z. PGC-1α plays a functional role in exercise-induced mitochondrial biogenesis and angiogenesis but not fiber-type transformation in mouse skeletal muscle. *Am. J. Physiol. Physiol.* **2010**, *298*, C572–C579. [CrossRef]
77. Jäger, S.; Handschin, C.; St.-Pierre, J.; Spiegelman, B.M. AMP-activated protein kinase (AMPK) action in skeletal muscle via direct phosphorylation of PGC-1. *Proc. Natl. Acad. Sci. USA* **2007**, *104*, 12017–12022. [CrossRef]
78. Gerhart-Hines, Z.; Rodgers, J.T.; Bare, O.; Lerin, C.; Kim, S.-H.; Mostoslavsky, R.; Alt, F.W.; Wu, Z.; Puigserver, P. Metabolic control of muscle mitochondrial function and fatty acid oxidation through SIRT1/PGC-1α. *EMBO J.* **2007**, *26*, 1913–1923. [CrossRef]
79. Hardie, D.G. AMP-activated protein kinase–an energy sensor that regulates all aspects of cell function. *Genes Dev.* **2011**, *25*, 1895–1908. [CrossRef]
80. Cantó, C.; Auwerx, J. PGC-1α, SIRT1 and AMPK, an energy sensing network that controls energy expenditure. *Curr. Opin. Lipidol.* **2009**, *20*, 98–105. [CrossRef]
81. Cerutti, R.; Pirinen, E.; Lamperti, C.; Marchet, S.; Sauve, A.A.; Li, W.; Leoni, V.; Schon, E.A.; Dantzer, F.; Auwerx, J.; et al. NAD+-Dependent Activation of Sirt1 Corrects the Phenotype in a Mouse Model of Mitochondrial Disease. *Cell Metab.* **2014**, *19*, 1042–1049. [CrossRef] [PubMed]
82. Peralta, S.; Garcia, S.; Yin, H.Y.; Arguello, T.; Diaz, F.; Moraes, C.T. Sustained AMPK activation improves muscle function in a mitochondrial myopathy mouse model by promoting muscle fiber regeneration. *Hum. Mol. Genet.* **2016**, *25*, 3178–3191. [CrossRef] [PubMed]
83. Saada, A.; Dan, P.; Weissman, S.; Link, G.; Wikstrom, J.D.; Saada, A. Screening for Active Small Molecules in Mitochondrial Complex I Deficient Patient's Fibroblasts, Reveals AICAR as the Most Beneficial Compound. *PLoS ONE* **2011**, *6*, e26883. [CrossRef]
84. Lefebvre, P.; Chinetti, G.; Fruchart, J.-C.; Staels, B. Sorting out the roles of PPAR in energy metabolism and vascular homeostasis. *J. Clin. Investig.* **2006**, *116*, 571–580. [CrossRef]
85. Kersten, S. Integrated physiology and systems biology of PPARα. *Mol. Metab.* **2014**, *3*, 354–371. [CrossRef]
86. Djouadi, F.; Bastin, J. Mitochondrial Genetic Disorders: Cell Signaling and Pharmacological Therapies. *Cells* **2019**, *8*, 289. [CrossRef]
87. Bastin, J.; Aubey, F.; Rötig, A.; Munnich, A.; Djouadi, F. Activation of Peroxisome Proliferator-Activated Receptor Pathway Stimulates the Mitochondrial Respiratory Chain and Can Correct Deficiencies in Patients' Cells Lacking Its Components. *J. Clin. Endocrinol. Metab.* **2008**, *93*, 1433–1441. [CrossRef]
88. Casarin, A.; Giorgi, G.; Pertegato, V.; Siviero, R.; Cerqua, C.; Doimo, M.; Basso, G.; Sacconi, S.; Cassina, M.; Rizzuto, R.; et al. Copper and bezafibrate cooperate to rescue cytochrome c oxidase deficiency in cells of patients with sco2 mutations. *Orphanet J. Rare Dis.* **2012**, *7*, 21. [CrossRef]
89. Douiev, L.; Sheffer, R.; Horvath, G.A.; Saada, A. Bezafibrate Improves Mitochondrial Fission and Function in DNM1L-Deficient Patient Cells. *Cells* **2020**, *9*, 301. [CrossRef]

90. Yatsuga, S.; Suomalainen, A. Effect of bezafibrate treatment on late-onset mitochondrial myopathy in mice. *Hum. Mol. Genet.* **2011**, *21*, 526–535. [CrossRef]
91. Dillon, L.M.; Hida, A.; Garcia, S.; Prolla, T.A.; Moraes, C.T. Long-Term Bezafibrate Treatment Improves Skin and Spleen Phenotypes of the mtDNA Mutator Mouse. *PLoS ONE* **2012**, *7*, e44335. [CrossRef] [PubMed]
92. Steele, H.; Gomez-Duran, A.; Pyle, A.; Hopton, S.; Newman, J.; Stefanetti, R.J.; Charman, S.J.; Parikh, J.D.; He, L.; Viscomi, C.; et al. Metabolic effects of bezafibrate in mitochondrial disease. *EMBO Mol. Med.* **2020**, *12*, e11589. [CrossRef] [PubMed]
93. Hondares, E.; Mora, O.; Yubero, P.; De La Concepción, M.R.; Iglesias, R.; Giralt, M.; Villarroya, F. Thiazolidinediones and Rexinoids Induce Peroxisome Proliferator-Activated Receptor-Coactivator (PGC)-1α Gene Transcription: An Autoregulatory Loop Controls PGC-1α Expression in Adipocytes via Peroxisome Proliferator-Activated Receptor-γ Coactivation. *Endocrinology* **2006**, *147*, 2829–2838. [CrossRef] [PubMed]
94. Miglio, G.; Rosa, A.C.; Rattazzi, L.; Collino, M.; Lombardi, G.; Fantozzi, R. PPARγ stimulation promotes mitochondrial biogenesis and prevents glucose deprivation-induced neuronal cell loss. *Neurochem. Int.* **2009**, *55*, 496–504. [CrossRef]
95. Wilson-Fritch, L.; Burkart, A.; Bell, G.; Mendelson, K.; Leszyk, J.D.; Nicoloro, S.M.; Czech, M.P.; Corvera, S. Mitochondrial Biogenesis and Remodeling during Adipogenesis and in Response to the Insulin Sensitizer Rosiglitazone. *Mol. Cell. Biol.* **2003**, *23*, 1085–1094. [CrossRef]
96. Rong, J.X.; Klein, J.-L.D.; Qiu, Y.; Xie, M.; Johnson, J.H.; Waters, K.M.; Zhang, V.; Kashatus, J.A.; Remlinger, K.S.; Bing, N.; et al. Rosiglitazone Induces Mitochondrial Biogenesis in Differentiated Murine 3T3-L1 and C3H/10T1/2 Adipocytes. *PPAR Res.* **2011**, *2011*, 1–11. [CrossRef]
97. Strum, J.C.; Shehee, R.; Virley, D.; Richardson, J.; Mattie, M.; Selley, P.; Ghosh, S.; Nock, C.; Saunders, A.; Roses, A. Rosiglitazone Induces Mitochondrial Biogenesis in Mouse Brain. *J. Alzheimers Dis.* **2007**, *11*, 45–51. [CrossRef]
98. Andreux, P.A.; Houtkooper, R.H.; Auwerx, J. Pharmacological approaches to restore mitochondrial function. *Nat. Rev. Drug Discov.* **2013**, *12*, 465–483. [CrossRef]
99. Bieganowski, P.; Brenner, C. Discoveries of Nicotinamide Riboside as a Nutrient and Conserved NRK Genes Establish a Preiss-Handler Independent Route to NAD+ in Fungi and Humans. *Cell* **2004**, *117*, 495–502. [CrossRef]
100. Cantó, C.; Menzies, K.J.; Auwerx, J. NAD+ Metabolism and the Control of Energy Homeostasis: A Balancing Act between Mitochondria and the Nucleus. *Cell Metab.* **2015**, *22*, 31–53. [CrossRef]
101. Bai, P.; Cantó, C.; Oudart, H.; Brunyánszki, A.; Cen, Y.; Thomas, C.; Yamamoto, H.; Huber, A.; Kiss, B.; Houtkooper, R.H.; et al. PARP-1 Inhibition Increases Mitochondrial Metabolism through SIRT1 Activation. *Cell Metab.* **2011**, *13*, 461–468. [CrossRef] [PubMed]
102. Pirinen, E.; Cantó, C.; Jo, Y.S.; Morato, L.; Zhang, H.; Menzies, K.J.; Williams, E.G.; Mouchiroud, L.; Moullan, N.; Hagberg, C.; et al. Pharmacological Inhibition of Poly(ADP-Ribose) Polymerases Improves Fitness and Mitochondrial Function in Skeletal Muscle. *Cell Metab.* **2014**, *19*, 1034–1041. [CrossRef] [PubMed]
103. Katsyuba, E.; Mottis, A.; Zietak, M.; De Franco, F.; Van Der Velpen, V.; Gariani, K.; Ryu, D.; Cialabrini, L.; Matilainen, O.; Liscio, P.; et al. De novo NAD+ synthesis enhances mitochondrial function and improves health. *Nature* **2018**, *563*, 354–359. [CrossRef] [PubMed]
104. Belenky, P.; Bogan, K.L.; Brenner, C. NAD+ metabolism in health and disease. *Trends Biochem. Sci.* **2007**, *32*, 12–19. [CrossRef]
105. Pirinen, E.; Auranen, M.; Khan, N.A.; Brilhante, V.; Urho, N.; Pessia, A.; Hakkarainen, A.; Kuula, J.; Heinonen, U.; Schmidt, M.S.; et al. Niacin Cures Systemic NAD+ Deficiency and Improves Muscle Performance in Adult-Onset Mitochondrial Myopathy. *Cell Metab.* **2020**, *31*, 1078–1090.e5. [CrossRef]
106. Khan, N.A.; Auranen, M.; Paetau, I.; Pirinen, E.; Euro, L.; Forsström, S.; Pasila, L.; Velagapudi, V.; Carroll, C.J.; Auwerx, J.; et al. Effective treatment of mitochondrial myopathy by nicotinamide riboside, a vitamin B 3. *EMBO Mol. Med.* **2014**, *6*, 721–731. [CrossRef]
107. Schöndorf, D.C.; Ivanyuk, D.; Baden, P.; Sanchez-Martinez, A.; De Cicco, S.; Yu, C.; Giunta, I.; Schwarz, L.K.; Di Napoli, G.; Panagiotakopoulou, V.; et al. The NAD+ Precursor Nicotinamide Riboside Rescues Mitochondrial Defects and Neuronal Loss in iPSC and Fly Models of Parkinson's Disease. *Cell Rep.* **2018**, *23*, 2976–2988. [CrossRef]
108. Lee, C.F.; Caudal, A.; Abell, L.; Gowda, G.A.N.; Tian, R. Targeting NAD+ Metabolism as Interventions for Mitochondrial Disease. *Sci. Rep.* **2019**, *9*, 1–10. [CrossRef]

109. Airhart, S.E.; Shireman, L.M.; Risler, L.J.; Anderson, G.D.; Gowda, G.A.N.; Raftery, D.; Tian, R.; Shen, D.D.; O'Brien, K.D. An open-label, non-randomized study of the pharmacokinetics of the nutritional supplement nicotinamide riboside (NR) and its effects on blood NAD+ levels in healthy volunteers. *PLoS ONE* **2017**, *12*, e0186459. [CrossRef]
110. Barrow, J.J.; Balsa, E.; Verdeguer, F.; Tavares, C.D.J.; Soustek, M.S.; Hollingsworth, L.R.; Jedrychowski, M.; Vogel, R.; Paulo, J.A.; Smeitink, J.; et al. Bromodomain Inhibitors Correct Bioenergetic Deficiency Caused by Mitochondrial Disease Complex I Mutations. *Mol. Cell* **2016**, *64*, 163–175. [CrossRef]
111. Baratta, M.G.; Schinzel, A.C.; Zwang, Y.; Bandopadhayay, P.; Bowman-Colin, C.; Kutt, J.; Curtis, J.; Piao, H.; Wong, L.C.; Kung, A.L.; et al. An in-tumor genetic screen reveals that the BET bromodomain protein, BRD4, is a potential therapeutic target in ovarian carcinoma. *Proc. Natl. Acad. Sci. USA* **2015**, *112*, 232–237. [CrossRef] [PubMed]
112. Howitz, K.T.; Bitterman, K.J.; Cohen, H.Y.; Lamming, D.W.; Lavu, S.; Wood, J.G.; Zipkin, R.E.; Chung, P.; Kisielewski, A.; Zhang, L.-L.; et al. Small molecule activators of sirtuins extend Saccharomyces cerevisiae lifespan. *Nat. Cell Biol.* **2003**, *425*, 191–196. [CrossRef] [PubMed]
113. Price, N.L.; Gomes, A.P.; Ling, A.J.; Duarte, F.V.; Martin-Montalvo, A.; North, B.J.; Agarwal, B.; Ye, L.; Ramadori, G.; Teodoro, J.S.; et al. SIRT1 Is Required for AMPK Activation and the Beneficial Effects of Resveratrol on Mitochondrial Function. *Cell Metab.* **2012**, *15*, 675–690. [CrossRef] [PubMed]
114. Lagouge, M.; Argmann, C.; Gerhart-Hines, Z.; Meziane, H.; Lerin, C.; Daussin, F.; Messadeq, N.; Milne, J.; Lambert, P.; Elliott, P.; et al. Resveratrol Improves Mitochondrial Function and Protects against Metabolic Disease by Activating SIRT1 and PGC-1α. *Cell* **2006**, *127*, 1109–1122. [CrossRef] [PubMed]
115. Cantó, C.; Gerhart-Hines, Z.; Feige, J.N.; Lagouge, M.; Noriega, L.; Milne, J.C.; Elliott, P.J.; Puigserver, P.; Auwerx, J. AMPK regulates energy expenditure by modulating NAD+ metabolism and SIRT1 activity. *Nat. Cell Biol.* **2009**, *458*, 1056–1060. [CrossRef] [PubMed]
116. Dasgupta, B.; Milbrandt, J. Resveratrol stimulates AMP kinase activity in neurons. *Proc. Natl. Acad. Sci. USA* **2007**, *104*, 7217–7222. [CrossRef]
117. Borra, M.T.; Smith, B.C.; Denu, J.M. Mechanism of Human SIRT1 Activation by Resveratrol. *J. Biol. Chem.* **2005**, *280*, 17187–17195. [CrossRef]
118. Beher, D.; Wu, J.; Cumine, S.; Kim, K.W.; Lu, S.-C.; Atangan, L.; Wang, M. Resveratrol is Not a Direct Activator of SIRT1 Enzyme Activity. *Chem. Biol. Drug Des.* **2009**, *74*, 619–624. [CrossRef]
119. Kaeberlein, M.; McDonagh, T.; Heltweg, B.; Hixon, J.; Westman, E.A.; Caldwell, S.D.; Napper, A.; Curtis, R.; Distefano, P.S.; Fields, S.; et al. Substrate-specific Activation of Sirtuins by Resveratrol. *J. Biol. Chem.* **2005**, *280*, 17038–17045. [CrossRef]
120. Um, J.-H.; Park, S.-J.; Kang, H.; Yang, S.; Foretz, M.; McBurney, M.W.; Kim, M.K.; Viollet, B.; Chung, J.H. AMP-Activated Protein Kinase-Deficient Mice Are Resistant to the Metabolic Effects of Resveratrol. *Diabetes* **2010**, *59*, 554–563. [CrossRef]
121. Hou, X.; Xu, S.; Maitland-Toolan, K.A.; Sato, K.; Jiang, B.; Ido, Y.; Lan, F.; Walsh, K.; Wierzbicki, M.; Verbeuren, T.J.; et al. SIRT1 Regulates Hepatocyte Lipid Metabolism through Activating AMP-activated Protein Kinase. *J. Biol. Chem.* **2008**, *283*, 20015–20026. [CrossRef] [PubMed]
122. Lan, F.; Cacicedo, J.M.; Ruderman, N.; Ido, Y. SIRT1 Modulation of the Acetylation Status, Cytosolic Localization, and Activity of LKB1. *J. Biol. Chem.* **2008**, *283*, 27628–27635. [CrossRef] [PubMed]
123. Akyuva, Y.; Nazıroğlu, M. Resveratrol attenuates hypoxia-induced neuronal cell death, inflammation and mitochondrial oxidative stress by modulation of TRPM2 channel. *Sci. Rep.* **2020**, *10*, 1–16. [CrossRef] [PubMed]
124. Revin, V.V.; Pinyaev, S.; Parchaykina, M.V.; Revina, E.S.; Maksimov, G.V.; Kuzmenko, T.P. The Effect of Resveratrol on the Composition and State of Lipids and the Activity of Phospholipase A2 During the Excitation and Regeneration of Somatic Nerves. *Front. Physiol.* **2019**, *10*. [CrossRef]
125. De Paepe, B.; Van Coster, R. A Critical Assessment of the Therapeutic Potential of Resveratrol Supplements for Treating Mitochondrial Disorders. *Nutrients* **2017**, *9*, 1017. [CrossRef]
126. Davis, J.M.; Murphy, E.A.; Carmichael, M.D.; Davis, B. Quercetin increases brain and muscle mitochondrial biogenesis and exercise tolerance. *Am. J. Physiol. Integr. Comp. Physiol.* **2009**, *296*, R1071–R1077. [CrossRef]
127. Koshinaka, K.; Honda, A.; Masuda, H.; Sato, A. Effect of Quercetin Treatment on Mitochondrial Biogenesis and Exercise-Induced AMP-Activated Protein Kinase Activation in Rat Skeletal Muscle. *Nutrients* **2020**, *12*, 729. [CrossRef]

128. Wang, D.-M.; Li, S.-Q.; Wu, W.-L.; Zhu, X.-Y.; Wang, Y.; Yuan, H.-Y. Effects of Long-Term Treatment with Quercetin on Cognition and Mitochondrial Function in a Mouse Model of Alzheimer's Disease. *Neurochem. Res.* **2014**, *39*, 1533–1543. [CrossRef]
129. Karuppagounder, S.; Madathil, S.; Pandey, M.; Haobam, R.; Rajamma, U.; Mohanakumar, K. Quercetin up-regulates mitochondrial complex-I activity to protect against programmed cell death in rotenone model of Parkinson's disease in rats. *Neuroscience* **2013**, *236*, 136–148. [CrossRef]
130. Zhu, L.; Liu, Z.; Feng, Z.; Hao, J.; Shen, W.; Li, X.; Sun, L.; Sharman, E.; Wang, Y.; Wertz, K.; et al. Hydroxytyrosol protects against oxidative damage by simultaneous activation of mitochondrial biogenesis and phase II detoxifying enzyme systems in retinal pigment epithelial cells. *J. Nutr. Biochem.* **2010**, *21*, 1089–1098. [CrossRef]
131. Feng, Z.; Bai, L.; Yan, J.; Li, Y.; Shen, W.; Wang, Y.; Wertz, K.; Weber, P.; Zhang, Y.; Chen, Y.; et al. Mitochondrial dynamic remodeling in strenuous exercise-induced muscle and mitochondrial dysfunction: Regulatory effects of hydroxytyrosol. *Free Radic. Biol. Med.* **2011**, *50*, 1437–1446. [CrossRef] [PubMed]
132. Casuso, R.A.; Al-Fazazi, S.; Hidalgo-Gutierrez, A.; López, L.C.; Plaza-Díaz, J.; Rueda-Robles, A.; Huertas, J.R. Hydroxytyrosol influences exercise-induced mitochondrial respiratory complex assembly into supercomplexes in rats. *Free Radic. Biol. Med.* **2019**, *134*, 304–310. [CrossRef] [PubMed]
133. Zheng, A.; Li, H.; Xu, J.; Cao, K.; Li, H.; Pu, W.; Yang, Z.; Peng, Y.; Long, J.; Liu, J.; et al. Hydroxytyrosol improves mitochondrial function and reduces oxidative stress in the brain of db/db mice: Role of AMP-activated protein kinase activation. *Br. J. Nutr.* **2015**, *113*, 1667–1676. [CrossRef] [PubMed]
134. Brunetti, G.; Di Rosa, G.; Scuto, M.; Leri, M.; Stefani, M.; Schmitz-Linneweber, C.; Calabrese, V.; Saul, N. Healthspan Maintenance and Prevention of Parkinson's-like Phenotypes with Hydroxytyrosol and Oleuropein Aglycone in C. elegans. *Int. J. Mol. Sci.* **2020**, *21*, 2588. [CrossRef]
135. Eckert, G.P.; Schiborr, C.; Hagl, S.; Abdel-Kader, R.; Müller, W.E.; Rimbach, G.; Frank, J. Curcumin prevents mitochondrial dysfunction in the brain of the senescence-accelerated mouse-prone 8. *Neurochem. Int.* **2013**, *62*, 595–602. [CrossRef]
136. Chin, D.; Hagl, S.; Hoehn, A.; Huebbe, P.; Pallauf, K.; Grune, T.; Frank, J.; Eckert, G.P.; Rimbach, G. Adenosine triphosphate concentrations are higher in the brain of APOE3- compared to APOE4-targeted replacement mice and can be modulated by curcumin. *Genes Nutr.* **2014**, *9*, 397. [CrossRef]
137. Kalpravidh, R.W.; Siritanaratkul, N.; Insain, P.; Charoensakdi, R.; Panichkul, N.; Hatairaktham, S.; Srichairatanakool, S.; Phisalaphong, C.; Rachmilewitz, E.; Fucharoen, S. Improvement in oxidative stress and antioxidant parameters in β-thalassemia/Hb E patients treated with curcuminoids. *Clin. Biochem.* **2010**, *43*, 424–429. [CrossRef]
138. Nasseri, E.; Mohammadi, E.; Tamaddoni, A.; Qujeq, D.; Zayeri, F.; Zand, H. Benefits of Curcumin Supplementation on Antioxidant Status in β-Thalassemia Major Patients: A Double-Blind Randomized Controlled Clinical Trial. *Ann. Nutr. Metab.* **2017**, *71*, 136–144. [CrossRef]
139. Musi, N.; Goodyear, L.J. Targeting the AMP-activated protein kinase for the treatment of type 2 diabetes. *Curr. Drug Targets Immune Endocr. Metab. Disord.* **2002**, *2*, 119–127. [CrossRef]
140. Goodyear, L.J. The Exercise Pill—Too Good to Be True? *N. Engl. J. Med.* **2008**, *359*, 1842–1844. [CrossRef]
141. Bundred, N.J.; Gardovskis, J.; Jaskiewicz, J.; Eglitis, J.; Paramonov, V.; McCormack, P.; Swaisland, H.; Cavallin, M.; Parry, T.; Carmichael, J.; et al. Evaluation of the pharmacodynamics and pharmacokinetics of the PARP inhibitor olaparib: A Phase I multicentre trial in patients scheduled for elective breast cancer surgery. *Investig. New Drugs* **2013**, *31*, 949–958. [CrossRef] [PubMed]
142. Conze, D.; Brenner, C.; Kruger, C.L. Safety and Metabolism of Long-term Administration of NIAGEN (Nicotinamide Riboside Chloride) in a Randomized, Double-Blind, Placebo-controlled Clinical Trial of Healthy Overweight Adults. *Sci. Rep.* **2019**, *9*, 1–13. [CrossRef] [PubMed]
143. Conze, D.B.; Crespo-Barreto, J.; Kruger, C.L. Safety assessment of nicotinamide riboside, a form of vitamin B3. *Hum. Exp. Toxicol.* **2016**, *35*, 1149–1160. [CrossRef] [PubMed]
144. Marinescu, A.G.; Chen, J.; Holmes, H.E.; Guarente, L.; Mendes, O.; Morris, M.; Dellinger, R.W. Safety Assessment of High-Purity, Synthetic Nicotinamide Riboside (NR-E) in a 90-Day Repeated Dose Oral Toxicity Study, With a 28-Day Recovery Arm. *Int. J. Toxicol.* **2020**, *39*, 307–320. [CrossRef]
145. Lacza, Z.; Pankotai, E.; Csordás, A.; Gero, D.; Kiss, L.; Horváth, E.M.; Kollai, M.; Busija, D.W.; Szabó, C. Mitochondrial NO and reactive nitrogen species production: Does mtNOS exist? *Nitric Oxide* **2006**, *14*, 162–168. [CrossRef]

146. Leite, A.C.R.; Oliveira, H.C.; Utino, F.L.; Garcia, R.; Alberici, L.C.; Fernandes, M.P.; Castilho, R.F.; Vercesi, A.E. Mitochondria generated nitric oxide protects against permeability transition via formation of membrane protein S-nitrosothiols. *Biochim. Biophys. Acta (BBA) Bioenerg.* **2010**, *1797*, 1210–1216. [CrossRef]
147. Ghafourifar, P.; Cadenas, E. Mitochondrial nitric oxide synthase. *Trends Pharmacol. Sci.* **2005**, *26*, 190–195. [CrossRef]
148. Eqian, J.; Fulton, D.J. Post-translational regulation of endothelial nitric oxide synthase in vascular endothelium. *Front. Physiol.* **2013**, *4*, 347. [CrossRef]
149. Francis, S.H.; Busch, J.L.; Corbin, J.D. cGMP-Dependent Protein Kinases and cGMP Phosphodiesterases in Nitric Oxide and cGMP Action. *Pharmacol. Rev.* **2010**, *62*, 525–563. [CrossRef]
150. Kaupp, U.B.; Seifert, R. Cyclic Nucleotide-Gated Ion Channels. *Physiol. Rev.* **2002**, *82*, 769–824. [CrossRef]
151. Fischmeister, R.; Méry, P.-F. Regulation of cardiac Ca2+ channels by cGMP and NO. In *Molecular Physiology and Pharmacology of Cardiac Ion Channels and Transporters*; Springer: Dordrecht, The Netherlands, 1996; pp. 93–105. [CrossRef]
152. White, R.E. Cyclic GMP and Ion Channel Regulation. In *Adv. Second Messenger and Phosphoprotein Res.*; Elsevier: London, UK, 1999; Volume 33, pp. 251–277. [CrossRef]
153. Brown, G.C. CELL BIOLOGY: Enhanced: NO Says Yes to Mitochondria. *Science* **2003**, *299*, 838–839. [CrossRef] [PubMed]
154. Gureev, A.P.; Shaforostova, E.A.; Popov, V.N. Regulation of Mitochondrial Biogenesis as a Way for Active Longevity: Interaction Between the Nrf2 and PGC-1α Signaling Pathways. *Front. Genet.* **2019**, *10*, 435. [CrossRef] [PubMed]
155. Gutsaeva, D.R.; Carraway, M.S.; Suliman, H.B.; Demchenko, I.T.; Shitara, H.; Yonekawa, H.; Piantadosi, C.A. Transient Hypoxia Stimulates Mitochondrial Biogenesis in Brain Subcortex by a Neuronal Nitric Oxide Synthase-Dependent Mechanism. *J. Neurosci.* **2008**, *28*, 2015–2024. [CrossRef] [PubMed]
156. Sanders, O. Sildenafil for the Treatment of Alzheimer's Disease: A Systematic Review. *J. Alzheimers Dis. Rep.* **2020**, *4*, 91–106. [CrossRef] [PubMed]
157. Ohama, E.; Ohara, S.; Ikuta, F.; Tanaka, K.; Nishizawa, M.; Miyatake, T. Mitochondrial angiopathy in cerebral blood vessels of mitochondrial eneephalomyopathy. *Acta Neuropathol.* **1987**, *74*, 226–233. [CrossRef] [PubMed]
158. Vattemi, G.; Mechref, Y.; Marini, M.; Tonin, P.; Minuz, P.; Grigoli, L.; Guglielmi, V.; Klouckova, I.; Chiamulera, C.; Meneguzzi, A.; et al. Increased Protein Nitration in Mitochondrial Diseases: Evidence for Vessel Wall Involvement. *Mol. Cell. Proteom.* **2010**, *10*, 110 002964. [CrossRef] [PubMed]
159. Sarti, P.; Forte, E.; Giuffrè, A.; Mastronicola, D.; Magnifico, M.C.; Arese, M. The Chemical Interplay between Nitric Oxide and Mitochondrial Cytochrome c Oxidase: Reactions, Effectors and Pathophysiology. *Int. J. Cell Biol.* **2012**, *2012*, 1–11. [CrossRef]
160. El-Hattab, A.W.; Hsu, J.W.; Emrick, L.T.; Wong, L.-J.C.; Craigen, W.J.; Jahoor, F.; Scaglia, F. Restoration of impaired nitric oxide production in MELAS syndrome with citrulline and arginine supplementation. *Mol. Genet. Metab.* **2012**, *105*, 607–614. [CrossRef]
161. Naini, A.; Kaufmann, P.; Shanske, S.; Engelstad, K.; De Vivo, D.C.; Schon, E.A. Hypocitrullinemia in patients with MELAS: An insight into the "MELAS paradox". *J. Neurol. Sci.* **2005**, *229*, 187–193. [CrossRef]
162. Koga, Y.; Akita, Y.; Junko, N.; Yatsuga, S.; Povalko, N.; Fukiyama, R.; Ishii, M.; Matsuishi, T. Endothelial dysfunction in MELAS improved by l-arginine supplementation. *Neurology* **2006**, *66*, 1766–1769. [CrossRef]
163. Tengan, C.H.; Kiyomoto, B.H.; Godinho, R.O.; Gamba, J.; Neves, A.C.; Schmidt, B.; Oliveira, A.S.; Gabbai, A.A. The role of nitric oxide in muscle fibers with oxidative phosphorylation defects. *Biochem. Biophys. Res. Commun.* **2007**, *359*, 771–777. [CrossRef] [PubMed]
164. El-Hattab, A.W.; Emrick, L.T.; Craigen, W.J.; Scaglia, F. Citrulline and arginine utility in treating nitric oxide deficiency in mitochondrial disorders. *Mol. Genet. Metab.* **2012**, *107*, 247–252. [CrossRef] [PubMed]
165. Koga, Y.; Akita, Y.; Nishioka, J.; Yatsuga, S.; Povalko, N.; Tanabe, Y.; Fujimoto, S.; Matsuishi, T. L-Arginine improves the symptoms of strokelike episodes in MELAS. *Neurology* **2005**, *64*, 710–712. [CrossRef] [PubMed]
166. El-Hattab, A.W.; Emrick, L.T.; Chanprasert, S.; Craigen, W.J.; Scaglia, F. Mitochondria: Role of citrulline and arginine supplementation in MELAS syndrome. *Int. J. Biochem. Cell Biol.* **2014**, *48*, 85–91. [CrossRef] [PubMed]
167. El-Hattab, A.W.; Emrick, L.T.; Williamson, K.C.; Craigen, W.J.; Scaglia, F. The effect of citrulline and arginine supplementation on lactic acidemia in MELAS syndrome. *Meta Gene* **2013**, *1*, 8–14. [CrossRef]

168. Koga, Y.; Povalko, N.; Nishioka, J.; Katayama, K.; Kakimoto, N.; Matsuishi, T. MELAS and l-arginine therapy: Pathophysiology of stroke-like episodes. *Ann. N. Y. Acad. Sci.* **2010**, *1201*, 104–110. [CrossRef]
169. El-Hattab, A.W.; Emrick, L.T.; Hsu, J.W.; Chanprasert, S.; Almannai, M.; Craigen, W.J.; Jahoor, F.; Scaglia, F. Impaired nitric oxide production in children with MELAS syndrome and the effect of arginine and citrulline supplementation. *Mol. Genet. Metab.* **2016**, *117*, 407–412. [CrossRef]
170. Potter, L.R.; Yoder, A.R.; Flora, D.R.; Antos, L.K.; Dickey, D.M. Natriuretic Peptides: Their Structures, Receptors, Physiologic Functions and Therapeutic Applications. In *cGMP: Generators, Effectors and Therapeutic Implications*; Schmidt, H.H.H.W., Hofmann, F., Stasch, J.-P., Eds.; Springer: Berlin/Heidelberg, Germany, 2009; pp. 341–366.
171. Miyashita, K.; Itoh, H.; Tsujimoto, H.; Tamura, N.; Fukunaga, Y.; Sone, M.; Yamahara, K.; Taura, D.; Inuzuka, M.; Sonoyama, T.; et al. Natriuretic Peptides/cGMP/cGMP-Dependent Protein Kinase Cascades Promote Muscle Mitochondrial Biogenesis and Prevent Obesity. *Diabetes* **2009**, *58*, 2880–2892. [CrossRef]
172. Engeli, S.; Birkenfeld, A.L.; Badin, P.-M.; Bourlier, V.; Louche, K.; Viguerie, N.; Thalamas, C.; Montastier, E.; Larrouy, D.; Harant, I.; et al. Natriuretic peptides enhance the oxidative capacity of human skeletal muscle. *J. Clin. Investig.* **2012**, *122*, 4675–4679. [CrossRef]
173. Whitaker, R.M.; Wills, L.P.; Stallons, L.J.; Schnellmann, R.G. cGMP-Selective Phosphodiesterase Inhibitors Stimulate Mitochondrial Biogenesis and Promote Recovery from Acute Kidney Injury. *J. Pharmacol. Exp. Ther.* **2013**, *347*, 626–634. [CrossRef]
174. Corbin, J.D. Mechanisms of action of PDE5 inhibition in erectile dysfunction. *Int. J. Impot. Res.* **2004**, *16*, S4–S7. [CrossRef] [PubMed]
175. Mitschke, M.M.; Hoffmann, L.S.; Gnad, T.; Scholz, D.; Kruithoff, K.; Mayer, P.; Haas, B.; Sassmann, A.; Pfeifer, A.; Kilić, A. Increased cGMP promotes healthy expansion and browning of white adipose tissue. *FASEB J.* **2013**, *27*, 1621–1630. [CrossRef] [PubMed]
176. Lorenz, C.; Lesimple, P.; Bukowiecki, R.; Zink, A.; Inak, G.; Mlody, B.; Singh, M.; Semtner, M.; Mah, N.; Auré, K.; et al. Human iPSC-Derived Neural Progenitors Are an Effective Drug Discovery Model for Neurological mtDNA Disorders. *Cell Stem Cell* **2017**, *20*, 659–674.e9. [CrossRef] [PubMed]
177. Percival, J.M.; Siegel, M.P.; Knowels, G.; Marcinek, D.J. Defects in mitochondrial localization and ATP synthesis in the mdx mouse model of Duchenne muscular dystrophy are not alleviated by PDE5 inhibition. *Hum. Mol. Genet.* **2013**, *22*, 153–167. [CrossRef] [PubMed]
178. Tetsi, L.; Charles, A.-L.; Georg, I.; Goupilleau, F.; Lejay, A.; Talha, S.; Maumy-Bertrand, M.; Lugnier, C.; Geny, B. Effect of the Phosphodiesterase 5 Inhibitor Sildenafil on Ischemia-Reperfusion-Induced Muscle Mitochondrial Dysfunction and Oxidative Stress. *Antioxidants* **2019**, *8*, 93. [CrossRef] [PubMed]
179. Cornish, K.S.; Barras, C. Leber's Hereditary Optic Neuropathy Precipitated by Tadalafil Use for Erectile Dysfunction. *Semin. Ophthalmol.* **2011**, *26*, 7–10. [CrossRef]
180. Choi, M.H.; Lee, I.K.; Kim, G.W.; Kim, B.U.; Han, Y.-H.; Yu, D.-Y.; Park, H.S.; Kim, K.Y.; Lee, J.S.; Choi, C.; et al. Regulation of PDGF signalling and vascular remodelling by peroxiredoxin II. *Nat. Cell Biol.* **2005**, *435*, 347–353. [CrossRef]
181. Sena, L.A.; Chandel, N.S. Physiological Roles of Mitochondrial Reactive Oxygen Species. *Mol. Cell* **2012**, *48*, 158–167. [CrossRef]
182. Balaban, R.S.; Nemoto, S.; Finkel, T. Mitochondria, Oxidants, and Aging. *Cell* **2005**, *120*, 483–495. [CrossRef]
183. Wallace, D.C.; Fan, W. The pathophysiology of mitochondrial disease as modeled in the mouse. *Genes Dev.* **2009**, *23*, 1714–1736. [CrossRef]
184. Guo, C.; Sun, L.; Chen, X.; Zhang, D. Oxidative stress, mitochondrial damage and neurodegenerative diseases. *Neural Regen. Res.* **2013**, *8*, 2003–2014. [PubMed]
185. Polyak, E.; Ostrovsky, J.; Peng, M.; Dingley, S.D.; Tsukikawa, M.; Kwon, Y.J.; McCormack, S.E.; Bennett, M.; Xiao, R.; Seiler, C.; et al. N-acetylcysteine and vitamin E rescue animal longevity and cellular oxidative stress in pre-clinical models of mitochondrial complex I disease. *Mol. Genet. Metab.* **2018**, *123*, 449–462. [CrossRef] [PubMed]
186. Enns, G.M.; Moore, T.; Le, A.; Atkuri, K.; Shah, M.K.; Cusmano-Ozog, K.; Niemi, A.-K.; Cowan, T.M. Degree of Glutathione Deficiency and Redox Imbalance Depend on Subtype of Mitochondrial Disease and Clinical Status. *PLoS ONE* **2014**, *9*, e100001. [CrossRef] [PubMed]
187. Salmi, H.; Leonard, J.V.; Rahman, S.; Lapatto, R. Plasma thiol status is altered in children with mitochondrial diseases. *Scand. J. Clin. Lab. Investig.* **2012**, *72*, 152–157. [CrossRef]

188. Mancuso, M.; Orsucci, D.; LoGerfo, A.; Rocchi, A.; Petrozzi, L.; Nesti, C.; Galetta, F.; Santoro, G.; Murri, L.; Siciliano, G. Oxidative stress biomarkers in mitochondrial myopathies, basally and after cysteine donor supplementation. *J. Neurol.* **2009**, *257*, 774–781. [CrossRef] [PubMed]
189. Bartsakoulia, M.; Müller, J.S.; Gomez-Duran, A.; Yu-Wai-Man, P.; Boczonadi, V.; Horváth, H.R. Cysteine Supplementation May be Beneficial in a Subgroup of Mitochondrial Translation Deficiencies. *J. Neuromuscul. Dis.* **2016**, *3*, 363–379. [CrossRef] [PubMed]
190. Nesterova, G.; Gahl, W.A. Cystinosis. In *GeneReviews®*; Adam, M.P., Ardinger, H.H., Pagon, R.A., Wallace, S.E., Bean, L.J., Stephens, K., Amemiya, A., Eds.; University of Washington: Seattle, WA, USA, 1993.
191. Besouw, M.; Masereeuw, R.; Heuvel, L.V.D.; Levtchenko, E. Cysteamine: An old drug with new potential. *Drug Discov. Today* **2013**, *18*, 785–792. [CrossRef] [PubMed]
192. Guha, S.; Konkwo, C.; Lavorato, M.; Mathew, N.D.; Peng, M.; Ostrovsky, J.; Kwon, Y.-J.; Polyak, E.; Lightfoot, R.; Seiler, C.; et al. Pre-clinical evaluation of cysteamine bitartrate as a therapeutic agent for mitochondrial respiratory chain disease. *Hum. Mol. Genet.* **2019**, *28*, 1837–1852. [CrossRef]
193. Dohil, R.; Rioux, P. Pharmacokinetic Studies of Cysteamine Bitartrate Delayed-Release. *Clin. Pharmacol. Drug Dev.* **2013**, *2*, 178–185. [CrossRef]
194. Ferreira, L.F.; Campbell, K.S.; Reid, M.B. N-acetylcysteine in handgrip exercise: Plasma thiols and adverse reactions. *Int. J. Sport Nutr. Exerc. Metab.* **2011**, *21*, 146–154. [CrossRef]
195. Viscomi, C.; Burlina, A.B.; Dweikat, I.; Savoiardo, M.; Lamperti, C.; Hildebrandt, T.M.; Tiranti, V.; Zeviani, M. Combined treatment with oral metronidazole and N-acetylcysteine is effective in ethylmalonic encephalopathy. *Nat. Med.* **2010**, *16*, 869–871. [CrossRef] [PubMed]
196. Tiranti, V.; Viscomi, C.; Hildebrandt, T.; Di Meo, I.; Mineri, R.; Tiveron, C.; Levitt, M.D.; Prelle, A.; Fagiolari, G.; Rimoldi, M.; et al. Loss of ETHE1, a mitochondrial dioxygenase, causes fatal sulfide toxicity in ethylmalonic encephalopathy. *Nat. Med.* **2009**, *15*, 200–205. [CrossRef] [PubMed]
197. Di Meo, I.; Fagiolari, G.; Prelle, A.; Viscomi, C.; Zeviani, M.; Tiranti, V. Chronic Exposure to Sulfide Causes Accelerated Degradation of Cytochrome c Oxidase in Ethylmalonic Encephalopathy. *Antioxid. Redox Signal.* **2011**, *15*, 353–362. [CrossRef] [PubMed]
198. Kitzler, T.M.; Gupta, I.R.; Osterman, B.; Poulin, C.; Trakadis, Y.; Waters, P.J.; Buhas, D.C. Acute and Chronic Management in an Atypical Case of Ethylmalonic Encephalopathy. *JIMD Rep.* **2018**, *45*, 57–63. [CrossRef] [PubMed]
199. Kılıç, M.; Dedeoğlu, Ö.; Göçmen, R.; Kesici, S.; Yüksel, D. Successful treatment of a patient with ethylmalonic encephalopathy by intravenous N-acetylcysteine. *Metab. Brain Dis.* **2017**, *32*, 293–296. [CrossRef]
200. Boyer, M.; Sowa, M.; Di Meo, I.; Eftekharian, S.; Steenari, M.; Tiranti, V.; Abdenur, J. Response to medical and a novel dietary treatment in newborn screen identified patients with ethylmalonic encephalopathy. *Mol. Genet. Metab.* **2018**, *124*, 57–63. [CrossRef]
201. Bustamante, J. α-Lipoic Acid in Liver Metabolism and Disease. *Free Radic. Biol. Med.* **1998**, *24*, 1023–1039. [CrossRef]
202. Smith, A.R.; Shenvi, S.V.; Widlansky, M.; Suh, J.H.; Hagen, T.M. Lipoic Acid as a Potential Therapy for Chronic Diseases Associated with Oxidative Stress. *Curr. Med. Chem.* **2004**, *11*, 1135–1146. [CrossRef]
203. Kozlov, A.V.; Gille, L.; Staniek, K.; Nohl, H. Dihydrolipoic Acid Maintains Ubiquinone in the Antioxidant Active Form by Two-Electron Reduction of Ubiquinone and One-Electron Reduction of Ubisemiquinone. *Arch. Biochem. Biophys.* **1999**, *363*, 148–154. [CrossRef]
204. Teichert, J.; Hermann, R.; Ruus, P.; Preiss, R. Plasma Kinetics, Metabolism, and Urinary Excretion of Alpha-Lipoic Acid following Oral Administration in Healthy Volunteers. *J. Clin. Pharmacol.* **2003**, *43*, 1257–1267. [CrossRef]
205. El-Hattab, A.W.; Zarante, A.M.; Almannai, M.; Scaglia, F. Therapies for mitochondrial diseases and current clinical trials. *Mol. Genet. Metab.* **2017**, *122*, 1–9. [CrossRef] [PubMed]
206. Rodriguez, M.C.; Macdonald, J.R.; Mahoney, D.J.; Parise, G.; Beal, M.F.; Tarnopolsky, M.A. Beneficial effects of creatine, CoQ10, and lipoic acid in mitochondrial disorders. *Muscle Nerve* **2007**, *35*, 235–242. [CrossRef] [PubMed]
207. Beltran, R.S.; Coker, S.B. Familial Spastic Paraparesis: A Case of a Mitochondrial Disorder. *Pediatr. Neurosurg.* **1990**, *16*, 40–42. [CrossRef] [PubMed]
208. Eleff, S.; Kennaway, N.G.; Buist, N.R.; Darley-Usmar, V.M.; Capaldi, R.A.; Bank, W.J.; Chance, B. 31P NMR study of improvement in oxidative phosphorylation by vitamins K3 and C in a patient with a defect in electron transport at complex III in skeletal muscle. *Proc. Natl. Acad. Sci. USA* **1984**, *81*, 3529–3533. [CrossRef]

209. Mowat, D.; Kirby, D.M.; Kamath, K.R.; Kan, A.; Thorburn, D.R.; Christodoulou, J. Respiratory chain complex III deficiency with pruritus: A novel vitamin responsive clinical feature. *J. Pediatr.* **1999**, *134*, 352–354. [CrossRef]
210. Andreu, A.L.; Hanna, M.G.; Reichmann, H.; Bruno, C.; Penn, A.S.; Tanji, K.; Pallotti, F.; Iwata, S.; Bonilla, E.; Lach, B.; et al. Exercise Intolerance Due to Mutations in the CytochromebGene of Mitochondrial DNA. *N. Engl. J. Med.* **1999**, *341*, 1037–1044. [CrossRef]
211. Koopman, W.J.H.; Verkaart, S.; Vries, S.E.V.E.-D.; Grefte, S.; Smeitink, J.A.; Nijtmans, L.G.; Willems, P.H. Mitigation of NADH: Ubiquinone oxidoreductase deficiency by chronic Trolox treatment. *Biochim. Biophys. Acta (BBA) Bioenerg.* **2008**, *1777*, 853–859. [CrossRef]
212. Distelmaier, F.; Visch, H.-J.; Smeitink, J.A.M.; Mayatepek, E.; Koopman, W.J.H.; Willems, P.H.G.M. The antioxidant Trolox restores mitochondrial membrane potential and Ca2+-stimulated ATP production in human complex I deficiency. *J. Mol. Med.* **2009**, *87*, 515–522. [CrossRef]
213. Bentinger, M.; Brismar, K.; Dallner, G. The antioxidant role of coenzyme Q. *Mitochondrion* **2007**, *7*, S41–S50. [CrossRef]
214. Musumeci, O.; Naini, A.; Slonim, A.E.; Skavin, N.; Hadjigeorgiou, G.L.; Krawiecki, N.; Weissman, B.M.; Tsao, C.-Y.; Mendell, J.R.; Shanske, S.; et al. Familial cerebellar ataxia with muscle coenzyme Q10 deficiency. *Neurology* **2001**, *56*, 849–855. [CrossRef]
215. Lamperti, C.; Naini, A.; Hirano, M.; De Vivo, D.; Bertini, E.; Servidei, S.; Valeriani, M.; Lynch, D.; Banwell, B.; Berg, M.; et al. Cerebellar ataxia and coenzyme Q10 deficiency. *Neurology* **2003**, *60*, 1206–1208. [CrossRef] [PubMed]
216. Argov, Z.; Bank, W.J.; Maris, J.; Eleff, S.; Kennaway, N.G.; Olson, R.E.; Chance, B. Treatment of mitochondrial myopathy due to complex III deficiency with vitamins K3 and C: A31P-NMR follow-up study. *Ann. Neurol.* **1986**, *19*, 598–602. [CrossRef] [PubMed]
217. Turunen, M.; Olsson, J.; Dallner, G. Metabolism and function of coenzyme Q. *Biochim. Biophys. Acta (BBA) Biomembr.* **2004**, *1660*, 171–199. [CrossRef] [PubMed]
218. Geromel, V.; Darin, N.; Chrétien, D.; Bénit, P.; Delonlay, P.; Rötig, A.; Munnich, A.; Rustin, P. Coenzyme Q10 and idebenone in the therapy of respiratory chain diseases: Rationale and comparative benefits. *Mol. Genet. Metab.* **2002**, *77*, 21–30. [CrossRef]
219. Neergheen, V.; Chalasani, A.; Wainwright, L.; Yubero, D.; Montero, R.; Artuch, R.; Hargreaves, I. Coenzyme Q10 in the Treatment of Mitochondrial Disease. *J. Inborn Errors Metab. Screen.* **2017**, *5*, 232640981770777. [CrossRef]
220. Villanueva-Paz, M.; Povea-Cabello, S.; Villalón-García, I.; Álvarez-Córdoba, M.; Suárez-Rivero, J.M.; Talaverón-Rey, M.; Jackson, S.; Falcón-Moya, R.; Rodríguez-Moreno, A.; Sánchez-Alcázar, J.A. Parkin-mediated mitophagy and autophagy flux disruption in cellular models of MERRF syndrome. *Biochim. Biophys. Acta (BBA) Mol. Basis Dis.* **2020**, *1866*, 165726. [CrossRef]
221. Ogasahara, S.; Nishikawa, Y.; Yorifuji, S.; Soga, F.; Nakamura, Y.; Takahashi, M.; Hashimoto, S.; Kono, N.; Tarui, S. Treatment of Kearns-Sayre syndrome with coenzyme Q10. *Neurology* **1986**, *36*, 45. [CrossRef]
222. Chan, A.; Reichmann, H.; Kögel, A.; Beck, A.; Gold, R. Metabolic changes in patients with mitochondrial myopathies and effects of coenzyme Q10 therapy. *J. Neurol.* **1998**, *245*, 681–685. [CrossRef]
223. Bendahan, D.; Desnuelle, C.; Vanuxem, D.; Confort-Gouny, S.; Figarella-Branger, D.; Pellissier, J.-F.; Kozak-Ribbens, G.; Pouget, J.; Serratrice, G.; Cozzone, P.J. 31P NMR spectroscopy and ergometer exercise test as evidence for muscle oxidative performance improvement with coenzyme Q in mitochondrial myopathies. *Neurology* **1992**, *42*, 1203. [CrossRef]
224. Goda, S.; Hamada, T.; Ishimoto, S.; Kobayashi, T.; Goto, I.; Kuroiwa, Y. Clinical improvement after administration of coenzyme Q10 in a patient with mitochondrial encephalomyopathy. *J. Neurol.* **1987**, *234*, 62–63. [CrossRef]
225. Nishikawa, Y.; Takahashi, M.; Yorifuji, S.; Nakamura, Y.; Ueno, S.; Tarui, S.; Kozuka, T.; Nishimura, T. Long-term coenzyme Q10 therapy for a mitochondrial encephalomyopathy with cytochrome c oxidase deficiency: A 31P NMR study. *Neurology* **1989**, *39*, 399. [CrossRef] [PubMed]
226. Zierz, S.; Jahns, G.; Jerusalem, F. Coenzyme Q in serum and muscle of 5 patients with Kearns-Sayre syndrome and 12 patients with ophthalmoplegia plus. *J. Neurol.* **1989**, *236*, 97–101. [CrossRef] [PubMed]

227. Barbiroli, B.; Iotti, S.; Lodi, R. Improved brain and muscle mitochondrial respiration with CoQ. An in vivo study by 31P-MR spectroscopy in patients with mitochondrial cytopathies. *BioFactors* **1999**, *9*, 253–260. [CrossRef] [PubMed]
228. Shoffner, J.M.; Lott, M.T.; Voljavec, A.S.; Soueidan, S.A.; Costigan, D.A.; Wallace, D.C. Spontaneous Kearns-Sayre/chronic external ophthalmoplegia plus syndrome associated with a mitochondrial DNA deletion: A slip-replication model and metabolic therapy. *Proc. Natl. Acad. Sci. USA* **1989**, *86*, 7952–7956. [CrossRef]
229. Matthews, P.M.; Ford, B.; Dandurand, R.J.; Eidelman, D.H.; O'Connor, D.; Sherwin, A.; Karpati, G.; Andermann, F.; Arnold, D.L. Coenzyme Q10 with multiple vitamins is generally ineffective in treatment of mitochondrial disease. *Neurology* **1993**, *43*, 884. [CrossRef]
230. Bresolin, N.; Bet, L.; Binda, A.; Moggio, M.; Comi, G.; Nador, F.; Ferrante, C.; Carenzi, A.; Scarlato, G. Clinical and biochemical correlations in mitochondrial myopathies treated with coenzyme Q10. *Neurology* **1988**, *38*, 892. [CrossRef]
231. Marriage, B.; Clandinin, M.; Macdonald, I.M.; Glerum, D. Cofactor treatment improves ATP synthetic capacity in patients with oxidative phosphorylation disorders. *Mol. Genet. Metab.* **2004**, *81*, 263–272. [CrossRef]
232. Glover, E.I.; Martin, J.; Maher, A.; Thornhill, R.E.; Moran, G.R.; Tarnopolsky, M.A. A randomized trial of coenzyme Q10 in mitochondrial disorders. *Muscle Nerve* **2010**, *42*, 739–748. [CrossRef]
233. Sacconi, S.; Trevisson, E.; Salviati, L.; Aymé, S.; Rigal, O.; Redondo, A.G.; Mancuso, M.; Siciliano, G.; Tonin, P.; Angelini, C.; et al. Coenzyme Q10 is frequently reduced in muscle of patients with mitochondrial myopathy. *Neuromuscul. Disord.* **2010**, *20*, 44–48. [CrossRef]
234. Stacpoole, P.W.; Degrauw, T.J.; Feigenbaum, A.S.; Hoppel, C.; Kerr, D.S.; McCandless, S.E.; Miles, M.V.; Robinson, B.H.; Tang, P.H. Design and implementation of the first randomized controlled trial of coenzyme Q10 in children with primary mitochondrial diseases. *Mitochondrion* **2012**, *12*, 623–629. [CrossRef]
235. Zs.-Nagy, I. Chemistry, toxicology, pharmacology and pharmacokinetics of idebenone: A review. *Arch. Gerontol. Geriatr.* **1990**, *11*, 177–186. [CrossRef]
236. Di Prospero, N.A.; Sumner, C.J.; Penzak, S.R.; Ravina, B.; Fischbeck, K.H.; Taylor, J.P. Safety, Tolerability, and Pharmacokinetics of High-Dose Idebenone in Patients With Friedreich Ataxia. *Arch. Neurol.* **2007**, *64*, 803–808. [CrossRef] [PubMed]
237. Angebault, C.; Gueguen, N.; Desquiret-Dumas, V.; Chevrollier, A.; Guillet, V.; Verny, C.; Cassereau, J.; Ferré, M.; Milea, D.; Amati-Bonneau, P.; et al. Idebenone increases mitochondrial complex I activity in fibroblasts from LHON patients while producing contradictory effects on respiration. *BMC Res. Notes* **2011**, *4*, 557. [CrossRef] [PubMed]
238. Morvan, D.; Demidem, A. NMR metabolomics of fibroblasts with inherited mitochondrial Complex I mutation reveals treatment-reversible lipid and amino acid metabolism alterations. *Metabolomics* **2018**, *14*, 1–10. [CrossRef]
239. Heitz, F.D.; Erb, M.; Anklin, C.; Robay, D.; Pernet, V.; Gueven, N. Idebenone Protects against Retinal Damage and Loss of Vision in a Mouse Model of Leber's Hereditary Optic Neuropathy. *PLoS ONE* **2012**, *7*, e45182. [CrossRef]
240. Klopstock, T.; Yu-Wai-Man, P.; Dimitriadis, K.; Rouleau, J.; Heck, S.; Bailie, M.; Atawan, A.; Chattopadhyay, S.; Schubert, M.; Garip, A.; et al. A randomized placebo-controlled trial of idebenone in Leber's hereditary optic neuropathy. *Brain* **2011**, *134*, 2677–2686. [CrossRef]
241. Rudolph, G.; Dimitriadis, K.; Büchner, B.; Heck, S.; Al-Tamami, J.; Seidensticker, F.; Rummey, C.; Leinonen, M.; Meier, T.; Klopstock, T. Effects of Idebenone on Color Vision in Patients With Leber Hereditary Optic Neuropathy. *J. Neuro Ophthalmol.* **2013**, *33*, 30–36. [CrossRef]
242. Klopstock, T.; Metz, G.; Yu-Wai-Man, P.; Büchner, B.; Gallenmüller, C.; Bailie, M.; Nwali, N.; Griffiths, P.G.; Von Livonius, B.; Reznicek, L.; et al. Persistence of the treatment effect of idebenone in Leber's hereditary optic neuropathy. *Brain* **2013**, *136*, e230. [CrossRef]
243. Holzerova, E.; Danhauser, K.; Haack, T.B.; Kremer, L.S.; Melcher, M.; Ingold, I.; Kobayashi, S.; Terrile, C.; Wolf, P.; Schaper, J.; et al. Human thioredoxin 2 deficiency impairs mitochondrial redox homeostasis and causes early-onset neurodegeneration. *Brain* **2015**, *139*, 346–354. [CrossRef]

244. Alexander, C.; Votruba, M.; Pesch, U.E.; Thiselton, D.L.; Mayer, S.; Moore, A.; Rodriguez, M.; Kellner, U.; Leo-Kottler, B.; Auburger, G.; et al. OPA1, encoding a dynamin-related GTPase, is mutated in autosomal dominant optic atrophy linked to chromosome 3q28. *Nat. Genet.* **2000**, *26*, 211–215. [CrossRef]
245. Smith, T.; Seto, S.; Ganne, P.; Votruba, M. A randomized, placebo-controlled trial of the benzoquinone idebenone in a mouse model of OPA1-related dominant optic atrophy reveals a limited therapeutic effect on retinal ganglion cell dendropathy and visual function. *Neuroscience* **2016**, *319*, 92–106. [CrossRef] [PubMed]
246. Barboni, P.; Valentino, M.L.; La Morgia, C.; Carbonelli, M.; Savini, G.; De Negri, A.; Simonelli, F.; Sadun, F.; Caporali, L.; Maresca, A.; et al. Idebenone treatment in patients with OPA1-mutant dominant optic atrophy. *Brain* **2013**, *136*, e231. [CrossRef] [PubMed]
247. Romagnoli, M.; La Morgia, C.; Carbonelli, M.; Di Vito, L.; Amore, G.; Zenesini, C.; Cascavilla, M.L.; Barboni, P.; Carelli, V. Idebenone increases chance of stabilization/recovery of visual acuity in OPA1-dominant optic atrophy. *Ann. Clin. Transl. Neurol.* **2020**, *7*, 590–594. [CrossRef] [PubMed]
248. Smith, R.A.; Murphy, M.P. Animal and human studies with the mitochondria-targeted antioxidant MitoQ. *Ann. N. Y. Acad. Sci. USA* **2010**, *1201*, 96–103. [CrossRef]
249. Asin-Cayuela, J.; Manas, A.-R.B.; James, A.M.; Smith, R.A.J.; Murphy, M.P. Fine-tuning the hydrophobicity of a mitochondria-targeted antioxidant. *FEBS Lett.* **2004**, *571*, 9–16. [CrossRef]
250. James, A.M.; Sharpley, M.S.; Manas, A.-R.B.; Frerman, F.E.; Hirst, J.; Smith, R.A.J.; Murphy, M.P. Interaction of the Mitochondria-targeted Antioxidant MitoQ with Phospholipid Bilayers and Ubiquinone Oxidoreductases. *J. Biol. Chem.* **2007**, *282*, 14708–14718. [CrossRef]
251. Jauslin, M.L.; Meier, T.; Smith, R.A.J.; Murphy, P.M. Mitochondria-targeted antioxidants protect Friedreich Ataxia fibroblasts from endogenous oxidative stress more effectively than untargeted antioxidants. *FASEB J.* **2003**, *17*, 1–10. [CrossRef]
252. Rodriguez-Cuenca, S.; Cochemé, H.M.; Logan, A.; Abakumova, I.; Prime, T.A.; Rose, C.; Vidal-Puig, A.; Smith, A.C.; Rubinsztein, D.C.; Fearnley, I.M.; et al. Consequences of long-term oral administration of the mitochondria-targeted antioxidant MitoQ to wild-type mice. *Free Radic. Biol. Med.* **2010**, *48*, 161–172. [CrossRef]
253. Smith, R.A.J.; Porteous, C.M.; Gane, A.M.; Murphy, M.P. Delivery of bioactive molecules to mitochondria in vivo. *Proc. Natl. Acad. Sci. USA* **2003**, *100*, 5407–5412. [CrossRef]
254. Snow, B.; Rolfe, F.L.; Lockhart, M.M.; Frampton, C.M.; O'Sullivan, J.D.; Fung, V.; Smith, R.A.; Murphy, M.P.; Taylor, K.M. A double-blind, placebo-controlled study to assess the mitochondria-targeted antioxidant MitoQ as a disease-modifying therapy in Parkinson's disease. *Mov. Disord.* **2010**, *25*, 1670–1674. [CrossRef]
255. Rossman, M.J.; Santos-Parker, J.R.; Steward, C.A.; Bispham, N.Z.; Cuevas, L.M.; Rosenberg, H.L.; Woodward, K.A.; Chonchol, M.; Gioscia-Ryan, R.A.; Murphy, M.P.; et al. Chronic Supplementation With a Mitochondrial Antioxidant (MitoQ) Improves Vascular Function in Healthy Older Adults. *Hypertension* **2018**, *71*, 1056–1063. [CrossRef] [PubMed]
256. MacKenzie, R.M.; Salt, I.P.; Miller, W.H.; Logan, A.; Ibrahim, H.A.; Degasperi, A.; Dymott, J.A.; Hamilton, C.A.; Murphy, M.P.; Delles, C.; et al. Mitochondrial reactive oxygen species enhance AMP-activated protein kinase activation in the endothelium of patients with coronary artery disease and diabetes. *Clin. Sci.* **2012**, *124*, 403–411. [CrossRef] [PubMed]
257. Gioscia-Ryan, R.A.; Battson, M.L.; Cuevas, L.M.; Eng, J.S.; Murphy, M.P.; Seals, D.R. Mitochondria-targeted antioxidant therapy with MitoQ ameliorates aortic stiffening in old mice. *J. Appl. Physiol.* **2018**, *124*, 1194–1202. [CrossRef] [PubMed]
258. Junior, R.F.R.; Dabkowski, E.R.; Shekar, K.C.; O'connell, K.A.; Hecker, P.A.; Murphy, M.P. MitoQ improves mitochondrial dysfunction in heart failure induced by pressure overload. *Free Radic. Biol. Med.* **2018**, *117*, 18–29. [CrossRef]
259. Enns, G.M.; Kinsman, S.L.; Perlman, S.L.; Spicer, K.M.; Abdenur, J.E.; Cohen, B.H.; Amagata, A.; Barnes, A.; Kheifets, V.; Shrader, W.D.; et al. Initial experience in the treatment of inherited mitochondrial disease with EPI-743. *Mol. Genet. Metab.* **2012**, *105*, 91–102. [CrossRef]
260. Martinelli, D.; Catteruccia, M.; Piemonte, F.; Pastore, A.; Tozzi, G.; Dionisi-Vici, C.; Pontrelli, G.; Corsetti, T.; Livadiotti, S.; Kheifets, V.; et al. EPI-743 reverses the progression of the pediatric mitochondrial disease—Genetically defined Leigh Syndrome. *Mol. Genet. Metab.* **2012**, *107*, 383–388. [CrossRef]

261. Pastore, A.; Petrillo, S.; Tozzi, G.; Carrozzo, R.; Martinelli, D.; Dionisi-Vici, C.; Di Giovamberardino, G.; Ceravolo, F.; Klein, M.B.; Miller, G.; et al. Glutathione: A redox signature in monitoring EPI-743 therapy in children with mitochondrial encephalomyopathies. *Mol. Genet. Metab.* **2013**, *109*, 208–214. [CrossRef]
262. Kouga, T.; Takagi, M.; Miyauchi, A.; Shimbo, H.; Iai, M.; Yamashita, S.; Murayama, K.; Klein, M.B.; Miller, G.; Goto, T.; et al. Japanese Leigh syndrome case treated with EPI-743. *Brain Dev.* **2018**, *40*, 145–149. [CrossRef]
263. Sadun, A.A.; Chicani, C.F.; Ross-Cisneros, F.N.; Barboni, P.; Thoolen, M.; Shrader, W.D.; Kubis, K.; Carelli, V.; Miller, G. Effect of EPI-743 on the Clinical Course of the Mitochondrial Disease Leber Hereditary Optic Neuropathy. *Arch. Neurol.* **2012**, *69*, 331–338. [CrossRef]
264. Lynch, D.R.; Willi, S.M.; Wilson, R.B.; Cotticelli, M.G.; Brigatti, K.W.; Deutsch, E.C.; Kucheruk, O.; Shrader, W.; Rioux, P.; Miller, G.; et al. A0001 in Friedreich ataxia: Biochemical characterization and effects in a clinical trial. *Mov. Disord.* **2012**, *27*, 1026–1033. [CrossRef]
265. Frantz, M.-C.; Skoda, E.M.; Sacher, J.R.; Epperly, M.W.; Goff, J.P.; Greenberger, J.S.; Wipf, P. Synthesis of analogs of the radiation mitigator JP4-039 and visualization of BODIPY derivatives in mitochondria. *Org. Biomol. Chem.* **2013**, *11*, 4147–4153. [CrossRef] [PubMed]
266. Leipnitz, G.; Mohsen, A.-W.; Karunanidhi, A.; Seminotti, B.; Roginskaya, V.Y.; Markantone, D.M.; Grings, M.; Mihalik, S.J.; Wipf, P.; Van Houten, B.; et al. Evaluation of mitochondrial bioenergetics, dynamics, endoplasmic reticulum-mitochondria crosstalk, and reactive oxygen species in fibroblasts from patients with complex I deficiency. *Sci. Rep.* **2018**, *8*, 1–14. [CrossRef] [PubMed]
267. Seminotti, B.; Leipnitz, G.; Karunanidhi, A.; Kochersperger, C.; Roginskaya, V.Y.; Basu, S.; Wang, Y.; Wipf, P.; Van Houten, B.; Mohsen, A.-W.; et al. Mitochondrial energetics is impaired in very long-chain acyl-CoA dehydrogenase deficiency and can be rescued by treatment with mitochondria-targeted electron scavengers. *Hum. Mol. Genet.* **2019**, *28*, 928–941. [CrossRef] [PubMed]
268. Beyrath, J.; Pellegrini, M.; Renkema, H.; Houben, L.; Pecheritsyna, S.; Van Zandvoort, P.; Broek, P.V.D.; Bekel, A.; Eftekhari, P.; Smeitink, J.A.M. KH176 Safeguards Mitochondrial Diseased Cells from Redox Stress-Induced Cell Death by Interacting with the Thioredoxin System/Peroxiredoxin Enzyme Machinery. *Sci. Rep.* **2018**, *8*, 1–14. [CrossRef]
269. De Haas, R.; Das, D.; Garanto, A.; Renkema, H.G.; Greupink, R.; Broek, P.V.D.; Pertijs, J.; Collin, R.W.J.; Willems, P.; Beyrath, J.; et al. Therapeutic effects of the mitochondrial ROS-redox modulator KH176 in a mammalian model of Leigh Disease. *Sci. Rep.* **2017**, *7*, 1–11. [CrossRef]
270. Frambach, S.J.; Van De Wal, M.A.; Broek, P.H.V.D.; Smeitink, J.A.; Russel, F.G.; De Haas, R.; Schirris, T.J.J. Effects of clofibrate and KH176 on life span and motor function in mitochondrial complex I-deficient mice. *Biochim. Biophys. Acta (BBA) Mol. Basis Dis.* **2020**, *1866*, 165727. [CrossRef]
271. Koene, S.; Spaans, E.; Van Bortel, L.M.; Van Lancker, G.; Delafontaine, B.; Badilini, F.; Beyrath, J.; Smeitink, J. KH176 under development for rare mitochondrial disease: A first in man randomized controlled clinical trial in healthy male volunteers. *Orphanet J. Rare Dis.* **2017**, *12*, 163. [CrossRef]
272. Janssen, M.C.; Koene, S.; De Laat, P.; Hemelaar, P.; Pickkers, P.; Spaans, E.; Beukema, R.; Beyrath, J.; Groothuis, J.; Verhaak, C.; et al. The KHENERGY Study: Safety and Efficacy of KH 176 in Mitochondrial m.3243A>G Spectrum Disorders. *Clin. Pharmacol. Ther.* **2019**, *105*, 101–111. [CrossRef]
273. Khondrion Receives Rare Pediatric Disease Designation for Sonlicromanol from US FDA. GlobeNewswire News Room. 28 September 2020. Available online: http://www.globenewswire.com/news-release/2020/09/28/2099659/0/en/Khondrion-Receives-Rare-Pediatric-Disease-Designation-for-Sonlicromanol-from-US-FDA.html (accessed on 6 October 2020).
274. Antonenko, Y.N.; Avetisyan, A.V.; Bakeeva, L.E.; Chernyak, B.V.; Chertkov, V.A.; Domnina, L.V.; Ivanova, O.Y.; Izyumov, D.S.; Khailova, L.S.; Klishin, S.S.; et al. Mitochondria-targeted plastoquinone derivatives as tools to interrupt execution of the aging program. 1. Cationic plastoquinone derivatives: Synthesis and in vitro studies. *Biochemistry* **2008**, *73*, 1273–1287. [CrossRef]
275. Severin, F.F.; Severina, I.I.; Antonenko, Y.N.; Rokitskaya, T.I.; Cherepanov, D.A.; Mokhova, E.N.; Vyssokikh, M.Y.; Pustovidko, A.V.; Markova, O.V.; Yaguzhinsky, L.S.; et al. Penetrating cation/fatty acid anion pair as a mitochondria-targeted protonophore. *Proc. Natl. Acad. Sci. USA* **2010**, *107*, 663–668. [CrossRef]

276. Lyamzaev, K.G.; Panteleeva, A.A.; Karpukhina, A.A.; Galkin, I.I.; Popova, E.N.; Pletjushkina, O.Y.; Rieger, B.; Busch, K.B.; Mulkidjanian, A.Y.; Chernyak, B.V. Novel Fluorescent Mitochondria-Targeted Probe MitoCLox Reports Lipid Peroxidation in Response to Oxidative Stress In Vivo. *Oxidative Med. Cell. Longev.* **2020**, *2020*, 1–11. [CrossRef] [PubMed]
277. Stefanova, N.A.; Ershov, N.I.; Kolosova, N.G. Suppression of Alzheimer's Disease-Like Pathology Progression by Mitochondria-Targeted Antioxidant SkQ1: A Transcriptome Profiling Study. *Oxidative Med. Cell. Longev.* **2019**, *2019*, 3984906-17. [CrossRef] [PubMed]
278. Kolosova, N.G.; Tyumentsev, M.A.; Muraleva, N.A.; Kiseleva, E.; Vitovtov, A.O.; Stefanova, N.A. Antioxidant SkQ1 Alleviates Signs of Alzheimer's Disease-like Pathology in Old OXYS Rats by Reversing Mitochondrial Deterioration. *Curr. Alzheimer Res.* **2017**, *14*, 1283–1292. [CrossRef] [PubMed]
279. Fetisova, E.K.; Muntyan, M.S.; Lyamzaev, K.G.; Chernyak, B.V. Therapeutic Effect of the Mitochondria-Targeted Antioxidant SkQ1 on the Culture Model of Multiple Sclerosis. *Oxidative Med. Cell. Longev.* **2019**, *2019*, 1–10. [CrossRef]
280. Veretinskaya, A.G.; Podshivalova, L.S.; Frolova, O.Y.; Belopolskaya, M.V.; Averina, O.A.; Kushnir, E.A.; Marmiy, N.V.; Lovat, M.L. Effects of mitochondrial antioxidant SkQ1 on biochemical and behavioral parameters in a Parkinsonism model in mice. *Biochemistry* **2017**, *82*, 1513–1520. [CrossRef]
281. Shabalina, I.G.; Vyssokikh, M.Y.; Gibanova, N.; Csikasz, R.I.; Edgar, D.; Hallden-Waldemarson, A.; Rozhdestvenskaya, Z.; Bakeeva, L.E.; Vays, V.B.; Pustovidko, A.V.; et al. Improved health-span and lifespan in mtDNA mutator mice treated with the mitochondrially targeted antioxidant SkQ1. *Aging* **2017**, *9*, 315–339. [CrossRef]
282. Edgar, D.; Trifunovic, A. The mtDNA mutator mouse: Dissecting mitochondrial involvement in aging. *Aging* **2009**, *1*, 1028–1032. [CrossRef]
283. Tilokani, L.; Nagashima, S.; Paupe, V.; Prudent, J. Mitochondrial dynamics: Overview of molecular mechanisms. *Essays Biochem.* **2018**, *62*, 341–360. [CrossRef]
284. Friedman, J.R.; Nunnari, J. Mitochondrial form and function. *Nat. Cell Biol.* **2014**, *505*, 335–343. [CrossRef]
285. Frezza, C.; Cipolat, S.; De Brito, O.M.; Micaroni, M.; Beznoussenko, G.V.; Rudka, T.; Bartoli, D.; Polishuck, R.S.; Danial, N.N.; De Strooper, B.; et al. OPA1 Controls Apoptotic Cristae Remodeling Independently from Mitochondrial Fusion. *Cell* **2006**, *126*, 177–189. [CrossRef]
286. Lapuente-Brun, E.; Moreno-Loshuertos, R.; Acín-Pérez, R.; Latorre-Pellicer, A.; Colás, C.; Balsa, E.; Perales-Clemente, E.; Quirós, P.M.; Calvo, E.; Rodríguez-Hernández, Á.; et al. Supercomplex Assembly Determines Electron Flux in the Mitochondrial Electron Transport Chain. *Science* **2013**, *340*, 1567–1570. [CrossRef] [PubMed]
287. Cogliati, S.; Frezza, C.; Soriano, M.E.; Varanita, T.; Quintana-Cabrera, R.; Corrado, M.; Cipolat, S.; Costa, V.; Casarin, A.; Gomes, L.C.; et al. Mitochondrial Cristae Shape Determines Respiratory Chain Supercomplexes Assembly and Respiratory Efficiency. *Cell* **2013**, *155*, 160–171. [CrossRef] [PubMed]
288. Delettre, C.; Lenaers, G.; Pelloquin, L.; Belenguer, P.; Hamel, C.P. OPA1 (Kjer type) dominant optic atrophy: A novel mitochondrial disease. *Mol. Genet. Metab.* **2002**, *75*, 97–107. [CrossRef] [PubMed]
289. Delettre, C.; Lenaers, G.; Griffoin, J.-M.; Gigarel, N.; Lorenzo, C.; Belenguer, P.; Pelloquin, L.; Grosgeorge, J.; Turc-Carel, C.; Perret, E.; et al. Nuclear gene OPA1, encoding a mitochondrial dynamin-related protein, is mutated in dominant optic atrophy. *Nat. Genet.* **2000**, *26*, 207–210. [CrossRef]
290. Züchner, S.; Mersiyanova, I.V.; Muglia, M.; Bissar-Tadmouri, N.; Rochelle, J.M.; Dadali, E.L.; Zappia, M.; Nelis, E.; Patitucci, A.; Senderek, J.P.; et al. Mutations in the mitochondrial GTPase mitofusin 2 cause Charcot-Marie-Tooth neuropathy type 2A. *Nat. Genet.* **2004**, *36*, 449–451. [CrossRef]
291. Waterham, H.R.; Koster, J.; Van Roermund, C.W.T.; Mooyer, P.A.W.; Wanders, R.J.A.; Leonard, J.V. A Lethal Defect of Mitochondrial and Peroxisomal Fission. *N. Engl. J. Med.* **2007**, *356*, 1736–1741. [CrossRef]
292. Shamseldin, H.E.; Alshammari, M.; Al-Sheddi, T.; Salih, M.A.; Alkhalidi, H.; Kentab, A.; Repetto, G.M.; Hashem, M.; Alkuraya, F.S. Genomic analysis of mitochondrial diseases in a consanguineous population reveals novel candidate disease genes. *J. Med. Genet.* **2012**, *49*, 234–241. [CrossRef]
293. Civiletto, G.; Varanita, T.; Cerutti, R.; Gorletta, T.; Barbaro, S.; Marchet, S.; Lamperti, C.; Viscomi, C.; Scorrano, L.; Zeviani, M. Opa1 Overexpression Ameliorates the Phenotype of Two Mitochondrial Disease Mouse Models. *Cell Metab.* **2015**, *21*, 845–854. [CrossRef]
294. Zeviani, M.; Luna-Sanchez, M.; Scorrano, L.; Viscomi, C.; Calvo, G.B. Opa1 overexpression protects from early onset Mpv17-/-related mouse kidney disease. *Mol. Ther.* **2020**. [CrossRef]

295. Cassidy-Stone, A.; Chipuk, J.E.; Ingerman, E.; Song, C.; Yoo, C.; Kuwana, T.; Kurth, M.J.; Shaw, J.T.; Hinshaw, J.E.; Green, D.R.; et al. Chemical Inhibition of the Mitochondrial Division Dynamin Reveals Its Role in Bax/Bak-Dependent Mitochondrial Outer Membrane Permeabilization. *Dev. Cell* **2008**, *14*, 193–204. [CrossRef]
296. Wang, D.; Wang, J.; Bonamy, G.M.C.; Meeusen, S.; Brusch, R.G.; Turk, C.; Yang, P.-Y.; Schultz, P.G. A Small Molecule Promotes Mitochondrial Fusion in Mammalian Cells. *Angew. Chem. Int. Ed.* **2012**, *51*, 9302–9305. [CrossRef]
297. Qi, X.; Qvit, N.; Su, Y.-C.; Mochly-Rosen, D. A novel Drp1 inhibitor diminishes aberrant mitochondrial fission and neurotoxicity. *J. Cell Sci.* **2013**, *126*, 789–802. [CrossRef] [PubMed]
298. Bartolák-Suki, E.; Imsirovic, J.; Nishibori, Y.; Krishnan, R.; Suki, B. Regulation of Mitochondrial Structure and Dynamics by the Cytoskeleton and Mechanical Factors. *Int. J. Mol. Sci.* **2017**, *18*, 1812. [CrossRef] [PubMed]
299. Flatau, G.; Lemichez, E.; Gauthier, M.J.; Chardin, P.; Paris, S.; Fiorentini, C.; Boquet, P. Toxin-induced activation of the G protein p21 Rho by deamidation of glutamine. *Nat. Cell Biol.* **1997**, *387*, 729–733. [CrossRef] [PubMed]
300. Fabbri, A.; Travaglione, S.; Maroccia, Z.; Guidotti, M.; Pierri, C.; Primiano, G.; Servidei, S.; Loizzo, S.; Fiorentini, C. The Bacterial Protein CNF1 as a Potential Therapeutic Strategy against Mitochondrial Diseases: A Pilot Study. *Int. J. Mol. Sci.* **2018**, *19*, 1825. [CrossRef] [PubMed]
301. Karaa, A.; Haas, R.; Goldstein, A.; Vockley, J.; Weaver, W.D.; Cohen, B.H. Randomized dose-escalation trial of elamipretide in adults with primary mitochondrial myopathy. *Neurology* **2018**, *90*, e1212–e1221. [CrossRef] [PubMed]
302. Schlame, M.; Ren, M. The role of cardiolipin in the structural organization of mitochondrial membranes. *Biochim. Biophys. Acta (BBA) Biomembr.* **2009**, *1788*, 2080–2083. [CrossRef] [PubMed]
303. Zhang, M.; Mileykovskaya, E.; Dowhan, W. Cardiolipin is essential for organization of complexes III and IV into a supercomplex in intact yeast mitochondria. *J. Biol. Chem.* **2005**, *280*, 29403–29408. [CrossRef]
304. Manczak, M.; Mao, P.; Calkins, M.J.; Cornea, A.; Reddy, A.P.; Murphy, M.P.; Szeto, H.H.; Park, B.; Reddy, P.H. Mitochondria-Targeted Antioxidants Protect Against Amyloid-β Toxicity in Alzheimer's Disease Neurons. *J. Alzheimers Dis.* **2010**, *20*, S609–S631. [CrossRef]
305. Birk, A.V.; Liu, S.; Soong, Y.; Mills, W.; Singh, P.; Warren, J.D.; Seshan, S.V.; Pardee, J.D.; Szeto, H.H. The Mitochondrial-Targeted Compound SS-31 Re-Energizes Ischemic Mitochondria by Interacting with Cardiolipin. *J. Am. Soc. Nephrol.* **2013**, *24*, 1250–1261. [CrossRef]
306. Dai, D.-F.; Hsieh, E.J.; Chen, T.; Menendez, L.G.; Basisty, N.B.; Tsai, L.; Beyer, R.P.; Crispin, D.A.; Shulman, N.J.; Szeto, H.H.; et al. Global Proteomics and Pathway Analysis of Pressure-Overload–Induced Heart Failure and Its Attenuation by Mitochondrial-Targeted Peptides. *Circ. Heart Fail.* **2013**, *6*, 1067–1076. [CrossRef]
307. Neil, E.E.; Bisaccia, E.K. Nusinersen: A Novel Antisense Oligonucleotide for the Treatment of Spinal Muscular Atrophy. *J. Pediatr. Pharmacol. Ther.* **2019**, *24*, 194–203. [CrossRef] [PubMed]
308. Siegel, M.P.; Kruse, S.E.; Percival, J.M.; Goh, J.; White, C.C.; Hopkins, H.C.; Kavanagh, T.J.; Szeto, H.H.; Rabinovitch, P.S.; Marcinek, D.J. Mitochondrial-targeted peptide rapidly improves mitochondrial energetics and skeletal muscle performance in aged mice. *Aging Cell* **2013**, *12*, 763–771. [CrossRef] [PubMed]
309. Kloner, R.A.; Shi, J.; Dai, W. New therapies for reducing post-myocardial left ventricular remodeling. *Ann. Transl. Med.* **2015**, *3*. [CrossRef]
310. Karaa, A.; Haas, R.; Goldstein, A.; Vockley, J.; Cohen, B.H. A randomized crossover trial of elamipretide in adults with primary mitochondrial myopathy. *J. Cachex Sarcopenia Muscle* **2020**, *11*, 909–918. [CrossRef] [PubMed]
311. Bento, C.F.; Renna, M.; Ghislat, G.; Puri, C.; Ashkenazi, A.; Vicinanza, M.; Menzies, F.M.; Rubinsztein, D.C. Mammalian Autophagy: How Does It Work? *Annu. Rev. Biochem.* **2016**, *85*, 685–713. [CrossRef]
312. Saxton, R.A.; Sabatini, D.M. mTOR Signaling in Growth, Metabolism, and Disease. *Cell* **2017**, *168*, 960–976. [CrossRef]
313. Johnson, S.C.; Yanos, M.E.; Kayser, E.-B.; Quintana, A.; Sangesland, M.; Castanza, A.; Uhde, L.; Hui, J.; Wall, V.Z.; Gagnidze, A.; et al. mTOR Inhibition Alleviates Mitochondrial Disease in a Mouse Model of Leigh Syndrome. *Science* **2013**, *342*, 1524–1528. [CrossRef]
314. Civiletto, G.; Dogan, S.A.; Cerutti, R.; Fagiolari, G.; Moggio, M.; Lamperti, C.; Benincá, C.; Viscomi, C.; Zeviani, M. Rapamycin rescues mitochondrial myopathy via coordinated activation of autophagy and lysosomal biogenesis. *EMBO Mol. Med.* **2018**, *10*, e8799. [CrossRef]

315. Wang, A.; Mouser, J.; Pitt, J.; Promislow, D.; Kaeberlein, M. Rapamycin enhances survival in a Drosophila model of mitochondrial disease. *Oncotarget* **2016**, *7*, 80131–80139. [CrossRef]
316. Zheng, X.; Boyer, L.; Jin, M.; Kim, Y.; Fan, W.; Bardy, C.; Berggren, T.; Evans, R.M.; Gage, F.H.; Hunter, T. Alleviation of neuronal energy deficiency by mTOR inhibition as a treatment for mitochondria-related neurodegeneration. *eLife* **2016**, *5*. [CrossRef]
317. Peng, M.; Ostrovsky, J.; Kwon, Y.J.; Polyak, E.; Licata, J.; Tsukikawa, M.; Marty, E.; Thomas, J.; Felix, C.A.; Xiao, R.; et al. Inhibiting cytosolic translation and autophagy improves health in mitochondrial disease. *Hum. Mol. Genet.* **2015**, *24*, 4829–4847. [CrossRef] [PubMed]
318. Johnson, S.C.; Martinez, F.; Bitto, A.; Gonzalez, B.; Tazaerslan, C.; Cohen, C.; Delaval, L.; Timsit, J.; Knebelmann, B.; Terzi, F.; et al. mTOR inhibitors may benefit kidney transplant recipients with mitochondrial diseases. *Kidney Int.* **2019**, *95*, 455–466. [CrossRef] [PubMed]
319. Sage-Schwaede, A.; Engelstad, K.; Salazar, R.; Curcio, A.; Khandji, A.; Jr, J.H.G.; De Vivo, D.C. Exploring mTOR inhibition as treatment for mitochondrial disease. *Ann. Clin. Transl. Neurol.* **2019**, *6*, 1877–1881. [CrossRef] [PubMed]
320. Barriocanal-Casado, E.; Hidalgo-Gutiérrez, A.; Raimundo, N.; González-García, P.; Acuña-Castroviejo, D.; Escames, G.; López, L.C. Rapamycin administration is not a valid therapeutic strategy for every case of mitochondrial disease. *EBioMedicine* **2019**, *42*, 511–523. [CrossRef] [PubMed]
321. Opelz, G.; Unterrainer, C.; Süsal, C.; Döhler, B. Immunosuppression with mammalian target of rapamycin inhibitor and incidence of post-transplant cancer in kidney transplant recipients. *Nephrol. Dial. Transplant.* **2016**, *31*, 1360–1367. [CrossRef]
322. Seo, B.B.; Matsuno-Yagi, A.; Yagi, T. Modulation of oxidative phosphorylation of human kidney 293 cells by transfection with the internal rotenone-insensitive NADH-quinone oxidoreductase (NDI1) gene of Saccharomyces cerevisiae. *Biochim. Biophys. Acta (BBA) Bioenerg.* **1999**, *1412*, 56–65. [CrossRef]
323. Rasmusson, A.G.; Soole, K.L.; Elthon, T.E. ALTERNATIVE NAD(P)H DEHYDROGENASES OF PLANT MITOCHONDRIA. *Annu. Rev. Plant Biol.* **2004**, *55*, 23–39. [CrossRef]
324. Sanz, A.; Soikkeli, M.; Portero-Otín, M.; Wilson, A.; Kemppainen, E.; McIlroy, G.; Ellilä, S.; Kemppainen, K.K.; Tuomela, T.; Lakanmaa, M.; et al. Expression of the yeast NADH dehydrogenase Ndi1 in Drosophila confers increased lifespan independently of dietary restriction. *Proc. Natl. Acad. Sci. USA* **2010**, *107*, 9105–9110. [CrossRef]
325. Perales-Clemente, E.; Bayona-Bafaluy, M.P.; Pérez-Martos, A.; Barrientos, A.; Fernández-Silva, P.; Enriquez, J.A. Restoration of electron transport without proton pumping in mammalian mitochondria. *Proc. Natl. Acad. Sci. USA* **2008**, *105*, 18735–18739. [CrossRef]
326. Dassa, E.P.; Dufour, E.; Goncalves, S.; Paupe, V.; Hakkaart, G.A.J.; Jacobs, H.T.; Rustin, P. Expression of the alternative oxidase complements cytochrome c oxidase deficiency in human cells. *EMBO Mol. Med.* **2009**, *1*, 30–36. [CrossRef]
327. Fernandez-Ayala, D.J.; Sanz, A.; Vartiainen, S.; Kemppainen, K.K.; Babusiak, M.; Mustalahti, E.; Costa, R.; Tuomela, T.; Zeviani, M.; Chung, J.; et al. Expression of the Ciona intestinalis Alternative Oxidase (AOX) in Drosophila Complements Defects in Mitochondrial Oxidative Phosphorylation. *Cell Metab.* **2009**, *9*, 449–460. [CrossRef] [PubMed]
328. Chadderton, N.; Palfi, A.; Millington-Ward, S.; Gobbo, O.; Overlack, N.; Carrigan, M.; O'Reilly, M.; Campbell, M.T.; Ehrhardt, C.; Wolfrum, U.; et al. Intravitreal delivery of AAV-NDI1 provides functional benefit in a murine model of Leber hereditary optic neuropathy. *Eur. J. Hum. Genet.* **2013**, *21*, 62–68. [CrossRef] [PubMed]
329. McElroy, G.S.; Reczek, C.R.; Reyfman, P.A.; Mithal, D.S.; Horbinski, C.M.; Chandel, N.S. NAD+ Regeneration Rescues Lifespan, but Not Ataxia, in a Mouse Model of Brain Mitochondrial Complex I Dysfunction. *Cell Metab.* **2020**, *32*, 301–308.e6. [CrossRef] [PubMed]
330. Rapola, J.; Heikkilä, P.; Fellman, V. Pathology of lethal fetal growth retardation syndrome with aminoaciduria, iron overload, and lactic acidosis (GRACILE). *Pediatr. Pathol. Mol. Med.* **2002**, *21*, 183–193. [CrossRef] [PubMed]
331. Fellman, V.; Rapola, J.; Pihko, H.; Varilo, T.; Raivio, K.O. Iron-overload disease in infants involving fetal growth retardation, lactic acidosis, liver haemosiderosis, and aminoaciduria. *Lancet* **1998**, *351*, 490–493. [CrossRef]

332. Dogan, S.A.; Cerutti, R.; Benincá, C.; Brea-Calvo, G.; Jacobs, H.T.; Zeviani, M.; Szibor, M.; Viscomi, C. Perturbed Redox Signaling Exacerbates a Mitochondrial Myopathy. *Cell Metab.* **2018**, *28*, 764–775.e5. [CrossRef]
333. Catania, A.; Iuso, A.; Bouchereau, J.; Kremer, L.S.; Paviolo, M.; Terrile, C.; Bénit, P.; Rasmusson, A.G.; Schwarzmayr, T.; Tiranti, V.; et al. Arabidopsis thaliana alternative dehydrogenases: A potential therapy for mitochondrial complex I deficiency? Perspectives and pitfalls. *Orphanet J. Rare Dis.* **2019**, *14*, 236. [CrossRef]
334. Houshmand, M.; Holme, E.; Oldfors, A.; Holmberg, E. De novo mutation in the mitochondrial ATP synthase subunit 6 gene (T8993G) with rapid segregation resulting in Leigh syndrome in the offspring. *Qual. Life Res.* **1995**, *96*, 290–294. [CrossRef]
335. Carling, P.J.; Cree, L.M.; Chinnery, P.F. The implications of mitochondrial DNA copy number regulation during embryogenesis. *Mitochondrion* **2011**, *11*, 686–692. [CrossRef]
336. Wei, W.; Chinnery, P.F. Inheritance of mitochondrial DNA in humans: Implications for rare and common diseases. *J. Intern. Med.* **2020**, *287*, 634–644. [CrossRef]
337. Rai, P.K.; Craven, L.; Hoogewijs, K.; Russell, O.M.; Chrzanowska-Lightowlers, Z. Advances in methods for reducing mitochondrial DNA disease by replacing or manipulating the mitochondrial genome. *Essays Biochem.* **2018**, *62*, 455–465. [CrossRef] [PubMed]
338. Sallevelt, S.C.E.H.; Dreesen, J.C.F.M.; Coonen, E.; Paulussen, A.D.C.; El Hellebrekers, D.M.; Die-Smulders, C.E.M.D.; Smeets, H.J.M.; Lindsey, P. Preimplantation genetic diagnosis for mitochondrial DNA mutations: Analysis of one blastomere suffices. *J. Med. Genet.* **2017**, *54*, 693–697. [CrossRef] [PubMed]
339. Treff, N.R.; Campos, J.; Tao, X.; Levy, B.; Ferry, K.M.; Scott, R.T. Blastocyst preimplantation genetic diagnosis (PGD) of a mitochondrial DNA disorder. *Fertil. Steril.* **2012**, *98*, 1236–1240. [CrossRef]
340. Craven, L.; Tuppen, H.A.; Greggains, G.D.; Harbottle, S.J.; Murphy, J.L.; Cree, L.M.; Murdoch, A.P.; Chinnery, P.F.; Taylor, R.W.; Lightowlers, R.N.; et al. Pronuclear transfer in human embryos to prevent transmission of mitochondrial DNA disease. *Nat. Cell Biol.* **2010**, *465*, 82–85. [CrossRef] [PubMed]
341. Herbert, M.; Turnbull, D. Progress in mitochondrial replacement therapies. *Nat. Rev. Mol. Cell Biol.* **2018**, *19*, 71–72. [CrossRef]
342. Craven, L.; Tang, M.-X.; Gorman, G.S.; De Sutter, P.; Heindryckx, B. Novel reproductive technologies to prevent mitochondrial disease. *Hum. Reprod. Update* **2017**, *23*, 501–519. [CrossRef]
343. Ishii, T.; Hibino, Y. Mitochondrial manipulation in fertility clinics: Regulation and responsibility. *Reprod. Biomed. Soc. Online* **2018**, *5*, 93–109. [CrossRef]
344. Tachibana, M.; Sparman, M.; Sritanaudomchai, H.; Ma, H.; Clepper, L.; Woodward, J.; Li, Y.; Ramsey, C.; Kolotushkina, O.; Mitalipov, S. Mitochondrial gene replacement in primate offspring and embryonic stem cells. *Nat. Cell Biol.* **2009**, *461*, 367–372. [CrossRef]
345. Kang, E.; Wu, J.; Gutierrez, N.M.; Koski, A.; Tippner-Hedges, R.; Agaronyan, K.; Platero-Luengo, A.; Martinez-Redondo, P.; Ma, H.; Lee, Y.; et al. Mitochondrial replacement in human oocytes carrying pathogenic mitochondrial DNA mutations. *Nat. Cell Biol.* **2016**, *540*, 270–275. [CrossRef]
346. Zhang, J.; Liu, H.; Luo, S.; Chavez-Badiola, A.; Liu, Z.; Yang, M.; Munne, S.; Konstantinidis, M.; Wells, D.; Huang, T. First live birth using human oocytes reconstituted by spindle nuclear transfer for mitochondrial DNA mutation causing Leigh syndrome. *Fertil. Steril.* **2016**, *106*, e375–e376. [CrossRef]
347. Hudson, G.; Takeda, Y.; Herbert, M. Reversion after replacement of mitochondrial DNA. *Nature* **2019**, *574*. [CrossRef]
348. Zhang, J.; Liu, H.; Luo, S.; Lu, Z.; Chávez-Badiola, A.; Liu, Z.; Yang, M.; Merhi, Z.; Silber, S.J.; Munné, S.; et al. Live birth derived from oocyte spindle transfer to prevent mitochondrial disease. *Reprod. Biomed. Online* **2017**, *34*, 361–368. [CrossRef] [PubMed]
349. Sato, A.; Kono, T.; Nakada, K.; Ishikawa, K.; Inoue, S.-I.; Yonekawa, H.; Hayashi, J.-I. Gene therapy for progeny of mito-mice carrying pathogenic mtDNA by nuclear transplantation. *Proc. Natl. Acad. Sci. USA* **2005**, *102*, 16765–16770. [CrossRef] [PubMed]
350. Hyslop, L.A.; Blakeley, P.; Craven, L.; Richardson, J.; Fogarty, N.M.E.; Fragouli, E.; Lamb, M.; Wamaitha, S.E.; Prathalingam, N.; Zhang, Q.; et al. Towards clinical application of pronuclear transfer to prevent mitochondrial DNA disease. *Nat. Cell Biol.* **2016**, *534*, 383–386. [CrossRef] [PubMed]
351. Yasuzaki, Y.; Yamada, Y.; Harashima, H. Mitochondrial matrix delivery using MITO-Porter, a liposome-based carrier that specifies fusion with mitochondrial membranes. *Biochem. Biophys. Res. Commun.* **2010**, *397*, 181–186. [CrossRef]

352. Yamada, Y.; Harashima, H. Targeting the Mitochondrial Genome via a Dual Function MITO-Porter: Evaluation of mtDNA Levels and Mitochondrial Function. *Methods Mol. Biol.* **2015**, *1265*, 123–133. [CrossRef]
353. Lyrawati, D.; Trounson, A.; Cram, D. Expression of GFP in the Mitochondrial Compartment Using DQAsome-Mediated Delivery of an Artificial Mini-mitochondrial Genome. *Pharm. Res.* **2011**, *28*, 2848–2862. [CrossRef]
354. Mahata, B.; Mukherjee, S.; Mishra, S.; Bandyopadhyay, A.; Adhya, S. Functional Delivery of a Cytosolic tRNA into Mutant Mitochondria of Human Cells. *Science* **2006**, *314*, 471–474. [CrossRef]
355. Kawamura, E.; Maruyama, M.; Abe, J.; Sudo, A.; Takeda, A.; Takada, S.; Yokota, T.; Kinugawa, S.; Harashima, H.; Yamada, Y. Validation of Gene Therapy for Mutant Mitochondria by Delivering Mitochondrial RNA Using a MITO-Porter. *Mol. Ther. Nucleic Acids* **2020**, *20*, 687–698. [CrossRef]
356. Yamada, Y.; Somiya, K.; Miyauchi, A.; Osaka, H.; Harashima, H. Validation of a mitochondrial RNA therapeutic strategy using fibroblasts from a Leigh syndrome patient with a mutation in the mitochondrial ND3 gene. *Sci. Rep.* **2020**, *10*, 1–13. [CrossRef]
357. Weissig, V. DQAsomes as the Prototype of Mitochondria-Targeted Pharmaceutical Nanocarriers: Preparation, Characterization, and Use. *Methods Mol. Biol.* **2015**, *1265*, 1–11. [CrossRef] [PubMed]
358. Adhya, S. Leishmania mitochondrial tRNA importers. *Int. J. Biochem. Cell Biol.* **2008**, *40*, 2681–2685. [CrossRef] [PubMed]
359. Tanaka, M.; Borgeld, H.-J.; Zhang, J.; Muramatsu, S.-I.; Gong, J.-S.; Yoneda, M.; Maruyama, W.; Naoi, M.; Ibi, T.; Sahashi, K.; et al. Gene Therapy for Mitochondrial Disease by Delivering Restriction Endonuclease SmaI into Mitochondria. *J. Biomed. Sci.* **2002**, *9*, 534–541. [CrossRef] [PubMed]
360. Comte, C.; Tonin, Y.; Heckel-Mager, A.-M.; Boucheham, A.; Smirnov, A.; Auré, K.; Lombès, A.; Martin, R.P.; Entelis, N.; Tarassov, I. Mitochondrial targeting of recombinant RNAs modulates the level of a heteroplasmic mutation in human mitochondrial DNA associated with Kearns Sayre Syndrome. *Nucleic Acids Res.* **2013**, *41*, 418–433. [CrossRef]
361. Jo, A.; Ham, S.; Lee, G.H.; Lee, Y.-S.; Kim, S.; Shin, J.-H.; Lee, Y. Efficient Mitochondrial Genome Editing by CRISPR/Cas9. *BioMed Res. Int.* **2015**, *2015*, 1–10. [CrossRef]
362. Moretton, A.; Morel, F.; Macao, B.; Lachaume, P.; Ishak, L.; Lefebvre, M.; Garreau-Balandier, I.; Vernet, P.; Falkenberg, M.; Farge, G. Selective mitochondrial DNA degradation following double-strand breaks. *PLoS ONE* **2017**, *12*, e0176795. [CrossRef]
363. Hussain, S.-R.A.; Yalvac, M.E.; Khoo, B.; Eckardt, S.; McLaughlin, K.J. Adapting CRISPR/Cas9 System for Targeting Mitochondrial Genome. *BioRxiv* **2020**. [CrossRef]
364. Gammage, P.A.; Moraes, C.T.; Minczuk, M. Mitochondrial Genome Engineering: The Revolution May Not Be CRISPR-Ized. *Trends Genet.* **2018**, *34*, 101–110. [CrossRef]
365. Kauppila, J.H.; Baines, H.L.; Bratic, A.; Simard, M.-L.; Freyer, C.; Mourier, A.; Stamp, C.; Filograna, R.; Larsson, N.-G.; Greaves, L.C.; et al. A Phenotype-Driven Approach to Generate Mouse Models with Pathogenic mtDNA Mutations Causing Mitochondrial Disease. *Cell Rep.* **2016**, *16*, 2980–2990. [CrossRef]
366. Gammage, P.A.; Viscomi, C.; Simard, M.-L.; Costa, A.S.H.; Gaude, E.; Powell, C.A.; Van Haute, L.; McCann, B.J.; Rebelo-Guiomar, P.; Cerutti, R.; et al. Genome editing in mitochondria corrects a pathogenic mtDNA mutation in vivo. *Nat. Med.* **2018**, *24*, 1691–1695. [CrossRef]
367. Bacman, S.R.; Kauppila, J.H.K.; Pereira, C.V.; Nissanka, N.; Miranda, M.; Pinto, M.; Williams, S.L.; Larsson, N.-G.; Stewart, J.B.; Moraes, C.T. MitoTALEN reduces mutant mtDNA load and restores tRNAAla levels in a mouse model of heteroplasmic mtDNA mutation. *Nat. Med.* **2018**, *24*, 1696–1700. [CrossRef] [PubMed]
368. Mok, B.Y.; De Moraes, M.H.; Zeng, J.; Yeh, M.M.; Kotrys, A.V.; Raguram, A.; Hsu, F.; Radey, M.C.; Peterson, S.B.; Mootha, V.K.; et al. A bacterial cytidine deaminase toxin enables CRISPR-free mitochondrial base editing. *Nat. Cell Biol.* **2020**, *583*, 631–637. [CrossRef] [PubMed]
369. Manfredi, G.; Fu, J.; Ojaimi, J.; Sadlock, J.E.; Kwong, J.Q.; Guy, J.; Schon, E.A. Rescue of a deficiency in ATP synthesis by transfer of MTATP6, a mitochondrial DNA-encoded gene, to the nucleus. *Nat. Genet.* **2002**, *30*, 394–399. [CrossRef] [PubMed]
370. Ellouze, S.; Augustin, S.; Bouaita, A.; Bonnet, C.; Simonutti, M.; Forster, V.; Picaud, S.; Sahel, J.-A.; Corral-Debrinski, M. Optimized Allotopic Expression of the Human Mitochondrial ND4 Prevents Blindness in a Rat Model of Mitochondrial Dysfunction. *Am. J. Hum. Genet.* **2008**, *83*, 373–387. [CrossRef] [PubMed]

371. Guy, J.; Feuer, W.J.; Davis, J.L.; Porciatti, V.; Gonzalez, P.J.; Koilkonda, R.D.; Yuan, H.; Hauswirth, W.W.; Lam, B.L. Gene Therapy for Leber Hereditary Optic Neuropathy. *Ophthalmology* **2017**, *124*, 1621–1634. [CrossRef]
372. Wan, X.; Pei, H.; Zhao, M.-J.; Yang, S.; Hu, W.-K.; He, H.; Ma, S.-Q.; Zhang, G.; Dong, X.-Y.; Chen, C.; et al. Efficacy and Safety of rAAV2-ND4 Treatment for Leber's Hereditary Optic Neuropathy. *Sci. Rep.* **2016**, *6*, 21587. [CrossRef]
373. Spees, J.L.; Olson, S.D.; Whitney, M.J.; Prockop, D.J. Mitochondrial transfer between cells can rescue aerobic respiration. *Proc. Natl. Acad. Sci. USA* **2006**, *103*, 1283–1288. [CrossRef]
374. Ahmad, T.; Mukherjee, S.; Pattnaik, B.; Kumar, M.; Singh, S.; Rehman, R.; Tiwari, B.K.; Jha, K.A.; Barhanpurkar, A.P.; Wani, M.R.; et al. Miro1 regulates intercellular mitochondrial transport & enhances mesenchymal stem cell rescue efficacy. *EMBO J.* **2014**, *33*, 994–1010. [CrossRef]
375. Yosef, O.B.; Jacoby, E.; Gruber, N.; Varda-Bloom, N.; Azaria, E.; Eisenstein, E.; Barak, S.; Ahonniska-Assa, J.; Anikster, Y.; Toren, A. Promising Results for Kearns-Sayre Syndrome of First in Man Treatment by Mitochondrial Augmentation Therapy (457). *Neurology* **2020**, *94*, 457.
376. Mingozzi, F.; High, K.A. Therapeutic in vivo gene transfer for genetic disease using AAV: Progress and challenges. *Nat. Rev. Genet.* **2011**, *12*, 341–355. [CrossRef]
377. Gao, G.-P.; Alvira, M.R.; Wang, L.; Calcedo, R.; Johnston, J.; Wilson, J.M. Novel adeno-associated viruses from rhesus monkeys as vectors for human gene therapy. *Proc. Natl. Acad. Sci. USA* **2002**, *99*, 11854–11859. [CrossRef] [PubMed]
378. Pebay-Peyroula, E.; Dahout-Gonzalez, C.; Kahn, R.; Trézéguet, V.; Lauquin, G.J.-M.; Brandolin, G. Structure of mitochondrial ADP/ATP carrier in complex with carboxyatractyloside. *Nat. Cell Biol.* **2003**, *426*, 39–44. [CrossRef] [PubMed]
379. Gropp, T.; Brustovetsky, N.; Klingenberg, M.; Müller, V.; Fendler, K.; Bamberg, E. Kinetics of electrogenic transport by the ADP/ATP carrier. *Biophys. J.* **1999**, *77*, 714–726. [CrossRef]
380. Walter, M.C.; Czermin, B.; Müller-Ziermann, S.; Bulst, S.; Stewart, J.D.; Hudson, G.; Schneiderat, P.; Abicht, A.; Holinski-Feder, E.; Lochmuller, H.; et al. Late-onset ptosis and myopathy in a patient with a heterozygous insertion in POLG2. *J. Neurol.* **2010**, *257*, 1517–1523. [CrossRef]
381. Flierl, A.; Chen, Y.; Coskun, P.E.; Samulski, R.J.; Wallace, D.C. Adeno-associated virus-mediated gene transfer of the heart/muscle adenine nucleotide translocator (ANT) in mouse. *Gene Ther.* **2005**, *12*, 570–578. [CrossRef]
382. Di Meo, I.; Marchet, S.; Lamperti, C.; Zeviani, M.; Viscomi, C. AAV9-based gene therapy partially ameliorates the clinical phenotype of a mouse model of Leigh syndrome. *Gene Ther.* **2017**, *24*, 661–667. [CrossRef]
383. Parikh, S.; Karaa, A.; Goldstein, A.; Ng, Y.S.; Gorman, G.; Feigenbaum, A.; Christodoulou, J.; Haas, R.; Tarnopolsky, M.; Cohen, B.K.; et al. Solid organ transplantation in primary mitochondrial disease: Proceed with caution. *Mol. Genet. Metab.* **2016**, *118*, 178–184. [CrossRef]
384. Spinazzola, A.; Viscomi, C.; Fernandez-Vizarra, E.; Carrara, F.; D'Adamo, P.; Calvo, S.E.; Marsano, R.M.; Donnini, C.; Weiher, H.; Strisciuglio, P.; et al. MPV17 encodes an inner mitochondrial membrane protein and is mutated in infantile hepatic mitochondrial DNA depletion. *Nat. Genet.* **2006**, *38*, 570–575. [CrossRef]
385. Shimura, M.; Kuranobu, N.; Ogawa-Tominaga, M.; Akiyama, N.; Sugiyama, Y.; Ebihara, T.; Fushimi, T.; Ichimoto, K.; Matsunaga, A.; Tsuruoka, T.; et al. Clinical and molecular basis of hepatocerebral mitochondrial DNA depletion syndrome in Japan: Evaluation of outcomes after liver transplantation. *Orphanet J. Rare Dis.* **2020**, *15*, 1–9. [CrossRef]
386. Hassan, S.; Mahmoud, A.; Mohammed, T.O.; Mohammad, S. Pediatric liver transplantation from a living donor in mitochondrial disease: Good outcomes in DGUOK deficiency? *Pediatr. Transplant.* **2020**, *24*, 13714. [CrossRef]
387. Tiranti, V.; Briem, E.; Lamantea, E.; Mineri, R.; Papaleo, E.; De Gioia, L.; Forlani, F.; Rinaldo, P.; Dickson, P.; Abu-Libdeh, B.; et al. ETHE1 mutations are specific to ethylmalonic encephalopathy. *J. Med. Genet.* **2005**, *43*, 340–346. [CrossRef] [PubMed]
388. Viscomi, C.; Bottani, E.; Zeviani, M. Emerging concepts in the therapy of mitochondrial disease. *Biochim. Biophys. Acta (BBA) Bioenerg.* **2015**, *1847*, 544–557. [CrossRef] [PubMed]
389. Di Meo, I.; Auricchio, A.; Lamperti, C.; Burlina, A.; Viscomi, C.; Zeviani, M. Effective AAV-mediated gene therapy in a mouse model of ethylmalonic encephalopathy. *EMBO Mol. Med.* **2012**, *4*, 1008–1014. [CrossRef] [PubMed]

390. Torres-Torronteras, J.; Viscomi, C.; Cabrera-Pérez, R.; Cámara, Y.; Di Meo, I.; Barquinero, J.; Auricchio, A.; Pizzorno, G.; Hirano, M.; Zeviani, M.; et al. Gene Therapy Using a Liver-targeted AAV Vector Restores Nucleoside and Nucleotide Homeostasis in a Murine Model of MNGIE. *Mol. Ther.* **2014**, *22*, 901–907. [CrossRef] [PubMed]

391. Chan, K.Y.; Jang, M.J.; Yoo, B.B.; Greenbaum, A.; Ravi, N.; Wu, W.-L.; Sánchez-Guardado, L.; Lois, C.; Mazmanian, S.K.; Deverman, B.E.; et al. Engineered AAVs for efficient noninvasive gene delivery to the central and peripheral nervous systems. *Nat. Neurosci.* **2017**, *20*, 1172–1179. [CrossRef] [PubMed]

392. Nishino, I. MNGIE (mitochondrial neurogastrointestinal encephalomyopathy). *Ryoikibetsu Shokogun Shirizu* **2001**, *47*, 792–800.

393. Hirano, M.; Garone, C.; Quinzii, C.M. CoQ10 deficiencies and MNGIE: Two treatable mitochondrial disorders. *Biochim. Biophys. Acta (BBA) Gen. Subj.* **2012**, *1820*, 625–631. [CrossRef]

394. Spinazzola, A.; Marti, R.; Nishino, I.; Andreu, A.L.; Naini, A.; Tadesse, S.; Pela, I.; Zammarchi, E.; Donati, M.A.; Oliver, J.A.; et al. Altered Thymidine Metabolism Due to Defects of Thymidine Phosphorylase. *J. Biol. Chem.* **2001**, *277*, 4128–4133. [CrossRef]

395. De Giorgio, R.; Pironi, L.; Rinaldi, R.; Boschetti, E.; Caporali, L.; Capristo, M.; Casali, C.; Cenacchi, G.; Contin, M.; D'Angelo, R.; et al. Liver transplantation for mitochondrial neurogastrointestinal encephalomyopathy. *Ann. Neurol.* **2016**, *80*, 448–455. [CrossRef]

396. Dionisi-Vici, C.; Diodato, D.; Torre, G.; Picca, S.; Pariante, R.; Picardo, S.G.; Di Meo, I.; Rizzo, C.; Tiranti, V.; Zeviani, M.; et al. Liver transplant in ethylmalonic encephalopathy: A new treatment for an otherwise fatal disease. *Brain* **2016**, *139*, 1045–1051. [CrossRef]

397. Tam, A.; Aldhaheri, N.S.; Mysore, K.; Tessier, M.E.; Goss, J.; Fernandez, L.A.; D'Alessandro, A.M.; Schwoerer, J.S.; Rice, G.M.; Elsea, S.H.; et al. Improved clinical outcome following liver transplant in patients with ethylmalonic encephalopathy. *Am. J. Med. Genet. Part A* **2019**, *179*, 1015–1019. [CrossRef]

398. Grabhorn, E.; Tsiakas, K.; Herden, U.; Fischer, L.; Freisinger, P.; Marquardt, T.; Ganschow, R.; Briem-Richter, A.; Santer, R. Long-term outcomes after liver transplantation for deoxyguanosine kinase deficiency: A single-center experience and a review of the literature. *Liver Transplant.* **2014**, *20*, 464–472. [CrossRef]

399. Lindvall, O.; Kokaia, Z.; Martinez-Serrano, A. Stem cell therapy for human neurodegenerative disorders—how to make it work. *Nat. Med.* **2004**, *10*, S42–S50. [CrossRef]

400. Hirano, M.; Martí, R.; Casali, C.; Tadesse, S.; Uldrick, T.; Fine, B.; Escolar, D.M.; Valentino, M.L.; Nishino, I.; Hesdorffer, C.; et al. Allogeneic stem cell transplantation corrects biochemical derangements in MNGIE. *Neurology* **2006**, *67*, 1458–1460. [CrossRef]

401. Filosto, M.; Scarpelli, M.; Tonin, P.; Lucchini, G.; Pavan, F.; Santus, F.; Parini, R.; Donati, M.A.; Cotelli, M.S.; Vielmi, V.; et al. Course and management of allogeneic stem cell transplantation in patients with mitochondrial neurogastrointestinal encephalomyopathy. *J. Neurol.* **2012**, *259*, 2699–2706. [CrossRef]

402. Garone, C.; Viscomi, C. Towards a therapy for mitochondrial disease: An update. *Biochem. Soc. Trans.* **2018**, *46*, 1247–1261. [CrossRef]

403. Wang, L.; Saada, A.; Eriksson, S. Kinetic Properties of Mutant Human Thymidine Kinase 2 Suggest a Mechanism for Mitochondrial DNA Depletion Myopathy. *J. Biol. Chem.* **2002**, *278*, 6963–6968. [CrossRef]

404. Taanman, J.-W.; Muddle, J.R.; Muntau, A.C. Mitochondrial DNA depletion can be prevented by dGMP and dAMP supplementation in a resting culture of deoxyguanosine kinase-deficient fibroblasts. *Hum. Mol. Genet.* **2003**, *12*, 1839–1845. [CrossRef]

405. Rampazzo, C.; Miazzi, C.; Franzolin, E.; Pontarin, G.; Ferraro, P.; Frangini, M.; Reichard, P.; Bianchi, V. Regulation by degradation, a cellular defense against deoxyribonucleotide pool imbalances. *Mutat. Res. Toxicol. Environ. Mutagen.* **2010**, *703*, 2–10. [CrossRef]

406. Garone, C.; García-Díaz, B.; Emmanuele, V.; López, L.C.; Tadesse, S.; Akman, H.O.; Tanji, K.; Quinzii, C.M.; Hirano, M. Deoxypyrimidine monophosphate bypass therapy for thymidine kinase 2 deficiency. *EMBO Mol. Med.* **2014**, *6*, 1016–1027. [CrossRef]

407. Lopez-Gomez, C.; Levy, R.J.; Sanchez-Quintero, M.J.; Juanola-Falgarona, M.; Barca, E.; Garcia-Diaz, B.; Tadesse, S.; Garone, C.; Hirano, M. Deoxycytidine and Deoxythymidine Treatment for Thymidine Kinase 2 Deficiency. *Ann. Neurol.* **2017**, *81*, 641–652. [CrossRef] [PubMed]

408. Bulst, S.; Abicht, A.; Holinski-Feder, E.; Müller-Ziermann, S.; Koehler, U.; Thirion, C.; Walter, M.C.; Stewart, J.D.; Chinnery, P.F.; Lochmuller, H.; et al. In vitro supplementation with dAMP/dGMP leads to partial restoration of mtDNA levels in mitochondrial depletion syndromes. *Hum. Mol. Genet.* **2009**, *18*, 1590–1599. [CrossRef] [PubMed]
409. Munro, B.; Horvath, R.; Müller, J.S. Nucleoside supplementation modulates mitochondrial DNA copy number in the dguok -/- zebrafish. *Hum. Mol. Genet.* **2019**, *28*, 796–803. [CrossRef] [PubMed]
410. Domínguez-González, C.; Madruga-Garrido, M.; Mavillard, F.; Garone, C.; Aguirre-Rodríguez, F.J.; Donati, M.A.; Kleinsteuber, K.; Martí, I.; Martín-Hernández, E.; Morealejo-Aycinena, J.P.; et al. Deoxynucleoside Therapy for Thymidine Kinase 2–Deficient Myopathy. *Ann. Neurol.* **2019**, *86*, 293–303. [CrossRef] [PubMed]
411. Carrabba, G.; Macchini, F.; Fabietti, I.; Schisano, L.; Meccariello, G.; Campanella, R.; Bertani, G.; Locatelli, M.; Boito, S.; Porro, G.A.; et al. Minimally invasive fetal surgery for myelomeningocele: Preliminary report from a single center. *Neurosurg. Focus* **2019**, *47*, E12. [CrossRef] [PubMed]
412. Lindenburg, I.T.M.; Van Kamp, I.L.; Oepkes, D. Intrauterine Blood Transfusion: Current Indications and Associated Risks. *Fetal Diagn. Ther.* **2014**, *36*, 263–271. [CrossRef] [PubMed]
413. Rashnonejad, A.; Chermahini, G.A.; Gündüz, C.; Onay, H.; Aykut, A.; Durmaz, B.; Baka, M.; Su, Q.; Gao, G.; Özkınay, F. Fetal Gene Therapy Using a Single Injection of Recombinant AAV9 Rescued SMA Phenotype in Mice. *Mol. Ther.* **2019**, *27*, 2123–2133. [CrossRef]
414. Peranteau, W.H.; Flake, A.W. The Future of In Utero Gene Therapy. *Mol. Diagn. Ther.* **2020**, *24*, 135–142. [CrossRef]
415. Visapää, I.; Fellman, V.; Vesa, J.; Dasvarma, A.; Hutton, J.L.; Kumar, V.; Payne, G.S.; Makarow, M.; Van Coster, R.; Taylor, R.W.; et al. GRACILE Syndrome, a Lethal Metabolic Disorder with Iron Overload, Is Caused by a Point Mutation in BCS1L. *Am. J. Hum. Genet.* **2002**, *71*, 863–876. [CrossRef]
416. Inak, G.; Rybak-Wolf, A.; Lisowski, P.; Juettner, R.; Zink, A.; Mlody, B.; Glazar, P.; Secker, C.; Ciptasari, U.H.; Stenzel, W.; et al. SURF1 mutations causative of Leigh syndrome impair human neurogenesis. *bioRxiv* **2019**, 551390. [CrossRef]
417. Quadalti, C.; Brunetti, D.; Lagutina, I.; Duchi, R.; Perota, A.; Lazzari, G.; Cerutti, R.; Di Meo, I.; Johnson, M.; Bottani, E.; et al. SURF1 knockout cloned pigs: Early onset of a severe lethal phenotype. *Biochim. Biophys. Acta (BBA) Mol. Basis Dis.* **2018**, *1864*, 2131–2142. [CrossRef] [PubMed]
418. Romero-Morales, A.I.; Rastogi, A.; Temuri, H.; Rasmussen, M.L.; McElroy, G.S.; Hsu, L.; Almonacid, P.M.; Millis, B.A.; Chandel, N.S.; Cartailler, J.P.; et al. Human iPSC-derived cerebral organoids model features of Leigh Syndrome and reveal abnormal corticogenesis. *bioRxiv* **2020**. [CrossRef]
419. Massaro, G.; Mattar, C.N.Z.; Wong, A.M.S.; Sirka, E.; Buckley, S.M.K.; Herbert, B.R.; Karlsson, S.; Perocheau, D.P.; Burke, D.; Heales, S.; et al. Fetal gene therapy for neurodegenerative disease of infants. *Nat. Med.* **2018**, *24*, 1317–1323. [CrossRef] [PubMed]
420. MacKenzie, T.C. Future AAVenues for In Utero Gene Therapy. *Cell Stem Cell* **2018**, *23*, 320–321. [CrossRef]
421. Zheng, X.; Boyer, L.; Jin, M.; Mertens, J.; Kim, Y.; Mandel, G.; Hamm, M.; Gage, F.H.; Hunter, T. Metabolic reprogramming during neuronal differentiation from aerobic glycolysis to neuronal oxidative phosphorylation. *eLife* **2016**, *5*, 13374. [CrossRef]
422. Bifari, F.; Dolci, S.; Bottani, E.; Pino, A.; Di Chio, M.; Zorzin, S.; Ragni, M.; Zamfir, R.G.; Brunetti, D.; Bardelli, D.; et al. Complete neural stem cell (NSC) neuronal differentiation requires a branched chain amino acids-induced persistent metabolic shift towards energy metabolism. *Pharmacol. Res.* **2020**, *158*, 104863. [CrossRef]
423. Brunetti, D.; Bottani, E.; Segala, A.; Marchet, S.; Rossi, F.; Orlando, F.; Malavolta, M.; Carruba, M.O.; Lamperti, C.; Provinciali, M.; et al. Targeting Multiple Mitochondrial Processes by a Metabolic Modulator Prevents Sarcopenia and Cognitive Decline in SAMP8 Mice. *Front. Pharmacol.* **2020**, *11*, 1171. [CrossRef]
424. Langer, Y.; Aran, A.; Gulsuner, S.; Abu Libdeh, B.; Renbaum, P.; Brunetti, D.; Teixeira, P.-F.; Walsh, T.; Zeligson, S.; Ruotolo, R.; et al. Mitochondrial PITRM1 peptidase loss-of-function in childhood cerebellar atrophy. *J. Med. Genet.* **2018**, *55*, 599–606. [CrossRef]

425. Pérez, M.J.; Ivanyuk, D.; Panagiotakopoulou, V.; Di Napoli, G.; Kalb, S.; Brunetti, D.; Al-Shaana, R.; Kaeser, S.A.; Fraschka, S.A.-K.; Jucker, M.; et al. Loss of function of the mitochondrial peptidase PITRM1 induces proteotoxic stress and Alzheimer's disease-like pathology in human cerebral organoids. *Mol. Psychiatry* **2020**, 1–18. [CrossRef]
426. Motori, E.; Atanassov, I.; Kochan, S.M.V.; Folz-Donahue, K.; Sakthivelu, V.; Giavalisco, P.; Toni, N.; Puyal, J.; Larsson, N.-G. Neuronal metabolic rewiring promotes resilience to neurodegeneration caused by mitochondrial dysfunction. *Sci. Adv.* **2020**, *6*, eaba8271. [CrossRef]

Publisher's Note: MDPI stays neutral with regard to jurisdictional claims in published maps and institutional affiliations.

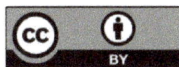

© 2020 by the authors. Licensee MDPI, Basel, Switzerland. This article is an open access article distributed under the terms and conditions of the Creative Commons Attribution (CC BY) license (http://creativecommons.org/licenses/by/4.0/).

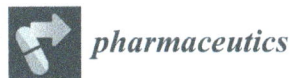

Review

Mitochondria-Targeted Drug Delivery in Cardiovascular Disease: A Long Road to Nano-Cardio Medicine

Francesca Forini [1,*], Paola Canale [1,2], Giuseppina Nicolini [1] and Giorgio Iervasi [1]

1. CNR Intitute of Clinical Physiology, Via G.Moruzzi 1, 56124 Pisa, Italy; p.canale@studenti.unipi.it (P.C.); nicolini@ifc.cnr.it (G.N.); iervasi@ifc.cnr.it (G.I.)
2. Department of Biology, University of Pisa, Via Volta 4 bis, 56126 Pisa, Italy
* Correspondence: simona@ifc.cnr.it

Received: 1 November 2020; Accepted: 18 November 2020; Published: 20 November 2020

Abstract: Cardiovascular disease (CVD) represents a major threat for human health. The available preventive and treatment interventions are insufficient to revert the underlying pathological processes, which underscores the urgency of alternative approaches. Mitochondria dysfunction plays a key role in the etiopathogenesis of CVD and is regarded as an intriguing target for the development of innovative therapies. Oxidative stress, mitochondrial permeability transition pore opening, and excessive fission are major noxious pathways amenable to drug therapy. Thanks to the advancements of nanotechnology research, several mitochondria-targeted drug delivery systems (DDS) have been optimized with improved pharmacokinetic and biocompatibility, and lower toxicity and antigenicity for application in the cardiovascular field. This review summarizes the recent progress and remaining obstacles in targeting mitochondria as a novel therapeutic option for CVD. The advantages of nanoparticle delivery over un-targeted strategies are also discussed.

Keywords: cardiovascular disease; drug delivery; mitochondria dysfunctions; nanocarriers

1. Introduction

Cardiovascular disease (CVD), including atherosclerosis, ischemic heart disease, hypertension, metabolic syndrome, and heart failure (HF), is a leading cause of morbidity and mortality worldwide. In most cases, the available one-target therapies relieve symptoms but do not fully address the molecular mechanisms that are often complex and interconnected.

In the last decades, mitochondria have become the fulcrum of an intense research activity aimed at developing innovative therapeutic strategies. Within the cardiovascular system (CVS), mitochondria exert key functions involved in energy production and catabolic and anabolic processes. In addition, mitochondria occupy a central position in the regulation of calcium (Ca^{2+}) handling, reactive oxygen species (ROS) homeostasis, and integration of cell death or survival pathways [1,2]. Therefore, mitochondrial dysfunctions are increasingly recognized to play a major role in the pathogenesis of multiple CVDs. Alterations of mitochondrial function result in impaired electron transport chain activity with increased ROS formation, mitochondrial Ca^{2+} overload, and aberrant mitochondrial quality control, which ultimately leads to diverse forms of cell death [1,2]. In addition, damaged mitochondria trigger inflammatory responses that further contribute to the evolution of CVD.

One major determinant of the mitochondria-dependent cell loss is the opening of the mitochondrial permeability transition pore (MPTP), an unselective high conductance channel of the inner mitochondrial membrane (IMM). MTPT opening causes a collapse of the IMM potential, ATP depletion, energy crisis, and release of cytochrome c and other death factors resulting in lethal cardiomyocyte injury [2,3]. MPTP opening has been largely characterized as a key determinant of acute cardiac ischemia and reperfusion (IR) injuries but its crucial role in non-ischemic cardiomyopathy and HF has also been documented both in experimental models and in the clinical setting [4,5]. Therefore, mitochondria ROS and MPTP are primary targets for therapeutic intervention in CVD.

Attempts to limit ROS production and MPTP activation with generic antioxidants have proven ineffective in large clinical trials [6–8]. One of the main explanations is probably the insufficient drug delivery at the site of ROS production.

Since then, an intensive investigation effort has been dedicated to developing mitochondria-targeting agents with improved pharmacological features for preventing or treating CVD. Several drug delivery systems (DDS), based on nanocarriers, have been thus far formulated, having the ability to selectively accumulate in the mitochondria, avoiding off-target effects (Table 1).

Table 1. Main delivery strategies and protective cargos explored in the cardiovascular field.

Carrier	Delivery Strategy	Cargo	Cardioprotective Effect
TTP small molecules (lipophilic cation)	Negative IMM potential	Antioxidants, H$_2$S and NO donors, isosteviol	ROS scavenging [9–31] PTM [32–40] mitoKATP activation [41]
PH-sensitive polymeric NPs (chitosan, HA)	CD44-dependent cell targeting, SS31(Mito-targeting)	SS31	Cardiolipin binding [42]
Polymeric NPs (PLGA; PEG; PEG-PLGA)	EPR effect (injured tissue-targeting), RGD (endothelial cell targeting), SS31 (mito-targeting)	CsA, fission inhibitors, nutraceutics	Cyclophylin D binding [43,44], inhibition of MPTPO [45], pleiotropic [46,47]
Lipid/polymeric NP (TPGS-PLGA)	EPR (injured tissue targeting), TTP (mito-targeting)	Tanshinone	Pleiotropic [48]
Lipid/polymeric NPs (MCTD)	EPR effect (injured tissue targeting), IMTP (cell targeting), SS31 (mito-targeting)	Resveratrol	Pleiotropic [49]
Liposome (mito-porter)	R8 (cell targeting), fusogenic lipid (mito-targeting)	Multiple mitoprotective agents	Pleiotropic [50–53]

Abbreviations: CD44, extracellular matrix protein receptor; CsA, cyclosporine A; EPR, enhanced permeability and retention; HA, hyaluronic acid; IMPT, ischemic myocardium-targeting peptide MCTD, multistage continuous targeted drug delivery; MPTPO, mitochondrial permeability transition pore opening; NP, nanoparticle; PEG, polyethylene glycol; PLGA, poly(lactic-co-glycolic); PTM, post-translational protein modification; R8, octa-arginine peptide; RGD, arginyl-glycyl-aspartic acid; ROS, reactive oxygen species; SS31, Szeto–Schiller-tetra-peptide 31; TPGS, D-α-tocopheryl-PEG-succinate; TTP, triphenylphosphonium.

A widely adopted strategy exploits the negative membrane potential of the IMM ($\Delta\psi_m$) to concentrate bioactive cardioprotective molecules against their concentration gradient. The most utilized mitochondria-targeting vehicle in the cardiovascular (CV) field is triphenylphosphonium (TPP), whose strong lipophilic and delocalized cationic nature has gained much traction to target various pharmacophores (Table 1). An alternative approach takes advantage of small mitochondria-targeting cationic peptides. Among them, the Szeto–Schiller-tetra-peptide 31 (SS31) and its acetate salt MTP-131 (also known as Bendavia or Elamipretide) have found widespread application in CV research (Table 1). These carriers are composed of alternating aromatic-cationic motifs (D-Arg-2'6'-dimethylTyr-Lys-Phe-NH$_2$) that facilitate high solubility and uptake in a membrane potential-independent fashion [54]. Therefore, with respect to the membrane potential-dependent TPP-derivatives, SS-31 offers a greater capacity to act on both functional and diseased mitochondria.

A variety of DDSs for the treatment of CVD is based on the highly biodegradable and biocompatible poly(lactic-co-glycolic) acid (PLGA), a copolymer approved by the U.S. Food and Drug Administration (FDA) for the design of drug carriers (Table 1). Remarkably, in the setting of acute ischemic injuries, PLGA nanoparticles (NPs) ensure sustained and targeted delivery by virtue of the enhanced permeability and retention (EPR) effect that characterizes the injured tissue [43,44]. Composite polymeric PLGA delivery systems have further been developed to avoid some drawbacks associated with PLGA NPs, including poor drug encapsulation and polymer degradation. In example, coating with polyethylene glycol (PEG) copolymer is frequently adopted to form a hydrated ring that protect sensitive molecules from degradation and reduces opsonization, thus resulting in prolonged circulation time and lower degradation by the immune system [55]. Like PLGA, PEG conjugation enhances NP delivery to the injured tissue via the EPR effect. In addition to these passive targeting strategies, active drug delivery systems have also been generated by conjugating the bioactive compounds to cell-specific ligands attached to the NPs (Table 1).

Several combinations of the delivery approaches described above have been integrated in more complex formulations, leading to polymeric/lipidic NPs that are internalized via endocytosis. One of such system, called multistage continuous targeted drug delivery (MCTD), has been designed for the specific uptake of cargo by mitochondria of the ischemic myocardium [49] (Table 1). The selectivity for the ischemic left ventricle (LV) is conferred by an ischemic myocardium targeting peptide (IMTP) consisting of Ser-Thr-Ser-Met-Leu-Lys-Ala. The IMTP drives endocytosis and cellular uptake. Within the cells, the nanocarriers escape lysosome degradation and enter the mitochondria thanks to the addiction of SS31 moieties [49]. To facilitate accumulation at the ischemic tissue, the researchers also introduced PLGA and PEG modifications into the formulation (Table 1). Finally, liposome-based carriers have been developed for mitochondria delivery via membrane fusion. In one of these systems, called Mito-porter, the liposome particles carry on their surface a small octa-arginine peptide (R8) that drives cellular uptake via macropinocytosis and prevents lysosomal degradation [56] (Table 1). The lipid composition of this DDS has been designed to achieve the highest degree of fusion with the mitochondrial membrane and release of the cargo in the mitochondria [56]. A major advantage of the vesicular NPs is the ability to deliver a greater amount and wide variety of therapeutic compounds from small molecules to large macromolecules. In example, the Mito-porter system has been successfully employed to regulate mitochondrial function by driving mitochondrial uptake of several oligonucleotide species including mRNA, antisense RNA, and expression vector [50–52].

In light of such premises, the aim of this review is to provide an updated overview on the main mitochondria-targeted cardioprotective compounds thus far analyzed in the preclinical and clinical arena with a focus on the potentiality and pitfalls of the nanocarrier-based delivery strategies.

2. Mitochondria-Targeted Antioxidants

2.1. Coenzyme Q10 (CoQ10)

The mitochondria permeable coenzyme Q10 (CoQ10) (or ubiquinone) is the only endogenously synthesized liposoluble antioxidant. Besides its role in electron transfer chain, the fully reduced form (ubiquinol) exerts a well-characterized lipid peroxidation-inhibitory effect [57], whose therapeutic potential has largely been investigated in CVD [58].

In several animal models of acute cardiac ischemia and HF, CoQ10 treatment resulted in attenuation of mitochondria structural damage, increase of high energy substrates, improved endothelial function, and mitigation of adriamycin cardiotoxicity [58].

The clinical benefit of CoQ10 therapy is still under evaluation. If inconclusive findings have been reported in the setting of acute IR [58], a more defined cardioprotective effect has emerged with prolonged CoQ10 administration in chronic CVD. In the Q-SYMBIO randomized double blind trial, 106 weeks of CoQ10 treatment improved symptoms and reduced major adverse cardiovascular events in HF patients, while no substantial differences were observed in the short term [59]. In addition, in women with type II diabetes mellitus, long-term CoQ10 supplementation lowered major CVD risk factors including fasting blood sugar levels, insulin resistance index, and total and low density lipoprotein (LDL) cholesterol [60]. The overall data indicate a disease- and time-dependent efficacy of CoQ10 that needs to be further tested in large-scale studies. In this regard, an ongoing phase II clinical trial in a large study population is dedicated to comparison of the clinical benefits of up to 12 weeks of treatment with CoQ10 or D-ribose in patients with diastolic HF, or HF with preserved ejection fraction (HFPEF) (NCT03133793). The findings will help to better clarify the added therapeutic value of CoQ10 in HF.

2.2. Mitoquinone (MitoQ)

Owing to its lipophilic nature and large molecular weight, CoQ10 exhibits a rather poor bioavailability [61]. To achieve more successful mitochondria targeting and more efficient antioxidant treatment, CoQ10 has been linked to TPP vehicle to form mitoquinone (MitoQ).

Within the mitochondria, MitoQ localizes at the IMM where it acts as an effective antioxidant against lipid peroxidation and a scavenger of peroxynitrites. MitoQ treatment has been shown to confer cardioprotection in multiple in vitro and in vivo experimental models. In vitro, MitoQ prevented oxidative damage and cell death caused by hydrogen peroxide and chemically-induced IR [57–62]. MitoQ-mediated ROS scavenging was also involved in rescuing mitochondria function and cardiac performance in rodent models of acute IR [9]. In a mouse model of heterotopic heart transplantation, administration of MitoQ to the donor heart in the storage solution protected against IR injury by blocking graft oxidative damage and dampening the early pro-inflammatory response in the recipient [10]. In spontaneously hypertensive rats, 8 weeks of treatment with MitoQ reduced systolic blood pressure and attenuated cardiac hypertrophy [11]. Finally, in a mouse model of severe pressure overload, MitoQ ameliorated contractile dysfunction and improved mitochondrial network integrity and mitochondrial–sarcoplasmic reticulum (SR) alignment [12,13]. At the molecular level, MitoQ inhibited the noxious interplay between profibrotic factors and mitochondrially associated redox signaling while normalizing mitochondrial dynamics. Interestingly, MitoQ rescued the dysregulation of several redox-sensitive noncoding RNAs associated with cardiac remodeling such as the pro-hypertrophic long non-coding RNA cardiac hypertrophy-associated transcript (Chast), the anti-hypertrophic long non-coding RNA my-heart (Mhrt), and the long non-coding Plscr4/miRNA-214 axis [12,13]. Given the increasing importance of non-coding RNA species in the pathophysiology of the cardiovascular system, these findings highlight a previously unappreciated therapeutic potential of MitoQ to contrast the evolution of HF.

The promising results from preclinical studies have encouraged clinical research. In a small clinical trial in elderly subjects, 6 weeks of MitoQ treatment ameliorated age-related vascular dysfunction by improving endothelial function and reducing mitochondrial-derived oxidative stress and arterial stiffening [14]. The potential benefit of 4 weeks of MitoQ administration is also under evaluation in two ongoing clinical trials on age-dependent degenerative processes. The first pilot study will assess the effect and sex-related differences of MitoQ supplementation on mitochondrial activity, LV diastolic performance, and vascular function in elderly subjects (NCT03586414). A second phase IV study will address the role of MitoQ in ameliorating mitochondrial dysfunction, exercise intolerance, and large blood vessel hemodynamics in HFPEF patients with or without chronic kidney disease comorbidity (NCT03960073). The results of these projects may be of crucial importance to confirm the therapeutic indication of MitoQ in alleviating the age-dependent deterioration of the overall CV function.

2.3. 10-(6′-Plastoquinonyl)-Decyltriphenylphosphonium (SkQ1)

SkQ1 is another TPP-based lipophilic cation bearing the chloroplast-derived analogue plastoquinone instead of ubiquinone. Within the mitochondria, SkQ1 binds to cardiolipin, an IMM-specific phospholipid with a central role in the regulation of cristae architecture, respiratory chain complex integrity, and supercomplex organization [2,61]. It has been demonstrated that interaction of cardiolipin with cytochrome c converts the respiratory chain electron carrier into a peroxidase. Binding of SkQ1 to cardiolipin inhibits such a noxious interaction, thus preventing cytochrome c-mediated mitochondrial oxidative damage [15]. In several in vivo and ex vivo rat models, SkQ1 protected against hydrogen peroxide injury, cardiac arrhythmias, and myocardial infarction [16,17]. More recently, SkQ1 administration has been shown to prevent mitochondrial oxidative stress, heart hypertrophy, and diastolic dysfunction in a mouse model of high fructose-induced cardiac remodeling [18]. Moreover, SkQ1 favored antioxidant system activation in the heart and blood serum of rats with streptozotocin-induced type I diabetes mellitus [19], and alleviated heart pathology in a mouse model of premature aging [20].

SkQ1 antioxidant properties have been observed at very low concentrations, while at higher concentrations, SkQ1 becomes a prooxidant, similarly to what has been observed for MitoQ [61]. It is worth noting that the concentration range for SkQ1-induced favorable effects is greater than that of MitoQ, which may represent a potential advantage for SkQ1 implementation in the clinical arena [61].

In the clinical context, SkQ1 safety and beneficial effects have only been evaluated in patients with dry eye syndrome [63]. Given the high antioxidant property at a low dose observed in preclinical studies, testing the therapeutic potential of SkQ1 in patients with CVD may open new therapeutic perspectives.

2.4. Mito-Tempo (MT)

Mito-Tempo (MT) is a mimetic of the mitochondrial superoxide dismutase consisting of a TPP-conjugated piperidine nitroxide. Besides detoxifying superoxide radicals, it also limits hydroxyl radical production by oxidizing ferrous iron [64]. The protective effects of MT have been documented in a wide range of experimental animal models. In a rat setting of metabolic syndromes, elimination of the mitochondrial oxidative stress with MT rescued cardiac collateral growth after repetitive ischemia insults [21]. MT was also shown to attenuate cardiomyopathy and preserve cardiac function in streptozotocin and db/db mouse models of type I and type II diabetes as well as in high-fat diet-fed mice [22–24]. In mouse models of renin–angiotensin system activation, MT reduced cellular superoxide and improved endothelial function and NO bioavailability by decreasing nicotinamide adenine dinucleotide phosphate (NADPH) oxidase [25–27]. In these contexts, MT prevented ventricular tachycardia and sudden cardiac death by increasing the connexin-43 levels and gap junction organization [25–27]. Interestingly, MT was able to reduce blood pressure even after the onset of hypertension while non-mitochondrial targeted antioxidants were ineffective [25–27]. Similarly, in a HF mouse model with cardiac-restricted mitochondrial calpain overexpression, MT but not general antioxidants attenuated cardiac cell death, HF evolution, and mortality [28]. In the murine model of chronic pressure overload MT administration markedly improved both cardiac contractile performance and mitochondrial respiratory function by decreasing the oxidative post-translational modification to Lon protease homolog, a mitochondrial protease critically involved in the process of mitochondria quality control [29]. Finally, the cardioprotective action of MT was recently extended to a more clinically relevant pig model of severe pressure overload and β-adrenergic stimulation that better recapitulated important features of non-ischemic arrhythmogenic HF [30]. In such a large animal model, chronic administration of MT prevented HF and effectively reduced ROS production in both mitochondrial and cytosolic compartments of the failing myocytes, which was associated with the normalization of the perturbed mitochondrial proteome and phospho-proteome [30]. Analogous to the above-mentioned hypertension mice models, MT was also effective after the onset of cardiac hypertrophy, suggesting that MT administration can be exploited even to revert overt cardiac disease [30].

Accordingly, in an ex vivo study on arterioles and mononuclear cells from patients with type II diabetes, MT exposure significantly reduced mitochondrial ROS and improved endothelial and vascular function [31].

In summary, the available clinical data on TPP-derived antioxidants indicate a disease-dependent efficacy that is expected to guide future development (Figure 1). The disappointing results in acute ischemic insults are counterbalanced by the effectiveness of long-term treatments in reverting risk factors and chronic/degenerative CV alterations leading to HF progression. The disease-dependent behavior of these drug carriers is consistent with a different maintenance of the IMM potential that abruptly falls in the ischemia-reperfused cell, thus exhausting the driving force for lipophilic cation uptake. In the presence of better preserved IMM potential, such as in non-ischemic CVD, TPP-linked scavenging compounds could represent good candidates to overcome the permeability and targeting problems observed with general antioxidants (Figure 1). However, the clinical data are still very limited, and more work on large patient cohorts is needed in order to better understand the therapeutic efficacy of this mitochondria-targeting strategy.

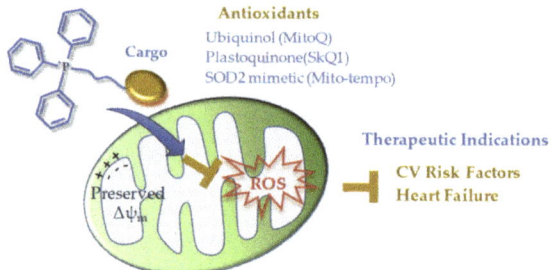

Figure 1. Mitochondria-targeted delivery of antioxidants based on triphenilphosphonium lipophilic cation.

2.5. *Szeto–Schiller 31 (SS31)*

Szeto–Schiller 31 (SS-31) and its acetate salt MTP-131 (also known as Bendavia or Elamipretide) are highly permeable mitochondria-targeted antioxidant peptides. SS31 was initially thought to exert its protective effect mainly through the ROS-scavenging activity of the dimethyltyrosine residue [65,66]. However, subsequent studies revealed a further mechanism of SS31 action. Similarly to SkQ1, SS31 binds to cardiolipin and modulates its hydrophobic interaction with cytochrome c to block the peroxidase activity of the carrier in favor of the electron transfer function [54,67]. More in depth insights on the SS31 activity within the cardiac mitochondria have been provided in a recent mass spectrometry analysis of the SS31-protein interaction landscape [68]. The identified SS31 interactors, all cardiolipin-binding proteins, play a key functional role in ATP production and transport, as well as in 2-oxoglutarate metabolism and signaling, which is consistent with improved mitochondrial function resulting from SS31 treatment [68].

The cardioprotective effect of SS31 has been documented in several experimental settings of cardiac disease. In small and large animal models of cardiac IR, the administration of SS31, either at the onset of ischemia or even just prior to reperfusion, limited myocardial damage and adverse remodeling and improved the recovery of cardiac function [69–71]. SS31 has also been shown to protect against pathological hypertrophy and fibrosis in mice models of hypertensive cardiomyopathy or transverse aortic constriction (TAC)-induced pressure overload [68,69]. Such beneficial effects were paralleled by reduced degree of mitochondria functional and structural alterations and by amelioration of proteomic profiling of either mitochondrial or non-mitochondrial proteins [72,73]. In a dog model of microembolism-induced HF, SS31 chronic treatment following the onset of HF preserved mitochondria function and bioenergetic, decreased ROS burden, improved systolic function, and reduced the plasmatic biomarkers of HF [74]. Finally, in a pig model of metabolic syndrome, SS31 administration attenuated the early alterations to cardiac function to cardiac mitochondria organization and to mitochondria–SR interaction [75].

Overall, these preclinical studies confirm that mitochondrial dysfunction and oxidative damage are crucial pathogenic mechanisms in CVD and that pharmacological interventions to preserve cardiolipin and cardiolipin–protein interactions would be of great therapeutic relevance even to revert overt pathologies.

However, translating the benefits of SS31 to the bedside has proven challenging either in acute ischemia and HF. The EMBRACE STEMI multicenter phase IIa trial evaluated the efficacy of SS31 in 297 patients with ST-segment elevation myocardial infarction (STEMI) [76]. While safe and well tolerated, SS31 infusion started before the onset of percutaneous coronary intervention and lasting for 1h after reperfusion, showed no significant impact on infarct size or LV function [76].

In the setting of HF with reduced ejection fraction (HFREF), a preliminary success was obtained in a proof-of-concept phase I randomized, placebo-controlled trial [77]. In this study, patients were treated with a single 4 h intravenous infusion of SS31 at different dosages with a 24h follow-up. The high-dose SS31 induced a significant decrease in LV end diastolic (LVEDV) and end systolic volumes (LVESV), suggesting that SS31 could improve cardiac function in HF. Of note, the maximal cardioprotective effect was observed at the peak of SS31 plasma concentration and decreased as the plasma concentration of SS31 disappeared (24h post-infusion). These findings highlight an important dose–effect relationship that is critically influenced by SS31 plasma half-life [77]. The positive results were not confirmed in a successive phase II clinical trial on HFREF patients. Although well tolerated, 4 weeks of daily subcutaneous infusion of SS31 did not produce the expected effects on primary and secondary endpoints including LVESV, Nt-proBNP plasma levels, and LV ejection fraction [78]. As a partial explanation, it has been postulated that 4 weeks treatment may be insufficient to correct cardiac remodeling and mitochondrial dynamics in HF [78]. These disappointing findings highlight the need to elucidate the optimal dosing, timing, and duration of drug administration to successfully move from the bench to the bedside. In addition, with SS31 being a cationic peptide, there may be some factors limiting its bioavailability in human myocardial mitochondria such as systemic proteases, rapid metabolism, and sequestration by blood products, which ultimately may result in a short half-life. The rapid clearance of uncojugated SS31 from plasma observed in patients supports this hypothesis [77]. In addition, direct incubation of freshly isolated myocardial mitochondria with SS31 effectively improved the organelle function and rescued the altered activity of supercomplexes CI, CII, and CIII [79], thus confirming that the negative results of clinical trials may have arisen, at least in part, from insufficient mitochondrial targeting within the cardiac tissue.

To overcome this limitation, Liu et al. [42] encapsulated SS31 in pH-sensitive NPs composed of cationic chitosan, a linear polysaccharide used for drug delivery [80], and anionic hyaluronic acid (HA), a compound with known selectivity for the receptor CD44. It is worth noting that CD44 is upregulated at the site of inflammation and cell injury [77,81]; therefore, this active DDS possesses diverse advantages: (i) the ability to protect SS31 from blood proteases, (ii) the ability to rapidly release SS31 in acidic pH conditions, and (iii) more specific cell targeting (Figure 2). The combination of such cell-targeted and organelle-targeted NP formulation has been successfully validated in human endothelial cells subjected to oxidative stress and in a rodent model of acute renal injury induced by ROS [64] (Figure 2).

Since CD44 is also overexpressed in acute and chronic CVD [81–83], the new formulation appears as a promising approach to concentrate the antioxidant and anti-inflammatory properties of SS31 at the site of cardiac injury. Of note, owing to the IMM potential-independent uptake of SS31, this DDS may also be ideal in particularly injured mitochondria such as in myocardial IR. Further studies are recommended to validate such an interesting hypothesis.

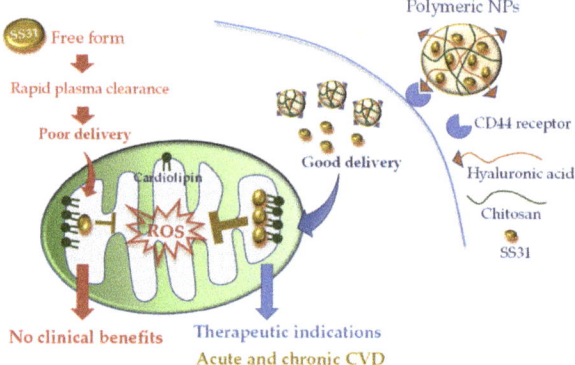

Figure 2. Mitochondria-targeted delivery of SS31 in free form versus nanoparticle (NP) formulation. Free SS31 is more prone to plasmatic degradation and rapid clearance, which might have undermined clinical benefit. NP formulation, with cell targeting moiety (hyaluronic acid) and higher mitochondrial uptake, is expected to confer promising therapeutic efficacy either in acute or chronic cardiovascular disease (CVD).

3. Inhibition of MPTP Opening

Another major target of cardioprotection is the mitochondrial permeability transition pore (MPTP) [84]. Although the molecular nature of the MPTP is still controversial, the matrix protein cyclophilin D (Cyp D) plays a crucial role in MPTP opening upon heart injury and has long been regarded as a target for limiting cell loss and improving heart performance in the post-ischemic setting [85,86]. Cyclosporin A (CsA), a lipophilic cyclic peptide initially developed as an immunosuppressant, has also been demonstrated to inhibit MPTP opening by binding to CypD [87]. Several experimental studies in small and large animal models have documented the myocardial infarct size-limiting properties of CsA administered at the time of reperfusion, when the MPTP opening is expected to occur [85]. CsA has also been reported to protect the heart in other experimental settings of acute IR injuries such as neonatal cardioplegic arrest and reperfusion and resuscitated cardiac arrest [85].

In accordance with the animal studies, CsA administration at the time of reperfusion has been shown to protect the heart against IR injury in patients undergoing aortic valve surgery [88] and to reduce infarct size and circulating injury biomarkers in a small proof-of-concept clinical trial on STEMI patients [89]. In contrast to the encouraging preliminary results, in the successive CIRCUS and CYCLE large multicenter clinical trials on STEMI patients, a single bolus CsA administration was unable to show any benefit on a variety of endpoints such as ST segment resolution, LV function, adverse remodeling, release of cardiac damage biomarkers, and clinical outcomes at 6 or 12 months [90,91]. Matching the results of the CIRCUS and CYCLE studies, in a more recent and smaller trial (CAPRI), a single CsA bolus did not affect infarct size or LV remodeling in STEMI patients [92]. Moreover, the characterization of the lymphocyte kinetics and plasmatic concentration of CsA during the 24 h period post-injection offered some putative explanations of the negative results: (i) CsA did not reach ischemic cardiomyocytes, (ii) CsA needed to be given at an earlier time point during myocardial ischemia, and (iii) 1 bolus of CsA is not sufficient to inhibit the proliferation of the pro-inflammatory CD4 T-lymphocyte during remodeling. Such indications may help to draw the direction of future studies.

Recently bioabsorbable PLGA-CsA NPs have been developed to improve the bioavailability and facilitate delivery of CsA to the injured cardiomyocyte, thus obtaining a more efficient inhibition of MPTP opening. The accumulation of PLGA-CsA NPs at the IR myocardium is favored by the EPR effect at injured tissue [43,44]. In line with the expectancy, in cardiomyocyte cultures, PLGA-CsA NPs demonstrated a greater propensity to accumulate in ROS-injured mitochondria and an improved cytoprotection at a dose lower than CsA alone [43]. In a murine model of IR, CsA loaded in PLGA NPs showed a more enhanced cardioprotective effect than CsA alone through the inhibition of MTPT opening [43]. However, PLGA-CsA NPs may also present unfavorable features such as the unspecific uptake by the mononuclear phagocyte system in the blood circulation, which is expected to reduce the accumulation of PLGA-CsA NPs in mitochondria of the ischemic cardiomyocytes [44,93]. To address this constraint and avoid extra-mitochondrial accumulation of CsA, researchers have formulated hybrid PLGA-CsA NPs by coating PEG on PLGA NP surface. Moreover, the mitochondriotropic SS31 peptide has been added to the formulation to increase mitochondrial delivery [43] (Figure 3). The resulting CsA-PLGA-PEG-SS31 DDS exhibited significant cardioprotective effects against IR in rats through accumulating in the injured mitochondria, protecting mitochondrial integrity and decreasing cardiomyocyte cell death and myocardial infarct area [43]. Alternatively, Mito-porter could potentially be used to deliver mitoprotective agents such as CsA to cardiac mitochondria in ischaemic cardiomyocytes following acute myocardial infarction [53].

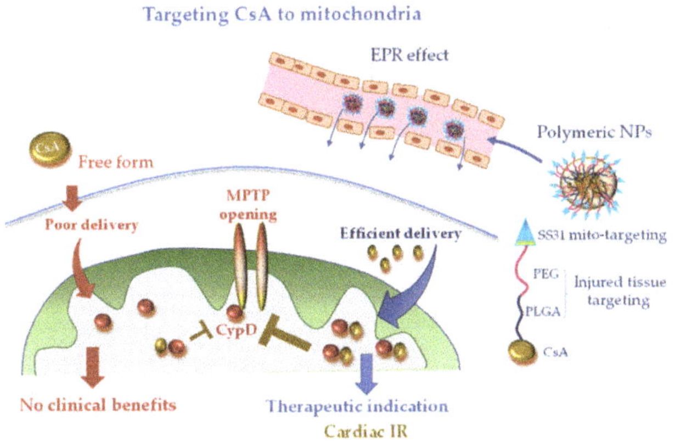

Figure 3. Mitochondria-targeted delivery of cyclosporine A (CsA) in free form versus nanoparticle (NP) formulation. Free CsA suffers of poor delivery at the injured tissue, which might have undermined clinical benefit. NP formulation, with tissue injury targeting moieties (polyethylene glycol (PEG) and poly(lactic-co-glycolic) acid (PLGA)) and mitochondriotropic SS31 moiety, is anticipated to confer promising therapeutic efficacy, especially in acute ischemic CVD. CydD, cyclophillin D; EPR, enhanced permeability and retention; IR, ischemia and reperfusion; MTPT, mitochondrial permeability transition pore; PEG, polyethylene glycol; PLGA, poly(lactic-co-glycolic).

These promising nanocarrier approaches may have great therapeutic potential to be tested in future large animal models of CVD and pilot clinical studies.

4. Mitochondria-Targeted Donors of Nitric Oxide (NO) and Hydrogen Sulfide (H_2S)

Nitric oxide (NO) and hydrogen sulfide (H_2S) at low concentrations exert well-documented cardioprotective actions against IR injuries by acting as signaling molecules and by inducing redox-based post-translational modifications on thiol groups of key mitochondrial proteins [94–98]. As a consequence, mitochondrial-targeted exogenous donors of NO or H_2S have been formulated as powerful tools for basic studies and innovative pharmacotherapeutic agents in ischemic cardiac disease (Table 2).

Table 2. Mitochondrial delivery of cardioprotective NO and H_2S donors and putative best therapeutic indications to be explored in humans.

Carrier	Function	Cardioprotective Mechanism	Therapeutic Indications
TTP-conjugation MitoSNO	NO donor	Reversible mitochondria protein nitrosilation	Cardiac IR Post ischemic HF
TTP-conjugation AP39	H_2S donor	MTPT opening inhibition	Cardioplegic solution Cardiac transplantation HF
4CPI	H_2S donor	MitoK-ATP activation	Cardioplegic solution Cardiac transplantation HF
3PI	H_2S donor	MitoK-ATP activation	Cardioplegic solution Cardiac transplantation HF

Abbreviations: AP39, [(10-oxo-10-(4-(3-thioxo-3H-1,2-dithiol-5yl)phenoxy)decyl) triphenylphosphonium bromide]; 4CPI, 4-carboxy-phenyl-isothiocyanate; HF, heart failure; MitoK-ATP, ATP sensitive mitochondrial potassium channel; 3PI, 3-pyridyl-isothiocyanate; TTP, triphenylphosphonium.

4.1. MitoSNO

The mitochondria-selective S-nitrosating agent (MitoSNO) is a TTP-linked S-nitrosothiol that selectively modulates and protects mitochondrial function from excessive ROS formation at the onset of myocardial reperfusion (Table 2). In several rodent models of IR, MitoSNO has been shown to limit infarct size, post-ischemic adverse cardiac remodeling, and HF evolution [32–35]. Mechanistically, MitoSNO transfers a nitric oxide moiety onto particular thiol proteins on respiratory complexes I and IV. In particular, selective S-nitrosation of complex I slows the reactivation of mitochondria during the crucial first minutes of the post-ischemic tissue reperfusion, thereby decreasing ROS production, oxidative damage, and tissue necrosis [32,34]. The study on MitoSNO-derived S-nitrosation in IR identified a number of other enzymes of central importance for mitochondrial metabolism, specifically those supplying electrons to the respiratory chain from the breakdown of carbohydrates and fatty acids [33]. The reversal of such post-translation modifications 5–10 mins after the onset of reperfusion is supposed to allow the mitochondria to return to full activity in a more physiological context and confer long-lasting protection against post-ischemic HF development [32–35].

4.2. AP39

AP39 is a mitochondrial-targeted, TPP-bound donor of H_2S, with cardioprotective effect documented either in vitro and in vivo (Table 2). AP39 has been shown to protect endothelial cells from hyperglycemia-induced mitochondrial-derived oxidative damage and has been proposed as a helpful agent against diabetic vascular complications [36]. In cardiomyocyte cultures, AP39 inhibited ROS-dependent mitochondria injuries and cell death by increasing the mitochondrial Ca^{2+} retention capacity and directly inhibiting MPTP opening [37]. In a mouse model of cardiac arrest and cardiopulmonary resuscitation, AP39 administration at the onset of resuscitation improved neurological outcomes by maintaining mitochondrial integrity and reducing oxidative stress [38]. In mice models of IR, AP39 injected at reperfusion provided direct mitochondria and cardiac protection through inhibition of MPTP opening at a site different than CypD and independently from the activation of cytosolic pro-death pathways [37,39]. In a recent work on mice, supplementing AP39 in the preservation solution protected cardiac grafts from prolonged ischemia, highlighting the therapeutic potential of this approach in preventing IR injury in heart transplant [40].

4.3. Isothiocyanate Derivatives

Isothiocyanate derivatives have also been synthetized as mito-protective H_2S-donor compounds (Table 2).

The 4-carboxy-phenyl-isothiocyanate (4CPI) is a slow H_2S-releasing molecule, endowed with vasorelaxant and hypotensive effects [99]. In isolated rat hearts subjected to IR, preconditioning with 4CPI inhibited ROS formation, improved the post-ischemic recovery of myocardial functional parameters, and limited tissue injury [100]. These effects were antagonized by a specific blocker of the mitochondria ATP-sensitive potassium channel (mitoKATP), a recently identified protein of the IMM, whose activation under anoxic condition exerts a series of well-documented cardioprotective actions [101,102].

In a similar work, 3-pyridyl-isothiocyanate (3PI) has been identified as a new promising cardioprotective agent by means of an isothyocianate library screen [103]. The beneficial pharmacological properties were successfully characterized in ex vivo and in vivo rat IR models in which 3PI administration before the IR procedure resulted in significant reduction of infarct size and attenuated the release of injury biomarkers [103]. The antioxidant and antiapoptotic responses to 3PI were largely dependent by the activation of mitoK-ATP channel, thus confirming the crucial involvement of this channel in the cardioprotective effects of isothiocyanate derivatives.

The clinical benefits of H_2S donors in IR patients has never been investigated. With the exception of MitoSNO, a major limitation of these compounds is the characteristic to confer the best protection when administered as a preconditioning strategy before the ischemic insult. A more feasible application of H_2S donors against IR injuries in patients could be supplementation in the cardioplegic solution during heart surgery or in the preservation medium before heart transplant (Table 2). As a final point, H_2S donors have been investigated only in the setting of IR; however, a recent finding opens novel possibilities extending the potential therapeutic effect of this strategy also to overt HF [104]. Further preclinical and clinical studies are indispensable to fix these critical aspects.

5. Inhibitors of Mitochondrial Fission

Altered mitochondrial morphology, with increased fission and fragmented mitochondria, is a hallmark of mitochondrial dysfunctions in a variety of human CVD, including acute ischemia and HF [105,106]. Since the GTPase dynamin-1-like protein (Drp1) is one main executor of mitochondria fission, specific inhibitors of Drp1 have been developed and tested in preclinical animal models of cardiac disease.

5.1. Mitochondrial Division Inhibitor 1 (Mdivi-1)

Mitochondrial division inhibitor 1 (Mdivi-1) is a quinazolinone derivative identified as a Drp1-selective inhibitor through a chemical library screen. Mdivi-1 has been firstly reported to inhibit Drp1-dependent mitochondrial fission, cytochrome c release, and apoptosis in yeast and non-cardiomyocyte mammalian stressed cells [107]. In in vitro and in vivo murine models of cardiac IR, Mdiv-1 prevented mitochondria fragmentation and dysfunction, limited cell death, attenuated the incidence of arrhythmia, and reduced infarct size [106,108,109]. In these studies, Mdivi-1 administration was protective either before or during the ischemic insult, even though the best results were obtained with the pre-ischemia treatment [106]. On the contrary, in a small pilot study on a more clinically relevant pig model of IR, administration of Mdivi-1 immediately prior to the onset of reperfusion did not reduce infarct size or preserve LV function [108]. The authors concluded that larger studies with different Mdivi1 dosages and more specific Drp1 inhibitors are required before translating the benefit of Drp1 targeting to patients.

The cardioprotective effects of Mdivi-1 have also been explored in non-ischemic settings of adverse cardiac remodeling [110,111]. In spontaneously hypertensive rats and mice with pressure overload-induced HF, daily injection of Mdivi for 7/8 days improved LV function and reduced the extent of myocardial fibrosis and cell death by mitigating mitophagy due to excessive mitochondrial fission [110,111].

To the best of our knowledge, thus far, human studies are limited to Mdivi-1 application in in vitro or ex vivo settings. In human endothelial cells in culture and in human arterioles, Mdivi-1 prevented mitochondria fragmentation and improved vascular function after a clinically relevant low-glucose exposure [112]. On the basis of these data, it has been suggested that Drp1 may represent a therapeutic target for improving cardiovascular complications among diabetic patients receiving intensive glucose control therapy [112]. Worthy of mention, Midivi1 also promoted cardiac differentiation of human induced pluripotent stem cells (iPSCs) in culture by shifting the balance of mitochondrial morphology toward fusion. According to these findings, Drp1 may represent a new molecular target to promote the differentiation of human iPSCs into cardiac lineages for future personalized cardiac-regenerative medicine [45].

Recently, a more precise mitochondrial-targeted delivery of Mdivi1 was developed by loading the drug in PLGA NPs [113]. Midivi1-PLGA NPs better protected rat neonatal cardiomyocytes against H_2O_2-induced oxidative stress in comparison with Mdivi-1 alone. The improved mitochondrial localization and greater beneficial effects of Midiv1-NP were also confirmed in Langhendorff and in vivo mouse models of cardiac IR treated with the DDS at the time of reperfusion [113]. These results raise the interesting working hypothesis that Midivi1 NPs may be used to overcome the limitation of un-targeted Midiv1 observed in large animal studies, shortening the road to clinical translation (Figure 4).

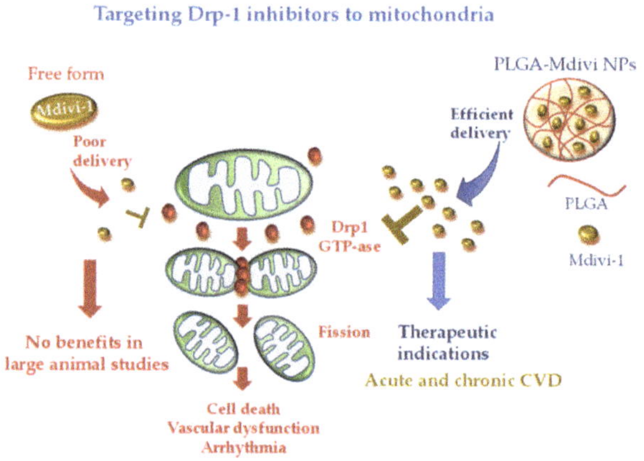

Figure 4. Mitochondria-targeted delivery of dynamin-1-like protein (Drp1) inhibitor (mitochondrial division inhibitor 1 (Mdivi-1)) in free form versus nanoparticle (NP) formulation. Free Mdivi-1 may suffer from poor delivery at the injured tissue in clinically relevant large animal models, which might abrogate the benefits observed in small animals. NP formulation, with tissue injury targeting moieties, is anticipated to confer promising therapeutic efficacy either in acute or chronic CVD.

5.2. Drp1 inhibitor 1 (Driptor1) and Drp1 inhibitor 1a (Driptor1a)

Novel Drp1 inhibitors have been recently identified by an in silico chemical screen. Among them, the ellipticine compound, termed Drp1 inhibitor 1 (Driptor1), and a congener of Driptor1, termed Drp1 inhibitor 1a (Driptor1a), were demonstrated to exert a more potent and specific Drp1 inhibitory effect than MDVI-1 [114]. In particular, Driptor1a offered cardioprotection in a rat Langendorff right ventricle IR model [114]. The full potential of these very preliminary findings needs to be further explored in small and large animal models of CVD.

6. Mitochondria-Targeting of Natural Compounds with Pleiotropic Effects

Cardiovascular diseases are complex multifactorial pathologies in which multiple components of mitochondrial physiology in different cell types concur to speed up the disease evolution. Therefore, strategies directed at a single target may be insufficient to ensure adequate protection [115]. Different natural bioactive compounds have thus far been described with pleiotropic beneficial effects on a plethora of CVD [116]. Among them, phenolic and terpenoid phytochemicals have been shown to protect the vascular and cardiac function against mitochondria-mediated pro-oxidant, pro-apoptotic, and pro-inflammatory injuries through the modulation of multiple cell signaling transduction pathways in different cell types [116]. Thanks to their multitargeted effects and good tolerability, natural molecules are promising candidates to counteract the development of multifaceted disorders such as CVD (Figure 5).

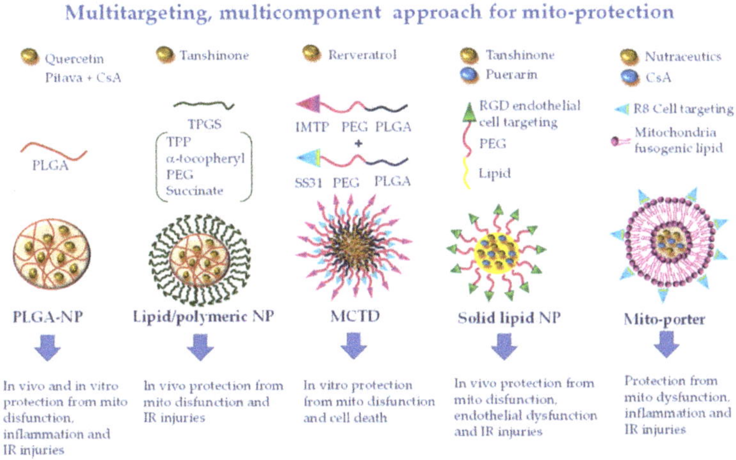

Figure 5. Multitargeting, multicomponent approaches for mito-protection exploiting the pleiotropic effects of several nutraceutics or the combination of more protective compounds with different mechanisms of action. NPs can be functionalized to achieve optimal targeting of specific tissue districts and cell types. Polyethylene glycol (PEG) and poly(lactic-co-glycolic) acid (PLGA) accumulate NPs at the injury site because of the enhanced permeability and retention effect. The ischemic myocardium-targeting peptide (IMPT) ensures vehiculation at the IR zone. The cell-targeting peptides RGD and R8 drive cell uptake. Finally, triphenilphosphonium (TPP), Szeto–Schiller 31 (SS31), and mitochondria fusogenic lipid moieties elicit greater mitochondrial uptake.

6.1. Resveratrol

Resveratrol (RES), a polyphenol contained in abundance in grape skins, exhibits attractive antithrombotic, anti-inflammatory, and antioxidant properties to be exploited in the context of acute and chronic CVD [117]. Increasing experimental evidence have demonstrated the cardioprotective effects of RES against LV dysfunction and adverse remodeling following IR injury, pharmacological agent-induced cardiotoxicity, obesity, and diabetes [118]. Mainly, RES improves vascular and cardiac performance via protection of endothelial and cardiac mitochondrial function [119,120]. Its beneficial effects largely derive from the intrinsic ROS scavenging activity, the ability to increase antioxidant defense, and the ability to modulate cytokine production and mitochondrial biogenesis [117,121].

More contrasting results have been reported in clinical studies [121]. Despite good tolerability and protective effects, especially at higher doses, available human studies indicate a rapid metabolism of RES, which may have limited its cardiac bioavailability in some cardiac patient cohorts [122,123].

This constraint has been addressed by a nano-formulation recently developed to specifically target resveratrol to cardiac mitochondria. In this study, resveratrol was delivered in the vesicular multistage continuous targeted drug delivery NPs (MCTD-NPs) either in rat cardiomyoblasts in culture or in a rat model of cardiac IR [49]. Thanks to the IMTP moiety, the intracellular uptake of MCTD-NPs was specifically enhanced in IR injured cells with a concomitant reduction of mitochondrial ROS, MPTP opening, and mitochondria-dependent apoptotic pathways (Figure 5). In vivo, MCTD-NP administration at the onset of reperfusion increased the distribution of RVS in the ischemic myocardium and reduced infarct size with an increased efficiency with respect to RVS alone or RVS delivered in PLGA NPs [49]. These results demonstrated the reliability of a novel platform for specific delivery of protective cargo to cardiac mitochondria in the setting of ischemic cardiac disease.

6.2. Quercetin

Quercetin (QUE) is a polyphenol extracted from various plants. Experimental in vivo and in vitro studies have shown that quercetin has a wide range of biological actions including anti-inflammatory activities as well as the ability to attenuate oxidative stress, lipid peroxidation, platelet aggregation, and capillary permeability [124,125]. Furthermore, QUE has a prominent protective action against mitochondrial dysfunction and mitochondria-dependent cell death [126,127]. In accordance, a meta-analysis of clinical trials evidenced a blood pressure-lowering activity of high dosage QUE intake [128].

Similarly to RES, QUE presents pharmacokinetic hurdles, with only 20% of the administered dose reaching the blood. To improve QUE bioavailability, NP-mediated delivery has been implemented. In a recent work, QUE was encapsulated in PLGA-NPs and tested in vitro in a surrogate model of cardiac cells [46]. The higher delivery degree of encapsulated QUE with respect to free QUE resulted in a superior protection capacity, as evidenced by improved antioxidant properties, decreasing cell death after IR injury and preserving mitochondrial membrane potential and ATP synthesis (Figure 5). The results point to the potential of this strategy for the treatment of oxidative stress in cardiac diseases [46]. Further works are necessary to confirm these findings in an in vivo model of CVD.

6.3. Isosteviol

Isosteviol (IST) is a bioactive diterpenoid extracted by *Stevia rebaudiana* that has a variety of biological activities targeted at the CVS, including anti-hypertensive, anti-hyperglycemic, antioxidant, and anti-inflammatory effects [129]. In cardiomyoblasts subjected to simulated IR or pro-hypertrophic injuries, IST restored mitochondrial membrane potential, morphological integrity, and biogenesis; decreased ROS levels; and upregulated the expression of antioxidant enzymes [130,131]. In addition, IST relieved IR injury in rodent hearts and isolated pig hearts [132,133]. At least some of the observed beneficial effects of IST can be attributed to stimulation of the mitoKATP channel, since a selective mitoKATP inhibitor abolished its protective action [133].

The key role of mitoKATP channels in the IST cardioprotective profile suggested a strategy for effectively driving diterpene compounds into the mitochondria to improve their pharmacokinetic profile and, consequently, their pharmacological effects. The mitochondriotropic properties of a TPP conjugate formulation of IST have been investigated in vitro and in vivo [41]. In a heart cell line, the mitochondrial uptake of TPP-IST was associated to mild IMM depolarization and inhibition of Ca^{2+} overload, which is compatible with activation of mitoKATP channel [41]. Administration of TPP-IST to a rat model of IR exerted significant cardioprotective effects at a 100-fold lower concentration with respect to the effective dose of free IST, suggesting that the mitochondrial delivery afforded by the TPP strategy led to a significant improvement of the cardioprotective effects [41].

6.4. Tanshinone

Tanshinone (TN) diterpene compound is a major active ingredient derived from the Chinese medical herb *Salvia miltiorrhiza* and is a widely investigated therapeutic agent for the treatment of CVD [134]. Thanks to its pleiotropic antioxidant, antihypertensive, anti-inflammatory, and lipid lowering activities, TN inhibits cardiac IR injury and adverse remodeling, blunts endothelial and vascular dysfunctions, and prevents platelet aggregation [134]. Its main mechanisms of action are inhibition of mitochondrial ROS production, MPTP opening, and mitochondria-mediated cell death. However, its poor water solubility and low oral bioavailability have hindered its clinical application.

To overcome this limitation, a lipid-polymeric nanocarrier (LPN) for mitochondrial-targeted delivery of TN has been recently developed. The formulation consists in a PLGA-TN mixture enclosed in a lipophilic shell formed by TPP linked to a D-α-tocopheryl-PEG-succinate (TPGS) moiety, an FDA-approved biocompatible excipient widely used for drug delivery [135] (Figure 5). The TN-LPN exhibited a better efficiency in terms of compatibility, biodistribution, and pharmacokinetic profile with respect to free TN and PLGA-TN NP formulations. It is worth noting that evident cardioprotective effects were observed in a rat model of IR, in which TN-LPN was added at the onset of reperfusion [48].

These results indicated that the TPP-TPGS/TN/LPNs represent promising nanocarriers for efficient delivery of cardiovascular drugs and other therapeutic agents for the treatment of CVD. However, future studies are needed to better evaluate the safety and efficacy of such an approach in different CVD settings and in large animal models.

7. Simultaneous Drug Delivery for a More Efficient Combination Therapy

Another promising multi-component and multi-targeted approach consists in the combined delivery of more than one cardioprotective agent. In a recent study by Gao et al., solid lipid nanocarriers made of DSPE (1,2-distearoyl-sn-glycero-3-phosphoethanolamine) were co-loaded with TN and puerarin (PUE)-prodrug [136] (Figure 5). PUE is a major active ingredient derived from the Chinese medical herb *Radix puerariae*, with significant mito-protective effects directed at the endothelial cells [137]. To favor a more precise targeting of PUE to endothelial cells of the ischemic myocardium, vesicular NPs have been developed with PEG-modified cyclic arginyl-glycyl-aspartic (RGD) acid peptide. The PEG particle drives the accumulation at the infarct site due to the EPR effect, while the RGD moiety is a specific ligand for the endothelial avb3 integrin receptor. This DDS has proven effective in reducing infarct size in a rat model of acute myocardial infarction [138]. The same approach used for the simultaneous administration of TAN and PUE resulted in greater cellular uptake and smaller infarct size with respect to the single phytochemicals delivered either in free or NP formulations [136]. The findings indicate the synergistic effect of the double drugs loaded in one system, suggesting a promising strategy for the treatment of myocardial infarction.

Along the same line, in another work, PLGA-based polymeric NPs containing CsA (CsA-NPs) and pitavastatin (Pitava-NPs) were simultaneously administered to target mitochondrial dysfunction and monocyte-mediated inflammation in a mouse model of acute cerebral IR [47]. Through blocking MPTP opening and chemokine receptor-2-dependent inflammation, concomitant administration of CsA-NPs and Pitava-NPs at the time of reperfusion decreased infarct size and attenuated neurological deficits as compared to single administration of CsA-NPs or Pitava-NPs (Figure 5). Given the crucial involvement of MPTP opening and inflammation in promoting cardiac injuries, it is conceivable that a similar NP-based combination therapy could also provide benefits in CVD [47]. Finally, the highly versatile Mito-porter DDS can potentially be employed to achieve mitochondria-targeted multiple delivery of protective agents, including nutraceutics and CsA, for a more efficient combination therapy in CVD (Figure 5).

8. Conclusions and Future Perspectives

As the central role of mitochondrial signaling in CVD has become clearer, research efforts have been oriented toward direct modulation of mitochondrial functions. CoQ10, SS31, and CsA are the better characterized unconjugated mito-drugs thus far tested. However, despite encouraging results emerging from animal models, no mitoprotective drugs have passed clinical trials in large patient cohorts [6–8,76,90–92]. One possible explanation may have been poor delivery to the diseased cells and tissue districts. In this regard, nanotechnology has made huge progress in recent years to address the current limitations and to offer sustained delivery to mitochondria. Nanopreparations can be optimized to achieve improved biodegradability, pharmacokinetic properties, and bio-distribution profiles.

A variety of promising new cardiovascular nanoformulations have been tested in in vitro and in vivo experimental models. Although exciting, most of these studies are still at an embryonic preclinical stage. On the road to nano-cardio medicine, several critical issues need to be addressed to accomplish a more realistic translatability to human health. The vast majority of experimental studies have been performed in small-sized young animals without comorbidities, which hardly recapitulates the conditions of elderly cardiovascular patients presenting with more than one pathology. Therefore, a more rigorous design of pre-clinical models, with accurate selection of dosage and mode of administration and taking into account aging, sex differences, comorbidities, and co-medications, is of paramount importance for the development of more successful clinical trials. As a second key point, efficacious DDS must face the multifactorial nature of CVD. Innovative therapeutic strategies should comprise a multi-faceted approach targeted at different mitochondrial noxious pathways, without disregarding non-cardiomyocyte cells including fibroblasts, endothelial cells, and inflammatory cells that critically contribute to CVD evolution. The emerging multifunctional, mitoprotective NPs might represent good candidates to enable such a paradigm shift in the future (Figure 5).

Author Contributions: Conceptualization, F.F.; writing—original draft preparation, F.F.; bibliographic search and analysis, P.C. and G.N.; writing—review and editing, F.F., P.C., G.N. and G.I.; supervision, G.I.; funding acquisition, G.I. All authors have read and agreed to the published version of the manuscript.

Funding: This research received no external funding.

Conflicts of Interest: The authors declare no conflict of interest.

References

1. Forini, F.; Nicolini, G.; Kusmic, C.; Iervasi, G. Protective Effects of Euthyroidism Restoration on Mitochondria Function and Quality Control in Cardiac Pathophysiology. *Int. J. Mol. Sci.* **2019**, *20*, 3377. [CrossRef]
2. Forini, F.; Pitto, L.; Nicolini, G. Thyroid hormone, mitochondrial function and cardioprotection. In *Thyroid and Heart. A comprehensive Translational Essay*; Iervasi, G., Pingitore, A., Gerdes, A.M., Razvi, S., Eds.; Springer: Cham, Switzerland, 2020; pp. 109–126.
3. Forini, F.; Nicolini, G.; Iervasi, G. Mitochondria as key targets of cardioprotection in cardiac ischemic disease: Role of thyroid hormone triiodothyronine. *Int. J. Mol. Sci.* **2015**, *16*, 6312–6336. [CrossRef]
4. Dhingra, R.; Guberman, M.; Rabinovich-Nikitin, I.; Gerstein, J.; Margulets, V.; Gang, H.; Madden, N.; Thliveris, J.; Kirshenbaum, L.A. Impaired NF-κB signalling underlies cyclophilin D-mediated mitochondrial permeability transition pore opening in doxorubicin cardiomyopathy. *Cardiovasc. Res.* **2020**, *116*, 1161–1174. [CrossRef]
5. Moon, S.H.; Liu, X.; Cedars, A.M.; Yang, K.; Kiebish, M.A.; Joseph, S.M.; Kelley, J.; Jenkins, C.M.; Gross, R.W. Heart failure-induced activation of phospholipase iPLA2γ generates hydroxyeicosatetraenoic acids opening the mitochondrial permeability transition pore. *J. Biol. Chem.* **2018**, *293*, 115–129. [CrossRef]
6. Sesso, H.D.; Buring, J.E.; Christen, W.G.; Kurth, T.; Belanger, C.; MacFadyen, J.; Bubes, V.; Manson, J.E.; Glynn, R.J.; Gaziano, J.M. Vitamins E and C in the prevention of cardiovascular disease in men: The Physicians' Health Study II randomized controlled trial. *JAMA* **2008**, *300*, 2123–2133. [CrossRef]
7. Song, Y.; Cook, N.R.; Albert, C.M.; Van Denburgh, M.; Manson, J.E. Effects of vitamins C and E and beta-carotene on the risk of type 2 diabetes in women at high risk of cardiovascular disease: A randomized controlled trial. *Am. J. Clin. Nutr.* **2009**, *90*, 429–437. [CrossRef]
8. Schmidt, H.H.; Stocker, R.; Vollbracht, C.; Paulsen, G.; Riley, D.; Daiber, A.; Cuadrado, A. Antioxidants in Translational Medicine. *Antioxid. Redox Signal.* **2015**, *23*, 1130–1143. [CrossRef]
9. Adlam, V.J.; Harrison, J.C.; Porteous, C.M.; James, A.M.; Smith, R.A.; Murphy, M.P.; Sammut, I.A. Targeting an antioxidant to mitochondria decreases cardiac ischemia-reperfusion injury. *FASEB J.* **2005**, *19*, 1088–1095. [CrossRef] [PubMed]
10. Dare, A.J.; Logan, A.; Prime, T.A.; Rogatti, S.; Goddard, M.; Bolton, E.M.; Bradley, J.A.; Pettigrew, G.J.; Murphy, M.P.; Saeb-Parsy, K. The mitochondria-targeted anti-oxidant MitoQ decreases ischemia-reperfusion injury in a murine syngeneic heart transplant model. *J. Heart Lung Transplant.* **2015**, *34*, 1471–1480. [CrossRef] [PubMed]
11. Graham, D.; Huynh, N.N.; Hamilton, C.A.; Beattie, E.; Smith, R.A.; Cochemé, H.M.; Murphy, M.P.; Dominiczak, A.F. Mitochondria-targeted antioxidant MitoQ10 improves endothelial function and attenuates cardiac hypertrophy. *Hypertension* **2009**, *54*, 322–328. [CrossRef] [PubMed]

12. Goh, K.Y.; He, L.; Song, J.; Jinno, M.; Rogers, A.J.; Sethu, P.; Halade, G.V.; Rajasekaran, N.S.; Liu, X.; Prabhu, S.D.; et al. Mitoquinone ameliorates pressure overload-induced cardiac fibrosis and left ventricular dysfunction in mice. *Redox Biol.* **2019**, *21*, 101100. [CrossRef] [PubMed]
13. Kim, S.; Song, J.; Ernst, P.; Latimer, M.N.; Ha, C.M.; Goh, K.Y.; Ma, W.; Rajasekaran, N.S.; Zhang, J.; Liu, X.; et al. MitoQ regulates redox-related noncoding RNAs to preserve mitochondrial network integrity in pressure-overload heart failure. *Am. J. Physiol. Heart Circ. Physiol.* **2020**, *318*, H682–H695. [CrossRef] [PubMed]
14. Rossman, M.J.; Santos-Parker, J.R.; Steward, C.A.C.; Bispham, N.Z.; Cuevas, L.M.; Rosenberg, H.L.; Woodward, K.A.; Chonchol, M.; Gioscia-Ryan, R.A.; Murphy, M.P.; et al. Chronic Supplementation with a Mitochondrial Antioxidant (MitoQ) Improves Vascular Function in Healthy Older Adults. *Hypertension* **2018**, *71*, 1056–1063. [CrossRef] [PubMed]
15. Firsov, A.M.; Kotova, E.A.; Orlov, V.N.; Antonenko, Y.N.; Skulachev, V.P. A mitochondria-targeted antioxidant can inhibit peroxidase activity of cytochrome c by detachment of the protein from liposomes. *FEBS Lett.* **2016**, *590*, 2836–2843. [CrossRef] [PubMed]
16. Antonenko, Y.N.; Avetisyan, A.V.; Bakeeva, L.E.; Chernyak, B.V.; Chertkov, V.A.; Domnina, L.V.; Ivanova, O.Y.; Izyumov, D.S.; Khailova, L.S.; Klishin, S.S.; et al. Mitochondria-targeted plastoquinone derivatives as tools to interrupt execution of the aging program. 1. Cationic plastoquinone derivatives: Synthesis and in vitro studies. *Biochemistry* **2008**, *73*, 1273–1287. [CrossRef] [PubMed]
17. Bakeeva, L.E.; Barskov, I.V.; Egorov, M.V.; Isaev, N.K.; Kapelko, V.I.; Kazachenko, A.V.; Kirpatovsky, V.I.; Kozlovsky, S.V.; Lakomkin, V.L.; Levina, S.B.; et al. Mitochondria-targeted plastoquinone derivatives as tools to interrupt execution of the aging program. 2. Treatment of some ROS- and age-related diseases (heart arrhythmia, heart infarctions, kidney ischemia, and stroke). *Biochemistry* **2008**, *73*, 1288–1299. [CrossRef] [PubMed]
18. Zhang, Y.B.; Meng, Y.H.; Chang, S.; Zhang, R.Y.; Shi, C. High fructose causes cardiac hypertrophy via mitochondrial signaling pathway. *Am. J. Transl. Res.* **2016**, *8*, 4869–4880.
19. Agarkov, A.A.; Popova, T.N.; Boltysheva, Y.G. Influence of 10-(6-plastoquinonyl) decyltriphenylphosphonium on free-radical homeostasis in the heart and blood serum of rats with streptozotocin-induced hyperglycemia. *World J. Diabetes* **2019**, *10*, 546–559. [CrossRef]
20. Shabalina, I.G.; Vyssokikh, M.Y.; Gibanova, N.; Csikasz, R.I.; Edgar, D.; Hallden-Waldemarson, A.; Rozhdestvenskaya, Z.; Bakeeva, L.E.; Vays, V.B.; Pustovidko, A.V.; et al. Improved health-span and lifespan in mtDNA mutator mice treated with the mitochondrially targeted antioxidant SkQ1. *Aging* **2017**, *9*, 315–339. [CrossRef]
21. Pung, Y.F.; Rocic, P.; Murphy, M.P.; Smith, R.A.; Hafemeister, J.; Ohanyan, V.; Guarini, G.; Yin, L.; Chilian, W.M. Resolution of mitochondrial oxidative stress rescues coronary collateral growth in Zucker obese fatty rats. *Arterioscler. Thromb. Vasc. Biol.* **2012**, *32*, 325–334. [CrossRef]
22. Luo, M.; Guan, X.; Luczak, E.D.; Lang, D.; Kutschke, W.; Gao, Z.; Yang, J.; Glynn, P.; Sossalla, S.; Swaminathan, P.D.; et al. Diabetes increases mortality after myocardial infarction by oxidizing CaMKII. *J. Clin. Investig.* **2013**, *123*, 1262–1274. [CrossRef] [PubMed]
23. Ni, R.; Cao, T.; Xiong, S.; Ma, J.; Fan, G.C.; Lacefield, J.C.; Lu, Y.; Le Tissier, S.; Peng, T. Therapeutic inhibition of mitochondrial reactive oxygen species with mito-TEMPO reduces diabetic cardiomyopathy. *Free Radic. Biol. Med.* **2016**, *90*, 12–23. [CrossRef] [PubMed]
24. Jeong, E.M.; Chung, J.; Liu, H.; Go, Y.; Gladstein, S.; Farzaneh-Far, A.; Lewandowski, E.D.; Dudley, S.C., Jr. Role of Mitochondrial Oxidative Stress in Glucose Tolerance, Insulin Resistance, and Cardiac Diastolic Dysfunction. *J. Am. Heart Assoc.* **2016**, *5*, e003046. [CrossRef] [PubMed]
25. Dikalova, A.E.; Bikineyeva, A.T.; Budzyn, K.; Nazarewicz, R.R.; McCann, L.; Lewis, W.; Harrison, D.G.; Dikalov, S.I. Therapeutic targeting of mitochondrial superoxide in hypertension. *Circ. Res.* **2010**, *107*, 106–116. [CrossRef]
26. Sovari, A.A.; Rutledge, C.A.; Jeong, E.M.; Dolmatova, E.; Arasu, D.; Liu, H.; Vahdani, N.; Gu, L.; Zandieh, S.; Xiao, L.; et al. Mitochondria oxidative stress, connexin43 remodeling, and sudden arrhythmic death. *Circ. Arrhythmia Electrophysiol.* **2013**, *6*, 623–631. [CrossRef]
27. Dikalov, S.I.; Nazarewicz, R.R.; Bikineyeva, A.; Hilenski, L.; Lassègue, B.; Griendling, K.K.; Harrison, D.G.; Dikalova, A.E. Nox2-induced production of mitochondrial superoxide in angiotensin II-mediated endothelial oxidative stress and hypertension. *Antioxid. Redox Signal.* **2014**, *20*, 281–294. [CrossRef]

28. Cao, T.; Fan, S.; Zheng, D.; Wang, G.; Yu, Y.; Chen, R.; Song, L.S.; Fan, G.C.; Zhang, Z.; Peng, T. Increased calpain-1 in mitochondria induces dilated heart failure in mice: Role of mitochondrial superoxide anion. *Basic Res. Cardiol.* **2019**, *114*, 17. [CrossRef]
29. Hoshino, A.; Okawa, Y.; Ariyoshi, M.; Kaimoto, S.; Uchihashi, M.; Fukai, K.; Iwai-Kanai, E.; Matoba, S. Oxidative post-translational modifications develop LONP1 dysfunction in pressure overload heart failure. *Circ. Heart Fail.* **2014**, *7*, 500–509. [CrossRef]
30. Dey, S.; DeMazumder, D.; Sidor, A.; Foster, D.B.; O'Rourke, B. Mitochondrial ROS Drive Sudden Cardiac Death and Chronic Proteome Remodeling in Heart Failure. *Circ Res.* **2018**, *123*, 356–371. [CrossRef]
31. Kizhakekuttu, T.J.; Wang, J.; Dharmashankar, K.; Ying, R.; Gutterman, D.D.; Vita, J.A.; Widlansky, M.E. Adverse alterations in mitochondrial function contribute to type 2 diabetes mellitus-related endothelial dysfunction in humans. *Arterioscler. Thromb. Vasc. Biol.* **2012**, *32*, 2531–2539. [CrossRef]
32. Prime, T.A.; Blaikie, F.H.; Evans, C.; Nadtochiy, S.M.; James, A.M.; Dahm, C.C.; Vitturi, D.A.; Patel, R.P.; Hiley, C.R.; Abakumova, I.; et al. A Mitochondria-Targeted S-Nitrosothiol Modulates Respiration, Nitrosates Thiols, and Protects against Ischemia-Reperfusion Injury. *Proc. Natl. Acad. Sci. USA* **2009**, *106*, 10764–10769. [CrossRef] [PubMed]
33. Chouchani, E.T.; Hurd, T.R.; Nadtochiy, S.M.; Brookes, P.S.; Fearnley, I.M.; Lilley, K.S.; Smith, R.A.; Murphy, M.P. Identification of S-nitrosated mitochondrial proteins by S-nitrosothiol difference in gel electrophoresis (SNO-DIGE): Implications for the regulation of mitochondrial function by reversible S-nitrosation. *Biochem. J.* **2010**, *430*, 49–59. [CrossRef] [PubMed]
34. Chouchani, E.T.; Methner, C.; Nadtochiy, S.M.; Logan, A.; Pell, V.R.; Ding, S.; James, A.M.; Cochemé, H.M.; Reinhold, J.; Lilley, K.S.; et al. Cardioprotection by S-nitrosation of a cysteine switch on mitochondrial complex I. *Nat. Med.* **2013**, *19*, 753–759. [CrossRef] [PubMed]
35. Methner, C.; Chouchani, E.T.; Buonincontri, G.; Pell, V.R.; Sawiak, S.J.; Murphy, M.P.; Krieg, T. Mitochondria selective S-nitrosation by mitochondria-targeted S-nitrosothiol protects against post-infarct heart failure in mouse hearts. *Eur. J. Heart Fail.* **2014**, *16*, 712–717. [CrossRef]
36. Gerő, D.; Torregrossa, R.; Perry, A.; Waters, A.; Le-Trionnaire, S.; Whatmore, J.L.; Wood, M.; Whiteman, M. The novel mitochondria-targeted hydrogen sulfide (H_2S) donors AP123 and AP39 protect against hyperglycemic injury in microvascular endothelial cells in vitro. *Pharmacol. Res.* **2016**, *113*, 186–198. [CrossRef]
37. Chatzianastasiou, A.; Bibli, S.I.; Andreadou, I.; Efentakis, P.; Kaludercic, N.; Wood, M.E.; Whiteman, M.; Di Lisa, F.; Daiber, A.; Manolopoulos, V.G.; et al. Cardioprotection by H_2S Donors: Nitric Oxide-Dependent and Independent Mechanisms. *J. Pharmacol. Exp. Ther.* **2016**, *358*, 431–440. [CrossRef]
38. Ikeda, K.; Marutani, E.; Hirai, S.; Wood, M.E.; Whiteman, M.; Ichinose, F. Mitochondria-targeted hydrogen sulfide donor AP39 improves neurological outcomes after cardiac arrest in mice. *Nitric Oxide* **2015**, *49*, 90–96. [CrossRef]
39. Karwi, Q.G.; Bornbaum, J.; Boengler, K.; Torregrossa, R.; Whiteman, M.; Wood, M.E.; Schulz, R.; Baxter, G.F. AP39, a mitochondria-targeting hydrogen sulfide (H_2S) donor, protects against myocardial reperfusion injury independently of salvage kinase signalling. *Br. J. Pharmacol.* **2017**, *174*, 287–301. [CrossRef]
40. Zhu, C.; Su, Y.; Juriasingani, S.; Zheng, H.; Veramkovich, V.; Jiang, J.; Sener, A.; Whiteman, M.; Lacefield, J.; Nagpal, D.; et al. Supplementing preservation solution with mitochondria-targeted H_2S donor AP39 protects cardiac grafts from prolonged cold ischemia-reperfusion injury in heart transplantation. *Am. J. Transplant.* **2019**, *19*, 3139–3148. [CrossRef]
41. Testai, L.; Strobykina, I.; Semenov, V.V.; Semenova, M.; Pozzo, E.D.; Martelli, A.; Citi, V.; Martini, C.; Breschi, M.C.; Kataev, V.E.; et al. Mitochondriotropic and Cardioprotective Effects of Triphenylphosphonium-Conjugated Derivatives of the Diterpenoid Isosteviol. *Int. J. Mol. Sci.* **2017**, *18*, 2060. [CrossRef]
42. Liu, D.; Jin, F.; Shu, G.; Xu, X.; Qi, J.; Kang, X.; Yu, H.; Lu, K.; Jiang, S.; Han, F.; et al. Enhanced efficiency of mitochondria-targeted peptide SS-31 for acute kidney injury by pH-responsive and AKI-kidney targeted nanopolyplexes. *Biomaterials* **2019**, *211*, 57–67. [CrossRef] [PubMed]
43. Ikeda, G.; Matoba, T.; Nakano, Y.; Nagaoka, K.; Ishikita, A.; Nakano, K.; Funamoto, D.; Sunagawa, K.; Egashira, K. Nanoparticle-Mediated Targeting of Cyclosporine A Enhances Cardioprotection Against Ischemia-Reperfusion Injury Through Inhibition of Mitochondrial Permeability Transition Pore Opening. *Sci. Rep.* **2016**, *6*, 20467. [CrossRef]

44. Zhang, C.X.; Cheng, Y.; Liu, D.Z.; Liu, M.; Cui, H.; Zhang, B.L.; Mei, Q.B.; Zhou, S.Y. Mitochondria-targeted cyclosporin A delivery system to treat myocardial ischemia reperfusion injury of rats. *J. Nanobiotechnology* **2019**, *17*, 18. [CrossRef] [PubMed]
45. Hoque, A.; Sivakumaran, P.; Bond, S.T.; Ling, N.X.Y.; Kong, A.M.; Scott, J.W.; Bandara, N.; Hernández, D.; Liu, G.S.; Wong, R.C.B.; et al. Mitochondrial fission protein Drp1 inhibition promotes cardiac mesodermal differentiation of human pluripotent stem cells. *Cell Death Discov.* **2018**, *4*, 39. [CrossRef]
46. Lozano, O.; Lázaro-Alfaro, A.; Silva-Platas, C.; Oropeza-Almazán, Y.; Torres-Quintanilla, A.; Bernal-Ramírez, J.; Alves-Figueiredo, H.; García-Rivas, G. Nanoencapsulated Quercetin Improves Cardioprotection during Hypoxia-Reoxygenation Injury through Preservation of Mitochondrial Function. *Oxidative Med. Cell. Longev.* **2019**, *2019*, 7683051. [CrossRef] [PubMed]
47. Okahara, A.; Koga, J.I.; Matoba, T.; Fujiwara, M.; Tokutome, M.; Ikeda, G.; Nakano, K.; Tachibana, M.; Ago, T.; Kitazono, T.; et al. Simultaneous targeting of mitochondria and monocytes enhances neuroprotection against ischemia-reperfusion injury. *Sci. Rep.* **2020**, *10*, 14435. [CrossRef] [PubMed]
48. Zhang, S.; Li, J.; Hu, S.; Wu, F.; Zhang, X. Triphenylphosphonium and D-α-tocopheryl polyethylene glycol 1000 succinate-modified, tanshinone IIA-loaded lipid-polymeric nanocarriers for the targeted therapy of myocardial infarction. *Int. J. Nanomed.* **2018**, *13*, 4045–4057. [CrossRef]
49. Cheng, Y.; Liu, D.Z.; Zhang, C.X.; Cui, H.; Liu, M.; Zhang, B.L.; Mei, Q.B.; Lu, Z.F.; Zhou, S.Y. Mitochondria-targeted antioxidant delivery for precise treatment of myocardial ischemia-reperfusion injury through a multistage continuous targeted strategy. *Nanomedicine* **2019**, *16*, 236–249. [CrossRef]
50. Kawamura, E.; Maruyama, M.; Abe, J.; Sudo, A.; Takeda, A.; Takada, S.; Yokota, T.; Kinugawa, S.; Harashima, H.; Yamada, Y. Validation of Gene Therapy for Mutant Mitochondria by Delivering Mitochondrial RNA Using a MITO-Porter. *Mol. Ther. Nucleic Acids* **2020**, *20*, 687–698. [CrossRef]
51. Furukawa, R.; Yamada, Y.; Kawamura, E.; Harashima, H. Mitochondrial delivery of antisense RNA by MITO-Porter results in mitochondrial RNA knockdown, and has a functional impact on mitochondria. *Biomaterials* **2015**, *57*, 107–115. [CrossRef]
52. Ishikawa, T.; Somiya, K.; Munechika, R.; Harashima, H.; Yamada, Y. Mitochondrial transgene expression via an artificial mitochondrial DNA vector in cells from a patient with a mitochondrial disease. *J. Control Release* **2018**, *274*, 109–117. [CrossRef] [PubMed]
53. Ramachandra, C.J.A.; Hernandez-Resendiz, S.; Crespo-Avilan, G.E.; Lin, Y.H.; Hausenloy, D.J. Mitochondria in acute myocardial infarction and cardioprotection. *EBioMedicine* **2020**, *57*, 102884. [CrossRef] [PubMed]
54. Szeto, H.H. First-in-class cardiolipin-protective compound as a therapeutic agent to restore mitochondrial bioenergetics. *Br. J. Pharmacol.* **2014**, *171*, 2029–2050. [CrossRef] [PubMed]
55. Suk, J.S.; Xu, Q.; Kim, N.; Hanes, J.; Ensign, L.M. PEGylation as a strategy for improving nanoparticle-based drug and gene delivery. *Adv. Drug Deliv. Rev.* **2016**, *99*, 28–51. [CrossRef]
56. Yamada, Y.; Akita, H.; Kamiya, H.; Kogure, K.; Yamamoto, T.; Shinohara, Y.; Yamashita, K.; Kobayashi, H.; Kikuchi, H.; Harashima, H. MITO-Porter: A liposome-based carrier system for delivery of macromolecules into mitochondria via membrane fusion. *Biochim. Biophys. Acta* **2008**, *1778*, 423–432. [CrossRef]
57. Kelso, G.F.; Porteous, C.M.; Coulter, C.V.; Hughes, G.; Porteous, W.K.; Ledgerwood, E.C.; Smith, R.A.; Murphy, M.P. Selective targeting of a redox-active ubiquinone to mitochondria within cells: Antioxidant and antiapoptotic properties. *J. Biol. Chem.* **2001**, *276*, 4588–4596. [CrossRef]
58. Ayer, A.; Macdonald, P.; Stocker, R. CoQ_{10} Function and Role in Heart Failure and Ischemic Heart Disease. *Annu. Rev. Nutr.* **2015**, *35*, 175–213. [CrossRef]
59. Mortensen, S.A.; Rosenfeldt, F.; Kumar, A.; Dolliner, P.; Filipiak, K.J.; Pella, D.; Alehagen, U.; Steurer, G.; Littarru, G.P. Q-SYMBIO Study Investigators. The effect of coenzyme Q10 on morbidity and mortality in chronic heart failure: Results from Q-SYMBIO: A randomized double-blind trial. *JACC Heart Fail.* **2014**, *2014*, 641–649. [CrossRef]
60. Gholami, M.; Rezvanfar, M.R.; Delavar, M.; Abdollahi, M.; Khosrowbeygi, A. Effects of Coenzyme Q10 Supplementation on Serum Values of Gamma-glutamyl transferase, Pseudocholinesterase, Bilirubin, Ferritin, and High-Sensitivity C-Reactive Protein in Women with Type 2 Diabetes. *Exp. Clin. Endocrinol. Diabetes* **2019**, *127*, 311–319. [CrossRef]

61. Zielonka, J.; Joseph, J.; Sikora, A.; Hardy, M.; Ouari, O.; Vasquez-Vivar, J.; Cheng, G.; Lopez, M.; Kalyanaraman, B. Mitochondria-Targeted Triphenylphosphonium-Based Compounds: Syntheses, Mechanisms of Action, and Therapeutic and Diagnostic Applications. *Chem. Rev.* **2017**, *117*, 10043–10120. [CrossRef]
62. Neuzil, J.; Widén, C.; Gellert, N.; Swettenham, E.; Zobalova, R.; Dong, L.F.; Wang, X.F.; Lidebjer, C.; Dalen, H.; Headrick, J.P.; et al. Mitochondria transmit apoptosis signalling in cardiomyocyte-like cells and isolated hearts exposed to experimental ischemia-reperfusion injury. *Redox Rep.* **2007**, *12*, 148–162. [CrossRef] [PubMed]
63. Zernii, E.Y.; Gancharova, O.S.; Baksheeva, V.E.; Golovastova, M.O.; Kabanova, E.I.; Savchenko, M.S.; Tiulina, V.V.; Sotnikova, L.F.; Zamyatnin, A.A., Jr.; Philippov, P.P.; et al. Mitochondria-Targeted Antioxidant SkQ1 Prevents Anesthesia-Induced Dry Eye Syndrome. *Oxid Med. Cell Longev.* **2017**, *2017*, 9281519. [CrossRef]
64. Trnka, J.; Blaikie, F.H.; Smith, R.A.; Murphy, M.P. A mitochondria-targeted nitroxide is reduced to its hydroxylamine by ubiquinol in mitochondria. *Free Radic. Biol. Med.* **2008**, *44*, 1406–1419. [CrossRef] [PubMed]
65. Zhao, K.; Luo, G.; Giannelli, S.; Szeto, H.H. Mitochondria-targeted peptide prevents mitochondrial depolarization and apoptosis induced by tert-butyl hydroperoxide in neuronal cell lines. *Biochem. Pharmacol.* **2005**, *70*, 1796–1806. [CrossRef] [PubMed]
66. Whiteman, M.; Spencer, J.P.; Szeto, H.H.; Armstrong, J.S. Do mitochondriotropic antioxidants prevent chlorinative stress-induced mitochondrial and cellular injury? *Antioxid. Redox Signal.* **2008**, *10*, 641–650. [CrossRef] [PubMed]
67. Birk, A.V.; Chao, W.M.; Bracken, C.; Warren, J.D.; Szeto, H.H. Targeting mitochondrial cardiolipin and the cytochrome c/cardiolipin complex to promote electron transport and optimize mitochondrial ATP synthesis. *Br. J. Pharmacol.* **2014**, *171*, 2017–2028. [CrossRef] [PubMed]
68. Chavez, J.D.; Tang, X.; Campbell, M.D.; Reyes, G.; Kramer, P.A.; Stuppard, R.; Keller, A.; Zhang, H.; Rabinovitch, P.S.; Marcinek, D.J.; et al. Mitochondrial protein interaction landscape of SS-31. *Proc. Natl. Acad. Sci. USA* **2020**, *117*, 15363–15373. [CrossRef]
69. Kloner, R.A.; Hale, S.L.; Dai, W.; Gorman, R.C.; Shuto, T.; Koomalsingh, K.J.; Gorman, J.H., III; Sloan, R.C.; Frasier, C.R.; Watson, C.A.; et al. Reduction of ischemia/reperfusion injury with bendavia, a mitochondria-targeting cytoprotective Peptide. *J. Am. Heart Assoc.* **2012**, *1*, e001644. [CrossRef]
70. Brown, D.A.; Hale, S.L.; Baines, C.P.; del Rio, C.L.; Hamlin, R.L.; Yueyama, Y.; Kijtawornrat, A.; Yeh, S.T.; Frasier, C.R.; Stewart, L.M.; et al. Reduction of early reperfusion injury with the mitochondria-targeting peptide bendavia. *J. Cardiovasc. Pharmacol. Ther.* **2014**, *19*, 121–132. [CrossRef]
71. Cho, J.; Won, K.; Wu, D.; Soong, Y.; Liu, S.; Szeto, H.H.; Hong, M.K. Potent mitochondria-targeted peptides reduce myocardial infarction in rats. *Coron. Artery Dis.* **2007**, *18*, 215–220. [CrossRef]
72. Dai, D.F.; Chen, T.; Szeto, H.; Nieves-Cintrón, M.; Kutyavin, V.; Santana, L.F.; Rabinovitch, P.S. Mitochondrial targeted antioxidant peptide ameliorates hypertensive cardiomyopathy. *J. Am. Coll. Cardiol.* **2011**, *58*, 73–82. [CrossRef] [PubMed]
73. Dai, D.F.; Hsieh, E.J.; Chen, T.; Menendez, L.G.; Basisty, N.B.; Tsai, L.; Beyer, R.P.; Crispin, D.A.; Shulman, N.J.; Szeto, H.H.; et al. Global proteomics and pathway analysis of pressure-overload-induced heart failure and its attenuation by mitochondrial-targeted peptides. *Circ. Heart Fail.* **2013**, *6*, 1067–1076. [CrossRef] [PubMed]
74. Sabbah, H.N.; Gupta, R.C.; Kohli, S.; Wang, M.; Hachem, S.; Zhang, K. Chronic Therapy with Elamipretide (MTP-131), a Novel Mitochondria-Targeting Peptide, Improves Left Ventricular and Mitochondrial Function in Dogs with Advanced Heart Failure. *Circ. Heart Fail.* **2016**, *9*, e002206. [CrossRef] [PubMed]
75. Yuan, F.; Woollard, J.R.; Jordan, K.L.; Lerman, A.; Lerman, L.O.; Eirin, A. Mitochondrial targeted peptides preserve mitochondrial organization and decrease reversible myocardial changes in early swine metabolic syndrome. *Cardiovasc. Res.* **2018**, *114*, 431–442. [CrossRef] [PubMed]
76. Gibson, C.M.; Giugliano, R.P.; Kloner, R.A.; Bode, C.; Tendera, M.; Jánosi, A.; Merkely, B.; Godlewski, J.; Halaby, R.; Korjian, S.; et al. EMBRACE STEMI study: A Phase 2a trial to evaluate the safety, tolerability, and efficacy of intravenous MTP-131 on reperfusion injury in patients undergoing primary percutaneous coronary intervention. *Eur. Heart J.* **2016**, *37*, 1296–1303. [CrossRef] [PubMed]

77. Daubert, M.A.; Yow, E.; Dunn, G.; Marchev, S.; Barnhart, H.; Douglas, P.S.; O'Connor, C.; Goldstein, S.; Udelson, J.E.; Sabbah, H.N. Novel Mitochondria-Targeting Peptide in Heart Failure Treatment: A Randomized, Placebo-Controlled Trial of Elamipretide. *Circ. Heart Fail.* **2017**, *10*, e004389. [CrossRef]
78. Butler, J.; Khan, M.S.; Anker, S.D.; Fonarow, G.C.; Kim, R.J.; Nodari, S.; O'Connor, C.M.; Pieske, B.; Pieske-Kraigher, E.; Sabbah, H.N.; et al. Effects of Elamipretide on Left Ventricular Function in Patients with Heart Failure with Reduced Ejection Fraction: The PROGRESS-HF Phase 2 Trial. *J. Card. Fail.* **2020**, *26*, 429–437. [CrossRef]
79. Chatfield, K.C.; Sparagna, G.C.; Chau, S.; Phillips, E.K.; Ambardekar, A.V.; Aftab, M.; Mitchell, M.B.; Sucharov, C.C.; Miyamoto, S.D.; Stauffer, B.L. Elamipretide Improves Mitochondrial Function in the Failing Human Heart. *JACC Basic Transl. Sci.* **2019**, *4*, 147–157. [CrossRef]
80. Agnihotri, S.A.; Mallikarjuna, N.N.; Aminabhavi, T.M. Recent advances on chitosan-based micro- and nanoparticles in drug delivery. *J. Control Release* **2004**, *100*, 5–28. [CrossRef]
81. Huebener, P.; Abou-Khamis, T.; Zymek, P.; Bujak, M.; Ying, X.; Chatila, K.; Haudek, S.; Thakker, G.; Frangogiannis, N.G. CD44 is critically involved in infarct healing by regulating the inflammatory and fibrotic response. *J. Immunol.* **2008**, *180*, 2625–2633. [CrossRef]
82. Dalal, S.; Zha, Q.; Daniels, C.R.; Steagall, R.J.; Joyner, W.L.; Gadeau, A.P.; Singh, M.; Singh, K. Osteopontin stimulates apoptosis in adult cardiac myocytes via the involvement of CD44 receptors, mitochondrial death pathway, and endoplasmic reticulum stress. *Am. J. Physiol. Heart Circ. Physiol.* **2014**, *306*, H1182–H1191. [CrossRef] [PubMed]
83. Suleiman, M.; Abdulrahman, N.; Yalcin, H.; Mraiche, F. The role of CD44, hyaluronan and NHE1 in cardiac remodeling. *Life Sci.* **2018**, *209*, 197–201. [CrossRef] [PubMed]
84. Javadov, S.; Karmazyn, M. Mitochondrial permeability transition pore opening as an endpoint to initiate cell death and as a putative target for cardioprotection. *Cell Physiol. Biochem.* **2007**, *20*, 1–22. [CrossRef] [PubMed]
85. Hausenloy, D.J.; Boston-Griffiths, E.A.; Yellon, D.M. Cyclosporin A and cardioprotection: From investigative tool to therapeutic agent. *Br. J. Pharmacol.* **2012**, *165*, 1235–1245. [CrossRef]
86. Mewton, N.; Cung, T.T.; Morel, O.; Cayla, G.; Bonnefoy-Cudraz, E.; Rioufol, G.; Angoulvant, D.; Guerin, P.; Elbaz, M.; Delarche, N.; et al. CIRCUS Study Investigators: Rationale and design of the Cyclosporine to ImpRove Clinical oUtcome in ST-elevation myocardial infarction patients (the CIRCUS trial). *Am. Heart J.* **2015**, *169*, 758–766. [CrossRef]
87. Halestrap, A.P.; Davidson, A.M. Inhibition of Ca2(+)-induced large-amplitude swelling of liver and heart mitochondria by cyclosporin is probably caused by the inhibitor binding to mitochondrial-matrix peptidyl-prolyl cis-trans isomerase and preventing it interacting with the adenine nucleotide translocase. *Biochem. J.* **1990**, *268*, 153–160. [CrossRef]
88. Chiari, P.; Angoulvant, D.; Mewton, N.; Desebbe, O.; Obadia, J.F.; Robin, J.; Farhat, F.; Jegaden, O.; Bastien, O.; Lehot, J.J.; et al. Cyclosporine protects the heart during aortic valve surgery. *Anesthesiology* **2014**, *121*, 232–238. [CrossRef]
89. Piot, C.; Croisille, P.; Staat, P.; Thibault, H.; Rioufol, G.; Mewton, N.; Elbelghiti, R.; Cung, T.T.; Bonnefoy, E.; Angoulvant, D.; et al. Effect of cyclosporine on reperfusion injury in acute myocardial infarction. *N. Engl. J. Med.* **2008**, *359*, 473–481. [CrossRef]
90. Cung, T.T.; Morel, O.; Cayla, G.; Rioufol, G.; Garcia-Dorado, D.; Angoulvant, D.; Bonnefoy-Cudraz, E.; Guérin, P.; Elbaz, M.; Delarche, N.; et al. Cyclosporine before PCI in Patients with Acute Myocardial Infarction. *N. Engl. J. Med.* **2015**, *373*, 1021–1031. [CrossRef]
91. Ottani, F.; Latini, R.; Staszewsky, L.; La Vecchia, L.; Locuratolo, N.; Sicuro, M.; Masson, S.; Barlera, S.; Milani, V.; Lombardi, M.; et al. Cyclosporine A in Reperfused Myocardial Infarction: The Multicenter, Controlled, Open-Label CYCLE Trial. *J. Am. Coll. Cardiol.* **2016**, *67*, 365–374. [CrossRef]
92. Cormack, S.; Mohammed, A.; Panahi, P.; Das, R.; Steel, A.J.; Chadwick, T.; Bryant, A.; Egred, M.; Stellos, K.; Spyridopoulos, I.; et al. Effect of ciclosporin on safety, lymphocyte kinetics and left ventricular remodelling in acute myocardial infarction. *Br. J. Clin. Pharmacol.* **2020**, *86*, 1387–1397. [CrossRef] [PubMed]
93. Pandita, D.; Kumar, S.; Lather, V. Hybrid poly(lactic-co-glycolic acid) nanoparticles: Design and delivery prospectives. *Drug Discov. Today* **2015**, *20*, 95–104. [CrossRef] [PubMed]

94. Andreadou, I.; Iliodromitis, E.K.; Rassaf, T.; Schulz, R.; Papapetropoulos, A.; Ferdinandy, P. The role of gasotransmitters NO, H₂S and CO in myocardial ischaemia/reperfusion injury and cardioprotection by preconditioning, postconditioning and remote conditioning. *Br. J. Pharmacol.* **2015**, *172*, 1587–1606. [CrossRef] [PubMed]
95. Bell, R.M.; Maddock, H.L.; Yellon, D.M. The cardioprotective and mitochondrial depolarising properties of exogenous nitric oxide in mouse heart. *Cardiovasc. Res.* **2003**, *57*, 405–415. [CrossRef]
96. Penna, C.; Perrelli, M.G.; Tullio, F.; Angotti, C.; Camporeale, A.; Poli, V.; Pagliaro, P. Diazoxide postconditioning induces mitochondrial protein S-nitrosylation and a redox-sensitive mitochondrial phosphorylation/translocation of RISK elements: No role for SAFE. *Basic Res. Cardiol.* **2013**, *108*, 371. [CrossRef]
97. Shimizu, Y.; Polavarapu, R.; Eskla, K.L.; Nicholson, C.K.; Koczor, C.A.; Wang, R.; Lewis, W.; Shiva, S.; Lefer, D.J.; Calvert, J.W. Hydrogen sulfide regulates cardiac mitochondrial biogenesis via the activation of AMPK. *J. Mol. Cell Cardiol.* **2018**, *116*, 29–40. [CrossRef]
98. Sun, J.; Aponte, A.M.; Menazza, S.; Gucek, M.; Steenbergen, C.; Murphy, E. Additive cardioprotection by pharmacological postconditioning with hydrogen sulfide and nitric oxide donors in mouse heart: S-sulfhydration vs. S-nitrosylation. *Cardiovasc. Res.* **2016**, *110*, 96–106. [CrossRef]
99. Martelli, A.; Testai, L.; Citi, V.; Marino, A.; Bellagambi, F.G.; Ghimenti, S.; Breschi, M.C.; Calderone, V. Pharmacological characterization of the vascular effects of aryl isothiocyanates: Is hydrogen sulfide the real player? *Vascul. Pharmacol.* **2014**, *60*, 32–41. [CrossRef]
100. Testai, L.; Marino, A.; Piano, I.; Brancaleone, V.; Tomita, K.; Di Cesare Mannelli, L.; Martelli, A.; Citi, V.; Breschi, M.C.; Levi, R.; et al. The novel H₂S-donor 4-carboxyphenyl isothiocyanate promotes cardioprotective effects against ischemia/reperfusion injury through activation of mitoKATP channels and reduction of oxidative stress. *Pharmacol. Res.* **2016**, *113*, 290–299. [CrossRef]
101. Xu, M.; Yigang, W.; Ahmar, A.; Muhammad, A. Mitochondrial KATP channel activation reduces anoxic injury by restoring mitochondrial membrane potential. *Am. J. Physiol. Heart Circ. Physiol.* **2001**, *281*, H1295–H1303. [CrossRef]
102. Paggio, A.; Checchetto, V.; Campo, A.; Menabò, R.; Di Marco, G.; Di Lisa, F.; Szabo, I.; Rizzuto, R.; De Stefani, D. Identification of an ATP-sensitive potassium channel in mitochondria. *Nature* **2019**, *572*, 609–613. [CrossRef] [PubMed]
103. Citi, V.; Corvino, A.; Fiorino, F.; Frecentese, F.; Magli, E.; Perissutti, E.; Santagada, V.; Brogi, S.; Flori, L.; Gorica, E.; et al. Structure-activity relationships study of isothiocyanates for H₂S releasing properties: 3-Pyridyl-isothiocyanate as a new promising cardioprotective agent. *J. Adv. Res.* **2020**. [CrossRef]
104. Wu, D.; Hu, Q.; Tan, B.; Rose, P.; Zhu, D.; Zhu, Y.Z. Amelioration of mitochondrial dysfunction in heart failure through S-sulfhydration of Ca²⁺/calmodulin-dependent protein kinase II. *Redox Biol.* **2018**, *19*, 250–262. [CrossRef] [PubMed]
105. Jhun, B.S.; O-Uchi, J.; Adaniya, S.M.; Cypress, M.W.; Yoon, Y. Adrenergic Regulation of Drp1-Driven Mitochondrial Fission in Cardiac Physio-Pathology. *Antioxidants* **2018**, *7*, 195. [CrossRef] [PubMed]
106. Maneechote, C.; Palee, S.; Chattipakorn, S.C.; Chattipakorn, N. Roles of mitochondrial dynamics modulators in cardiac ischaemia/reperfusion injury. *J. Cell Mol. Med.* **2017**, *21*, 2643–2653. [CrossRef]
107. Cassidy-Stone, A.; Chipuk, J.E.; Ingerman, E.; Song, C.; Yoo, C.; Kuwana, T.; Kurth, M.J.; Shaw, J.T.; Hinshaw, J.E.; Green, D.R.; et al. Chemical inhibition of the mitochondrial division dynamin reveals its role in Bax/Bak-dependent mitochondrial outer membrane permeabilization. *Dev. Cell* **2008**, *14*, 193–204. [CrossRef]
108. Ong, S.B.; Subrayan, S.; Lim, S.Y.; Yellon, D.M.; Davidson, S.M.; Hausenloy, D.J. Inhibiting mitochondrial fission protects the heart against ischemia/reperfusion injury. *Circulation* **2010**, *121*, 2012–2022. [CrossRef]
109. Sharp, W.W.; Fang, Y.H.; Han, M.; Zhang, H.J.; Hong, Z.; Banathy, A.; Morrow, E.; Ryan, J.J.; Archer, S.L. Dynamin-related protein 1 (Drp1)-mediated diastolic dysfunction in myocardial ischemia-reperfusion injury: Therapeutic benefits of Drp1 inhibition to reduce mitochondrial fission. *FASEB J.* **2014**, *28*, 316–326. [CrossRef]
110. Givvimani, S.; Munjal, C.; Tyagi, N.; Sen, U.; Metreveli, N.; Tyagi, S.C. Mitochondrial division/mitophagy inhibitor (Mdivi) ameliorates pressure overload induced heart failure. *PLoS ONE* **2012**, *7*, e32388. [CrossRef]
111. Qi, J.; Wang, F.; Yang, P.; Wang, X.; Xu, R.; Chen, J.; Yuan, Y.; Lu, J.; Duan, J. Mitochondrial Fission Is Required for Angiotensin II-Induced Cardiomyocyte Apoptosis Mediated by a Sirt1-p53 Signaling Pathway. *Front. Pharmacol.* **2018**, *9*, 176. [CrossRef]

112. Tanner, M.J.; Wang, J.; Ying, R.; Suboc, T.B.; Malik, M.; Couillard, A.; Branum, A.; Puppala, V.; Widlansky, M.E. Dynamin-related protein 1 mediates low glucose-induced endothelial dysfunction in human arterioles. *Am. J. Physiol. Heart Circ. Physiol.* **2017**, *312*, H515–H527. [CrossRef] [PubMed]
113. Ishikita, A.; Matoba, T.; Ikeda, G.; Koga, J.; Mao, Y.; Nakano, K.; Takeuchi, O.; Sadoshima, J.; Egashira, K. Nanoparticle-Mediated Delivery of Mitochondrial Division Inhibitor 1 to the Myocardium Protects the Heart From Ischemia-Reperfusion Injury Through Inhibition of Mitochondria Outer Membrane Permeabilization: A New Therapeutic Modality for Acute Myocardial Infarction. *J. Am. Heart Assoc.* **2016**, *5*, e003872. [CrossRef] [PubMed]
114. Wu, D.; Dasgupta, A.; Chen, K.H.; Neuber-Hess, M.; Patel, J.; Hurst, T.E.; Mewburn, J.D.; Lima, P.D.A.; Alizadeh, E.; Martin, A.; et al. Identification of novel dynamin-related protein 1 (Drp1) GTPase inhibitors: Therapeutic potential of Drpitor1 and Drpitor1a in cancer and cardiac ischemia-reperfusion injury. *FASEB J.* **2020**, *34*, 1447–1464. [CrossRef] [PubMed]
115. Davidson, S.M.; Ferdinandy, P.; Andreadou, I.; Bøtker, H.E.; Heusch, G.; Ibáñez, B.; Ovize, M.; Schulz, R.; Yellon, D.M.; Hausenloy, D.J.; et al. Multitarget Strategies to Reduce Myocardial Ischemia/Reperfusion Injury: JACC Review Topic of the Week. *J. Am. Coll. Cardiol.* **2019**, *73*, 89–99. [CrossRef] [PubMed]
116. Chang, X.; Zhang, T.; Zhang, W.; Zhao, Z.; Sun, J. Natural Drugs as a Treatment Strategy for Cardiovascular Disease through the Regulation of Oxidative Stress. *Oxidative Med. Cell. Longev.* **2020**, *2020*, 5430407. [CrossRef] [PubMed]
117. Wiciński, M.; Socha, M.; Walczak, M.; Wódkiewicz, E.; Malinowski, B.; Rewerski, S.; Górski, K.; Pawlak-Osińska, K. Beneficial Effects of Resveratrol Administration-Focus on Potential Biochemical Mechanisms in Cardiovascular Conditions. *Nutrients* **2018**, *10*, 1813. [CrossRef]
118. Arinno, A.; Apaijai, N.; Chattipakorn, S.C.; Chattipakorn, N. The roles of resveratrol on cardiac mitochondrial function in cardiac diseases. *Eur. J. Nutr.* **2020**. [CrossRef]
119. Lagouge, M.; Argmann, C.; Gerhart-Hines, Z.; Meziane, H.; Lerin, C.; Daussin, F.; Messadeq, N.; Milne, J.; Lambert, P.; Elliott, P.; et al. Resveratrol improves mitochondrial function and protects against metabolic disease by activating SIRT1 and PGC-1alpha. *Cell* **2006**, *127*, 1109–1122. [CrossRef]
120. Li, H.; Xia, N.; Hasselwander, S.; Daiber, A. Resveratrol and Vascular Function. *Int. J. Mol. Sci.* **2019**, *20*, 2155. [CrossRef]
121. Bagul, P.K.; Katare, P.B.; Bugga, P.; Dinda, A.K.; Banerjee, S.K. SIRT-3 Modulation by Resveratrol Improves Mitochondrial Oxidative Phosphorylation in Diabetic Heart through Deacetylation of TFAM. *Cells* **2018**, *7*, 235. [CrossRef]
122. Ramírez-Garza, S.L.; Laveriano-Santos, E.P.; Marhuenda-Muñoz, M.; Storniolo, C.E.; Tresserra-Rimbau, A.; Vallverdú-Queralt, A.; Lamuela-Raventós, R.M. Health Effects of Resveratrol: Results from Human Intervention Trials. *Nutrients* **2018**, *10*, 1892. [CrossRef] [PubMed]
123. De Ligt, M.; Bergman, M.; Fuentes, R.M.; Essers, H.; Moonen-Kornips, E.; Havekes, B.; Schrauwen-Hinderling, V.B.; Schrauwen, P. No effect of resveratrol supplementation after 6 months on insulin sensitivity in overweight adults: A randomized trial. *Am. J. Clin. Nutr.* **2020**, *112*, 1029–1038. [CrossRef] [PubMed]
124. Li, Y.; Yao, J.; Han, C.; Yang, J.; Chaudhry, M.T.; Wang, S.; Liu, H.; Yin, Y. Quercetin, Inflammation and Immunity. *Nutrients* **2016**, *8*, 167. [CrossRef] [PubMed]
125. Çelik, N.; Vurmaz, A.; Kahraman, A. Protective effect of quercetin on homocysteine-induced oxidative stress. *Nutrition* **2017**, *33*, 291–296. [CrossRef] [PubMed]
126. Khan, A.; Ali, T.; Rehman, S.U.; Khan, M.S.; Alam, S.I.; Ikram, M.; Muhammad, T.; Saeed, K.; Badshah, H.; Kim, M.O. Neuroprotective Effect of Quercetin Against the Detrimental Effects of LPS in the Adult Mouse Brain. *Front. Pharmacol.* **2018**, *9*, 1383. [CrossRef]
127. Qiu, L.; Luo, Y.; Chen, X. Quercetin attenuates mitochondrial dysfunction and biogenesis via upregulated AMPK/SIRT1 signaling pathway in OA rats. *Biomed. Pharmacother.* **2018**, *103*, 1585–1591. [CrossRef]
128. Serban, M.C.; Sahebkar, A.; Zanchetti, A.; Mikhailidis, D.P.; Howard, G.; Antal, D.; Andrica, F.; Ahmed, A.; Aronow, W.S.; Muntner, P.; et al. Lipid and Blood Pressure Meta-analysis Collaboration (LBPMC) Group. Effects of Quercetin on Blood Pressure: A Systematic Review and Meta-Analysis of Randomized Controlled Trials. *J. Am. Heart Assoc.* **2016**, *5*, e002713. [CrossRef]
129. Chatsudthipong, V.; Muanprasat, C. Stevioside and related compounds: Therapeutic benefits beyond sweetness. *Pharmacol. Ther.* **2009**, *121*, 41–54. [CrossRef]

130. Liu, F.; Su, H.; Liu, B.; Mei, Y.; Ke, Q.; Sun, X.; Tan, W. STVNa Attenuates Isoproterenol-Induced Cardiac Hypertrophy Response through the HDAC4 and Prdx2/ROS/Trx1 Pathways. *Int. J. Mol. Sci.* **2020**, *21*, 682. [CrossRef]
131. Mei, Y.; Liu, B.; Su, H.; Zhang, H.; Liu, F.; Ke, Q.; Sun, X.; Tan, W. Isosteviol sodium protects the cardiomyocyte response associated with the SIRT1/PGC-1α pathway. *J. Cell. Mol. Med.* **2020**, *24*, 10866–10875. [CrossRef]
132. Xu, D.; Li, Y.; Wang, J.; Davey, A.K.; Zhang, S.; Evans, A.M. The cardioprotective effect of isosteviol on rats with heart ischemia-reperfusion injury. *Life Sci.* **2007**, *80*, 269–274. [CrossRef] [PubMed]
133. Xu, D.; Zhang, S.; Foster, D.J.; Wang, J. The effects of isosteviol against myocardium injury induced by ischaemia-reperfusion in the isolated guinea pig heart. *Clin. Exp. Pharmacol. Physiol.* **2007**, *34*, 488–493. [CrossRef] [PubMed]
134. Li, Z.; Zou, J.; Cao, D.; Ma, X. Pharmacological basis of tanshinone and new insights into tanshinone as a multitarget natural product for multifaceted diseases. *Biomed. Pharmacother.* **2020**, *130*, 110599. [CrossRef]
135. Tan, S.; Zou, C.; Zhang, W.; Yin, M.; Gao, X.; Tang, Q. Recent developments in d-α-tocopheryl polyethylene glycol-succinate-based nanomedicine for cancer therapy. *Drug Deliv.* **2017**, *24*, 1831–1842. [CrossRef] [PubMed]
136. Gao, S.; Li, L.; Li, L.; Ni, J.; Guo, R.; Mao, J.; Fan, G. Effects of the combination of tanshinone IIA and puerarin on cardiac function and inflammatory response in myocardial ischemia mice. *J. Mol. Cell. Cardiol.* **2019**, *137*, 59–70. [CrossRef]
137. Gao, Y.; Wang, X.; He, C. An isoflavonoid-enriched extract from Pueraria lobata (kudzu) root protects human umbilical vein endothelial cells against oxidative stress induced apoptosis. *J. Ethnopharmacol.* **2016**, *193*, 524–530. [CrossRef]
138. Dong, Z.; Guo, J.; Xing, X.; Zhang, X.; Du, Y.; Lu, Q. RGD modified and PEGylated lipid nanoparticles loaded with puerarin: Formulation, characterization and protective effects on acute myocardial ischemia model. *Biomed. Pharmacother.* **2017**, *89*, 297–304. [CrossRef]

Publisher's Note: MDPI stays neutral with regard to jurisdictional claims in published maps and institutional affiliations.

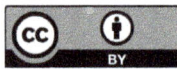

© 2020 by the authors. Licensee MDPI, Basel, Switzerland. This article is an open access article distributed under the terms and conditions of the Creative Commons Attribution (CC BY) license (http://creativecommons.org/licenses/by/4.0/).

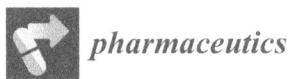

Review

Stem Cells as Drug-like Biologics for Mitochondrial Repair in Stroke

Jeffrey Farooq, You Jeong Park, Justin Cho, Madeline Saft, Nadia Sadanandan, Blaise Cozene and Cesar V. Borlongan *

Department of Neurosurgery and Brain Repair, University of South Florida Morsani College of Medicine, Tampa, FL 33612, USA; jfarooq@usf.edu (J.F.); youjeongpark@usf.edu (Y.J.P.); justincho@usf.edu (J.C.); saftmad@umich.edu (M.S.); nas146@georgetown.edu (N.S.); bcozene@tulane.edu (B.C.)
* Correspondence: cborlong@usf.edu

Received: 9 June 2020; Accepted: 26 June 2020; Published: 1 July 2020

Abstract: Stroke is a devastating condition characterized by widespread cell death after disruption of blood flow to the brain. The poor regenerative capacity of neural cells limits substantial recovery and prolongs disruptive sequelae. Current therapeutic options are limited and do not adequately address the underlying mitochondrial dysfunction caused by the stroke. These same mitochondrial impairments that result from acute cerebral ischemia are also present in retinal ischemia. In both cases, sufficient mitochondrial activity is necessary for cell survival, and while astrocytes are able to transfer mitochondria to damaged tissues to rescue them, they do not have the capacity to completely repair damaged tissues. Therefore, it is essential to investigate this mitochondrial transfer pathway as a target of future therapeutic strategies. In this review, we examine the current literature pertinent to mitochondrial repair in stroke, with an emphasis on stem cells as a source of healthy mitochondria. Stem cells are a compelling cell type to study in this context, as their ability to mitigate stroke-induced damage through non-mitochondrial mechanisms is well established. Thus, we will focus on the latest preclinical research relevant to mitochondria-based mechanisms in the treatment of cerebral and retinal ischemia and consider which stem cells are ideally suited for this purpose.

Keywords: retinal ischemia; blood–brain barrier; endothelial; reactive oxygen species; oxidative stress; tunneling nanotubules; neuron; central nervous system; inflammation; hypoxia

---

1. Stroke: A Trilogy of Cell Death Events

Stroke is currently the fifth leading cause of death in the United States and can cause disabling neurological deficits including cognitive impairment, hemiparesis, sensory disturbance, and aphasia [1]. Studies project that by 2030, 3.88% of the US population over the age of 18 will have a stroke and the total annual stroke-related costs will reach $240.67 billion [1]. Despite an emphasis on implementing effective acute and chronic stroke care made by the American Heart Association and American Stroke Association, there are only two FDA-approved treatment options available for acute stroke: tissue plasminogen activator (tPA) and endovascular thrombectomy. Unfortunately, their use is limited by the short therapeutic time window and risk for additional damage. Although rehabilitation is an option for chronic stroke care, functional recovery remains modest. Ischemic stroke comprises 87% of all stroke cases and involves inadequate blood perfusion to vital organs like the brain, which leads to oxygen and nutrient deprivation and subsequent cell death [2,3]. With the central nervous system's limited capability to recover after an injury, a treatment strategy to restore neurological function is an unmet need.

The ischemic cascade (Figure 1) triggered by stroke can be divided into three phases. During the acute phase—within the first few hours after stroke—blood flow, ATP, and energy stores in the tissue plummet, causing ionic disruption, mitochondrial dysfunction, and metabolic failure. The ionic imbalance and release of neurotransmitters spike the influx of sodium and calcium into the cell. This increased intracellular calcium activates phospholipases and proteases that degrade integral proteins, while the surplus of sodium leads to cellular swelling. [4] Furthermore, an increase in oxygen free radicals and other reactive oxygen species causes further damage and cell death during the acute phase [5,6]. The subacute phase follows, which lasts for the first few days after the ischemic event. Injured cerebral tissue releases cytokines, chemokines, cellular adhesion molecules, and matrix metalloproteases (MMPs), which increases the permeability of the blood–brain barrier (BBB) and attracts peripheral leukocytes to infiltrate and upregulate inflammation [4,7]. In the transition to the chronic phase, the inflammation resolves and tissue repair begins, but the endogenous repair process is not sufficient to confer functional recovery in stroke patients. Although the mechanism is not yet fully understood, the chronic phase is marked by the re-establishment of homeostasis and suppression of the inflammatory response. Like the neurological and cognitive deficit associated with cerebral stroke, retinal ischemia is characterized by visual impairment caused by lack of blood flow to the eye which results in a cascade of apoptotic events, oxidative stress, and mitochondria dysfunction in retinal ganglion cells [8]. Retinal ischemia is one of the major contributors to visual impairments caused by stroke and research suggests that mitochondria play a critical role in determining ganglion cell survival [9,10]. With the overlapping pathologic characteristics between cerebral and retinal ischemia in mind, the role of mitochondrial dysfunction in stroke offers a unique window to not only further the understanding of stroke pathology, but also to develop treatment strategies.

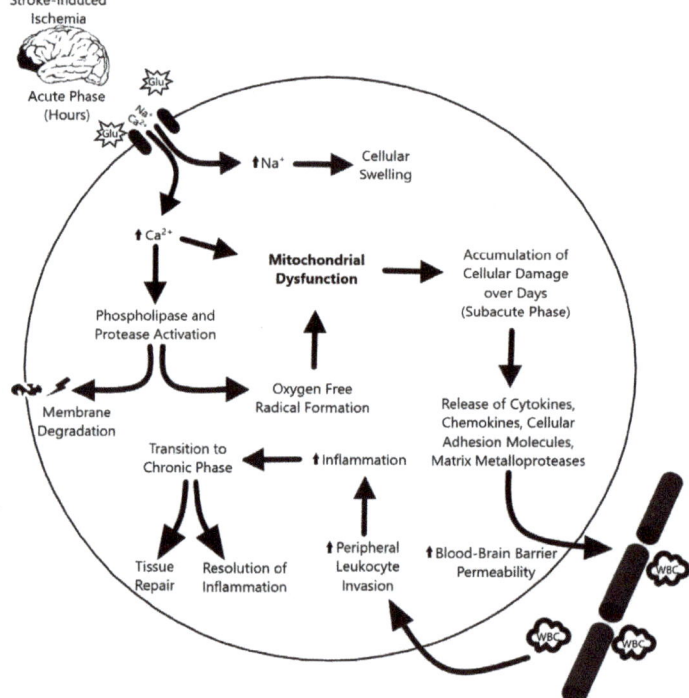

Figure 1. Overview of the three phases of the ischemic cascade. The acute phase following stroke-induced damaged precipitates ionic imbalances that ultimately propagate mitochondrial dysfunction. This progresses to subacute phase-based cellular damage, leukocyte invasion, and inflammation. Inflammation dissipates in the chronic phase, which culminates in tissue repair.

2. May the Force of Mitochondria Be with Stroke

Mitochondrial dysfunction plays a key role in the pathological progression of ischemic stroke [11]. Mitochondria are ubiquitous, double membrane-bound organelles that contain electron transport proteins, the ATP synthetase complex, and ATP/ADP transport proteins. They generate energy in the form of ATP by coupling the transfer of electrons from FADH2 and NADH through the electron transport chain with the phosphorylation of ADP. The majority of ATP generated in cerebral tissue is funneled into neuronal electrogenic activity [12]. Therefore, sufficient energy supply by the mitochondria is critical for neuronal excitability and survival. The mitochondria also produce reactive oxygen species (ROS) and play a role in regulating apoptosis—functions tightly linked to the pathology of ischemic stroke [11]. As in the case of many neurological disorders like amyotrophic lateral sclerosis and Parkinson's disease, cerebral ischemia leads to ROS overproduction, which compromises the functional and structural integrity of brain tissue [13,14]. During ischemic stroke, insufficient blood circulation deprives cerebral tissue of glucose and oxygen. This disruption prevents the mitochondria from performing oxidative phosphorylation, a process that generates 92% of the overall cellular ATP, and cells are no longer able to maintain their metabolic functions [11,15,16]. Furthermore, the defective oxidative metabolism leads to excess production of ROS and reactive nitrogen species (RNS) following the re-establishment of blood flow during reperfusion [11]. The oxidative stress overwhelms the neutralization capacity of the endogenous antioxidant system, and the overproduction of ROS and RNS ultimately results in cell death through the destruction of proteins, lipids, and DNA [11].

The body has multiple mechanisms to combat oxidative stress and clear damaged mitochondria. Cells can sequester functional mitochondria while degrading dysfunctional mitochondria via mitophagy [11,16]. In addition, increased permeability of damaged mitochondrial membranes allows the release of pro-apoptotic molecules into the cytoplasm and signals apoptotic cell death [11]. At the molecular level, creatine kinase (CK) enzymes transfer the phosphate from creatine phosphate to ADP, generating ATP and creatine. Cytosolic CK enzymes act as an intracellular energy buffer and expression of mitochondrial CK is upregulated during times of energy deprivation [16–18]. However, in the setting of ischemic stroke, the damage and oxidative stress are often beyond the scope of repair by endogenous mechanisms. For example, CK enzymes are also susceptible to damage by ROS and RNS, and post-stroke upregulation can lead to a buildup of crystalline mitochondrial CK inclusion bodies that exacerbate mitochondrial dysfunction [16,17,19,20]. Taken together, the role dysfunctional mitochondria play in the ischemic cascade presents opportunities to develop therapies for acute and chronic stroke. This review will cover the latest preclinical data that support stem cell-based approaches to repair dysfunctional mitochondria and restore/protect neurological function.

3. The Return of the Force: Enhancing Mitochondrial Function in Stroke

The discovery that stem cells can replace dysfunctional mitochondria in damaged cells has primed the field of stroke therapy for critical improvements in treatment outcomes [21]. In the presence of pathological stress, a series of cellular signals induce the formation of molecular bridges between stem cells and damaged cells through which mitochondria can travel [22]. Microvesicles, nanotubules, and gap junctions often form these intercellular connections, although transfer can also occur through direct uptake or cell fusion [23]. Regardless of the method of transit, stem cell-mediated mitochondrial replacement results in the restoration of cell function [24].

The ideal cell source to leverage the therapeutic benefits of mitochondrial transfer is bone marrow-derived mesenchymal stem cells (BM-MSCs). This cell type gives rise to endothelial progenitor cells (EPCs), which produce nearly all of the endothelial cells in the body [25]. In the context of stroke, EPCs repair damaged tissue and improve long-term outcomes by migrating through the blood–brain barrier (BBB) to the site of injury to promote angiogenesis [26,27]. This EPC-induced vascular regeneration is possibly due to mitochondrial transfer; however, there are other potential mechanisms through which the repair may occur, such as the release of pro-angiogenic factors from the EPCs themselves. To confirm the mechanism of repair is EPC-mediated mitochondrial transfer, three conditions must be true: EPCs must be able to export mitochondria, endothelial cells must take up those mitochondria, and the uptaken mitochondria must be able to restore endothelial cell function.

An in vitro stroke model proved that EPCs could successfully discharge their mitochondria [27]. Protein analysis of EPCs—identified via the cellular markers CD34, Flk-1, lectin-UEA, and vWF—showed enhanced expression of the mitochondrial membrane protein TOM40 and increased ATP concentration. The increased level of these two cellular components is an indication that mitochondrial production is upregulated in the post-stroke environment [27]. Additionally, the finding of mitochondria that exist within extracellular vesicles derived from EPCs demonstrates the presence of a mitochondrial export mechanism [27]. Furthermore, based on their oxygen consumption rates, the extracellular mitochondria function at a standard capacity [27]. Finally, the levels of extracellular mitochondria produced by EPC-derived cultures were similar to that of other cell types [27]. Taken together, this is strong evidence that EPCs can release sufficient amounts of active, viable mitochondria.

The next step in confirming a mechanism of EPC-mediated mitochondria transfer is to assess whether endothelial cells take up these extracellular mitochondria and whether this would aid the recipient cell. In that same study, confocal microscopy demonstrated evidence of mitochondria-containing, EPC-derived extracellular vesicles within endothelial cells in the cerebral vasculature [27]. Therefore, EPCs can release mitochondria, and brain endothelial cells can uptake them. There is also evidence that upon absorption of the EPC-derived mitochondria, capillary-like appendages form on the endothelial cells and assist in angiogenesis [27]. Another interesting observation in brain endothelial cells exposed to EPC-conditioned media is reduced membrane permeability and upregulated VE-cadherin production, a cytoskeletal stabilization protein that promotes cell-cell adhesions [27,28]. Exposure of these same endothelial cells to oxygen and glucose deprivation (OGD) conditions rescued intracellular mitochondrial DNA levels, supporting a mechanism where EPC-mediated mitochondrial transfer not only provides immediate benefit to the recipient cell via healthy donor mitochondria but also restores the ability of the recipient cell to produce mitochondria [27].

Although at this point there is considerable evidence for the role of EPCs in restoring mitochondrial function via a transfer mechanism, there was still much uncertainty surrounding the benefits of stem cell mitochondrial therapy. Additional studies on EPC-derived mitochondria addressed these concerns. FACS-assisted proteome analysis of OGD-exposed brain endothelial cells reveals that uptake of EPC-derived mitochondria enhances the production of angiogenic and BBB proteins, including Serpin E1, plasminogen, FGF-4, and bFGF [27]. These findings illustrate the tremendous therapeutic potential of EPCs in post-stroke recovery by improving mitochondrial function, restoring BBB function, and promoting angiogenesis.

The ischemic conditions brought about by stroke damage endothelial cells and predispose them towards undergoing intrinsic pathway apoptosis, which is mediated by mitochondrial dysfunction [29]. Integrating a stem cell-based mitochondria treatment ameliorates this issue. However, it does not further our understanding as to why the transfer of mitochondria provides neuroprotective effects against ischemia of neurons. Elucidating this mechanism will significantly advance the current understanding of stem cell mitochondrial therapy. Immunofluorescent imaging and the Seahorse or Clark electrode assays will be useful in evaluating the functionality of mitochondria transferred into neurons [16]. These techniques facilitate visual inspection of the mitochondria and quantification of the bioenergetic recovery associated with their intercellular transfer.

Importantly, astrocytes can also transfer their mitochondria to damaged neurons but do so in a transient fashion. Thus, they do not produce the same neuroprotective effects that occur via stem cell transplantation and cannot prevent secondary cell death [30]. Given the incredible therapeutic promise of stem cell treatment for stroke, it is essential to understand the mechanistic difference between these two approaches and why only stem cells confer neuroprotection.

Examination of the electron transport chain (ETC), specifically complexes I–IV, can be performed using ETC complex inhibitors to study each portion of the chain in isolation. Mouse models with mutated mitochondria are instrumental in this investigation in order to definitively determine whether it is the mitochondria themselves that confer the neuroprotection or whether a different characteristic of the stem cell is responsible [16]. When directly comparing EPC-cultured models to Rho0 (dysfunctional mitochondria) models, the results were similar. In both scenarios, graft survival was less than 1% in the first two weeks and was too low to measure between weeks four through twelve [27]. As neuroprotection is more vital than graft survival in EPC-mediated mitochondrial transfer, this corroborates the hypothesis that the Rho0-cultured cells did not gain any neuroprotective benefit.

The safety of BM-MSCs compared to other sources of stem cells is relatively well established [31]. Nevertheless, it is always valuable to deliberate on the safety profile compared to the therapeutic potential. There are three main concerns when discussing the use of EPCs as a stem cell transplant source. First, EPCs enhance vessel formation; therefore, the tumorigenicity is of particular concern in patients who have pre-existing tumors [32]. Second, the ability of EPCs to promote angiogenesis via endothelial growth factor signaling can cause cerebral edema [33]. Third, EPCs may encourage cerebral inflammation by recruiting monocytes and releasing interleukin-8, a proinflammatory cytokine, although this is controversial and is challenged by recent research that demonstrates the opposite phenomenon of inflammatory modulation [34,35]. Therefore, with mild exceptions, the use of EPCs appears to be a safe and promising avenue for stroke therapy.

4. Force in the Outer Rim: Stroke Extends to the Retina but may be Repaired by Stem Cell-Mediated Mitochondria Transfer

Up to this point, we concentrated on literature that characterizes the transfer of mitochondria from stem cells to endothelial cells and neurons in the context of the ischemic brain. However, stroke patients often suffer maladies that extend beyond the brain, and complete functional improvement must address these aspects of recovery as well. A prime example of this is that ischemic stroke may cause damage to the eye, leading to visual impairment and a significant delay in recovery [36,37]. Importantly, the same pathology-associated changes in mitochondrial activity that occur in the case of ischemic stroke also underlie cell survival and death in retinal ischemia [9,10].

It is valuable to understand the role of mitochondrial dysfunction in cerebral and ocular disease post-stroke due to the markedly similar pathology and treatment options between these two conditions [38]. In addition, given the benefits of MSC therapy in restoring mitochondrial function, it is plausible to infer that MSC treatment will have analogous effects in retinal ischemia, potentially diminishing the ischemia-induced cell death [38]. The use of a middle cerebral artery occlusion (MCAO) rat model and retinal pigment epithelium (RPE) cell culture model of OGD are beneficial for studying retinal ischemia, as they accurately reproduce the same symptomology in vivo and in vitro, respectively [38]. Following MCAO, blood perfusion to the ipsilateral hemisphere of the brain and ipsilateral eye decreases by 80%, a remarkably similar decrease to that seen in retinal and cerebral ischemia [38–40]. Upon resolution of the ischemia, blood flow returns to the ipsilateral eye and hemisphere nearly five minutes faster than the contralateral side due to angiogenesis and neovascularization of the affected tissues [38,41,42]. However, the perfusion rate stabilizes between the two eyes within three days of stroke, owing to the lack of collateral circulation [43–45]. On days 3 and 14 following MCAO, immunohistochemical analysis reveals insufficient blood flow to the retina, corresponding to a decrease in retinal ganglion cell survival and an increase in the rate of degeneration of the optic nerve [38]. Hemispheric blood flow post-stroke was also reduced [38]. RPE cell death is also increased in the in vitro OGD model [38]. Importantly, ischemic insult and the severe loss of healthy retinal cells coincides with mitochondrial dysfunction in both in vivo and in vitro models. Therefore, inducing ultrastructural defects in mitochondria is an effective model to study the pathological course of retinal ischemia [38].

There are considerable benefits to using MSC therapy to treat ischemia-induced eye damage, such as enhanced preservation of retinal ganglion cells. The decreased cell death is likely due to improved mitochondrial function, which may be due to MSC-derived mitochondrial transfer to the retinal ganglion cells [38]. MSC transplantation rescues the function of the electron transport chain within mitochondria, which also restores the energy balance of the cell. In addition, it ameliorates ganglion cell loss and optic nerve damage at the 14 days post-treatment [38]. RPE cells co-cultured with MSCs demonstrate improved survivability following OGD likely due to the restored network morphology, dynamics, and respiratory capacity of the mitochondria [38]. Sheltering mitochondrial DNA, improving respiration, and promoting mitochondrial signaling, the structure of mitochondrial networks is likely regulated by the balanced interaction between fission and fusion of the mitochondria [38]. However, when mitochondrial homeostasis is not present, typically when fission surpasses fusion, the mitochondria breaks apart into isolated, rounded mitochondria fragments [38]. The dynamics and configuration of the mitochondria and its network in vitro show that RPE cells co-cultured with MSCs possess much larger networks with less isolated, rounded mitochondrial fragments [38]. Additionally, stem cells that co-culture with MSCs reproduce standard expressive levels of the fusion protein mitofusin-2, which is downregulated by OGD insult [38,46,47]. MSC transplantation, however, does not increase the activity of OGD-induced fission protein dynamin-related protein-1 [39,48]. This is the first study to report about the ability of MSCs to regulate depolarization of the mitochondrial membrane by OGD [38].

The interaction of creatine and phosphocreatine conversion prevents lapses in cellular energy supplies under healthy conditions. However, it is still possible for the energy supply to be damaged under ischemic conditions, worsening mitochondrial dysfunction. Creatine supplementation possesses therapeutic characteristics in various neurodegenerative disorders that may address the lack of energy supply and the normal function of the mitochondria [49]. Therefore, creatine supplementation can rescue endangered mitochondria along with a host of other wide-reaching positive effects. Furthermore, stroke models that reveal the therapeutic benefits of creatine treatment also support this notion [50,51]. These non-clinical experiments highlight mitochondrial functioning as a key player for cerebral and retinal ischemia pathology. Consequently, the transfer of healthy mitochondria by stem cells moderates the restoration of mitochondrial function. By recovering the mitochondria, stem cells offer a potential treatment to restore the morphology and function of damaged neural and optic cells.

Based on previously mentioned studies, transferring healthy mitochondria by exogenous MSCs can potentially restore respiratory functions in ischemic retinal cells, reducing cell loss. Future studies should investigate how MSCs successfully transfer healthy mitochondria to retinal ganglion cells. Studies should also observe and describe the metabolic and proteomic properties of MSC-derived mitochondria post-transplantation into ischemic retinal cells. EPCs' affinity for BBB repair makes them a favorable MSC subtype. EPCs are known for being safe and effective to use in stem cell therapy. Additionally, their ability to donate healthy mitochondria justifies the need to further investigate its effects on retinal ischemia. However, the study presents a significant limitation. Specifically, no known study provides a detailed report regarding the physical characteristics of MSC that are involved in the mitochondrial transfer in retinal ischemia [38]. The function and phenotypic properties of EPC-derived mitochondria in cerebral stroke are explained in detail. However, the claim that EPCs are a key player in mitochondrial transfer in retinal ischemia lacks sufficient evidence. Future studies should focus on this distinct function of MSCs and EPCs to interconnect this gap in knowledge on mitochondria-mediated regenerative medicine of ischemic diseases.

5. The Rise of the Force: New Horizons in Mitochondrial Repair for Stroke

Stroke-induced ischemia results in insufficient oxygen delivery to cells and prevents mitochondria from performing cellular respiration. The ensuing loss of ATP is not compatible with cellular viability and ultimately precipitates mitochondrial dysfunction and cell death. In response to stroke and stroke-like lesions, cells upregulate mitochondrial synthesis to compensate for damaged mitochondria [52]. A variety of techniques can measure this new production of mitochondria, as well as the functional capacity of existing mitochondria. Therefore, mitochondria are potent biomarkers for stroke and ischemic brain injury. In addition, mitochondria are crucial organelles to target for therapeutic strategies due to their neuroprotective potential that helps bolster post-stroke recovery.

Despite the innovations in stroke therapy over the past decade, novel methods of research continue to elucidate fundamental information on the mechanistic role of mitochondria in stroke and enable the development of powerful new therapeutic strategies. A novel technology, Seahorse XFe24, measures mitochondrial respiration and allows investigators to directly detect changes in cellular energetics, rather than relying on cellular signaling [53]. This technique has the additional advantage of requiring only a small sample of mitochondria from each region of the brain for accurate analysis. Thus, Seahorse XFe24 is a convenient method to extract mechanistic data about mitochondrial function from experiments on mitochondrial repair in stroke. Along with novel technologies, several new strategies designed to target the mitochondria as therapeutics have emerged and are discussed below (Table 1).

Table 1. Recent Discoveries in Mitochondrial Repair for Stroke.

Milestone Discovery	Reference
Measuring mitochondrial respiration	[52,53]
Targeting mitochondria via pharmacological treatment	[54–57]
Normalizing autophagy	[58–60]
Enhancing mitophagy	[61–63]
Inhibiting MPTP	[64–68]
Inducing astrocyte-based transfer	[69,70]
Augmenting endogenous tissue repair	[71–80]

5.1. Pharmacological Treatment

Several pharmaceutical agents, such as the dopamine D2 receptor antagonist pramipexole (PPX), facilitate neuroprotection through the action of mitochondria. Administration of PPX to transient MCAO model rats after an ischemic stroke reduces infarct volume, neurological deficit severity, mitochondrial ROS formation, mitochondrial calcium concentration, and swelling of the mitochondrial membrane, while simultaneously increasing oxygen consumption and the respiratory control ratio [54]. Therefore, PPX is a promising treatment for ischemic stroke due to its ability to inhibit mitochondria-mediated cell death and improve neurological functions and motor strength.

The pharmacological administration of tetrahydrocurcumin (THC) also alleviates mitochondrial dysfunction and improves functional capacity and motor coordination. THC epigenetically reduces plasma and tissue homocysteine (Hcy) levels and Hcy-induced mitochondrial oxidative stress [55]. THC treatment of MCAO model mice compared to control mice significantly improves neuroscores, strengthens coordination and neuromuscular function, reduces cerebral blood flow, prevents damage from increased permeability in the brain interstitial parenchyma, decreases cerebrovascular permeability, modulates Hcy levels, and significantly reduces matrix metalloproteinase-9 levels [55]. Thus, THC's ability to alleviate oxidative stress and reverse ischemia-induced changes in mitochondria gives it potential as a treatment for ischemic stroke.

Another drug-based approach to mitochondrial dysfunction is the use of nicotinamide mononucleotide (NMN) to increase NAD+ levels. NMN extends the lifespan of mice with the mitochondrial disease Leigh Syndrome by normalizing NAD+ redox imbalance and lowering H1F1a accumulation in skeletal muscle [56]. Furthermore, NMN elevates alpha-ketoglutarate (KG) production and suppresses hypoxic signaling [56]. Direct administration of a cell-permeable form of KG also extends lifespan and delays the onset of neurological phenotype [56]. The encouraging results of NMN and KG treatment in Leigh Syndrome warrants their consideration for mitochondrial damage from stroke.

Cationic arginine-rich peptides (CARPs) are another candidate pharmacological therapeutic that specifically enhance mitochondria-mediated neuroprotection in stroke. CARPs are small peptides, composed of up to 30 amino acids, that cross the BBB and localize to mitochondria in neurons.

This property alone highlights their value as a pharmacologic treatment for stroke, as many other promising drugs do not effectively cross the BBB, making their administration difficult or ineffective. Once in the mitochondria, CARPs efficiently eliminate ROS that accumulate during ischemia and restore proper function of the mitochondria, rescuing the cell from free radical damage and reestablishing cellular viability [57].

5.2. Autophagy/Mitophagy

Although restoring the respiratory functions of mitochondria improves stroke outcomes, this is not the only strategy for recovery. Autophagy, the process of degrading and recycling damaged or unnecessary cellular components, can also mitigate mitochondrial dysfunction. A high salt diet is particularly dangerous because it increases the risk of hypertension-related stroke occurrence, reduces the efficiency of autophagy, and downregulates the production of the electron transport chain enzyme NDUFC2 [58]. However, the pharmacologic agent Tat-Beclin 1 restores autophagy activity, thereby mitigating stroke occurrences. This underscores the critical role of autophagy in normal mitochondrial function and suggests a possible pharmaceutical approach to treat hypertension-related stroke.

The proteins ULK1, NDP52, and TANK-Binding Kinase 1 (TBK1) are also meaningful targets for stroke therapies through targeting autophagy. TANK1 recruits the ULK1 complex to the NDP52 receptor to initiate autophagy under conditions of starvation [59]. Therefore, upregulating NDP52 on mitochondria enhances autophagy and can improve stroke outcomes by promoting the selective recycling of damaged mitochondria.

Another potential target of autophagy-based treatments involves the small molecule Compound R6 and its regulation of mitochondria-mediated apoptosis. The release of cytochrome c from damaged mitochondria activates the intrinsic apoptotic caspase-9/3 cascade and results in cell death [60]. Compound R6 represses apoptosis and activates autophagy by blocking cytochrome c release and restricting mammalian target of rapamycin (mTOR) activity, respectively [60]. It is also potentially a neuroprotective agent as it crosses the blood–brain barrier and accumulates in the brain after intravenous injection [60]. The capability of Compound R6 to improve retinal and cerebral cell survival post-stroke by inhibiting apoptosis and triggering autophagy of damaged mitochondria warrants its further study.

Along with autophagy, manipulating the discrete molecular mechanisms of mitochondria to enhance mitophagy is another approach to ameliorate stroke-induced mitochondrial dysfunction. Cell cycle progression in the presence of impaired mitochondria generates damaged daughter cells, further exacerbating tissue injury and delaying recovery. However, the serine/threonine kinase PINK1 and the E3 ubiquitin ligase Parkin mediate the elimination of these impaired mitochondria through induction of TBK1 to upregulate mitophagy, the targeted recycling of mitochondria. By directing TBK1 to the mitochondrial membrane, away from its role at the centromere during mitosis, PINK1 and Parkin halt the cell cycle at the G2/M phase [61]. Therefore, PINK1 and Parkin activation may mitigate ischemic injury and improve stroke outcomes.

In addition to enhancing TBK1-mediated mitophagy, PINK1 upregulates the Parkin-induced mitophagy pathway in the presence of damaged mitochondria. During an ischemic injury, the depleted mitochondrial membrane potential inhibits PINK1 importation to the inner mitochondrial membrane (IMM). Instead, PINK1 binds to Tom 7, accumulates on the outer mitochondrial membrane (OMM), then activates Parkin-induced mitophagy. However, the IMM-resident protease OMA1 cleaves PINK1 in the absence of Tom 7, abolishing mitophagy [62]. Hence, suppression of OMA1 promotes mitophagy and may act as a therapeutic tool in alleviating stroke-induced mitochondrial damage.

While the PINK1/Parkin pathway is valuable to preserve non-neuronal cells, Parkin-induced mitophagy is not as effective in neurons as only a small fraction of mitochondria in axons undergo mitophagy [63]. However, the Mul1/Mfn2 pathway is a valuable target to protect neuronal mitochondrial integrity under long-term stress. Mfn2, which normally mediates mitochondrial fusion and interaction with the endoplasmic reticulum (ER), is enhanced in the absence of Mul1, leading to hyperfusion and blockage of ER-Mito interactions. The loss of ER–mitochondria contact indirectly stimulates mitophagy. For this reason, regulating the Mul2–Mfn2 pathway, either by depleting Mul1 or overexpressing Mfn2, may be a useful therapeutic tool for stroke-induced mitochondrial damage.

5.3. Molecular and Other Mechanisms

Multiple cellular pathways spur mitochondrial deterioration in ischemic stroke. Apoptosis in mitochondria is upregulated during ischemic stroke and is associated with continuous mitochondrial permeability transition pore (MPTP) opening in the inner and outer mitochondrial membranes [64]. ROS production in the mitochondrial respiratory chain causes tissue damage during reperfusion. When oxygen returns to hypoxic brain tissues, it generates superoxide free radicals, which then cause oxidative damage and calcium accumulation. This leads to MPTP induction during ischemia that causes a decrease in mitochondrial membrane potential, depolarization of the mitochondria, swelling of the mitochondrial substances to the cytoplasm, and ultimately organ dysfunction and cell death [65,66]. Therefore, the key to protecting the mitochondria from oxidative damage is by using exogenous antioxidants during ischemic reperfusion (IR) injury and inhibiting MPTP induction. Specifically, using mitochondrial-targeted antioxidants protects against stroke-induced damage [67].

Mitochondrial transporters are also important in preventing atherosclerosis, the accumulation of fatty plaques on the inner wall of arteries, which is a significant risk factor for stroke. Poor metabolism or excess intake of lipids intensifies atherosclerotic plaque buildup and heightens the chance of stroke and ischemic brain injury. The mitochondrial calcium uniporter (MCU) prevents lipid accumulation and maintains appropriate bioenergetics by facilitating oxidative phosphorylation in the mitochondria [68]. However, the loss of MCU activity results in poor oxidative phosphorylation and the accretion of lipids on the arterial wall, thus promoting atherosclerosis and stroke [68]. Therefore, maintaining or enhancing the function of the MCU is another viable mitochondria-based strategy for anti-stroke therapeutics.

Another source of mitochondrial dysfunction that may exacerbate stroke pathology is the mitochondrial ADP/ATP carrier. Mitochondrial ADP/ATP carriers are located in the impermeable mitochondrial membrane and transport ADP into the mitochondrial matrix and ATP out for use as energy [69]. Inappropriate cellular energetics caused by ischemia may hinder the activity of the ADP/ATP carriers. Developing novel techniques to target these transporters may help maintain adequate ADP/ATP transport and improve stroke outcomes.

Astrocytes transfer their healthy mitochondria to neurons in the peri-infarct area post-stroke, and this endogenous neuroprotective mechanism is a candidate for stroke-therapy. In particular, the nuclear and desmosome-associated protein Pinin (Pnn) upregulates anti-apoptotic Bcl-2 expression, promotes ERK signaling, reduces pro-apoptotic cleaved caspase-3 production, and enhances astrocyte survival. Therefore, therapeutically augmenting Pnn expression may improve the endogenous capacity of astrocytes to protect neurons and repair ischemic tissue in the brain [70].

Hyperbaric oxygen therapy (HBOT), which delivers pure oxygen to patients in special high-pressure rooms, modulates inflammation in traumatic brain injury (TBI) when given after the onset of tissue damage. However, pretreatment with HBOT also reduces cell death and improves post-stroke outcomes by inducing endogenous astrocyte-based mitochondrial transfer to neuronal cells. The prophylactic use of HBOT to enhance neuroprotection circumvents the need for invasive surgical treatment and potentially toxic drug-based approaches [71]. Additionally, many hospitals already own HBOT chambers due to their therapeutic benefits in the treatment of various other ailments. Thus, there is already a strong framework for the use of HBOT-based mitochondrial transfer as a pretreatment for stroke to improve outcomes. Thus, there exists many unique and potentially efficacious pathways to augment mitochondrial repair for stroke therapy (Figure 2).

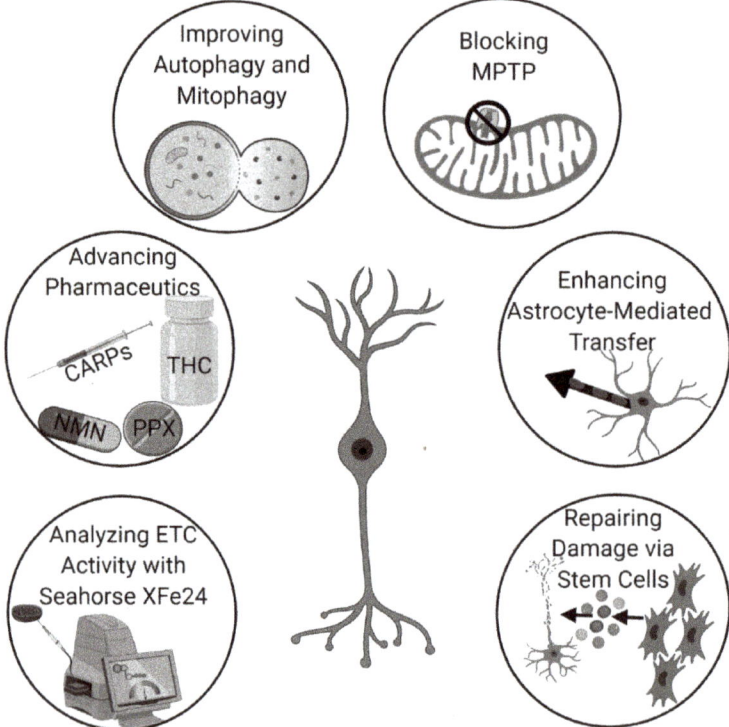

Figure 2. The use of mitochondrial repair for stroke is rapidly gaining momentum due to recent advancements in analytics, pharmaceutics, techniques that augment endogenous mechanisms, and stem cell therapy.

5.4. Stem Cells

Mitochondrial repair for stroke highlights the integral role of mitochondrial function on cell survival and neurological improvement. Mitochondrial dysfunction closely accompanies post-stroke secondary cell death. The hypoxic environment reduces energy production, further exacerbating stroke symptoms. Identifying a reliable method of mitochondrial transfer represents the first step towards developing an effective stroke treatment and is crucial to restoring cell function [72]. To this end, the transfer of healthy mitochondria from stem cells to areas of infarction stands as a potential avenue of therapy (Table 2). Stem cells transfer mitochondria via intercellular mechanisms to restore mitochondrial function in damaged cells, amplify cellular survival signals, and reprogram differentiated cells. Furthermore, they also mediate mitochondrial transfer from astrocytes into damaged neurons, enhancing neuronal vitality. Mitochondrial transfer thus serves as a viable means to reduce the chance of stroke-induced neuronal death and to restore the function of damaged cells [66].

While the benefits of stem cell therapy are clear, the mechanism is not. Determining the precise location of transfer between the donor and recipient cells will provide crucial insights into the mechanism and therapeutic actions of mitochondria. Such knowledge will guide efforts to optimize transfer conditions and maximize the beneficial effects of stem cells [73]. To this end, current research focuses on understanding the mechanism underlying mitochondrial transfer from stem cells into the stroke impacted brain. Cells utilize tunneling nanotubules (TNTs) or extracellular vesicles to transport mitochondria and other organelles between one another. Previous research has already shown that cell-to-cell signaling is involved in guiding healthy mitochondria from stem cells into damaged cells to rescue cell function. Intracellular quality of control helps maintain the functions of the mitochondria and combines fusion, fission, and degradation. For example, fusion of healthy and damaged mitochondria enables the exchange of DNA, proteins, and metabolites to prevent the buildup of damaged contents [66].

Although mitochondrial transfer is theoretically bidirectional, molecular signals released by damaged cells preferentially direct the movement of mitochondria and mtDNA from MSCs to damaged neurons [74]. One such signal is the activation of the pro-apoptotic protein caspase-3, which induces healthy mitochondria to move from MSCs to PC12 cells [64]. In addition, impaired retinal ganglion cells secrete proinflammatory cytokines, such as tumor necrosis factor-alpha and NF-kB, that initiate mitochondrial transfer from iPSC-MSCs [64]. Furthermore, extracellular vesicles that contain mitochondria released from the astrocytes help rescue neurons from ischemic stroke conditions and trigger CD38 to upregulate the release of mitochondria [66].

Deleting mitochondria from stem cells abolishes the regenerative benefits they confer to damaged endothelial cells, supporting the hypothesis that these organelles are responsible for repair. Furthermore, transferring mitochondria directly into ischemic brain tissue restores cellular energetics, facilitates homeostasis of the central nervous system (CNS), and resolves the inflammation that causes secondary cell death [38]. Stem cells afford vital protection to neurons and mitochondria in ischemic stroke, as well as in facilitating neuroprotection [75]. The following types of stem cells display a robust capacity to transfer healthy mitochondria to damaged neurons: Wharton's jelly MSCs, iPSCs, BM-MSCs, EPCs, and adipose-tissue-derived stem cells [64].

MSCs are the most common stem cell source for mitochondrial transfer and provide a protective mechanism to save damaged cells from mitochondrial dysfunction in response to stress. The transfer of MSC-derived mitochondria to endothelial cells can repress apoptosis after an IR injury by restoring aerobic respiration. The results of studies investigating this transfer are encouraging, paving the way for stem cell transplantation therapy for ischemic stroke [66]. An in vivo study co-cultured hypoxia-induced PC12 cells with MSCs. The treatment reduced apoptosis, swelling of mitochondria, and cristae dissipation. Interestingly, CoCl2 significantly improved the efficacy of the mitochondrial transfer [76].

Table 2. Overview of Stem Cell-Mediated Mitochondrial Repair for Stroke.

Experimentally Demonstrated Therapeutic Effect	Type of Stem Cell
Transfer of mitochondria via intracellular mechanisms to injured cells	MSC, iPSC, BM-MSC, EPC, ASC
Enhances astrocyte-based transfer	MSC, iPSC, BM-MSC, EPC, ASC
Represses apoptosis after IR injury	MSC
Reverses mitochondrial swelling	MSC
Diminishes mitochondrial cristae dissipation	MSC
Restores ischemic mitochondrial function	MSC
Ameliorates ganglion cell death within 14 days of stroke	MSC
Confers neuroprotection against OGD	MSC
Bolsters TNT formation after IR injury	MSC
Improves mitochondrial survival rate	hUC-MSC
Augments cell bioenergetics and locomotor function	BM-MSC
Rescues aerobic respiration in HUVECs	BM-MSC
Repairs dopaminergic neuron damage	iPSC

MSCs achieved efficacy of mitochondrial transplantation via intravenous transplantation into a middle cerebral artery occlusion (MCAO) mouse model. Here, retinal ischemia caused ganglion cells to deteriorate, impairing mitochondrial activity. These findings suggest that MSCs ameliorate mitochondrial dysfunction and ganglion cell death, as was observed 14 days after the stroke [38]. In vitro models produce similar results. Co-cultured retinal pigmented epithelium cells and MSCs displayed improved mitochondrial function and provided neuroprotection against OGD [38]. Additionally, the levels of phosphorylated AKT and BCL-XL increased following injection of mitochondria in the middle cerebral artery animal model. The rats injected with exogenous mitochondria demonstrated improved mitochondrial function and motor performance. Moreover, mitochondrial transfer in the MCAO mice triggered cell-surviving signals following ischemia and decreased energy deficits [66]. Therefore, the ability to restore mitochondrial function through mitochondrial transplantation provides insight into alleviating stroke-induced neuronal death.

The effect of OGD on MSCs derived from the perivascular region, cord lining, and Wharton's jelly of the human umbilical cord also implicated a key role of mitochondria in these specific MSC tissue sources. The mitochondria in the perivascular region MSCs showed the greatest activity while the MSCs from the cord lining demonstrated the highest survival rate. These findings suggest that hUC-MSCs may be a good source for mitochondrial transplantation for ischemic stroke treatment [77]. Additionally, co-culturing human umbilical vein endothelial (HUME) cells with MSCs improves aerobic respiration and TNT formation in in vitro IR injury models [66].

Human induced pluripotent stem cells (iPSCs) are also the subject of recent studies of mitochondrial transfer. PD model astrocytes derived from human iPSCs spontaneously release healthy mitochondria in damaged neuron cultures. This iPSC-induced mitochondrial transfer significantly ameliorates dopaminergic neuron damage and imparts neuroprotective effects [78]. iPSC's ability to attenuate neuronal damage through the intercellular transfer of mitochondria warrants further investigation into their therapeutic potential for ischemic stroke.

Spinal cord injury (SCI) models of mitochondrial transfer via bone marrow mesenchymal stem cells (BMSC) show promising results as well. Symptoms of both diseases are very similar: hypoxia, mitochondrial degeneration, oxidative stress, vascular injury, and axonal degeneration [79]. Healthy mitochondria are transferred from BMSCs to motor neurons when these cells are co-cultured in OGD conditions and transplanted into SCI rodents. The application of retinoic acid to this model increases gap junction intercellular communication (GJIC) and the release of mitochondria. In contrast, 18β glycyrrhetinic acid inhibits GJIC and decreases mitochondrial transfer. Mitochondrial transfer from BMSCs coincides with the induction and inhibition of GJIC. After the injured cells successfully integrate the mitochondria, locomotor function, cell survival, and bioenergetics improve [79]. Mitochondrial transfer via BMSCs is effective in treating and improving cardiovascular injury in animals and showcases the potential value of this cell type in stroke therapy. It is possible to transfer viable mitochondria to animal adults and embryonic cardiomyocytes. The transfer of mitochondria upregulates gene expression following an ischemic injury while simultaneously aiding in the reprogramming of adult animal cardiomyocytes. Moreover, treating ischemic human umbilical vein endothelial cells (HUVECs) with BMSC-based mitochondrial transfer therapy limits apoptosis and rescues aerobic respiration [80].

The omnipresent phenomenon of mitochondrial transfer allows for many applications in combination with stem cells. Contemporary literature details the efficacy of mitochondrial transfer in improving stroke, cardiovascular injury, spinal cord injury, and Parkinson's disease outcomes. The regenerative capacity demonstrated in a variety of tissues warrants its consideration as a primary therapeutic option. In particular, the physiological and pathological improvements seen in treating ischemic stroke illustrate the capability of mitochondrial transfer therapy. However, before moving into clinical trials, the optimal stem cell type must be identified to maximize the efficacy and potency of treatment. Further investigation is needed to discover the true potential of stem cell-based mitochondrial transfer therapy and improve long-term stroke outcomes.

Author Contributions: Conceptualization, J.F., Y.J.P., J.C., M.S., N.S., B.C., and C.V.B..; literature analysis, J.F., Y.J.P., J.C., M.S., N.S., B.C., and C.V.B.; resources, C.V.B.; writing—original draft preparation, J.F., Y.J.P., J.C., M.S., N.S., B.C., and C.V.B; writing—review and editing, J.F., Y.J.P., J.C., M.S., N.S., B.C., and C.V.B.; supervision, C.V.B.; project administration, C.V.B.; funding acquisition, C.V.B. All authors have read and agreed to the published version of the manuscript.

Funding: Cesar V. Borlongan is funded by National Institutes of Health (NIH) R01NS090962, NIH R01NS102395, and NIH R21NS109575.

Acknowledgments: The authors appreciate the excellent technical assistance of Grace Wei in rendering the graphical abstract, as well as Figure 2, which was created with biorender.com.

Conflicts of Interest: The authors declare no conflict of interest. C.V.B. declares patents and patent applications related to stem cell therapy. Additionally, C.V.B. was funded and received royalties and stock options from Astellas, Asterias, Sanbio, Athersys, KMPHC, and International Stem Cell Corporation; and also received consultant compensation for Chiesi Farmaceutici. The other authors have no other relevant affiliations or financial involvement with any organization or entity with a financial interest in or financial conflict with the subject matter or materials discussed in the manuscript apart from those disclosed.

References

1. Ovbiagele, B.; Goldstein, L.B.; Higashida, R.T.; Howard, V.J.; Johnston, S.C.; Khavjou, O.A.; Lackland, D.T.; Lichtman, J.H.; Mohl, S.; Sacco, R.L.; et al. Forecasting the Future of Stroke in the United States. *Stroke* **2013**, *44*, 2361–2375. [CrossRef] [PubMed]
2. Benjamin, E.J.; Muntner, P.; Alonso, A.; Bittencourt, M.S.; Callaway, C.W.; Carson, A.P.; Chamberlain, A.M.; Chang, A.R.; Cheng, S.; Das, S.R.; et al. Heart Disease Stroke Statistics—2019 Update: A Report From the American Heart Association. *Circulation* **2019**, *139*, e56–e528. [CrossRef]
3. Sacco, R.L.; Kasner, S.E.; Broderick, J.P.; Caplan, L.R.; Connors, J.J.; Culebras, A.; Elkind, M.S.V.; George, M.G.; Hamdan, A.D.; Higashida, R.T.; et al. An Updated Definition of Stroke for the 21st Century. *Stroke* **2013**, *44*, 2064–2089. [CrossRef] [PubMed]
4. Lo, E.H.; Dalkara, T.; Moskowitz, M.A. Mechanisms, challenges and opportunities in stroke. *Nat. Rev. Neurosci.* **2003**, *4*, 399–415. [CrossRef] [PubMed]
5. Hao, L.; Zou, Z.; Tian, H.; Zhang, Y.; Zhou, H.; Liu, L. Stem cell-based therapies for ischemic stroke. *Biomed. Res. Int.* **2014**, *2014*, 468748. [CrossRef]
6. Lakhan, S.E.; Kirchgessner, A.; Hofer, M. Inflammatory mechanisms in ischemic stroke: Therapeutic approaches. *J. Transl. Med.* **2009**, *7*, 97. [CrossRef]
7. Stonesifer, C.; Corey, S.; Ghanekar, S.; Diamandis, Z.; Acosta, S.A.; Borlongan, C.V. Stem cell therapy for abrogating stroke-induced neuroinflammation and relevant secondary cell death mechanisms. *Prog Neurobiol.* **2017**, *158*, 94–131. [CrossRef]
8. Kingsbury, C.; Heyck, M.; Bonsack, B.; Lee, J.Y.; Borlongan, C.V. Stroke gets in your eyes: Stroke-induced retinal ischemia and the potential of stem cell therapy. *Neural Regen. Res.* **2020**, *15*, 1014–1018. [CrossRef]
9. Osborne, N. Mitochondria: Their role in ganglion cell death and survival in primary open angle glaucoma. *Exp. Eye Res.* **2010**, *90*, 8. [CrossRef]
10. Park, S.W.; Kim, K.; Lindsey, J.; Dai, Y.; Heo, H.; Nguyen, D.; Ellisman, M.; Weinreb, R.; Ju, W. A selective inhibitor of drp1, mdivi-1, increases retinal ganglion cell survival in acute ischemic mouse retina. *Invest. Ophthalmol. Vis. Sci.* **2011**, *52*, 7. [CrossRef]
11. Yang, J.L.; Mukda, S.; Chen, S.D. Diverse roles of mitochondria in ischemic stroke. *Redox Biol.* **2018**, *16*, 263–275. [CrossRef] [PubMed]
12. Ames, A., 3rd. CNS energy metabolism as related to function. *Brain Res. Brain Res. Rev.* **2000**, *34*, 42–68. [CrossRef]
13. Cadenas, E.; Davies, K.J. Mitochondrial free radical generation, oxidative stress, and aging. *Free Radic Biol Med.* **2000**, *29*, 222–230. [CrossRef]
14. Valko, M.; Leibfritz, D.; Moncol, J.; Cronin, M.T.; Mazur, M.; Telser, J. Free radicals and antioxidants in normal physiological functions and human disease. *Int. J. Biochem Cell Biol.* **2007**, *39*, 44–84. [CrossRef] [PubMed]
15. Tarasov, A.I.; Griffiths, E.J.; Rutter, G.A. Regulation of ATP production by mitochondrial Ca(2+). *Cell Calcium* **2012**, *52*, 28–35. [CrossRef] [PubMed]
16. Heyck, M.; Bonsack, B.; Zhang, H.; Sadanandan, N.; Cozene, B.; Kingsbury, C.; Lee, J.Y.; Borlongan, C.V. The brain and eye: Treating cerebral and retinal ischemia through mitochondrial transfer. *Exp. Biol. Med. (Maywood)* **2019**, *244*, 1485–1492. [CrossRef]
17. Sims, N.R.; Muyderman, H. Mitochondria, oxidative metabolism and cell death in stroke. *Biochim. Biophys. Acta* **2010**, *1802*, 80–91. [CrossRef]
18. Saks, V.A.; Rosenshtraukh, L.V.; Smirnov, V.N.; Chazov, E.I. Role of creatine phosphokinase in cellular function and metabolism. *Can. J. Physiol. Pharmacol.* **1978**, *56*, 691–706. [CrossRef]
19. Schlattner, U.; Tokarska-Schlattner, M.; Wallimann, T. Mitochondrial creatine kinase in human health and disease. *Biochim. Biophys. Acta* **2006**, *1762*, 164–180. [CrossRef]

20. Stachowiak, O.; Dolder, M.; Wallimann, T.; Richter, C. Mitochondrial creatine kinase is a prime target of peroxynitrite-induced modification and inactivation. *J. Biol. Chem.* **1998**, *273*, 16694–16699. [CrossRef]
21. Li, X.; Zhang, Y.; Yeung, S.C.; Liang, Y.; Liang, X.; Ding, Y.; Ip, M.S.; Tse, H.F.; Mak, J.C.; Lian, Q. Mitochondrial transfer of induced pluripotent stem cell-derived mesenchymal stem cells to airway epithelial cells attenuates cigarette smoke-induced damage. *Am. J. Respir Cell Mol. Biol.* **2014**, *51*, 455–465. [CrossRef] [PubMed]
22. Spees, J.L.; Olson, S.D.; Whitney, M.J.; Prockop, D.J. Mitochondrial transfer between cells can rescue aerobic respiration. *Proc. Natl. Acad. Sci. USA* **2006**, *103*, 1283–1288. [CrossRef] [PubMed]
23. Abounit, S.; Zurzolo, C. Wiring through tunneling nanotubes–from electrical signals to organelle transfer. *J. Cell Sci.* **2012**, *125*, 1089–1098. [CrossRef] [PubMed]
24. Lin, H.Y.; Liou, C.W.; Chen, S.D.; Hsu, T.Y.; Chuang, J.H.; Wang, P.W.; Huang, S.T.; Tiao, M.M.; Chen, J.B.; Lin, T.K.; et al. Mitochondrial transfer from Wharton's jelly-derived mesenchymal stem cells to mitochondria-defective cells recaptures impaired mitochondrial function. *Mitochondrion* **2015**, *22*, 31–44. [CrossRef]
25. Hristov, M.; Erl, W.; Weber, P.C. Endothelial progenitor cells: Isolation and characterization. *Trends Cardiovasc. Med.* **2003**, *13*, 201–206. [CrossRef]
26. Fan, Y.; Shen, F.; Frenzel, T.; Zhu, W.; Ye, J.; Liu, J.; Chen, Y.; Su, H.; Young, W.L.; Yang, G.Y. Endothelial progenitor cell transplantation improves long-term stroke outcome in mice. *Ann. Neurol.* **2010**, *67*, 488–497. [CrossRef]
27. Hayakawa, K.; Chan, S.J.; Mandeville, E.T.; Park, J.H.; Bruzzese, M.; Montaner, J.; Arai, K.; Rosell, A.; Lo, E.H. Protective Effects of Endothelial Progenitor Cell-Derived Extracellular Mitochondria in Brain Endothelium. *Stem Cells* **2018**, *36*, 1404–1410. [CrossRef]
28. Meng, W.; Takeichi, M. Adherens junction: Molecular architecture and regulation. *Cold Spring Harb. Perspect. Biol.* **2009**, *1*, a002899. [CrossRef]
29. Wu, C.-C.; Bratton, S.B. Regulation of the intrinsic apoptosis pathway by reactive oxygen species. *Antioxid. Redox Signal.* **2013**, *19*, 546–558. [CrossRef]
30. Hayakawa, K.; Esposito, E.; Wang, X.; Terasaki, Y.; Liu, Y.; Xing, C.; Ji, X.; Lo, E.H. Transfer of mitochondria from astrocytes to neurons after stroke. *Nature* **2016**, *535*, 551–555. [CrossRef]
31. Aithal, A.P.; Bairy, L.K.; Seetharam, R.N. Safety Assessment of Human Bone Marrow-derived Mesenchymal Stromal Cells Transplantation in Wistar Rats. *J. Clin. Diagn. Res.* **2017**, *11*, FF01–FF03. [CrossRef]
32. Zhao, X.; Liu, H.-Q.; Li, J.; Liu, X.-L. Endothelial progenitor cells promote tumor growth and progression by enhancing new vessel formation. *Oncol. Lett.* **2016**, *12*, 793–799. [CrossRef] [PubMed]
33. Slevin, M.; Kumar, P.; Gaffney, J.; Kumar, S.; Krupinski, J. Can angiogenesis be exploited to improve stroke outcome? Mechanisms and therapeutic potential. *Clin. Sci. (Lond)* **2006**, *111*, 171–183. [CrossRef] [PubMed]
34. van der Strate, B.W.; Popa, E.R.; Schipper, M.; Brouwer, L.A.; Hendriks, M.; Harmsen, M.C.; van Luyn, M.J. Circulating human CD34+ progenitor cells modulate neovascularization and inflammation in a nude mouse model. *J. Mol. Cell Cardiol.* **2007**, *42*, 1086–1097. [CrossRef] [PubMed]
35. Acosta, S.A.; Lee, J.Y.; Nguyen, H.; Kaneko, Y.; Borlongan, C.V. Endothelial Progenitor Cells Modulate Inflammation-Associated Stroke Vasculome. *Stem Cell Rev. Rep.* **2019**, *15*, 256–275. [CrossRef] [PubMed]
36. Rowe, F. Stroke survivors' views and experiences on impact of visual impairment. *Brain Behav.* **2017**, *7*. [CrossRef]
37. Sand, K.M.; Midelfart, A.; Thomassen, L.; Melms, A.; Wilhelm, H.; Hoff, J. Visual impairment in stroke patients-a review. *Acta Neurol. Scand. Suppl.* **2013**, *196*, 5. [CrossRef]
38. Nguyen, H.; Lee, J.; Sanberg, P.; Napoli, E.; Borlongan, C. Eye opener in stroke. *Stroke* **2019**, *50*, 10. [CrossRef]
39. Borlongan, C.; Lind, J.; Dillon-Carter, O.; Yu, G.; Hadman, M.; Cheng, C.; Carroll, J.; Hess, D. Bone marrow grafts restore cerebral blood flow and blood brain barrier in stroke rats. *Brain Res.* **2004**, *1010*, 9. [CrossRef]
40. Taninishi, H.; Jung, J.; Izutsu, M.; Wang, Z.; Sheng, H.; Warner, D. A blinded randomized assessment of laser Doppler flowmetry efficacy in standardizing outcome from intraluminal filament MCAO in the rat. *J. Neurosci. Methods* **2015**, *241*, 10. [CrossRef]
41. Shih, Y.; De La Garza, B.; Huang, S.; Li, G.; Wang, L.; Duong, T. Comparison of retinal and cerebral blood flow between continuous arterial spin labeling MRI and fluorescent microsphere techniques. *J. Magn. Reson. Imaging* **2014**, *40*, 7. [CrossRef] [PubMed]
42. Hui, F.; Nguyen, C.; He, Z.; Vingrys, A.; Gurrell, R.; Fish, R.; Bui, B. Retinal and cortical blood flow dynamics following systemic blood-neural barrier disruption. *Front. Neurosci.* **2017**, *11*, 1. [CrossRef] [PubMed]

43. Ritzel, R.; Pan, S.; Verma, R.; Wizeman, J.; Crapser, J.; Patel, A.; Lieberman, R.; Mohan, R.; McCullough, L. Early retinal inflammatory biomarkers in the Middle cerebral artery occlusion model of ischemic stroke. *Mol. Vis.* **2016**, *22*, 14.
44. Allen, R.; Sayeed, I.; Oumarbaeva, Y.; Morrison, K.; Choi, P.; Pardue, M.; Stein, D. Progesterone treatment shows greater protection in brain vs. retina in a rat model of Middle cerebral artery occlusion: Progesterone receptor levels may play an important role. *Restor. Neurol. Neurosci.* **2016**, *34*, 17. [CrossRef]
45. Xiao, J.; Zhou, X.; Jiang, T.; Zhi, Z.; Li, Q.; Qu, J.; Chen, J. Unilateral cerebral ischemia inhibits optomotor responses of the ipsilateral eye in mice. *J. Integr. Neurosci.* **2012**, *11*, 8. [CrossRef]
46. Chen, X.; Zhang, G.; Guo, S.; Ding, J.; Lin, J.; Yang, Q.; Li, Z. Mfn2-mediated preservation of mitochondrial function contributes to the portective effects of BHAPI in response to ischemia. *J. Mol. Neurosci.* **2017**, *63*, 8. [CrossRef]
47. Shi, Y.; Yi, C.; Li, X.; Wang, J.; Zhou, F.; Chen, X. Overexpression of Mitofusin 2 decreased the reactive astrocytes proliferation in vitro induced by oxygen-glucose deprivation/reoxygenation. *Neurosci. Lett.* **2017**, *639*, 6. [CrossRef]
48. Zuo, W.; Zhang, S.; Xia, C.; Guo, X.; He, W.; Chen, N. Mitochondria autophagy is induced after hypoxic/ischemic stress in a Drp1 dependent manner: The role of inhibition of Drp1 in ischemic brain damage. *Neuropharmacology* **2014**, *86*, 13. [CrossRef]
49. Chaturvedi, R.K.; Flint Beal, M. Mitochondrial approaches for neuroprotection. *Ann. NY Acad. Sci.* **2008**, *1147*, 18. [CrossRef]
50. Prass, K.; Royl, G.; Lindauer, U.; Freyer, D.; Megow, D.; Dirnagl, U.; Stöckler-Ipsiroglu, G.; Wallimann, T.; Priller, J. Improved reperfusion and neuroprotection by creatine in a mouse model of stroke. *J. Cereb. Blood Flow Metab* **2007**, *27*, 8. [CrossRef]
51. Kitzenberg, D.; Colgan, S.; Glover, L. Creatine kinase in ischemic and inflammatory disorders. *Clin. Transl. Med.* **2016**, *5*, 1. [CrossRef] [PubMed]
52. Yamadera, M.; Fujimura, H.; Shimizu, Y.; Matsui, M.; Nakamichi, I.; Yokoe, M.; Sakoda, S. Increased number of mitochondria in capillaries distributed in stroke-like lesions of two patients with MELAS. *Neuropathology* **2019**, *39*, 404–410. [CrossRef] [PubMed]
53. Sperling, J.A.; Sakamuri, S.; Albuck, A.L.; Sure, V.N.; Evans, W.R.; Peterson, N.R.; Rutkai, I.; Mostany, R.; Satou, R.; Katakam, P.V.G. Measuring Respiration in Isolated Murine Brain Mitochondria: Implications for Mechanistic Stroke Studies. *Neuromol. Med.* **2019**, *21*, 493–504. [CrossRef] [PubMed]
54. Andrabi, S.S.; Ali, M.; Tabassum, H.; Parveen, S.; Parvez, S. Pramipexole prevents ischemic cell death via mitochondrial pathways in ischemic stroke. *Dis. Model. Mech.* **2019**, *12*. [CrossRef]
55. Mondal, N.K.; Behera, J.; Kelly, K.E.; George, A.K.; Tyagi, P.K.; Tyagi, N. Tetrahydrocurcumin epigenetically mitigates mitochondrial dysfunction in brain vasculature during ischemic stroke. *Neurochem. Int.* **2019**, *122*, 120–138. [CrossRef]
56. Lee, C.F.; Caudal, A.; Abell, L.; Nagana Gowda, G.A.; Tian, R. Targeting NAD(+) Metabolism as Interventions for Mitochondrial Disease. *Sci. Rep.* **2019**, *9*, 3073. [CrossRef]
57. MacDougall, G.; Anderton, R.S.; Mastaglia, F.L.; Knuckey, N.W.; Meloni, B.P. Mitochondria and neuroprotection in stroke: Cationic arginine-rich peptides (CARPs) as a novel class of mitochondria-targeted neuroprotective therapeutics. *Neurobiol. Dis.* **2019**, *121*, 17–33. [CrossRef]
58. Forte, M.; Bianchi, F.; Cotugno, M.; Marchitti, S.; De Falco, E.; Raffa, S.; Stanzione, R.; Di Nonno, F.; Chimenti, I.; Palmerio, S.; et al. Pharmacological restoration of autophagy reduces hypertension-related stroke occurrence. *Autophagy* **2019**. [CrossRef]
59. Vargas, J.; Wang, C.; Bunker, E.; Hao, L.; Maric, D.; Schiavo, G.; Randow, F.; Youle, R. Spatiotemporal Control of ULK1 Activation by NDP52 and TBK1 during Selective Autophagy. *Mol. Cell* **2019**, *74*, 16. [CrossRef]
60. Cao, R.; Li, L.; Ying, Z.; Cao, Z.; Ma, Y.; Mao, X.; Li, J.; Qi, X.; Zhang, Z.; Wang, X. A small molecule protects mitochondrial integrity by inhibiting mTOR activity. *Proc. Natl. Acad. Sci. USA* **2019**, *116*, 7. [CrossRef]
61. Sarraf, S.A.; Sideris, D.P.; Giagtzoglou, N.; Ni, L.; Kankel, M.W.; Sen, A.; Bochicchio, L.E.; Huang, C.H.; Nussenzweig, S.C.; Worley, S.H.; et al. PINK1/Parkin Influences Cell Cycle by Sequestering TBK1 at Damaged Mitochondria, Inhibiting Mitosis. *Cell Rep.* **2019**, *29*, 225–235.e225. [CrossRef] [PubMed]
62. Sekine, S.; Wang, C.; Sideris, D.P.; Bunker, E.; Zhang, Z.; Youle, R.J. Reciprocal Roles of Tom7 and OMA1 during Mitochondrial Import and Activation of PINK1. *Mol. Cell* **2019**, *73*, 1028–1043.e1025. [CrossRef]

63. Puri, R.; Cheng, X.T.; Lin, M.Y.; Huang, N.; Sheng, Z.H. Mul1 restrains Parkin-mediated mitophagy in mature neurons by maintaining ER-mitochondrial contacts. *Nat. Commun.* **2019**, *10*, 3645. [CrossRef] [PubMed]
64. Li, Y.; Sun, J.; Wu, R.; Bai, J.; Hou, Y.; Zeng, Y.; Zhang, Y.; Wang, X.; Wang, Z.; Meng, X. Mitochondrial MPTP: A Novel Target of Ethnomedicine for Stroke Treatment by Apoptosis Inhibition. *Front. Pharmacol.* **2020**, *11*, 352. [CrossRef] [PubMed]
65. Andrabi, S.S.; Tabassum, H.; Parveen, S.; Parvez, S. Ropinirole induces neuroprotection following reperfusion-promoted mitochondrial dysfunction after focal cerebral ischemia in Wistar rats. *Neurotoxicology* **2020**, *77*, 94–104. [CrossRef]
66. He, Z.; Ning, N.; Zhou, Q.; Khoshnam, S.E.; Farzaneh, M. Mitochondria as a therapeutic target for ischemic stroke. *Free Radic. Biol. Med.* **2020**, *146*, 45–58. [CrossRef]
67. Cabral-Costa, J.V.; Kowaltowski, A.J. Neurological disorders and mitochondria. *Mol. Aspects Med.* **2020**, *71*, 100826. [CrossRef]
68. Tomar, D.; Jaña, F.; Dong, Z.; Quinn, W.J., 3rd; Jadiya, P.; Breves, S.L.; Daw, C.C.; Srikantan, S.; Shanmughapriya, S.; Nemani, N.; et al. Blockade of MCU-Mediated Ca(2+) Uptake Perturbs Lipid Metabolism via PP4-Dependent AMPK Dephosphorylation. *Cell Rep.* **2019**, *26*, 3709–3725.e3707. [CrossRef]
69. Ruprecht, J.J.; King, M.S.; Zögg, T.; Aleksandrova, A.A.; Pardon, E.; Crichton, P.G.; Steyaert, J.; Kunji, E.R.S. The Molecular Mechanism of Transport by the Mitochondrial ADP/ATP Carrier. *Cell* **2019**, *176*, 435–447.e415. [CrossRef]
70. Mukda, S.; Tsai, C.Y.; Leu, S.; Yang, J.L.; Chan, S.H.H. Pinin protects astrocytes from cell death after acute ischemic stroke via maintenance of mitochondrial anti-apoptotic and bioenergetics functions. *J. Biomed. Sci* **2019**, *26*, 43. [CrossRef]
71. Lippert, T.; Borlongan, C.V. Prophylactic treatment of hyperbaric oxygen treatment mitigates inflammatory response via mitochondria transfer. *CNS Neurosci. Ther.* **2019**, *25*, 815–823. [CrossRef] [PubMed]
72. Borlongan, C.V.; Nguyen, H.; Lippert, T.; Russo, E.; Tuazon, J.; Xu, K.; Lee, J.Y.; Sanberg, P.R.; Kaneko, Y.; Napoli, E. May the force be with you: Transfer of healthy mitochondria from stem cells to stroke cells. *J. Cereb. Blood Flow Metab* **2019**, *39*, 367–370. [CrossRef] [PubMed]
73. Liu, K.; Guo, L.; Zhou, Z.; Pan, M.; Yan, C. Mesenchymal stem cells transfer mitochondria into cerebral microvasculature and promote recovery from ischemic stroke. *Microvasc. Res.* **2019**, *123*, 74–80. [CrossRef]
74. Surugiu, R.; Olaru, A.; Hermann, D.M.; Glavan, D.; Catalin, B.; Popa-Wagner, A. Recent Advances in Mono- and Combined Stem Cell Therapies of Stroke in Animal Models and Humans. *Int. J. Mol. Sci.* **2019**, *20*, 6029. [CrossRef]
75. Sarmah, D.; Kaur, H.; Saraf, J.; Vats, K.; Pravalika, K.; Wanve, M.; Kalia, K.; Borah, A.; Kumar, A.; Wang, X.; et al. Mitochondrial Dysfunction in Stroke: Implications of Stem Cell Therapy. *Transl. Stroke Res.* **2019**, *10*, 121–136. [CrossRef] [PubMed]
76. Yang, Y.; Ye, G.; Zhang, Y.-L.; He, H.-W.; Yu, B.-Q.; Hong, Y.-M.; You, W.; Li, X. Transfer of mitochondria from mesenchymal stem cells derived from induced pluripotent stem cells attenuates hypoxia-ischemia-induced mitochondrial dysfunction in PC12 cells. *Neural Regen. Res.* **2020**, *15*, 464–472. [CrossRef] [PubMed]
77. Russo, E.; Lee, J.Y.; Nguyen, H.; Corrao, S.; Anzalone, R.; La Rocca, G.; Borlongan, C.V. Energy Metabolism Analysis of Three Different Mesenchymal Stem Cell Populations of Umbilical Cord Under Normal and Pathologic Conditions. *Stem Cell Rev. Rep.* **2020**, *16*, 585–595. [CrossRef]
78. Cheng, X.-Y.; Biswas, S.; Li, J.; Mao, C.-J.; Chechneva, O.; Chen, J.; Li, K.; Li, J.; Zhang, J.-R.; Liu, C.-F.; et al. Human iPSCs derived astrocytes rescue rotenone-induced mitochondrial dysfunction and dopaminergic neurodegeneration in vitro by donating functional mitochondria. *Transl. Neurodegener.* **2020**, *9*, 13. [CrossRef]
79. Li, H.; Wang, C.; He, T.; Zhao, T.; Chen, Y.-Y.; Shen, Y.-L.; Zhang, X.; Wang, L.-L. Mitochondrial Transfer from Bone Marrow Mesenchymal Stem Cells to Motor Neurons in Spinal Cord Injury Rats via Gap Junction. *Theranostics* **2019**, *9*, 2017–2035. [CrossRef] [PubMed]
80. Li, C.; Cheung, M.K.H.; Han, S.; Zhang, Z.; Chen, L.; Chen, J.; Zeng, H.; Qiu, J. Mesenchymal stem cells and their mitochondrial transfer: A double-edged sword. *Biosci. Rep.* **2019**, *39*. [CrossRef]

© 2020 by the authors. Licensee MDPI, Basel, Switzerland. This article is an open access article distributed under the terms and conditions of the Creative Commons Attribution (CC BY) license (http://creativecommons.org/licenses/by/4.0/).

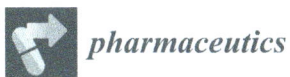

Review

Protective Effect of Mitochondria-Targeted Antioxidants against Inflammatory Response to Lipopolysaccharide Challenge: A Review

Ekaterina M. Fock and Rimma G. Parnova *

Sechenov Institute of Evolutionary Physiology and Biochemistry of the Russian Academy of Sciences, Saint-Petersburg 194223, Russia; efock@mail.ru
* Correspondence: rimma_parnova@mail.ru

Citation: Fock, E.M.; Parnova, R.G. Protective Effect of Mitochondria-Targeted Antioxidants against Inflammatory Response to Lipopolysaccharide Challenge: A Review. *Pharmaceutics* **2021**, *13*, 144. https://doi.org/10.3390/pharmaceutics13020144

Academic Editor: Joanna Kopecka
Received: 18 December 2020
Accepted: 17 January 2021
Published: 22 January 2021

Publisher's Note: MDPI stays neutral with regard to jurisdictional claims in published maps and institutional affiliations.

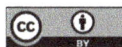

Copyright: © 2021 by the authors. Licensee MDPI, Basel, Switzerland. This article is an open access article distributed under the terms and conditions of the Creative Commons Attribution (CC BY) license (https://creativecommons.org/licenses/by/4.0/).

Abstract: Lipopolysaccharide (LPS), the major component of the outer membrane of Gram-negative bacteria, is the most abundant proinflammatory agent. Considerable evidence indicates that LPS challenge inescapably causes oxidative stress and mitochondrial dysfunction, leading to cell and tissue damage. Increased mitochondrial reactive oxygen species (mtROS) generation triggered by LPS is known to play a key role in the progression of the inflammatory response. mtROS at excessive levels impair electron transport chain functioning, reduce the mitochondrial membrane potential, and initiate lipid peroxidation and oxidative damage of mitochondrial proteins and mtDNA. Over the past 20 years, a large number of mitochondria-targeted antioxidants (mito-AOX) of different structures that can accumulate inside mitochondria and scavenge free radicals have been synthesized. Their protective role based on the prevention of oxidative stress and the restoration of mitochondrial function has been demonstrated in a variety of common diseases and pathological states. This paper reviews the current data on the beneficial application of different mito-AOX in animal endotoxemia models, in either in vivo or in vitro experiments. The results presented in our review demonstrate the promising potential of approaches based on mito-AOX in the development of new treatment strategies against Gram-negative infections and LPS per se.

Keywords: mitochondria-targeted antioxidants; inflammation; LPS; mitochondrial ROS

1. Introduction

Multiple diseases and pathological states caused by or associated with Gram-negative bacteria are accompanied by inflammation, local or systemic. Among them are respiratory and urogenital tract infections, endocarditis, gastritis, arthritis, meningitis, periodontal and endodontic diseases, diarrhea, and many other disorders [1,2]. Inflammatory processes that commonly accompany various noncommunicable diseases such as neurodegeneration, heart failure, cancer, diabetes mellitus, and others are exacerbated by the presence of Gram-negative infection. An extreme manifestation of inflammation is systemic inflammatory response syndrome, which is commonly observed in microbial infection-induced sepsis triggered by dysregulated inflammatory reactions and immunosuppression [3,4].

The most important virulent factor of Gram-negative bacteria that elicits the host's innate immune response and causes acute inflammation is lipopolysaccharide (LPS), the major component of the outer membrane of bacteria. In eukaryotes, LPS is mainly recognized by membrane-bound Toll-like receptor 4 (TLR4) expressed in immune and other cell types. As an experimental tool, this endotoxin is widely used in both in vitro experiments on different cell types and in vivo animal models to mimic Gram-negative infection or sepsis. The development of effective therapeutic approaches against LPS is highly important. Even if bacteria are killed by antibiotics, the inflammation induced by LPS itself commonly remains clinically relevant [5]. Recent data have found that disruption of the paracellular intestine barrier due to gut dysbiosis can provoke the release of bacterial LPS into the systemic circulation, causing chronic, low-grade inflammation in different organs, including the brain [6–8]. This makes explorations with LPS particularly important, not only as a simulator of Gram-negative infection, but also as a toxic agent per se.

Considerable evidence indicates that oxidative stress and mitochondrial dysfunction are common features in the majority of inflammatory states and diseases, acute or chronic [9–11]. It is generally accepted that excessive generation of reactive oxygen/nitrogen species and mitochondrial injury driven by an uncontrolled inflammatory response play a central role in the genesis of multiple-organ failure observed in sepsis (for review, see [12–16]). Mitochondrial damage and imbalanced generation of reactive oxygen species (ROS) have been shown to contribute to local inflammatory pathologies induced by LPS of Gram-negative bacteria [17,18].

Mitochondria are a major source of cellular reactive oxygen species (ROS) and, at the same time, a vulnerable target of ROS damage. In addition, endogenous oxidant defense mechanisms that protect the cell from excess ROS generation can be overwhelmed in different pathological states. Impairment of mitochondria plays a critical role in inducing cell apoptosis and tissue damage in different inflammatory states. Evidence indicates that endotoxemia is accompanied by a significant elevation in mitochondrial ROS (mtROS) generation, impairment of the electron transfer chain (ETC) and oxygen consumption, reduction in the mitochondrial membrane potential (MMP), deficiency in ATP production, decline in the endogenous antioxidant capacity, and accumulation of lipid peroxidation products [19–23]. mtROS are also able to stimulate NADPH oxidase activity, enhancing the cytosolic ROS level [24]. Recent data have highlighted the role of LPS-triggered mtROS in NLRP3 inflammasome assembly on the surface of the mitochondrial outer membrane, leading to the maturation of proinflammatory cytokines [25,26]. Since a critical step in mitochondria disturbances is known to be associated with harmful ETC-mediated ROS generation [27–31], their scavenging by antioxidants delivered specifically to mitochondria can be beneficial for restoration of mitochondrial function, preventing the development of inflammation and tissue damage. Over the past 20 years, a large number of mitochondria-targeted antioxidants (mito-AOX) that can accumulate inside mitochondria and scavenge free radicals have been synthesized and tested in different in vitro and in vivo models (for review, see [9,32–35]).

The most studied mito-AOX (MitoQ, SkQ, MitoTEMPO, and others) are conjugates of an antioxidant moiety with the triphenylphosphonium (TPP^+) lipophilic cation, which enables the rapid uptake of the chimeric molecule within mitochondria due to the negatively charged membrane potential across the inner mitochondrial membrane [36–38]. Another class of mito-AOX is Szeto–Schiller (SS) tetrapeptides, which have antioxidant properties attributed to their tyrosine or dimethyltyrosine residue. They accumulate within IMM independently of the mitochondrial membrane potential, binding with high affinity to cardiolipin [39,40]. The protective role of these and other mito-AOX based on the prevention of oxidative stress and the restoration of mitochondrial function has been demonstrated in a variety of common diseases and pathological states, such as atherosclerosis, metabolic diseases, ischemia/reperfusion injury, hypertension, degenerative neurological disorders, aging, and others (for review, see [9,31,32,41,42]).

This paper reviews the current data on the beneficial application of different mito-AOX in animal endotoxemia models, in either in vivo or in vitro experiments. We focused mainly on LPS challenge, although the cecal ligation and puncture (CLP) model mimicking polymicrobial sepsis was also considered. The anti-inflammatory action of mito-AOX observed at the cellular or the tissue level in LPS-induced inflammatory models, as well as challenges concerning mito-AOX application and their therapeutic potential, was discussed. In addition, we summarized the current knowledge on the anti-inflammatory benefits of competitive inhibitors of succinate oxidation, such as itaconate and malonate, which indirectly reduce mtROS generation. The schematic representation of inflammatory pathways triggered by LPS and the mechanisms of mito-AOX protection is presented in Figure 1.

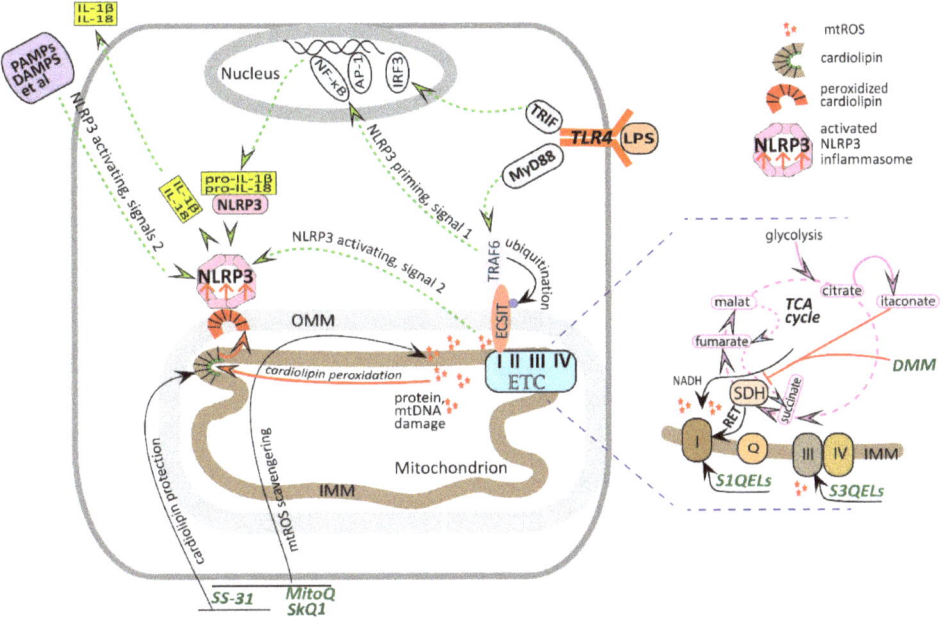

Figure 1. Diagram illustrating the protective mechanisms of mito-AOX against the LPS-induced cell inflammatory response. Activation of TLR4 by LPS triggers MyD88- or TRIF-dependent signaling pathways, resulting in the translocation of nuclear transcription factors NF-κB, AP-1, and IRF3 into the nucleus. This leads to the initiation of transcription of a wide range of pro- and anti-inflammatory mediators. LPS-induced priming of the NLRP3 inflammasome mediated by the adapter protein TRAF6 and NF-κB results in transcription of NLRP3 and inactive pro-IL-1β and pro-IL-18 proteins. In addition, TRAF6 is translocated to the mitochondria and ubiquitinates ECSIT, a protein implicated in complex I assembly and stability, resulting in its enrichment at the mitochondrial periphery and facilitation of mtROS production. Complexes I and III of the ETC are the main sites of mtROS production. In conditions of low forward electron transport, complex I can generate mtROS via NADH oxidation as well as via reverse electron transport (RET) from SDH to complex I (see the text). Inhibition of SDH by the TCA cycle derivative itaconate, as well as malonate or cell-permeable dimethyl malonate (DMM), attenuates RET and consequently diminishes mtROS production. mtROS serve as one of the numerous NLRP3 activating signals that cause the assembly and activation of the NLRP3 inflammasome complex and maturation and secretion of IL-1β and IL-18. In addition, mtROS damage proteins and mtDNA and induce lipid peroxidation. Oxidized cardiolipin is translocated from the IMM to the OMM, where it serves as a docking station for NLRP3. Mito-AOX, such as MitoQ, SkQ1, or SS-31, accumulate within the IMM to scavenge mtROS. SS-31, besides its ROS-scavenging properties, binds selectively to cardiolipin, increasing lipid packing of the membrane and tightening membrane curvatures, thus protecting the ETC and mitochondrial function. S1QELs and S3QELs, small molecules from different chemical families, specifically suppress mtROS production at ETC sites I_Q and III_{Qo}, respectively. Abbreviations: DAMP—damage-associated molecular pattern; ECSIT—evolutionarily conserved signaling intermediate in Toll pathways; ETC—electron transport chain; LPS—lipopolysaccharide; IMM—inner mitochondrial membrane; NLRP3—NLR family pyrin domain containing receptor 3 inflammasome; OMM—outer mitochondrial membrane; PAMP—pathogen-associated molecular pattern; mtROS—mitochondrial reactive oxygen species; SDH—succinate dehydrogenase.

2. Mechanisms of LPS-Triggered Inflammation

Inflammatory reactions play a critical role in LPS-induced tissue injury, which is caused by the adhesion and migration of leucocytes through the epithelium, the production of a variety of proinflammatory mediators by monocytes/macrophages, and oxidative stress driven by excess generation of reactive oxygen and nitrogen species. As the most abundant proinflammatory agent, LPS activates the systemic and cellular inflammatory response largely due to signaling through Toll-like receptor 4 (TLR4), which is expressed not only in immune cells but also in almost all cell types [43–45]. In mammalian cells, LPS-induced activation of TLR4 occurs through a series of interactions with several adapter proteins to facilitate its recognition by the TLR4/MD-2 receptor complex, which causes TLR4 oligomerization and recruitment of its numerous downstream adaptors. LPS/TLR4 signaling can be divided into MyD88-dependent and MyD88-independent (TRIF-dependent) pathways, leading to nuclear transcription factors NF-κB-, AP-1-, and IRF3-mediated induction of a wide range of pro- and anti-inflammatory mediators, such as cytokines, chemokines, eicosanoids, and others [46,47]. Stimulation of immune, epithelial, endothelial, and other cells by pro-inflammatory mediators results in excessive ROS/RNS generation, which is potentially damaging to all cellular compartments.

Recently, TLR4-independent LPS sensing pathways have been described [48]. First, transient receptor potential (TRP) channels have been identified as non-TLR membrane-bound sensors of LPS, and second, caspase-4/5 (and caspase-11 in mice) have been established as cytoplasmic sensors for LPS [48].

LPS has been shown to activate inflammasomes—cytosolic multiprotein complexes that mediate the propagation of the inflammatory response within the innate and the adaptive immune system as well as in epithelial cells [25,26,49,50]. Inflammasome activation is evoked by extra- and intracellular pathogens, such as Gram-negative bacteria, and/or by danger signals to activate caspase-1, resulting in a caspase-1-dependent, highly inflammatory form of cell death—pyroptosis [49,50]. It is thought that in Gram-negative infections, pyroptosis plays a key role in the destruction of intracellular bacterial replication niches. Inflammasomes are responsible for the maturation of proinflammatory cytokines, including IL-1β and IL-18, and for their secretion through the formation of pores in the plasma membrane [49,51,52]. The most studied inflammasome, NLRP3, is implicated in many different pathologies such as cancer and metabolic, neurodegenerative, and inflammatory diseases. Activation of the NLRP3 inflammasome occurs in two steps via different activating signals. Through TLR4 activation, LPS participates in the priming of inflammasome activation to initiate the transcription of NLRP3, inactive pro-IL-1β, and pro-IL-18 via NF-κB [51]. The second signals, which are notably diverse, include mtROS, derived mainly from ETC electron leakage [51], and initiate assembly of the inflammasome complex and, among other things, maturation of pro-IL-1β and pro-IL-18.

3. Generation of mtROS and Their Role in Normal and Pathological Conditions

ROS is a general term encompassing oxygen-free radicals, including superoxide ion (O_2^-) and hydroxyl radical ($^{\cdot}OH$), and nonradical oxygen substrates, e.g., hydrogen peroxide (H_2O_2) and singlet oxygen ($^1O_2$). ROS are produced during a wide range of biochemical reactions within the cell and within different cell compartments (mitochondria, peroxisomes, and endoplasmic reticulum). There are many cell proteins, bearing thiols, catecholamines, hydroquinones, and flavins, that may participate in intracellular ROS production. Although ROS can be produced in the cytosol by NADPH oxidases and xanthine oxidase, the major sources of ROS are mitochondria [30,31]. Simultaneously, mitochondria are a major target for damages by their own ROS.

Mitochondria can contain more than a dozen enzymatic sources of mtROS [53,54]. However, there is a consensus now that the mitochondrial respiratory chain is a primary source of mtROS, which are generated by the leakage of electrons from the ETC, resulting in a partial reduction in molecular oxygen. Mitochondrial complexes I (NADH-ubiquinone oxidoreductase) and III (cytochrome C oxidoreductase) are assumed to be a predominant source of superoxide generation under pathological conditions [30,55–57]. In particular, superoxide is generated by the reaction of O_2 with electrons originating either from direct transport from NADH under conditions of a slow respiration rate (due to low ATP demand or mitochondrial damage) or from the reverse electron transport (RET) from complex II (succinate dehydrogenase) to complex I under conditions of a high protonmotive force or when there is a high NADH/NAD$^+$ ratio in the matrix [30,55–57].

In healthy tissues under physiological conditions, mtROS generation and their removal by endogenous scavenging compounds and enzymes are tightly controlled by a complex antioxidant defense network including superoxide dismutase (SOD), catalase, ascorbic acid, tocopherol, reduced glutathione (GSH), etc. SOD catalyzes the conversion of superoxide to hydrogen peroxide, which, in turn, is converted to water by glutathione peroxidase (GPx). Under oxidative stress, the expression of antioxidant genes is activated by translocation of nuclear factor E2-related factor 2 (Nrf2) from the cytoplasm to the nucleus [11,58].

mtROS are necessary for the cell due to their essential role in various intracellular signaling pathways, including mitochondrial quality control by autophagy [59,60]. Disturbance of the fine-tuning of the equilibrium between mtROS generation and scavenging leads to excessive ROS production, resulting in severe damage of single cells and whole organs, loss of function, and then organism failure [61,62]. Numerous pathological conditions and diseases such as sepsis, cancer, metabolic diseases, neurodegenerative diseases, and others are triggered or accompanied by an increased level of mtROS [16,63,64]. At the cellular level, the most harmful effects of mtROS are associated with oxidation-triggered sustained damage of mitochondrial nucleic acids, proteins, and lipids, resulting in the impairment of ETC functioning and ATP production [64–69]. For example, mtROS-induced oxidation of cardiolipin polyunsaturated fatty acids damages cristae curvatures, reduces ETC complex activity, initiates cardiolipin translocation from the inner to the outer mitochondrial membrane, and triggers cytochrome C release into the cytosol, which is critical for the mitochondrial cell death pathway [70]. Furthermore, mtROS can oxidize proteins of the mitochondrial permeability transition pore, enhancing cytochrome C and mitochondrial DNA (mtDNA) release. mtDNA is especially sensitive to damage by ROS due to a lack of protective histones and its proximity to the ETC [71,72]. mtROS-initiated release of mtDNA is an important trigger of systemic inflammation, which is recognized by cells as a virulent pathogen motive [68]. Inflammatory conditions are commonly accompanied by excessive NO production, which, in turn, can interact with superoxide to generate the highly toxic peroxynitrite (ONOO$^-$) [14,73].

4. LPS Triggers mtROS Generation

Enhancement of ROS generated in both the cytosol and the mitochondria is an important step in LPS signaling that links the activation of TLR4 with the NF-kB-driven expression of proinflammatory mediators. Numerous animal models of sepsis (LPS or CLP) have demonstrated common abnormalities: increased level of ROS, decreased antioxidant capacity, and mitochondrial oxidative damage [14,15,74]. LPS-triggered generation of mitochondrial superoxide measured usually with the fluorogenic dye MitoSOX was demonstrated in different cell types, such as microglia [75,76], muscle myoblasts [23], gingival fibroblasts [17], human pulmonary bronchial epithelial cells [77], macrophages [78], and others. In addition, the decline in antioxidative enzymes and glutathione content caused by LPS contributes to the impairment of endogenous antioxidant defense and the subsequent increase in mtROS generation [79–83].

In a wide range of cell types, LPS application disturbs cellular energetics, which manifests itself in a decline in respiratory complex activity, decline in the mitochondrial membrane potential, reduction in mitochondrial respiration, and suppression of ATP production in a tissue-, time-, and dose-dependent manner [19,22,28,84–89]. A critical step in these disturbances is associated with excessive ROS generation [27–31]. In innate immune cells, LPS has been shown to switch the metabolic reprogramming from oxidative phosphorylation to aerobic glycolysis as a survival response maintaining the cellular ATP level [75,78,90,91], which results in the slowing or reversing of electron transport through respiratory complex I and a subsequent increase in ROS production.

The intrinsic mechanisms linking TLR4 signaling and mtROS have been studied mainly in phagocytic cells such as macrophages in which both cytosolic and mitochondrial

ROS generation is also related to their bactericidal activity [92,93]. Thus, it has been shown that LPS-triggered induction of mtROS is mediated by a complex I-associated protein evolutionarily conserved signaling intermediate in Toll pathways (ECSIT), which plays a key role in complex I assembly and stability [93,94]. Upon LPS stimulation, the TLR signaling adapter tumor necrosis factor receptor-associated factor 6 (TRAF6) is translocated to the mitochondria and ubiquitinates ECSIT, resulting in its enrichment at the mitochondrial periphery, thus leading to the augmentation of mitochondrial and cellular ROS generation [93]. TRAF6 also mediates the ubiquitination of the small GTPase Rac, maintaining it in an active GTP-loaded state, which is necessary for the full activation of the ROS-producing machinery [95]. In addition, it was demonstrated in macrophages that LPS activates mitochondrial mitofusin2 (Mfn2) expression, which has been shown to be a required step for mtROS generation. $Mfn2^{-/-}$ macrophages are not be able to produce mtROS and proinflammatory mediators in response to LPS [96]. Whether the above mechanisms exist in other cell types remains unknown.

5. Mitochondria-Targeted Antioxidants and Their Application against LPS-Triggered Inflammation

Generally, antioxidants are substances that can accept or donate electron(s) to eliminate the unpaired condition of free radicals, thus neutralizing them. Antioxidant drugs can either scavenge free radicals or turn into new free radicals, which in some cases are less active and dangerous than initial ones [97]. Antioxidants can also break chain reactions [98] as well as affect ROS-regulated enzymes through controlling the cellular level of free radicals [99–102]. The natural defense mechanisms are supplied by enzymatic and non-enzymatic antioxidants, which are distributed within the cell cytoplasm and organelles (such as SOD, GPx and reductase, catalase, vitamins, minerals, polyphenols, albumin, transferrin, ferritin, and a variety of others), whereas foods and supplements provide a wide variety of exogenous natural ones (e.g., vitamins B, C, and E; ions Zn, Cu, and Se; flavonoids; omega-3 fatty acids; L-carnitine; and Q-enzyme Q10).

5.1. Conjugates with Lipophilic Cations

An era of investigations applying mito-AOX conjugates began half a century ago when V. Skulachev and colleagues demonstrated the ability of lipophilic cations, such as triphenylphosphonium (TPP^+), to accumulate within mitochondria due to the large MMP (negative inside) [103]. In numerous chimeric mito-AOX compounds synthesized later, lipophilic cations, which provide drug accumulation several hundred-fold in the mitochondrial matrix, were grafted to antioxidant moieties, which quenched electrons from the respiratory chain, thus diminishing ROS elevation [104]. Conjugates designed in such a way are widely used as a tool for research, as well as for diagnostic and therapeutic purposes, including drug delivery (for review, see [105,106].

Triphenylphosphonium derivatives have been mainly used as a mitochondrial targeting moiety. They are conjugated with quinone derivatives (ubiquinone in MitoQs [36] or plastoquinone in SkQs [31,37]); with superoxide dismutase and catalase mimetics in MitoTEMPO and MitoTEMPOL, respectively [38]; and with vitamin E in MitoVitE [107], etc. Inside mitochondria, these chimeric mito-AOX undergo red/ox cycling: they not only quench radicals but also can be reduced afterward by the ETC.

Most of the in vivo studies and clinical trials were performed with MitoQ and SkQ1. As both compounds are found to be localized at the matrix-facing side of the inner mitochondrial membrane with their antioxidant portion and alkyl chain, their main protective activity is to prevent lipid peroxidation [108,109]. TPP-based mito-AOX accumulate preferentially in healthy and hyperpolarized mitochondria but not within injured mitochondria, which carry a lower membrane potential and therefore are capable of taking up lower doses of therapeutic antioxidants than normal ones [110,111].

TPP-based antioxidants have been widely used in both in vitro experiments on various types of cells exposed to LPS (Table 1) and in vivo experiments on typical animal models of inflammation or sepsis (administration of LPS or cecal ligation and puncture; Table 2).

Each cellular model mimics a specific pathological state or disorder associated with mtROS-induced inflammation. Among examples in Table 1 is LPS- or bacteria-induced mitochondrial dysfunction in oligodendrocytes (model of multiple sclerosis) [109], renal tubular cells (pyelonephritis and acute kidney injury) [18,112], microglia (neurodegeneration) [76], hepatocytes (liver failure) [113], endothelial cells (vascular abnormalities) [89,114], muscle myoblasts (diaphragm weakness) [23], gingival fibroblasts (periodontitis) [17], intestinal epithelial cells (impaired gut barrier function) [11], and others.

Table 1. In vitro effects of mitochondria-targeted antioxidants.

Inflammatory Model	Cells	Mito-AOX	Major Findings	Reference
LPS E. coli	Macrophages	MitoQ 50–100 nM	↓ Cellular ROS; ↓ IL-1β mRNA and protein expression	[92]
LPS E. coli	BV-2 murine microglial cells	MitoTEMPO 200 μM	↓ Mitochondrial and cellular ROS; ↓ iNOS and COX-2 expression; ↓ TNF-α, IL-1β, IL-6 content; ↓ NF-kB activation	[76]
LPS E. coli	Primary cultured frog urinary bladder epithelial cells	MitoQ 25 nM	↓ Cellular ROS; prevention of fatty acid oxidation decline and lipid droplet accumulation	[85]
LPS E. coli	Intestinal epithelial cell line-6 (IEC-6)	MitoQ 1 μM	Stimulation of nuclear translocation of Nrf2	[11]
LPS E. coli	NRK-52E (rat renal proximal tubular cell line)	MitoQ 1 μM	↓ Cellular ROS; ↓NLRP3 inflammasome activation; ↓ IL-1β, IL-18, and caspase-1	[112]
Mixture of cytokines + LPS E. coli	C2C12 muscle myoblasts	MitoTEMPOL 10 mg/L	↓ Mitochondrial superoxide generation; prevention of reduction in cell width	[23]
LPS E. coli + PepG S. aureus	HUVEC-C	MitoQ 1 μM	↓ Cellular ROS; restoration of MMP; ↓ IL-1β, IL-6, and IL-8	[114]
LPS E. coli + PepG S. aureus	HUVEC-C	Melatonin, 0.1, 1.0, 10, 100, and 500 μM; MitoVitE, 5 μM	↓ IL-6 and IL-8; ↓ NF-kB activation; ↓ loss of MMP; ↑ GSH level; ↓ decline in metabolic activity	[80,115]
LPS P. gingivalis	Human gingival fibroblasts	MitoTEMPO 50 μM	↓ Mitochondrial ROS; ↓ IL-6, IL-1β, and TNF-α production; ↓ activation of NF-B	[17]
Inflammatory mediators generated by incubation of white blood cells with LPS E. coli	Buffalo rat liver cell line-3A (BRL-3A)	MitoTEMPO, 500 nM	↓ Mitochondrial and cellular ROS; ↓iNOS mRNA; ↓ IL-6	[113]
LPS E. coli + IFN-γ + TNFα	HUVEC	Mitoquinone (MQ) 1 μM	↓ Cellular ROS; ↓ tyrosine nitration and iNOS protein expression; recovery of O_2 consumption and complex I activity	[89]
LPS E. coli + succinate	Bone marrow-derived macrophages	Dimethyl malonate, 10 mM; MitoQ, 500 nM; MitoTEMPO, 0.5–1 mM	↓ Cellular ROS, IL-1β, and HIF-1α; ↑ IL-1RA and IL-10	[78]
E. coli lysate + activated leucocytes	Primary culture rat kidney cells	SKQR1 10 nM	↓ Cellular ROS; ↓ cell dearth	[18]
LPS E. coli	Primary oligodendrocytes	SkQ1 5–10 nM	Restoration of myelin synthesis	[109]
LPS E. coli	Cardiomyocytes	Melatonin 100 μM	↓ Cellular ROS; ↓ loss of MMP; ↑ content of GSH, SOD; ↓ decline in BAP31 expression; ↑ cell viability	[79]

Table 1. Cont.

Inflammatory Model	Cells	Mito-AOX	Major Findings	Reference
LPS E. coli	Primary neonatal rat cardiomyocytes	Melatonin 100 μM	↓ IL-6, TNF-α, mRNA levels; ↓Bax and ↑ Bcl-2 expression; ↑ autophagy;	[116]
LPS E. coli	Human alveolar epithelial cells	Melatonin, 800 μM	↓ cellular ROS; ↓ MDA; ↑ SOD and GPx levels; prevention of LPS-induced epithelial–mesenchymal transition through Nrf2 activation	[81]
LPS E. coli	Macrophages RAW 264.7	Mn-porphyrin-oligopeptide conjugate, 10 μM	↓ LPS-induced cell dearth	[117]
LPS E. coli	Cardiomyocytes (H9C2 cell line)	SS-31, 10 μM	↓ ROS; ↓ MDA; ↓ mRNA level of IL-6, IL-1β, and TNF-α; normalized activity of GPx and SOD; ↓ MMP decline; ↑ ATP	[82]
LPS E. coli	Murine microglial cells (BV-2)	SS-31, 100 nM	↓ ROS; effect is mediated by Fis1; ↓ Fis1 expression; ↓ COX-2 and iNOS expression	[118]
LPS E. coli	Macrophages RAW 264.7	XJB-5-131 2 μmol/kg	↓ NO and inflammatory cytokines	[119]
E. coli 0157:H7	Human colonic epithelial cell line (Caco-2)	MitoTEMPO	↓ Cellular ROS; ↓NLRP3 inflammasome activation; ↓ IL-1β and IL-18	[120]

Table 2. In vivo effects of mitochondria-targeted antioxidants.

Model of Infection	Species	Organ Investigated	Mito-AOX	Mode of Antioxidant Application	Major Findings	Reference
LPS E. coli	Rat, mouse	Heart	MitoQ 500 μM	Given water orally for 2 days	↓ Oxidative stress; ↓ mitochondrial dysfunction; ↓ cardiac TNF-α level; ↓ reductions in cardiac pressure generation; ↓ caspase 3 and 9 activity	[21]
LPS E. coli	Mouse	Gut, serum	MitoQ 4 mg/kg	i.v. injection 15 min before LPS	↓ Gut barrier dysfunction, restoration of the level of tight junction proteins (ZO-1 and occludin); ↓ intestinal inflammatory response; ↑ SOD and GSH level; ↓TNF-α, IL-1, IL-6, and NO in intestines and plasma	[11]
LPS E. coli	Rat	Liver, serum	MitoTEMPO 50 nmol/kg; SKQ1 5 nmol/kg	i.p., 24 and 1 h before LPS	↓ iNOS expression; ↓ plasma NO; ↓liver damage	[113]
LPS E. coli	Rat (7-day-old pups)	Kidney	SkQR1 100 nmol/kg	i.p., 3 h before LPS	↓Acute kidney injury; preservation of cell proliferative activity	[121]
E. coli lysate	Rat	Kidney	SkQR1 500 nmol/kg in total	i.p., 1, 12, 24, 36, and 48 h after intraurethral bacteria injection	↓ Renal cell dearth and animal mortality, restoration of Bcl-2 level in kidney; ↓TNF-α in kidney	[18]

Table 2. Cont.

Model of Infection	Species	Organ Investigated	Mito-AOX	Mode of Antioxidant Application	Major Findings	Reference
LPS E. coli + PepG S. aureus	Rat	Liver, kidney, lungs, heart, gut	7.5 μmol/kg MitoQ, then 5 μmol/kg/h MitoQ	As a bolus i.v. infusion for 6 h after LPS+PepG	↓ Acute liver and renal dysfunction; ↑ MMP in most organs	[114]
LPS E. coli + PepG S. aureus	Rat	Liver, kidney	1.5 μmol/kg MitoQ or MitoVitE or melatonin, then 1 μmol/kg/h MitoQ, MitoVitE, or melatonin	As a bolus i.v. infusion for 5 h after LPS+PepG	↓ Mitochondrial damage; ↓ organ dysfunction; ↓ inflammatory response	[122]
CLP	Mouse	Kidney	MitoTEMPO 10 mg/kg	i.p., 6 h after operation	↓ Mitochondrial ROS, protection of complex I and II/III respiration; ↑ SOD; ↓ renal dysfunction (improved renal microcirculation and GFR); ↑ survival of animals	[22]
CLP	Mouse	Diaphragm	MitoTEMPOL 10 mg/kg/d	i.p., immediately after operation and 24 h later or only 6 h after operation	↓ Diaphragm weakness; ↓ mitochondrial superoxide generation; prevention of mitochondrial dysfunction; ↓ proteolytic enzyme activities; ↓ depletion of myosin heavy-chain protein content	[23]
LPS E. coli	Mouse	Heart	Melatonin 20 mg/kg/d	i.p., 48 h before LPS	↓ Cardiomyopathy; ↓ caspase 3 activation and cardiomyocyte apoptosis	[79]
LPS E. coli	Mouse	Heart	Melatonin 20 mg/kg/d	i.p., for 7 days before LPS	↓ Myocardial dysfunction and inflammation; ↓ cardiomyocyte apoptosis; ↑ AMPK activity and autophagy	[116]
LPS E. coli	Mouse (pregnant)	Placenta	Melatonin 5.0 mg/kg	i.p., 30 min before and 150 min after LPS	↓ Placental oxidative stress, hypoxic stress, and ER stress	[123]
CLP	Mouse	Diaphragm	Melatonin 30 mg/kg	i.p., four doses: 30 min before operation, just after operation, and 4 and 8 h after operation	↓ Respiratory chain failure; restoration of the redox status	[124]
CLP	Rat	Liver, kidney, lung, heart, diaphragm	Melatonin 10 mg/kg	i.p. 30 min before and 6 h after operation	↑ Level of GSH; ↓ MDA; ↓ tissue oxidative damage	[83]
LPS E. coli	Mouse	Heart	SS-31 5 mg/kg	i.p., 30 min after LPS	↓ ROS; restoration of myocardial damage; ↑ ATP; ↓ mRNA level of IL-6, IL-1β, and TNF-α; ↓ apoptosis; ↑ SOD and GPx	[82]
LPS E. coli	Mouse	Liver, serum	XJB-5-131 2 μmol/kg	i.v. 1 h before LPS	↓ Hepatic iNOS expression, ↓ blood nitrite level	[119]
LPS E. coli	Mouse	Hippocampus	SS-31 5 mg/kg	LPS microinjection in the hippocampi SS-31 i.p. 30 min before LPS and then once daily for 3 days thereafter	↓ ROS, MDA, IL-6, and TNF-α; ↑ SOD; ↓ hippocampal cell apoptosis; ↑ BDNF expression and synaptic protein levels, maintenance of hippocampal neuron morphology; ↓ memory impairment	[125]

Table 2. Cont.

Model of Infection	Species	Organ Investigated	Mito-AOX	Mode of Antioxidant Application	Major Findings	Reference
CLP	Mouse	Lung, kidney, liver	SS-31 5 mg/kg	i.p, immediately and 5 h after operation	↓ ROS, MDA, TNF-α, MPO activity, iNOS, and NF-κB p65; ↑ ATP; ↓ apoptosis, ↓ the histological damage; ↓ organ dysfunction, no result on mouse survival rate	[126]
CLP	Mouse	Hippocampus	SS-31 5 mg/kg	i.p, immediately after operation and once daily for 6 days thereafter	↓ ROS; ↓ NLRP3 and IL-1β; ↑ ATP; ↓ mitochondrial dysfunction; ↓ apoptosis; ↓ behavior and cognitive deficits; ↓ mortality rate	[127]
Live *E. coli* bacteria	Rat	Serum	M40401 (SOD mimetic) 0.25, 2.5, 25 μmol/kg/h	i.v. infusion 0.5 and 3 h after bacterial challenge	Maintenance of a normal mean arterial pressure; ↓ TNF-α and IL-1β; ↓ mortality	[128]

The application of different TPP-based mito-AOX (MitoQ, MitoVitE, MitoTEMPO, or MitoTEMPOL) to primary cultured cells or to cell lines exposed to LPS convincingly evidences their antioxidant and mitochondria-protective properties. As shown in Table 1, TPP-based compounds commonly demonstrate a decrease in mitochondrial/cellular ROS generation, the enhancement of the content of GSH and antioxidant enzymes such as SOD and GPx, and decreased accumulation of lipid peroxidation products such as MDA, as well as restoration of mitochondrial function. These antioxidants decrease the production of proinflammatory cytokines such as IL-1β and IL-18 and prevent NF-kB and caspase activation, leading to the inhibition of apoptosis and the increase in cell survival. MitoTEMPO or MitoQ application highlights the critical role of mtROS in LPS/*E. coli*-induced inflammasome activation, as shown in colonic epithelial cells [120] and renal proximal tubular cells [112].

Examples of the beneficial application of TPP-based antioxidants in different murine and rat acute inflammation models are summarized in Table 2. TPP-based antioxidants have been shown to accumulate in all major animal organs, such as the heart, kidney, liver, lung, and others, after oral, i.v., or i.p. administration [104,129].

The heart and the cardiovascular system suffer seriously during sepsis. MitoQ administration largely prevents LPS-induced cardiac mitochondrial dysfunction and reduction in cardiac pressure-generating capacity, inhibiting caspase 9 and 3 activity [21]. The septic response is well known to be related to widespread vascular endothelial injury, which plays a key role in the progression of multiple-organ failure [130]. Results obtained on human endothelial cells (HUVECs) exposed to LPS+PepG showed that MitoQ decreases cellular ROS generation, restores the MMP, and attenuates pro-inflammatory mediator production [114] (Table 1). A protective effect of mito-AOX has been demonstrated in an animal model of acute kidney injury caused by CLP following MitoTEMPO i.p. injection six hours after operation [22] or by LPS administration following i.p. injection of SKQR1 (plastoquinol conjugated with decylrhodamine) three hours before LPS administration [121]. In both protocols, despite their differences, mito-AOX were nephroprotective (Table 2). SKQR1 was also highly protective against acute pyelonephritis induced by intraurethral infection [18]. In the frog urinary bladder epithelium, which possesses the characteristics of the mammalian kidney collecting duct, MitoQ effectively inhibited LPS-induced ROS generation, the decline in fatty acid oxidation, and subsequent accumulation of lipid droplets, demonstrating a key role of mtROS in the shift of intracellular lipid metabolism under the influence of bacterial stimuli [85].

The impairment of gut permeability is a serious consequence of dysbiosis. MitoQ has been shown to improve intestinal permeability and inhibit LPS-induced bacterial translocation via a decrease in oxidative stress and restoration of the level of tight junction proteins (occludin and ZO-1) in the gut epithelium [11]. The authors showed that MitoQ alleviates LPS-induced oxidative stress in intestinal epithelial cells, triggering the nuclear translocation of the nuclear factor Nrf2, which, in turn, stimulates the expression of its downstream antioxidant genes [11].

Data presented in Table 2 indicate that the protective effect of mito-AOX can be observed independently on the differences in the administration protocol (application of mito-AOX before, immediately after LPS administration /CLP or some time later). Even a six-hour delay in therapy with a single dose of MitoTEMPO significantly increased mitochondrial respiration and improved renal function and survival of animals [22]. Both immediate and delayed administration of the dismutase mimetic MitoTEMPOL was found to prevent sepsis-induced diaphragm weakness in a similar mode [74]. These observations are very important due to their clinical relevance.

However, some studies have reported that TPP-conjugated compounds fail to inhibit mtROS-mediated injuries [131] or even have a detrimental effect on mitochondrial function. For example, in cultured mesangial cells, MitoQ, MitoTEMPOL, and MitoVitE at a dose of 1 µM inhibited oxidative phosphorylation [132]. Application of MitoQ (500 nM) to proximal tubule cells led to mitochondrial swelling and depolarization [133]. Both MitoQ (500 nM) and MitoTEMPOL (10 µM) had a marked negative effect on the respiration of myoblasts compared to controls [134]. The studies mentioned above revealed that the negative effect of TPP-conjugated compounds on mitochondrial function is related to the toxicity of the carbon alkyl chain of the cation moiety itself [132–134]. Another reason for TPP-conjugated mito-AOX toxicity is their ability to be pro-oxidants that generate superoxide via redox cycling [108,135]. A high concentration of antioxidants as well as other factors (the redox potential of matrix environments, the presence of Cu, Fe, and Zn ions) could reverse their behavior from anti- to pro-oxidant, subsequently causing toxic effects [111,136]. The pro-oxidant effect of MitoQ and other related compounds applied at high concentrations (more than 1 µM) has been shown to kill tumor cells, considering mito-AOX as potential chemotherapeutic drugs [111,137,138]. However, no pro-oxidant effect of MitoQ and other targeted quinones was demonstrated in mice who were fed antioxidants [139].

Since the probability of an adverse side effect of cation-conjugated mito-AOX provided by either a cation moiety or pro-oxidative behavior depends critically on their concentration; when dealing with this type of mito-AOX, it is particularly important to choose the relevant concentration, which, in turn, depends on a given cell type. For example, our experiments revealed that frog urinary bladder epithelial cells, demonstrating high tolerance to LPS, are very sensitive to the toxic effect of MitoQ (IC$_{50}$ = 400 nM) [85]. At doses higher than 25 nM, it reduced the oxygen consumption rate and cell viability, whereas the antioxidant potency of MitoQ and the ability to restore the LPS-induced decline in fatty acids oxidation were observed at a dose of 25 nM [85], which is much less than that in most other in vitro works [92,140–142]. Of note, the concentrations of mito-AOX used in in vitro experiments were much higher than those that can be achieved pharmacologically and were associated with protective effects in vivo [9].

5.2. Other Mitochondria-Targeted Conjugates

There was an attempt to design mito-AOX using the mitochondrial protein import machinery, which delivers nuclear-encoded mitochondrial proteins inside the mitochondria via translocase through the outer and inner membranes (TOM and TIM complexes, respectively). A mitochondria-targeted macrocyclic SOD mimetic was synthesized by attaching the mitochondria-targeting sequence peptide to the porphyrin ring of the manganese porphyrin complex MnMPy4P. The resulting construct MnMPy3P–MTS reportedly demonstrated a decrease in LPS-induced cell death in activated macrophages [117].

Another example of the successful application of mito-AOX against LPS is the hemigramicidin–TEMPO conjugate XJB-5-131, which consists of a stable nitroxide radical and a portion of the membrane-active cyclopeptide antibiotic gramicidin S. The gramicidin segment was used to target the nitroxide payload to mitochondria because antibiotics of this type have a high affinity for bacterial membranes [119]. XJB-5-131 limited the LPS-induced inflammatory response both in vitro in macrophages and in vivo in a mice septic model [119].

5.3. Melatonin

Melatonin is a natural antioxidant produced mainly by the pineal gland as well as by most of the organs and tissues. Frequent use of melatonin for treatment of insomnia is based on its traditionally accepted role as a hormonal regulator of the circadian rhythm. Besides this, melatonin possesses antiapoptotic, anti-inflammatory, and antitumor activity, as well as powerful antioxidant properties. These facts alongside its profoundly safe side-effect profile make it possible to propose melatonin as a promising adjunctive drug for different pathological states, including inflammation and sepsis (for review, see [143–147]).

Melatonin was first reported as a potent, broad-spectrum antioxidant and free-radical scavenger in the early 1990s [148]. The electron-rich melatonin molecule provides its antioxidant power via a cascade of scavenging reactions. Unlike classical antioxidants that have the potential to act as anti- and pro-oxidants via redox cycling [149], melatonin forms several stable end products excreted in the urine, which is believed to exclude its pro-oxidant effect [150]. Although the high lipid solubility of melatonin favors its entering all cells and subcellular compartments, melatonin is specifically targeted to mitochondria, where it enters via the oligopeptide transporters PEPT1 and PEPT2 [151]. In addition, melatonin is produced within mitochondria, and its generation can be inducible [152,153]. For these reasons, mitochondria have the highest level of melatonin.

Melatonin is one of the most important endogenous factors in limiting oxidative stress. It provides antioxidant defense via a plethora of mechanisms. Melatonin by itself and also its endogenous metabolites directly scavenge free radicals, bind heavy metals associated with radical production, reduce the membrane potential, and stimulate ETC complex activity and ATP synthesis [154–156]. Moreover, melatonin potentiates the activity of a wide variety of antioxidant enzymes. It inhibits the ubiquitination of Nrf2, allowing its binding with the antioxidant response element, which, in turn, activates the transcription of antioxidant genes [157,158]. Melatonin augments the SIRT3 signaling pathway, which protects mitochondria from oxidative damage, upregulates the synthesis of GSH, and acts synergistically with vitamin C, vitamin E, and GSH to scavenge free radicals [149,159].

Numerous experimental studies have revealed the antioxidant and anti-inflammatory properties of melatonin, both in vitro and in vivo. Typical examples are presented in Tables 1 and 2. On different cells challenged with LPS (HUVECs, cardiomyocytes, alveolar epithelial cells), it was shown that melatonin decreases ROS generation [79,81] and production of proinflammatory cytokines [80,81,116] and increases cellular antioxidant content (SOD, GSH) [79,80,115] through upregulation of Nrf2 expression [81]. Interestingly, not only melatonin but also its structurally related indolamine compounds (6-hydroxymelatonin, tryptamine or indole-3-carboxylic acid) possess antioxidant properties [80].

The beneficial application of melatonin was demonstrated in two animal models of sepsis—administration of LPS and CLP. Melatonin, being commonly injected i.p. before or after sepsis initiation, significantly improved sepsis-induced organ dysfunction (heart, kidney, liver, lung, placenta) by decreasing oxidative tissue damage and the inflammatory response, preserving mitochondrial function [79,83,116,122,123,160]. In the latest works on the septic cardiomyopathy model, it was shown that LPS suppresses the expression of B cell receptor-associated protein 31 (BAP31), a key regulator of endoplasmic reticulum stress, and melatonin could restore BAP31 expression. The knockdown of BAP31 attenuated the beneficial effects of melatonin on mitochondrial function and endoplasmic reticulum homeostasis under LPS [79], suggesting that, at least in part, melatonin contributes to the preservation of cardiac function in septic cardiomyopathy via regulation of BAP31 expression and stability. Another work demonstrated that autophagy plays a critical role in melatonin-induced myocardial protection. Thus, melatonin protects against LPS-induced septic myocardial injury by activating the AMPK-mediated autophagy pathway and further inhibiting mitochondrial injury and myocardial apoptosis [116].

5.4. Cell-Permeable Peptide Antioxidants

In the middle of the 2000s, a family of cell-permeable small synthetic tetrapeptides (Szeto–Schiller peptides (SS peptides)) was introduced as mitochondria-targeted antioxidants. The electron-scavenging abilities of SS peptides were provided by aromatic–cationic motifs in their molecules [39,161,162]. SS peptides readily penetrate the cell via diffusion, selectively accumulate within mitochondria, and concentrate in the IMM without reaching the mitochondrial matrix. In contrast to the MMP-driven entry of triphenylphosphonium-based conjugates into the mitochondria, the accumulation of SS peptides is independent of the MMP and does not depolarize the mitochondrial membrane. For this reason, SS peptides can penetrate not only normal mitochondria but also damaged ones with a low MMP [39].

The most studied peptide of this family is SS-31 (elamipretide, Bendavia™, MTP-131, D-Arg-Dmt-Lys-Phe-NH$_2$), which, in addition to its mtROS-scavenging ability, links selectively to cardiolipin by electrostatic and hydrophobic interactions [40,163]. Thus, SS-31 is now positioned more as a cardiolipin stabilizer/protector than as a mtROS scavenger.

Cardiolipin is readily oxidized by mtROS, which leads to multiple injuries. Oxidized cardiolipin disrupts the structure of respiratory supercomplexes to inhibit electron transfer and oxidative phosphorylation [70]. Translocation of oxidized cardiolipin from the IMM into the OMM provides a docking station for NLRP3 inflammasome assembly, and it can trigger mitochondrial fission and initiate mitophagy [164]. Binding of SS-31 to cardiolipin inhibits cardiolipin peroxidation, stabilizes cristae curvatures [40,163,165,166], and restores the stability and activity of respiratory complexes [167].

The linking of SS-31 to cardiolipin also inhibits the peroxidase activity of cytochrome C to result in decreasing mtROS production and improving the coupling between oxygen consumption and ATP synthesis [163]. SS-31 enhances ATP levels even under conditions of low substrate and oxygen supply, such as ischemia [40,165], or in increased energy demand states, such as sepsis and others pathologies [82,168,169]. The restoration of mitochondrial functioning by SS-31 can prevent a wide range of downstream cellular events, e.g., inflammasome activation and cytokine expression, autophagy, apoptosis, and necrosis. The beneficial effects of SS-31 were reported in different disease models (for review, see [32]), demonstrating the existence of a common mechanism mediating its action in different pathological conditions.

The protective effect of SS-31 against LPS was demonstrated in several in vitro and in vivo models (see Tables 1 and 2). In LPS-treated cells and CPL/LPS-challenged mice, SS-31 decreased apoptosis, improved sepsis-induced organ dysfunction, restored morphological damage, and reversed mitochondrial dysfunction [82,125–127]. It also attenuated ROS and MDA levels [82,125–127], maintained ATP production [82,126,127], and suppressed pro-inflammatory cytokine expression [82,125–127].

Several successive clinical trials in phases 1-3 were conducted in patients with cardiac, renal, skeletal muscle, and ophthalmic problems, as well as in mitochondrial myopathy patients (for review, see [32]). No adverse side effects of SS-31 were found until now. The safety of using SS-31, a drug with multiple beneficial pharmacological properties, for organs most affected by sepsis is particularly important. Very promising preclinical and clinical trial findings encourage to develop SS-31-based therapeutic approaches for the treatment of sepsis and other pathologies.

5.5. Suppressors of Site IQ and IIIQ Electron Leakage

Recently, small molecules from different chemical families that specifically suppress mitochondrial superoxide/H_2O_2 production (S1QELs for site I_Q [170] and S3QELs for site III_{Qo} [171]) were identified by chemical screening. They bind directly to complex I or III and selectively suppress electron leakage without inhibiting oxidative phosphorylation [170,171], as well as inhibit the reverse electron flow through complex I [172]. They do not cause cytotoxicity at their effective concentrations [171] and do not participate in redox recycling [173].

The cytoprotective effect of S1QELs against oxidative damage has been demonstrated in animal (rat, mouse), human, and different cellular models [171,174,175]. S1QELs protected against ischemia-reperfusion injury in a perfused mouse heart [176]. In a murine model of asystolic cardiac arrest, S1QELs diminished myocardial ROS, as well as improved myocardial function after cardiopulmonary resuscitation, neurologic outcomes, and survival [177]. In recent papers, S1QELs and S3QELs have been offered as promising investigation tools for elucidating the functioning of I_Q and III_{Qo} sites in normal and pathological conditions, opening up new possibilities for better therapy [173,178]. Given the fact that LPS-driven mtROS are generated predominantly by mitochondrial complex I, S1QELs can potentially be specific suppressors of LPS-induced mtROS production, gently withstanding LPS-induced oxidative stress. However, the efficiency of S1QELs and S3QELs in a sepsis animal model or LPS-induced injury remains poorly investigated and warrants further research.

6. Indirect Control of mtROS by Competitive Inhibitors of Succinate Dehydrogenase (SDH)

The accumulation of the citric acid cycle intermediate succinate, tightly connected with mtROS generation, has been shown to be a common cellular response to different pathological challenges such as ischemia/reperfusion, cancer, and inflammation [179–182]. An increase in the succinate level arises from SDH, operating in its opposite direction, which, in turn, is driven by fumarate overflow from purine nucleotide breakdown and partial reversal of the malate/aspartate shuttle [182]. Significant LPS-induced succinate accumulation was observed in macrophages [183], in which SDH activity is critical for determining the inflammatory phenotype of macrophages [78]. Subsequent rapid oxidation of succinate to fumarate by SDH under a large proton-motive force fuels RET, resulting in substantial generation of mtROS [78,179,180], which enhances pro-inflammatory cytokine expression by stabilizing hypoxia-inducible factor 1-alpha (HIF-1α) and suppresses the production of anti-inflammatory factors [78,183,184].

This pro-inflammatory scenario and metabolic reprogramming of immune cells are switched off by the generation of itaconate, another derivate of the citric acid cycle [185,186]. Itaconate produced from cis-aconitate is one of the most highly induced metabolites in LPS-activated macrophages, being an endogenous SDH inhibitor [78,185,186]. A significant decrease in LPS-stimulated mtROS and ROS-mediated cell damage was demonstrated in bone marrow-derived macrophages in the presence of 4-octyl itaconate or dimethyl itaconate, cell-permeable derivatives of itaconate [185,187]. In addition, in the cytosol, itaconate promotes the expression of anti-inflammatory and antioxidant genes by modifying the protein KEAP1, resulting in nuclear factor Nrf2 activation [188], as well as through the induction of an anti-inflammatory IkappaBzeta/ATF3 axis [186] to inhibit inflammasome activation. Thus, exposure to LPS not only promotes pro-inflammatory signaling via the succinate/mtROS pathway but also triggers a negative-feedback loop through itaconate-mediated induction of an anti-inflammatory program by SDH inhibition, as well as transcriptional factor Nrf2 and IkappaBzet/ATF3 activation. Dimethyl itaconate and 4-octyl itaconate were protective against LPS-induced injury in vivo [187,189]. Nevertheless, no substantial de-esterification of ester derivatives of itaconate was observed in activated macrophages, and only itaconate, but not its ester derivatives, led to increased intracellular succinate accumulation [189]. Further research is required to clarify this contradiction.

Another potent endogenous competitive inhibitor of SDH, malonate, also acts as an indirect mitochondrial antioxidant by inhibiting succinate-driven RET. Dimethyl malonate (DMM), a cell-permeable malonate derivative, which is rapidly hydrolyzed in the cell to generate malonate, was used in both in vitro and in vivo models as an indirect mitochondria-targeted antioxidant [78,190]. In bone marrow-derived macrophages treated by LPS+succinate, DMM increased basal and LPS-induced cytosolic succinate levels and decreased the production of cellular ROS and proinflammatory cytokines. Mice treated i.p. with DMM before stimulation with LPS demonstrated a decrease in serum IL-1β and an increase in IL-10 [78]. The potential anti-inflammatory benefits of DMM were investigated in a mouse model with LPS/d-galactosamine-induced acute hepatic damage. DMM significantly alleviated hepatic damage and systemic inflammation [190]. In macrophages, it was also found that DMM suppresses the expression of gene sets associated with inflammation, including IL-1β and other HIF-1α-dependent genes, wherein many genes that were upregulated by succinate were reciprocally downregulated by DMM [78,190].

7. Conclusions

In recent years, the worldwide spread of Gram-negative infections, both chronic and acute up to sepsis, common and nosocomial, continues to pose a threat to human health. The abundance of Gram-negative infections is closely related to the overuse of antibiotics, immunosuppressive therapy applied in cancer, organ transplantation, heart surgery, etc., as well as to the prevalence of invasive devices and procedures, opening the gate for infection [191]. The most serious problem of recent decades has become the failure of conventional antibiotics to fight against multidrug-resistant Gram-negative bacteria. Moreover, LPS, the endotoxin of Gram-negative bacteria, inevitably triggers the host's innate immune response and acute inflammation regardless of whether it remains in the membrane of alive or dead bacteria or is in cell-free form. The potential contribution of LPS and other toxins secreted by the gastrointestinal tract microbiome to human inflammatory disease is becoming increasingly acknowledged [6]. Thus, it has been shown that a particularly pro-inflammatory LPS subtype from the intestinal microbiome can penetrate the systemic circulation, cross the blood–brain barrier, and accumulate within CNS neurons, complicating or accelerating the development of neurodegenerative disorders such as Alzheimer's disease [7]. In this connection, the development of new therapeutic approaches directed to the resolution of LPS-driven inflammation and to the improvement of the outcome of the pathology is very important. For this reason, the introduction of anti-inflammatory strategies employing mito-AOX into clinical practice promises to be especially attractive.

The development of mito-AOX was based on approaches that allow one to limit excessive ROS production inside mitochondria via different mechanisms. Up to now, our knowledge of mtROS generation, their role in cell signaling and their impact on cellular antioxidant and pro- and anti-inflammatory mechanisms, is still insufficient and scant [10]. Nevertheless, besides the beneficial application of mito-AOX in numerous animal pathogenic models mentioned above, many clinical studies demonstrated the protective efficacy of mito-AOX in different pathological conditions wherever inflammation as well as mitochondria damage are involved. Thus, several successive SS-31 clinical trials in phases 1–3 were conducted in patients with cardiac, renal, skeletal muscle, and ophthalmic problems, as well as in mitochondrial myopathy patients (for review, see [32]). The safety of melatonin, which is widely used for counteracting sleep disturbances, was confirmed in a set of trials (for example, see Identifier: ChiCTR-TRC-13003997, ISRCTN15529655). Meta-analysis of randomized controlled trials demonstrated the effectiveness of melatonin in suppression of oxidative stress, which accompanies different pathological states [192]. In addition, melatonin was effective in newborns as an adjunctive therapy for sepsis [193] as well as in patients with *H. pylori*-associated dyspepsia [194].

MitoQ is now ubiquitously available as a dietary supplement. In clinical trials, it has shown efficiency in improving vascular function in middle-aged and elderly people and significantly decreased liver enzymes raised due to hepatitis C. Although it had no effect on Parkinson's disease progression, no adverse side effects of MitoQ have been observed when it was daily administered to patients for a year [195]. SkQ1-based Visomitin eye drops were approved for clinical use in Russia, and their safety and efficacy were confirmed in phase 2 US clinical trials. Interestingly, the direct suppression activity of SkQ1 at micromolar concentrations toward the growth of different Gram-positive and Gram-negative bacteria has been found recently [196], suggesting that SkQ1 lowering the bacterial membrane potential may also be effective in the protection of infected mammalian organs by killing invading bacteria. In recent years, exploration of the development of SDH inhibitors and clarification of the intrinsic mechanisms of their action has been also intensified, promising novel therapeutic strategies to limit inflammation.

Despite successful clinical trials, as mentioned above, the development of drugs based on mito-AOX and their application to Gram-negative infection are still in their infancy. Although numerous in vitro and in vivo studies have clearly demonstrated the protective effects of mito-AOX in different infection models, these results have not been translated to the clinic up to now. Future studies are needed to elucidate the time dependence and especially the long-term impact of mito-AOX application during chronic infection. Nevertheless, we believe that mtROS-targeted approaches possess great treatment potential and are worthy of being incorporated into preventive and therapeutic strategies against inflammation driven by Gram-negative infection. More research efforts are needed in the future to achieve this goal.

Author Contributions: R.G.P. and E.M.F. contributed equally to this work. All authors have read and agreed to the published version of the manuscript.

Funding: This research was funded by the Russian Government program (no. 075-00776-19-02).

Institutional Review Board Statement: Not applicable.

Informed Consent Statement: Not applicable.

Data Availability Statement: Not applicable.

Conflicts of Interest: The authors declare no conflict of interest.

Abbreviations

AMPK	5′ AMP-activated protein kinase
BAP31	B-cell receptor-associated protein 31
BDNF	Brain-derived neurotrophic factor
CLP	Cecal ligation puncture
COX2	Cyclo-oxygenase 2
DMM	Dimethyl malonate
GSH	Glutathione
GPx	Glutathione peroxidase
ETC	Electron transport chain
Fis1	Fission protein 1
IL-1β	Interleukin 1 beta
IL-18	Interleukin 18
iNOS	Inducible NO-synthase
IMM	Inner mitochondrial membrane
LPS	Lipopolysaccharide
MDA	Malondialdehyde
Mito-AOX	Mitochondria-targeted antioxidants
MMP	Membrane mitochondrial potential
MPO	Myeloperoxidase
mtDNA	Mitochondrial DNA
mtROS	Mitochondrial reactive oxygen species
NADH	Nicotinamide adenine dinucleotide
NLRP3	Inflammasome, NLR family pyrin domain containing receptor 3
NF-kB	Nuclear factor kappa B
Nrf2	Nuclear factor E2-related factor 2
OMM	Outer mitochondrial membrane
RET	Reverse electron transport

RNS	Reactive nitrogen species	
ROS	Reactive oxygen species	
TLR4	Toll-like receptor 4	
TPP+	Triphenylphosphonium	
SDH	Succinate dehydrogenase	
SOD	Superoxide dismutase	

References

1. Oliveira, J.; Reygaert, W.C. Gram Negative Bacteria. In *StatPearls*; StatPearls Publishing: Treasure Island, FL, USA, 2020.
2. Kaye, K.S.; Pogue, J.M. Infections Caused by Resistant Gram-Negative Bacteria: Epidemiology and Management. *Pharmacotherapy* **2015**, *35*, 949–962. [CrossRef]
3. Taeb, A.M.; Hooper, M.H.; Marik, P.E. Sepsis: Current Definition, Pathophysiology, Diagnosis, and Management. *Nutr. Clin. Pract.* **2017**, *32*, 296–308. [CrossRef] [PubMed]
4. Iskander, K.N.; Osuchowski, M.F.; Stearns-Kurosawa, D.J.; Kurosawa, S.; Stepien, D.; Valentine, C.; Remick, D.G. Sepsis: Multiple abnormalities, heterogeneous responses, and evolving understanding. *Physiol. Rev.* **2013**, *93*, 1247–1288. [CrossRef] [PubMed]
5. Brandenburg, K.; Schromm, A.B.; Weindl, G.; Heinbockel, L.; Correa, W.; Mauss, K.; Martinez de Tejada, G.; Garidel, P. An update on endotoxin neutralization strategies in Gram-negative bacterial infections. *Expert Rev. Anti Infect. Ther.* **2020**, 1–23. [CrossRef] [PubMed]
6. Lukiw, W.J. Gastrointestinal (GI) Tract Microbiome-Derived Neurotoxins-Potent Neuro-Inflammatory Signals From the GI Tract via the Systemic Circulation Into the Brain. *Front. Cell Infect. Microbiol.* **2020**, *10*, 22. [CrossRef] [PubMed]
7. Zhao, Y.H.; Jaber, V.; Lukiw, W.J. Secretory Products of the Human GI Tract Microbiome and Their Potential Impact on Alzheimer's Disease (AD): Detection of Lipopolysaccharide (LPS) in AD Hippocampus. *Front. Cell Infect. Microbiol.* **2017**, *7*, 318. [CrossRef]
8. Alexandrov, P.N.; Hill, J.M.; Zhao, Y.; Bond, T.; Taylor, C.M.; Percy, M.E.; Li, W.; Lukiw, W.J. Aluminum-induced generation of lipopolysaccharide (LPS) from the human gastrointestinal (GI)-tract microbiome-resident Bacteroides fragilis. *J. Inorg. Biochem.* **2020**, *203*, 110886. [CrossRef]
9. Murphy, M.P.; Hartley, R.C. Mitochondria as a therapeutic target for common pathologies. *Nat. Rev. Drug Discov.* **2018**, *17*, 865–886. [CrossRef]
10. Silwal, P.; Kim, J.K.; Kim, Y.J.; Jo, E.K. Mitochondrial Reactive Oxygen Species: Double-Edged Weapon in Host Defense and Pathological Inflammation During Infection. *Front. Immunol.* **2020**, *11*, 1649. [CrossRef]
11. Zhang, S.; Zhou, Q.; Li, Y.; Zhang, Y.; Wu, Y. MitoQ Modulates Lipopolysaccharide-Induced Intestinal Barrier Dysfunction via Regulating Nrf2 Signaling. *Mediat. Inflamm.* **2020**, *2020*, 3276148. [CrossRef]
12. Sygitowicz, G.; Sitkiewicz, D. Molecular mechanisms of organ damage in sepsis: An overview. *Braz. J. Infect. Dis.* **2020**, *24*, 552–560. [CrossRef] [PubMed]
13. Duran-Bedolla, J.; Montes de Oca-Sandoval, M.A.; Saldana-Navor, V.; Villalobos-Silva, J.A.; Rodriguez, M.C.; Rivas-Arancibia, S. Sepsis, mitochondrial failure and multiple organ dysfunction. *Clin. Investig. Med.* **2014**, *37*, E58–E69. [CrossRef] [PubMed]
14. Galley, H.F. Oxidative stress and mitochondrial dysfunction in sepsis. *Br. J. Anaesth.* **2011**, *107*, 57–64. [CrossRef] [PubMed]
15. Rocha, M.; Herance, R.; Rovira, S.; Hernandez-Mijares, A.; Victor, V.M. Mitochondrial dysfunction and antioxidant therapy in sepsis. *Infect. Disord. Drug Targets* **2012**, *12*, 161–178. [CrossRef]
16. Prauchner, C.A. Oxidative stress in sepsis: Pathophysiological implications justifying antioxidant co-therapy. *Burns* **2017**, *43*, 471–485. [CrossRef]
17. Li, X.; Wang, X.; Zheng, M.; Luan, Q.X. Mitochondrial reactive oxygen species mediate the lipopolysaccharide-induced pro-inflammatory response in human gingival fibroblasts. *Exp. Cell Res.* **2016**, *347*, 212–221. [CrossRef]
18. Plotnikov, E.Y.; Morosanova, M.A.; Pevzner, I.B.; Zorova, L.D.; Manskikh, V.N.; Pulkova, N.V.; Galkina, S.I.; Skulachev, V.P.; Zorov, D.B. Protective effect of mitochondria-targeted antioxidants in an acute bacterial infection. *Proc. Natl. Acad. Sci. USA* **2013**, *110*, E3100–E3108. [CrossRef]
19. Vanasco, V.; Magnani, N.D.; Cimolai, M.C.; Valdez, L.B.; Evelson, P.; Boveris, A.; Alvarez, S. Endotoxemia impairs heart mitochondrial function by decreasing electron transfer, ATP synthesis and ATP content without affecting membrane potential. *J. Bioenerg. Biomembr.* **2012**, *44*, 243–252. [CrossRef]
20. Chuang, Y.C.; Tsai, J.L.; Chang, A.Y.; Chan, J.Y.; Liou, C.W.; Chan, S.H. Dysfunction of the mitochondrial respiratory chain in the rostral ventrolateral medulla during experimental endotoxemia in the rat. *J. Biomed. Sci.* **2002**, *9*, 542–548. [CrossRef]
21. Supinski, G.S.; Murphy, M.P.; Callahan, L.A. MitoQ administration prevents endotoxin-induced cardiac dysfunction. *Am. J. Physiol. Regul. Integr. Comp. Physiol.* **2009**, *297*, R1095–R1102. [CrossRef]
22. Patil, N.K.; Parajuli, N.; MacMillan-Crow, L.A.; Mayeux, P.R. Inactivation of renal mitochondrial respiratory complexes and manganese superoxide dismutase during sepsis: Mitochondria-targeted antioxidant mitigates injury. *Am. J. Physiol. Renal. Physiol.* **2014**, *306*, F734–F743. [CrossRef] [PubMed]
23. Supinski, G.S.; Wang, L.; Schroder, E.A.; Callahan, L.A.P. MitoTEMPOL, a mitochondrial targeted antioxidant, prevents sepsis-induced diaphragm dysfunction. *Am. J. Physiol. Lung Cell Mol. Physiol.* **2020**, *319*, L228–L238. [CrossRef] [PubMed]

24. Dikalov, S.I.; Li, W.; Doughan, A.K.; Blanco, R.R.; Zafari, A.M. Mitochondrial reactive oxygen species and calcium uptake regulate activation of phagocytic NADPH oxidase. *Am. J. Physiol. Regul. Integr. Comp. Physiol.* **2012**, *302*, R1134–R1142. [CrossRef] [PubMed]
25. Tschopp, J. Mitochondria: Sovereign of inflammation? *Eur. J. Immunol.* **2011**, *41*, 1196–1202. [CrossRef]
26. Evavold, C.L.; Kagan, J.C. How Inflammasomes Inform Adaptive Immunity. *J. Mol. Biol.* **2018**, *430*, 217–237. [CrossRef]
27. Qiu, Z.; He, Y.; Ming, H.; Lei, S.; Leng, Y.; Xia, Z.Y. Lipopolysaccharide (LPS) Aggravates High Glucose- and Hypoxia/Reoxygenation-Induced Injury through Activating ROS-Dependent NLRP3 Inflammasome-Mediated Pyroptosis in H9C2 Cardiomyocytes. *J. Diabetes Res.* **2019**, *2019*, 8151836. [CrossRef]
28. Chandel, N.S.; McClintock, D.S.; Feliciano, C.E.; Wood, T.M.; Melendez, J.A.; Rodriguez, A.M.; Schumacker, P.T. Reactive oxygen species generated at mitochondrial Complex III stabilize HIF-1-alpha during hypoxia: A mechanism of O2 sensing. *J. Biol. Chem.* **2000**, *275*, 25130–25138. [CrossRef]
29. Zhang, H.; Zhang, W.; Jiao, F.; Li, X.; Zhang, H.; Wang, L.; Gong, Z. The nephroprotective effect of MS-275 on lipopolysaccharide (LPS)-induced acute kidney injury by inhibiting reactive oxygen species (ROS)-oxidative stress and endoplasmic reticulum stress. *Med. Sci. Mon. Int. Med. J. Exp. Clin. Res.* **2018**, *24*, 2620. [CrossRef]
30. Murphy, M.P. How mitochondria produce reactive oxygen species. *Biochem. J.* **2009**, *417*, 1–13. [CrossRef]
31. Skulachev, V.P. Cationic antioxidants as a powerful tool against mitochondrial oxidative stress. *Biochem. Biophys. Res. Commun.* **2013**, *441*, 275–279. [CrossRef]
32. Szeto, H.H. Stealth Peptides Target Cellular Powerhouses to Fight Rare and Common Age-Related Diseases. *Protein. Pept. Lett.* **2018**, *25*, 1108–1123. [CrossRef] [PubMed]
33. Kagan, V.E.; Wipf, P.; Stoyanovsky, D.; Greenberger, J.S.; Borisenko, G.; Belikova, N.A.; Yanamala, N.; Samhan Arias, A.K.; Tungekar, M.A.; Jiang, J.; et al. Mitochondrial targeting of electron scavenging antioxidants: Regulation of selective oxidation vs random chain reactions. *Adv. Drug Deliv. Rev.* **2009**, *61*, 1375–1385. [CrossRef] [PubMed]
34. Feniouk, B.A.; Skulachev, V.P. Cellular and Molecular Mechanisms of Action of Mitochondria-Targeted Antioxidants. *Curr. Aging Sci.* **2017**, *10*, 41–48. [CrossRef] [PubMed]
35. Oyewole, A.O.; Birch-Machin, M.A. Mitochondria-targeted antioxidants. *FASEB J.* **2015**, *29*, 4766–4771. [CrossRef] [PubMed]
36. Murphy, M.P.; Smith, R.A. Targeting antioxidants to mitochondria by conjugation to lipophilic cations. *Annu. Rev. Pharmacol. Toxicol.* **2007**, *47*, 629–656. [CrossRef]
37. Skulachev, M.V.; Antonenko, Y.N.; Anisimov, V.N.; Chernyak, B.V.; Cherepanov, D.A.; Chistyakov, V.A.; Egorov, M.V.; Kolosova, N.G.; Korshunova, G.A.; Lyamzaev, K.G.; et al. Mitochondrial-targeted plastoquinone derivatives. Effect on senescence and acute age-related pathologies. *Curr. Drug Targets* **2011**, *12*, 800–826. [CrossRef]
38. Trnka, J.; Blaikie, F.H.; Smith, R.A.; Murphy, M.P. A mitochondria-targeted nitroxide is reduced to its hydroxylamine by ubiquinol in mitochondria. *Free Radic. Biol. Med.* **2008**, *44*, 1406–1419. [CrossRef]
39. Zhao, K.; Zhao, G.M.; Wu, D.; Soong, Y.; Birk, A.V.; Schiller, P.W.; Szeto, H.H. Cell-permeable peptide antioxidants targeted to inner mitochondrial membrane inhibit mitochondrial swelling, oxidative cell death, and reperfusion injury. *J. Biol. Chem.* **2004**, *279*, 34682–34690. [CrossRef]
40. Birk, A.V.; Liu, S.; Soong, Y.; Mills, W.; Singh, P.; Warren, J.D.; Seshan, S.V.; Pardee, J.D.; Szeto, H.H. The mitochondrial-targeted compound SS-31 re-energizes ischemic mitochondria by interacting with cardiolipin. *J. Am. Soc. Nephrol.* **2013**, *24*, 1250–1261. [CrossRef]
41. Zinovkin, R.A.; Zamyatnin, A.A. Mitochondria-Targeted Drugs. *Curr. Mol. Pharmacol.* **2019**, *12*, 202–214. [CrossRef]
42. Murphy, M.P. Understanding and preventing mitochondrial oxidative damage. *Biochem. Soc. Trans.* **2016**, *44*, 1219–1226. [CrossRef] [PubMed]
43. Miller, S.I.; Ernst, R.K.; Bader, M.W. LPS, TLR4 and infectious disease diversity. *Nat. Rev. Microbiol.* **2005**, *3*, 36–46. [CrossRef] [PubMed]
44. Nikolaeva, S.; Bachteeva, V.; Fock, E.; Herterich, S.; Lavrova, E.; Borodkina, A.; Gambaryan, S.; Parnova, R. Frog urinary bladder epithelial cells express TLR4 and respond to bacterial LPS by increase of iNOS expression and L-arginine uptake. *Am. J. Physiol. Regul. Integr. Comp. Physiol.* **2012**, *303*, R1042–R1052. [CrossRef] [PubMed]
45. Lien, E.; Ingalls, R.R. Toll-like receptors. *Crit. Care Med.* **2002**, *30*, S1–S11. [CrossRef] [PubMed]
46. Lu, Y.C.; Yeh, W.C.; Ohashi, P.S. LPS/TLR4 signal transduction pathway. *Cytokine* **2008**, *42*, 145–151. [CrossRef] [PubMed]
47. Takeda, K.; Akira, S. TLR signaling pathways. *Semin. Immunol.* **2004**, *16*, 3–9. [CrossRef] [PubMed]
48. Mazgaeen, L.; Gurung, P. Recent Advances in Lipopolysaccharide Recognition Systems. *Int. J. Mol. Sci* **2020**, *21*, 379. [CrossRef] [PubMed]
49. Dagenais, M.; Skeldon, A.; Saleh, M. The inflammasome: In memory of Dr. Jurg Tschopp. *Cell Death Differ.* **2012**, *19*, 5–12. [CrossRef] [PubMed]
50. Demirel, I.; Persson, A.; Brauner, A.; Sarndahl, E.; Kruse, R.; Persson, K. Activation of the NLRP3 Inflammasome Pathway by Uropathogenic Escherichia coli Is Virulence Factor-Dependent and Influences Colonization of Bladder Epithelial Cells. *Front. Cell Infect. Microbiol.* **2018**, *8*, 81. [CrossRef] [PubMed]
51. Swanson, K.V.; Deng, M.; Ting, J.P. The NLRP3 inflammasome: Molecular activation and regulation to therapeutics. *Nat. Rev. Immunol.* **2019**, *19*, 477–489. [CrossRef] [PubMed]

52. Liu, X.; Zhang, Z.; Ruan, J.; Pan, Y.; Magupalli, V.G.; Wu, H.; Lieberman, J. Inflammasome-activated gasdermin D causes pyroptosis by forming membrane pores. *Nature* **2016**, *535*, 153–158. [CrossRef] [PubMed]
53. Sies, H.; Berndt, C.; Jones, D.P. Oxidative Stress. *Annu. Rev. Biochem.* **2017**, *86*, 715–748. [CrossRef] [PubMed]
54. Andreyev, A.Y.; Kushnareva, Y.E.; Murphy, A.N.; Starkov, A.A. Mitochondrial ROS Metabolism: 10 Years Later. *Biochemistry (Moscow)* **2015**, *80*, 517–531. [CrossRef] [PubMed]
55. Robb, E.L.; Hall, A.R.; Prime, T.A.; Eaton, S.; Szibor, M.; Viscomi, C.; James, A.M.; Murphy, M.P. Control of mitochondrial superoxide production by reverse electron transport at complex I. *J. Biol. Chem.* **2018**, *293*, 9869–9879. [CrossRef]
56. Treberg, J.R.; Quinlan, C.L.; Brand, M.D. Evidence for two sites of superoxide production by mitochondrial NADH-ubiquinone oxidoreductase (complex I). *J. Biol. Chem.* **2011**, *286*, 27103–27110. [CrossRef]
57. Hirst, J.; King, M.S.; Pryde, K.R. The production of reactive oxygen species by complex I. *Biochem. Soc. Trans.* **2008**, *36*, 976–980. [CrossRef]
58. Bellezza, I.; Giambanco, I.; Minelli, A.; Donato, R. Nrf2-Keap1 signaling in oxidative and reductive stress. *Biochim. Biophys. Acta Mol. Cell Res.* **2018**, *1865*, 721–733. [CrossRef]
59. Zorov, D.B.; Bannikova, S.Y.; Belousov, V.V.; Vyssokikh, M.Y.; Zorova, L.D.; Isaev, N.K.; Krasnikov, B.F.; Plotnikov, E.Y. Reactive oxygen and nitrogen species: Friends or foes? *Biochemistry (Moscow)* **2005**, *70*, 215–221. [CrossRef]
60. Droge, W. Free radicals in the physiological control of cell function. *Physiol. Rev.* **2002**, *82*, 47–95. [CrossRef]
61. Kozlov, A.V.; Bahrami, S.; Calzia, E.; Dungel, P.; Gille, L.; Kuznetsov, A.V.; Troppmair, J. Mitochondrial dysfunction and biogenesis: Do ICU patients die from mitochondrial failure? *Ann. Intensive Care* **2011**, *1*, 41. [CrossRef]
62. Zorov, D.B.; Juhaszova, M.; Sollott, S.J. Mitochondrial reactive oxygen species (ROS) and ROS-induced ROS release. *Physiol. Rev.* **2014**, *94*, 909–950. [CrossRef] [PubMed]
63. Di Meo, S.; Reed, T.; Venditti, P.; Victor, V. Role of ROS and RNS sources in physiological and pathological conditions. *Oxidative Med. Cell Longev.* **2016**, *2016*, 1245049. [CrossRef] [PubMed]
64. Yang, Y.; Karakhanova, S.; Hartwig, W.; D'Haese, J.G.; Philippov, P.P.; Werner, J.; Bazhin, A.V. Mitochondria and Mitochondrial ROS in Cancer: Novel Targets for Anticancer Therapy. *J. Cell. Physiol.* **2016**, *231*, 2570–2581. [CrossRef]
65. Robinson, A.R.; Yousefzadeh, M.J.; Rozgaja, T.A.; Wang, J.; Li, X.; Tilstra, J.S.; Feldman, C.H.; Gregg, S.Q.; Johnson, C.H.; Skoda, E.M.; et al. Spontaneous DNA damage to the nuclear genome promotes senescence, redox imbalance and aging. *Redox Biol.* **2018**, *17*, 259–273. [CrossRef] [PubMed]
66. Zhang, D.; Li, Y.; Heims-Waldron, D.; Bezzerides, V.; Guatimosim, S.; Guo, Y.; Gu, F.; Zhou, P.; Lin, Z.; Ma, Q.; et al. Mitochondrial Cardiomyopathy Caused by Elevated Reactive Oxygen Species and Impaired Cardiomyocyte Proliferation. *Circ. Res.* **2018**, *122*, 74–87. [CrossRef] [PubMed]
67. De, I.; Dogra, N.; Singh, S. The Mitochondrial Unfolded Protein Response: Role in Cellular Homeostasis and Disease. *Curr. Mol. Med.* **2017**, *17*, 587–597. [CrossRef]
68. Yao, X.; Carlson, D.; Sun, Y.; Ma, L.; Wolf, S.E.; Minei, J.P.; Zang, Q.S. Mitochondrial ROS Induces Cardiac Inflammation via a Pathway through mtDNA Damage in a Pneumonia-Related Sepsis Model. *PLoS ONE* **2015**, *10*, e0139416. [CrossRef]
69. Callahan, L.A.; Supinski, G.S. Sepsis induces diaphragm electron transport chain dysfunction and protein depletion. *Am. J. Respir. Crit. Care Med.* **2005**, *172*, 861–868. [CrossRef]
70. Paradies, G.; Petrosillo, G.; Paradies, V.; Ruggiero, F.M. Role of cardiolipin peroxidation and Ca^{2+} in mitochondrial dysfunction and disease. *Cell Calcium.* **2009**, *45*, 643–650. [CrossRef]
71. Orrenius, S.; Gogvadze, V.; Zhivotovsky, B. Calcium and mitochondria in the regulation of cell death. *Biochem. Biophys. Res. Commun.* **2015**, *460*, 72–81. [CrossRef]
72. Williamson, J.; Davison, G. Targeted Antioxidants in Exercise-Induced Mitochondrial Oxidative Stress: Emphasis on DNA Damage. *Antioxidants (Basel)* **2020**, *9*, 142. [CrossRef] [PubMed]
73. Poderoso, J.J. The formation of peroxynitrite in the applied physiology of mitochondrial nitric oxide. *Arch. Biochem. Biophys.* **2009**, *484*, 214–220. [CrossRef] [PubMed]
74. Supinski, G.S.; Schroder, E.A.; Callahan, L.A. Mitochondria and Critical Illness. *Chest* **2020**, *157*, 310–322. [CrossRef] [PubMed]
75. Voloboueva, L.A.; Emery, J.F.; Sun, X.; Giffard, R.G. Inflammatory response of microglial BV-2 cells includes a glycolytic shift and is modulated by mitochondrial glucose-regulated protein 75/mortalin. *FEBS Lett.* **2013**, *587*, 756–762. [CrossRef]
76. Park, J.; Min, J.S.; Kim, B.; Chae, U.B.; Yun, J.W.; Choi, M.S.; Kong, I.K.; Chang, K.T.; Lee, D.S. Mitochondrial ROS govern the LPS-induced pro-inflammatory response in microglia cells by regulating MAPK and NF-kappaB pathways. *Neurosci. Lett.* **2015**, *584*, 191–196. [CrossRef] [PubMed]
77. Jiao, P.; Li, W.; Shen, L.; Li, Y.; Yu, L.; Liu, Z. The protective effect of doxofylline against lipopolysaccharides (LPS)-induced activation of NLRP3 inflammasome is mediated by SIRT1 in human pulmonary bronchial epithelial cells. *Artif. Cells Nanomed. Biotechnol.* **2020**, *48*, 687–694. [CrossRef]
78. Mills, E.L.; Kelly, B.; Logan, A.; Costa, A.S.; Varma, M.; Bryant, C.E.; Tourlomousis, P.; Däbritz, J.H.M.; Gottlieb, E.; Latorre, I. Succinate dehydrogenase supports metabolic repurposing of mitochondria to drive inflammatory macrophages. *Cell* **2016**, *167*, 457–470.e413. [CrossRef] [PubMed]
79. Zhang, J.; Wang, L.; Xie, W.; Hu, S.; Zhou, H.; Zhu, P.; Zhu, H. Melatonin attenuates ER stress and mitochondrial damage in septic cardiomyopathy: A new mechanism involving BAP31 upregulation and MAPK-ERK pathway. *J. Cell. Physiol.* **2020**, *235*, 2847–2856. [CrossRef]

80. Lowes, D.A.; Almawash, A.M.; Webster, N.R.; Reid, V.L.; Galley, H.F. Melatonin and structurally similar compounds have differing effects on inflammation and mitochondrial function in endothelial cells under conditions mimicking sepsis. *Br. J. Anaesth.* **2011**, *107*, 193–201. [CrossRef]
81. Ding, Z.; Wu, X.; Wang, Y.; Ji, S.; Zhang, W.; Kang, J.; Li, J.; Fei, G. Melatonin prevents LPS-induced epithelial-mesenchymal transition in human alveolar epithelial cells via the GSK-3beta/Nrf2 pathway. *Biomed. Pharmacother.* **2020**, *132*, 110827. [CrossRef]
82. Liu, Y.; Yang, W.; Sun, X.; Xie, L.; Yang, Y.; Sang, M.; Jiao, R. SS31 Ameliorates Sepsis-Induced Heart Injury by Inhibiting Oxidative Stress and Inflammation. *Inflammation* **2019**, *42*, 2170–2180. [CrossRef] [PubMed]
83. Sener, G.; Toklu, H.; Kapucu, C.; Ercan, F.; Erkanli, G.; Kacmaz, A.; Tilki, M.; Yegen, B.C. Melatonin protects against oxidative organ injury in a rat model of sepsis. *Surg. Today* **2005**, *35*, 52–59. [CrossRef] [PubMed]
84. Quoilin, C.; Mouithys-Mickalad, A.; Duranteau, J.; Gallez, B.; Hoebeke, M. Endotoxin-induced basal respiration alterations of renal HK-2 cells: A sign of pathologic metabolism down-regulation. *Biochem. Biophys. Res. Commun.* **2012**, *423*, 350–354. [CrossRef] [PubMed]
85. Fock, E.; Bachteeva, V.; Lavrova, E.; Parnova, R. Mitochondrial-Targeted Antioxidant MitoQ Prevents E. coli Lipopolysaccharide-Induced Accumulation of Triacylglycerol and Lipid Droplets Biogenesis in Epithelial Cells. *J. Lipids* **2018**, *2018*, 5745790. [CrossRef]
86. Jeger, V.; Brandt, S.; Porta, F.; Jakob, S.M.; Takala, J.; Djafarzadeh, S. Dose response of endotoxin on hepatocyte and muscle mitochondrial respiration in vitro. *Biomed. Res. Int.* **2015**, *2015*, 353074. [CrossRef] [PubMed]
87. Karlsson, M.; Hara, N.; Morata, S.; Sjovall, F.; Kilbaugh, T.; Hansson, M.J.; Uchino, H.; Elmer, E. Diverse and Tissue-Specific Mitochondrial Respiratory Response in a Mouse Model of Sepsis-Induced Multiple Organ Failure. *Shock* **2016**, *45*, 404–410. [CrossRef]
88. Frisard, M.I.; Wu, Y.; McMillan, R.P.; Voelker, K.A.; Wahlberg, K.A.; Anderson, A.S.; Boutagy, N.; Resendes, K.; Ravussin, E.; Hulver, M.W. Low levels of lipopolysaccharide modulate mitochondrial oxygen consumption in skeletal muscle. *Metabolism* **2015**, *64*, 416–427. [CrossRef]
89. Apostolova, N.; Garcia-Bou, R.; Hernandez-Mijares, A.; Herance, R.; Rocha, M.; Victor, V.M. Mitochondrial antioxidants alleviate oxidative and nitrosative stress in a cellular model of sepsis. *Pharm. Res.* **2011**, *28*, 2910–2919. [CrossRef]
90. Raulien, N.; Friedrich, K.; Strobel, S.; Rubner, S.; Baumann, S.; von Bergen, M.; Korner, A.; Krueger, M.; Rossol, M.; Wagner, U. Fatty Acid Oxidation Compensates for Lipopolysaccharide-Induced Warburg Effect in Glucose-Deprived Monocytes. *Front. Immunol.* **2017**, *8*, 609. [CrossRef]
91. Palsson-McDermott, E.M.; Curtis, A.M.; Goel, G.; Lauterbach, M.A.; Sheedy, F.J.; Gleeson, L.E.; van den Bosch, M.W.; Quinn, S.R.; Domingo-Fernandez, R.; Johnston, D.G. Pyruvate kinase M2 regulates Hif-1α activity and IL-1β induction and is a critical determinant of the warburg effect in LPS-activated macrophages. *Cell Metab.* **2015**, *21*, 65–80. [CrossRef]
92. Kelly, B.; Tannahill, G.M.; Murphy, M.P.; O'Neill, L.A. Metformin Inhibits the Production of Reactive Oxygen Species from NADH:Ubiquinone Oxidoreductase to Limit Induction of Interleukin-1β (IL-1β) and Boosts Interleukin-10 (IL-10) in Lipopolysaccharide (LPS)-activated Macrophages. *J. Biol. Chem.* **2015**, *290*, 20348–20359. [CrossRef] [PubMed]
93. West, A.P.; Brodsky, I.E.; Rahner, C.; Woo, D.K.; Erdjument-Bromage, H.; Tempst, P.; Walsh, M.C.; Choi, Y.; Shadel, G.S.; Ghosh, S. TLR signalling augments macrophage bactericidal activity through mitochondrial ROS. *Nature* **2011**, *472*, 476–480. [CrossRef] [PubMed]
94. Kopp, E.; Medzhitov, R.; Carothers, J.; Xiao, C.; Douglas, I.; Janeway, C.A.; Ghosh, S. ECSIT is an evolutionarily conserved intermediate in the Toll/IL-1 signal transduction pathway. *Genes Dev.* **1999**, *13*, 2059–2071. [CrossRef] [PubMed]
95. Geng, J.; Sun, X.; Wang, P.; Zhang, S.; Wang, X.; Wu, H.; Hong, L.; Xie, C.; Li, X.; Zhao, H.; et al. Kinases Mst1 and Mst2 positively regulate phagocytic induction of reactive oxygen species and bactericidal activity. *Nat. Immunol.* **2015**, *16*, 1142–1152. [CrossRef] [PubMed]
96. Tur, J.; Pereira-Lopes, S.; Vico, T.; Marin, E.A.; Munoz, J.P.; Hernandez-Alvarez, M.; Cardona, P.J.; Zorzano, A.; Lloberas, J.; Celada, A. Mitofusin 2 in Macrophages Links Mitochondrial ROS Production, Cytokine Release, Phagocytosis, Autophagy, and Bactericidal Activity. *Cell Rep.* **2020**, *32*, 108079. [CrossRef]
97. Williams, R.J.; Spencer, J.P.; Rice-Evans, C. Flavonoids: Antioxidants or signalling molecules? *Free Radic. Biol. Med.* **2004**, *36*, 838–849. [CrossRef]
98. Murphy, M.P. Antioxidants as therapies: Can we improve on nature? *Free Radical. Biol. Med.* **2014**, *66*, 20–23. [CrossRef]
99. Haddad, J.J.; Land, S.C. Redox/ROS regulation of lipopolysaccharide-induced mitogen-activated protein kinase (MAPK) activation and MAPK-mediated TNF-alpha biosynthesis. *Br. J. Pharmacol.* **2002**, *135*, 520–536. [CrossRef]
100. Runkel, E.D.; Liu, S.; Baumeister, R.; Schulze, E. Surveillance-activated defenses block the ROS-induced mitochondrial unfolded protein response. *PLoS Genet.* **2013**, *9*, e1003346. [CrossRef]
101. Martindale, J.L.; Holbrook, N.J. Cellular response to oxidative stress: Signaling for suicide and survival. *J. Cell. Physiol.* **2002**, *192*, 1–15. [CrossRef]
102. Chen, L.; Liu, P.; Feng, X.; Ma, C. Salidroside suppressing LPS-induced myocardial injury by inhibiting ROS-mediated PI3K/Akt/mTOR pathway in vitro and in vivo. *J. Cell. Mol. Med.* **2017**, *21*, 3178–3189. [CrossRef] [PubMed]
103. Liberman, E.A.; Topaly, V.P. Permeability of bimolecular phospholipid membranes for fat-soluble ions. *Biofizika* **1969**, *14*, 452–461. [PubMed]
104. Kelso, G.F.; Porteous, C.M.; Hughes, G.; Ledgerwood, E.C.; Gane, A.M.; Smith, R.A.; Murphy, M.P. Prevention of mitochondrial oxidative damage using targeted antioxidants. *Ann. N. Y. Acad. Sci.* **2002**, *959*, 263–274. [CrossRef]

105. Battogtokh, G.; Choi, Y.S.; Kang, D.S.; Park, S.J.; Shim, M.S.; Huh, K.M.; Cho, Y.Y.; Lee, J.Y.; Lee, H.S.; Kang, H.C. Mitochondria-targeting drug conjugates for cytotoxic, anti-oxidizing and sensing purposes: Current strategies and future perspectives. *Acta Pharm. Sin. B* **2018**, *8*, 862–880. [CrossRef] [PubMed]
106. Zielonka, J.; Joseph, J.; Sikora, A.; Hardy, M.; Ouari, O.; Vasquez-Vivar, J.; Cheng, G.; Lopez, M.; Kalyanaraman, B. Mitochondria-Targeted Triphenylphosphonium-Based Compounds: Syntheses, Mechanisms of Action, and Therapeutic and Diagnostic Applications. *Chem. Rev.* **2017**, *117*, 10043–10120. [CrossRef]
107. Smith, R.A.; Porteous, C.M.; Coulter, C.V.; Murphy, M.P. Selective targeting of an antioxidant to mitochondria. *Eur. J. Biochem.* **1999**, *263*, 709–716. [CrossRef]
108. James, A.M.; Cocheme, H.M.; Smith, R.A.; Murphy, M.P. Interactions of mitochondria-targeted and untargeted ubiquinones with the mitochondrial respiratory chain and reactive oxygen species. Implications for the use of exogenous ubiquinones as therapies and experimental tools. *J. Biol. Chem.* **2005**, *280*, 21295–21312. [CrossRef]
109. Fetisova, E.K.; Muntyan, M.S.; Lyamzaev, K.G.; Chernyak, B.V. Therapeutic Effect of the Mitochondria-Targeted Antioxidant SkQ1 on the Culture Model of Multiple Sclerosis. *Oxidative Med. Cell. Longev.* **2019**, *2019*, 2082561. [CrossRef]
110. Ross, M.F.; Da Ros, T.; Blaikie, F.H.; Prime, T.A.; Porteous, C.M.; Severina, I.I.; Skulachev, V.P.; Kjaergaard, H.G.; Smith, R.A.; Murphy, M.P. Accumulation of lipophilic dications by mitochondria and cells. *Biochem. J.* **2006**, *400*, 199–208. [CrossRef]
111. Plotnikov, E.Y.; Zorov, D.B. Pros and Cons of Use of Mitochondria-Targeted Antioxidants. *Antioxidants* **2019**, *8*, 316. [CrossRef]
112. Lei, X.; Li, S.; Luo, C.; Wang, Y.; Liu, Y.; Xu, Z.; Huang, Q.; Zou, F.; Chen, Y.; Peng, F.; et al. Micheliolide Attenuates Lipopolysaccharide-Induced Inflammation by Modulating the mROS/NF-kappaB/NLRP3 Axis in Renal Tubular Epithelial Cells. *Mediat. Inflamm.* **2020**, *2020*, 3934769. [CrossRef] [PubMed]
113. Weidinger, A.; Mullebner, A.; Paier-Pourani, J.; Banerjee, A.; Miller, I.; Lauterbock, L.; Duvigneau, J.C.; Skulachev, V.P.; Redl, H.; Kozlov, A.V. Vicious inducible nitric oxide synthase-mitochondrial reactive oxygen species cycle accelerates inflammatory response and causes liver injury in rats. *Antioxid. Redox Signal.* **2015**, *22*, 572–586. [CrossRef] [PubMed]
114. Lowes, D.A.; Thottakam, B.M.; Webster, N.R.; Murphy, M.P.; Galley, H.F. The mitochondria-targeted antioxidant MitoQ protects against organ damage in a lipopolysaccharide-peptidoglycan model of sepsis. *Free Radic. Biol. Med.* **2008**, *45*, 1559–1565. [CrossRef] [PubMed]
115. Minter, B.E.; Lowes, D.A.; Webster, N.R.; Galley, H.F. Differential Effects of MitoVitE, alpha-Tocopherol and Trolox on Oxidative Stress, Mitochondrial Function and Inflammatory Signalling Pathways in Endothelial Cells Cultured under Conditions Mimicking Sepsis. *Antioxidants* **2020**, *9*, 195. [CrossRef]
116. Di, S.; Wang, Z.; Hu, W.; Yan, X.; Ma, Z.; Li, X.; Li, W.; Gao, J. The Protective Effects of Melatonin Against LPS-Induced Septic Myocardial Injury: A Potential Role of AMPK-Mediated Autophagy. *Front. Endocrinol. (Lausanne)* **2020**, *11*, 162. [CrossRef] [PubMed]
117. Asayama, S.; Kawamura, E.; Nagaoka, S.; Kawakami, H. Design of manganese porphyrin modified with mitochondrial signal peptide for a new antioxidant. *Mol. Pharm.* **2006**, *3*, 468–470. [CrossRef]
118. Mo, Y.N.; Deng, S.Y.; Zhang, L.N.; Huang, Y.; Li, W.C.; Peng, Q.Y.; Liu, Z.Y.; Ai, Y.H. SS-31 reduces inflammation and oxidative stress through the inhibition of Fis1 expression in lipopolysaccharide-stimulated microglia. *Biochem. Biophys. Res. Commun.* **2019**, *520*, 171–178. [CrossRef]
119. Fink, M.P.; Macias, C.A.; Xiao, J.; Tyurina, Y.Y.; Delude, R.L.; Greenberger, J.S.; Kagan, V.E.; Wipf, P. Hemigramicidin-TEMPO conjugates: Novel mitochondria-targeted antioxidants. *Crit. Care Med.* **2007**, *35*, S461–S467. [CrossRef]
120. Xue, Y.; Du, M.; Zhu, M.J. Quercetin suppresses NLRP3 inflammasome activation in epithelial cells triggered by Escherichia coli O157:H7. *Free Radic. Biol. Med.* **2017**, *108*, 760–769. [CrossRef]
121. Plotnikov, E.Y.; Pevzner, I.B.; Zorova, L.D.; Chernikov, V.P.; Prusov, A.N.; Kireev, I.I.; Silachev, D.N.; Skulachev, V.P.; Zorov, D.B. Mitochondrial Damage and Mitochondria-Targeted Antioxidant Protection in LPS-Induced Acute Kidney Injury. *Antioxidants* **2019**, *8*, 176. [CrossRef]
122. Lowes, D.; Webster, N.; Murphy, M.; Galley, H. Antioxidants that protect mitochondria reduce interleukin-6 and oxidative stress, improve mitochondrial function, and reduce biochemical markers of organ dysfunction in a rat model of acute sepsis. *Br. J. Anaesth.* **2013**, *110*, 472–480. [CrossRef] [PubMed]
123. Wang, H.; Li, L.; Zhao, M.; Chen, Y.H.; Zhang, Z.H.; Zhang, C.; Ji, Y.L.; Meng, X.H.; Xu, D.X. Melatonin alleviates lipopolysaccharide-induced placental cellular stress response in mice. *J. Pineal. Res.* **2011**, *50*, 418–426. [CrossRef] [PubMed]
124. Lopez, L.C.; Escames, G.; Tapias, V.; Utrilla, P.; Leon, J.; Acuna-Castroviejo, D. Identification of an inducible nitric oxide synthase in diaphragm mitochondria from septic mice—Its relation with mitochondrial dysfunction and prevention by melatonin. *Int. J. Biochem. Cell B* **2006**, *38*, 267–278. [CrossRef] [PubMed]
125. Zhao, W.; Xu, Z.; Cao, J.; Fu, Q.; Wu, Y.; Zhang, X.; Long, Y.; Zhang, X.; Yang, Y.; Li, Y.; et al. Elamipretide (SS-31) improves mitochondrial dysfunction, synaptic and memory impairment induced by lipopolysaccharide in mice. *J. Neuroinflamm.* **2019**, *16*, 230. [CrossRef]
126. Li, G.; Wu, J.; Li, R.; Yuan, D.; Fan, Y.; Yang, J.; Ji, M.; Zhu, S. Protective Effects of Antioxidant Peptide SS-31 Against Multiple Organ Dysfunctions During Endotoxemia. *Inflammation* **2016**, *39*, 54–64. [CrossRef]
127. Wu, J.; Zhang, M.; Hao, S.; Jia, M.; Ji, M.; Qiu, L.; Sun, X.; Yang, J.; Li, K. Mitochondria-Targeted Peptide Reverses Mitochondrial Dysfunction and Cognitive Deficits in Sepsis-Associated Encephalopathy. *Mol. Neurobiol.* **2015**, *52*, 783–791. [CrossRef]

128. Macarthur, H.; Couri, D.M.; Wilken, G.H.; Westfall, T.C.; Lechner, A.J.; Matuschak, G.M.; Chen, Z.; Salvemini, D. Modulation of serum cytokine levels by a novel superoxide dismutase mimetic, M40401, in an Escherichia coli model of septic shock: Correlation with preserved circulating catecholamines. *Crit. Care Med.* **2003**, *31*, 237–245. [CrossRef]
129. Smith, R.A.; Porteous, C.M.; Gane, A.M.; Murphy, M.P. Delivery of bioactive molecules to mitochondria in vivo. *Proc. Natl. Acad. Sci. USA* **2003**, *100*, 5407–5412. [CrossRef]
130. Huet, O.; Dupic, L.; Harrois, A.; Duranteau, J. Oxidative stress and endothelial dysfunction during sepsis. *Front. Biosci. (Landmark Ed.)* **2011**, *16*, 1986–1995. [CrossRef]
131. Rademann, P.; Weidinger, A.; Drechsler, S.; Meszaros, A.; Zipperle, J.; Jafarmadar, M.; Dumitrescu, S.; Hacobian, A.; Ungelenk, L.; Rostel, F.; et al. Mitochondria-Targeted Antioxidants SkQ1 and MitoTEMPO Failed to Exert a Long-Term Beneficial Effect in Murine Polymicrobial Sepsis. *Oxid. Med. Cell Longev.* **2017**, *2017*, 6412682. [CrossRef]
132. Reily, C.; Mitchell, T.; Chacko, B.K.; Benavides, G.; Murphy, M.P.; Darley-Usmar, V. Mitochondrially targeted compounds and their impact on cellular bioenergetics. *Redox Biol.* **2013**, *1*, 86–93. [PubMed]
133. Gottwald, E.M.; Duss, M.; Bugarski, M.; Haenni, D.; Schuh, C.D.; Landau, E.M.; Hall, A.M. The targeted anti-oxidant MitoQ causes mitochondrial swelling and depolarization in kidney tissue. *Physiol. Rep.* **2018**, *6*, e13667. [CrossRef] [PubMed]
134. Patkova, J.; Andel, M.; Trnka, J. Palmitate-induced cell death and mitochondrial respiratory dysfunction in myoblasts are not prevented by mitochondria-targeted antioxidants. *Cell Physiol. Biochem.* **2014**, *33*, 1439–1451. [CrossRef] [PubMed]
135. Doughan, A.K.; Dikalov, S.I. Mitochondrial redox cycling of mitoquinone leads to superoxide production and cellular apoptosis. *Antioxid. Redox Signal.* **2007**, *9*, 1825–1836. [CrossRef] [PubMed]
136. James, A.M.; Smith, R.A.; Murphy, M.P. Antioxidant and prooxidant properties of mitochondrial Coenzyme Q. *Arch. Biochem. Biophys.* **2004**, *423*, 47–56. [CrossRef]
137. Pokrzywinski, K.L.; Biel, T.G.; Kryndushkin, D.; Rao, V.A. Therapeutic Targeting of the Mitochondria Initiates Excessive Superoxide Production and Mitochondrial Depolarization Causing Decreased mtDNA Integrity. *PLoS ONE* **2016**, *11*, e0168283. [CrossRef] [PubMed]
138. Cheng, G.; Zielonka, J.; McAllister, D.M.; Mackinnon, A.C., Jr.; Joseph, J.; Dwinell, M.B.; Kalyanaraman, B. Mitochondria-targeted vitamin E analogs inhibit breast cancer cell energy metabolism and promote cell death. *BMC Cancer* **2013**, *13*, 285. [CrossRef]
139. Smith, R.A.; Murphy, M.P. Animal and human studies with the mitochondria-targeted antioxidant MitoQ. *Ann. N. Y. Acad. Sci.* **2010**, *1201*, 96–103. [CrossRef]
140. Fink, B.D.; Herlein, J.A.; Yorek, M.A.; Fenner, A.M.; Kerns, R.J.; Sivitz, W.I. Bioenergetic effects of mitochondrial-targeted coenzyme Q analogs in endothelial cells. *J. Pharmacol. Exp. Ther.* **2012**, *342*, 709–719. [CrossRef]
141. Lowes, D.A.; Wallace, C.; Murphy, M.P.; Webster, N.R.; Galley, H.F. The mitochondria targeted antioxidant MitoQ protects against fluoroquinolone-induced oxidative stress and mitochondrial membrane damage in human Achilles tendon cells. *Free Radic. Res.* **2009**, *43*, 323–328. [CrossRef]
142. McManus, M.J.; Murphy, M.P.; Franklin, J.L. Mitochondria-derived reactive oxygen species mediate caspase-dependent and -independent neuronal deaths. *Mol. Cell Neurosci.* **2014**, *63*, 13–23. [CrossRef] [PubMed]
143. Socaciu, A.I.; Ionut, R.; Socaciu, M.A.; Ungur, A.P.; Barsan, M.; Chiorean, A.; Socaciu, C.; Rajnoveanu, A.G. Melatonin, an ubiquitous metabolic regulator: Functions, mechanisms and effects on circadian disruption and degenerative diseases. *Rev. Endocr. Metab. Disord.* **2020**, *21*, 465–478. [CrossRef] [PubMed]
144. Reiter, R.J.; Mayo, J.C.; Tan, D.X.; Sainz, R.M.; Alatorre-Jimenez, M.; Qin, L. Melatonin as an antioxidant: Under promises but over delivers. *J. Pineal Res.* **2016**, *61*, 253–278. [CrossRef] [PubMed]
145. Colunga Biancatelli, R.M.L.; Berrill, M.; Mohammed, Y.H.; Marik, P.E. Melatonin for the treatment of sepsis: The scientific rationale. *J. Thorac. Dis.* **2020**, *12*, S54–S65. [CrossRef] [PubMed]
146. Andersen, L.P.; Werner, M.U.; Rosenkilde, M.M.; Fenger, A.Q.; Petersen, M.C.; Rosenberg, J.; Gogenur, I. Pharmacokinetics of high-dose intravenous melatonin in humans. *J. Clin. Pharmacol.* **2016**, *56*, 324–329. [CrossRef] [PubMed]
147. Posadzki, P.P.; Bajpai, R.; Kyaw, B.M.; Roberts, N.J.; Brzezinski, A.; Christopoulos, G.I.; Divakar, U.; Bajpai, S.; Soljak, M.; Dunleavy, G.; et al. Melatonin and health: An umbrella review of health outcomes and biological mechanisms of action. *BMC Med.* **2018**, *16*, 18. [CrossRef]
148. Poeggeler, B.; Saarela, S.; Reiter, R.J.; Tan, D.X.; Chen, L.D.; Manchester, L.C.; Barlow-Walden, L.R. Melatonin—A highly potent endogenous radical scavenger and electron donor: New aspects of the oxidation chemistry of this indole accessed in vitro. *Ann. N. Y. Acad. Sci.* **1994**, *738*, 419–420. [CrossRef]
149. Tan, D.X.; Manchester, L.C.; Reiter, R.J.; Qi, W.B.; Karbownik, M.; Calvo, J.R. Significance of melatonin in antioxidative defense system: Reactions and products. *Biol. Sign. Recept* **2000**, *9*, 137–159. [CrossRef]
150. Tan, D.X.; Manchester, L.C.; Terron, M.P.; Flores, L.J.; Reiter, R.J. One molecule, many derivatives: A never-ending interaction of melatonin with reactive oxygen and nitrogen species? *J. Pineal Res.* **2007**, *42*, 28–42. [CrossRef]
151. Venegas, C.; Garcia, J.A.; Escames, G.; Ortiz, F.; Lopez, A.; Doerrier, C.; Garcia-Corzo, L.; Lopez, L.C.; Reiter, R.J.; Acuna-Castroviejo, D. Extrapineal melatonin: Analysis of its subcellular distribution and daily fluctuations. *J. Pineal Res.* **2012**, *52*, 217–227. [CrossRef]
152. Tan, D.-X.; Manchester, L.C.; Esteban-Zubero, E.; Zhou, Z.; Reiter, R.J. Melatonin as a potent and inducible endogenous antioxidant: Synthesis and metabolism. *Molecules* **2015**, *20*, 18886–18906. [CrossRef] [PubMed]

153. He, C.; Wang, J.; Zhang, Z.; Yang, M.; Li, Y.; Tian, X.; Ma, T.; Tao, J.; Zhu, K.; Song, Y.; et al. Mitochondria Synthesize Melatonin to Ameliorate Its Function and Improve Mice Oocyte's Quality under in Vitro Conditions. *Int. J. Mol. Sci.* **2016**, *17*, 939. [CrossRef] [PubMed]
154. Lopez, A.; Garcia, J.A.; Escames, G.; Venegas, C.; Ortiz, F.; Lopez, L.C.; Acuna-Castroviejo, D. Melatonin protects the mitochondria from oxidative damage reducing oxygen consumption, membrane potential, and superoxide anion production. *J. Pineal Res.* **2009**, *46*, 188–198. [CrossRef] [PubMed]
155. Paradies, G.; Paradies, V.; Ruggiero, F.M.; Petrosillo, G. Protective role of melatonin in mitochondrial dysfunction and related disorders. *Arch. Toxicol.* **2015**, *89*, 923–939. [CrossRef] [PubMed]
156. Acuna Castroviejo, D.; Lopez, L.C.; Escames, G.; López, A.; Garcia, J.A.; Reiter, R.J. Melatonin-mitochondria interplay in health and disease. *Curr. Top. Med. Chem.* **2011**, *11*, 221–240. [CrossRef] [PubMed]
157. Vriend, J.; Reiter, R.J. Melatonin, bone regulation and the ubiquitin-proteasome connection: A review. *Life Sci.* **2016**, *145*, 152–160. [CrossRef]
158. Janjetovic, Z.; Jarrett, S.G.; Lee, E.F.; Duprey, C.; Reiter, R.J.; Slominski, A.T. Melatonin and its metabolites protect human melanocytes against UVB-induced damage: Involvement of NRF2-mediated pathways. *Sci. Rep.* **2017**, *7*, 1–13. [CrossRef] [PubMed]
159. Zhai, M.; Li, B.; Duan, W.; Jing, L.; Zhang, B.; Zhang, M.; Yu, L.; Liu, Z.; Yu, B.; Ren, K.; et al. Melatonin ameliorates myocardial ischemia reperfusion injury through SIRT3-dependent regulation of oxidative stress and apoptosis. *J. Pineal Res.* **2017**, *63*, e12419. [CrossRef]
160. Wu, J.Y.; Tsou, M.Y.; Chen, T.H.; Chen, S.J.; Tsao, C.M.; Wu, C.C. Therapeutic effects of melatonin on peritonitis-induced septic shock with multiple organ dysfunction syndrome in rats. *J. Pineal Res.* **2008**, *45*, 106–116. [CrossRef]
161. Szeto, H.H. Mitochondria-targeted cytoprotective peptides for ischemia-reperfusion injury. *Antioxid. Redox Signal.* **2008**, *10*, 601–619. [CrossRef]
162. Szeto, H.H. Development of mitochondria-targeted aromatic-cationic peptides for neurodegenerative diseases. *Ann. N. Y. Acad. Sci.* **2008**, *1147*, 112–121. [CrossRef] [PubMed]
163. Birk, A.V.; Chao, W.M.; Bracken, C.; Warren, J.D.; Szeto, H.H. Targeting mitochondrial cardiolipin and the cytochrome c/cardiolipin complex to promote electron transport and optimize mitochondrial ATP synthesis. *Br. J. Pharmacol.* **2014**, *171*, 2017–2028. [CrossRef] [PubMed]
164. Iyer, S.S.; He, Q.; Janczy, J.R.; Elliott, E.I.; Zhong, Z.; Olivier, A.K.; Sadler, J.J.; Knepper-Adrian, V.; Han, R.Z.; Qiao, L.; et al. Mitochondrial Cardiolipin Is Required for Nlrp3 Inflammasome Activation. *Immunity* **2013**, *39*, 311–323. [CrossRef] [PubMed]
165. Birk, A.V.; Chao, W.M.; Liu, S.; Soong, Y.; Szeto, H.H. Disruption of cytochrome c heme coordination is responsible for mitochondrial injury during ischemia. *Biochim. Biophys. Acta* **2015**, *1847*, 1075–1084. [CrossRef] [PubMed]
166. Szeto, H.H. First-in-class cardiolipin-protective compound as a therapeutic agent to restore mitochondrial bioenergetics. *Br. J. Pharmacol.* **2014**, *171*, 2029–2050. [CrossRef] [PubMed]
167. Szeto, H.H. Pharmacologic Approaches to Improve Mitochondrial Function in AKI and CKD. *J. Am. Soc. Nephrol.* **2017**, *28*, 2856–2865. [CrossRef]
168. Sabbah, H.N.; Gupta, R.C.; Kohli, S.; Wang, M.; Hachem, S.; Zhang, K. Chronic Therapy With Elamipretide (MTP-131), a Novel Mitochondria-Targeting Peptide, Improves Left Ventricular and Mitochondrial Function in Dogs With Advanced Heart Failure. *Circ. Heart Fail.* **2016**, *9*, e002206. [CrossRef]
169. Righi, V.; Constantinou, C.; Mintzopoulos, D.; Khan, N.; Mupparaju, S.P.; Rahme, L.G.; Swartz, H.M.; Szeto, H.H.; Tompkins, R.G.; Tzika, A.A. Mitochondria-targeted antioxidant promotes recovery of skeletal muscle mitochondrial function after burn trauma assessed by in vivo 31P nuclear magnetic resonance and electron paramagnetic resonance spectroscopy. *FASEB J.* **2013**, *27*, 2521–2530. [CrossRef]
170. Orr, A.L.; Ashok, D.; Sarantos, M.R.; Shi, T.; Hughes, R.E.; Brand, M.D. Inhibitors of ROS production by the ubiquinone-binding site of mitochondrial complex I identified by chemical screening. *Free Radic. Biol. Med.* **2013**, *65*, 1047–1059. [CrossRef]
171. Orr, A.L.; Vargas, L.; Turk, C.N.; Baaten, J.E.; Matzen, J.T.; Dardov, V.J.; Attle, S.J.; Li, J.; Quackenbush, D.C.; Goncalves, R.L. Suppressors of superoxide production from mitochondrial complex III. *Nat. Chem. Biol.* **2015**, *11*, 834. [CrossRef]
172. Wong, H.S.; Monternier, P.A.; Brand, M.D. S1QELs suppress mitochondrial superoxide/hydrogen peroxide production from site IQ without inhibiting reverse electron flow through Complex I. *Free Radic. Biol. Med.* **2019**, *143*, 545–559. [CrossRef] [PubMed]
173. Watson, M.A.; Wong, H.S.; Brand, M.D. Use of S1QELs and S3QELs to link mitochondrial sites of superoxide and hydrogen peroxide generation to physiological and pathological outcomes. *Biochem. Soc. Trans.* **2019**, *47*, 1461–1469. [CrossRef] [PubMed]
174. Brand, M.D. Mitochondrial generation of superoxide and hydrogen peroxide as the source of mitochondrial redox signaling. *Free Radic. Biol. Med.* **2016**, *100*, 14–31. [CrossRef] [PubMed]
175. Fang, J.; Wong, H.S.; Brand, M.D. Production of superoxide and hydrogen peroxide in the mitochondrial matrix is dominated by site IQ of complex I in diverse cell lines. *Redox Biol.* **2020**, *37*, 101722. [CrossRef]
176. Brand, M.D.; Goncalves, R.L.; Orr, A.L.; Vargas, L.; Gerencser, A.A.; Borch Jensen, M.; Wang, Y.T.; Melov, S.; Turk, C.N.; Matzen, J.T.; et al. Suppressors of Superoxide-H2O2 Production at Site IQ of Mitochondrial Complex I Protect against Stem Cell Hyperplasia and Ischemia-Reperfusion Injury. *Cell Metab.* **2016**, *24*, 582–592. [CrossRef]

177. Piao, L.; Fang, Y.H.; Hamanaka, R.B.; Mutlu, G.M.; Dezfulian, C.; Archer, S.L.; Sharp, W.W. Suppression of Superoxide-Hydrogen Peroxide Production at Site IQ of Mitochondrial Complex I Attenuates Myocardial Stunning and Improves Postcardiac Arrest Outcomes. *Crit. Care Med.* **2020**, *48*, e133–e140. [CrossRef]
178. Goncalves, R.L.; Watson, M.A.; Wong, H.-S.; Orr, A.L.; Brand, M.D. The use of site-specific suppressors to measure the relative contributions of different mitochondrial sites to skeletal muscle superoxide and hydrogen peroxide production. *Redox Biol.* **2020**, *28*, 101341. [CrossRef]
179. Murphy, M.P.; O'Neill, L.A.J. Krebs Cycle Reimagined: The Emerging Roles of Succinate and Itaconate as Signal Transducers. *Cell* **2018**, *174*, 780–784. [CrossRef]
180. Su, W.; Shi, J.; Zhao, Y.; Yan, F.; Lei, L.; Li, H. Porphyromonas gingivalis triggers inflammatory responses in periodontal ligament cells by succinate-succinate dehydrogenase-HIF-1alpha axis. *Biochem. Biophys. Res. Commun.* **2020**, *522*, 184–190. [CrossRef]
181. Ge, X.; Wang, L.; Li, M.; Xu, N.; Yu, F.; Yang, F.; Li, R.; Zhang, F.; Zhao, B.; Du, J. Vitamin D/VDR signaling inhibits LPS-induced IFNgamma and IL-1beta in Oral epithelia by regulating hypoxia-inducible factor-1alpha signaling pathway. *Cell Commun. Signal.* **2019**, *17*, 18. [CrossRef]
182. Chouchani, E.T.; Pell, V.R.; Gaude, E.; Aksentijevic, D.; Sundier, S.Y.; Robb, E.L.; Logan, A.; Nadtochiy, S.M.; Ord, E.N.J.; Smith, A.C.; et al. Ischaemic accumulation of succinate controls reperfusion injury through mitochondrial ROS. *Nature* **2014**, *515*, 431–435. [CrossRef] [PubMed]
183. Tannahill, G.M.; Curtis, A.M.; Adamik, J.; Palsson-McDermott, E.M.; McGettrick, A.F.; Goel, G.; Frezza, C.; Bernard, N.J.; Kelly, B.; Foley, N.H.; et al. Succinate is an inflammatory signal that induces IL-1beta through HIF-1alpha. *Nature* **2013**, *496*, 238–242. [CrossRef] [PubMed]
184. Yang, N.; Liang, Y.; Yang, P.; Ji, F. Propofol suppresses LPS-induced nuclear accumulation of HIF-1α and tumor aggressiveness in non-small cell lung cancer. *Oncol. Rep.* **2017**, *37*, 2611–2619. [CrossRef] [PubMed]
185. Lampropoulou, V.; Sergushichev, A.; Bambouskova, M.; Nair, S.; Vincent, E.E.; Loginicheva, E.; Cervantes-Barragan, L.; Ma, X.; Huang, S.C.-C.; Griss, T. Itaconate links inhibition of succinate dehydrogenase with macrophage metabolic remodeling and regulation of inflammation. *Cell Metab.* **2016**, *24*, 158–166. [CrossRef] [PubMed]
186. Bambouskova, M.; Gorvel, L.; Lampropoulou, V.; Sergushichev, A.; Loginicheva, E.; Johnson, K.; Korenfeld, D.; Mathyer, M.E.; Kim, H.; Huang, L.H.; et al. Electrophilic properties of itaconate and derivatives regulate the IkappaBzeta-ATF3 inflammatory axis. *Nature* **2018**, *556*, 501–504. [CrossRef]
187. Mills, E.L.; Ryan, D.G.; Prag, H.A.; Dikovskaya, D.; Menon, D.; Zaslona, Z.; Jedrychowski, M.P.; Costa, A.S.H.; Higgins, M.; Hams, E.; et al. Itaconate is an anti-inflammatory metabolite that activates Nrf2 via alkylation of KEAP1. *Nature* **2018**, *556*, 113–117. [CrossRef]
188. Hayes, J.D.; Dinkova-Kostova, A.T. The Nrf2 regulatory network provides an interface between redox and intermediary metabolism. *Trends Biochem. Sci.* **2014**, *39*, 199–218. [CrossRef]
189. Swain, A.; Bambouskova, M.; Kim, H.; Andhey, P.S.; Duncan, D.; Auclair, K.; Chubukov, V.; Simons, D.M.; Roddy, T.P.; Stewart, K.M.; et al. Comparative evaluation of itaconate and its derivatives reveals divergent inflammasome and type I interferon regulation in macrophages. *Nat. Metab.* **2020**, *2*, 594–602. [CrossRef]
190. Yang, Y.; Shao, R.; Tang, L.; Li, L.; Zhu, M.; Huang, J.; Shen, Y.; Zhang, L. Succinate dehydrogenase inhibitor dimethyl malonate alleviates LPS/d-galactosamine-induced acute hepatic damage in mice. *Innate Immun.* **2019**, *25*, 522–529. [CrossRef]
191. Sasaki, T.; Harada, S.; Yamamoto, S.; Ohkushi, D.; Hayama, B.; Takeda, K.; Hoashi, K.; Shiotani, J.; Takehana, K.; Doi, Y. Clinical characteristics of peripheral venous catheter-associated gram-negative bloodstream infection among patients with malignancy. *PLoS ONE* **2020**, *15*, e0228396. [CrossRef]
192. Ghorbaninejad, P.; Sheikhhossein, F.; Djafari, F.; Tijani, A.J.; Mohammadpour, S.; Shab-Bidar, S. Effects of melatonin supplementation on oxidative stress: A systematic review and meta-analysis of randomized controlled trials. *Horm. Mol. Biol. Clin. Investig.* **2020**, *41*. [CrossRef] [PubMed]
193. Henderson, R.; Kim, S.; Lee, E. Use of melatonin as adjunctive therapy in neonatal sepsis: A systematic review and meta-analysis. *Complement. Ther. Med.* **2018**, *39*, 131–136. [CrossRef] [PubMed]
194. Chojnacki, C.; Medrek-Socha, M.; Konrad, P.; Chojnacki, J.; Blonska, A. The value of melatonin supplementation in postmenopausal women with Helicobacter pylori-associated dyspepsia. *BMC Womens Health* **2020**, *20*, 262. [CrossRef] [PubMed]
195. Snow, B.J.; Rolfe, F.L.; Lockhart, M.M.; Frampton, C.M.; O'Sullivan, J.D.; Fung, V.; Smith, R.A.; Murphy, M.P.; Taylor, K.M.; Group, P.S. A double-blind, placebo-controlled study to assess the mitochondria-targeted antioxidant MitoQ as a disease-modifying therapy in Parkinson's disease. *Mov. Disord.* **2010**, *25*, 1670–1674. [CrossRef] [PubMed]
196. Nazarov, P.A.; Osterman, I.A.; Tokarchuk, A.V.; Karakozova, M.V.; Korshunova, G.A.; Lyamzaev, K.G.; Skulachev, M.V.; Kotova, E.A.; Skulachev, V.P.; Antonenko, Y.N. Mitochondria-targeted antioxidants as highly effective antibiotics. *Sci. Rep.* **2017**, *7*, 1394. [CrossRef] [PubMed]

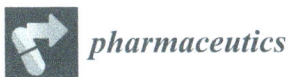

Review

Targeting Mitochondrial Oncometabolites: A New Approach to Overcome Drug Resistance in Cancer

Martina Godel, Giacomo Ortone, Dario Pasquale Anobile, Martina Pasino, Giulio Randazzo, Chiara Riganti [†] and Joanna Kopecka *,[†]

Department of Oncology, University of Torino, via Santena 5/bis, 10126 Torino, Italy; martina.godel@edu.unito.it (M.G.); giacomo.ortone@edu.unito.it (G.O.); dario.anobile@edu.unito.it (D.P.A.); martina.pasino530@edu.unito.it (M.P.); giulio.randazzo754@edu.unito.it (G.R.); chiara.riganti@unito.it (C.R.)
* Correspondence: joanna.kopecka@unito.it; Tel.: +39-670-5849
† Senior co-authorship.

Abstract: Drug resistance is the main obstacle for a successful cancer therapy. There are many mechanisms by which cancers avoid drug-mediated death, including alterations in cellular metabolism and apoptotic programs. Mitochondria represent the cell's powerhouse and the connection between carbohydrate, lipid and proteins metabolism, as well as crucial controllers of apoptosis, playing an important role not only in tumor growth and progression, but also in drug response. Alterations in tricarboxylic acid cycle (TCA) caused by mutations in three TCA enzymes—isocitrate dehydrogenase, succinate dehydrogenase and fumarate hydratase—lead to the accumulation of 2-hydroxyglutarate, succinate and fumarate respectively, collectively known as oncometabolites. Oncometabolites have pleiotropic effects on cancer biology. For instance, they generate a pseudohypoxic phenotype and induce epigenetic changes, two factors that may promote cancer drug resistance leading to disease progression and poor therapy outcome. This review sums up the most recent findings about the role of TCA-derived oncometabolites in cancer aggressiveness and drug resistance, highlighting possible pharmacological strategies targeting oncometabolites production in order to improve the efficacy of cancer treatment.

Keywords: mitochondrial oncometabolites; cancer drug resistance; cancer metabolism

Citation: Godel, M.; Ortone, G.; Anobile, D.P.; Pasino, M.; Randazzo, G.; Riganti, C.; Kopecka, J. Targeting Mitochondrial Oncometabolites: A New Approach to Overcome Drug Resistance in Cancer. *Pharmaceutics* 2021, *13*, 762. https://doi.org/10.3390/pharmaceutics13050762

Academic Editor: Tihomir Tomašič

Received: 12 April 2021
Accepted: 18 May 2021
Published: 20 May 2021

Publisher's Note: MDPI stays neutral with regard to jurisdictional claims in published maps and institutional affiliations.

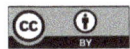

Copyright: © 2021 by the authors. Licensee MDPI, Basel, Switzerland. This article is an open access article distributed under the terms and conditions of the Creative Commons Attribution (CC BY) license (https://creativecommons.org/licenses/by/4.0/).

1. Introduction: Mitochondria in Cancer

Treating advanced tumors is still an important challenge because of the concomitant presence of intrinsic and acquired resistance to the commonly used anti-cancer drugs. Most advanced tumors share the ability to escape cell death mediated by anticancer drugs, while continuing their growth and progression. The main mechanisms responsible for drug resistance, often known as multidrug resistance since it involves multiple drugs with different mechanisms of action, are the reduced drug uptake and accumulation, the increased drug efflux via membrane transporters that decrease intratumor drug concentration and cytotoxicity, the efficient mechanisms of DNA repair, the bypass of the DNA damaging and the cell cycle arrest induced by many chemotherapeutics, the prevalence of survival pathways over apoptotic pathways, the metabolic reprograming [1]. Inhibition of apoptosis and metabolic rewiring are strongly correlated with altered mitochondria functions, protect cancer cells from drug-mediated death inducing drug resistance [2].

Traditionally, the shift from oxidative phosphorylation (OXPHOS) to aerobic glycolysis is considered a hallmark of cancer, postulated by Otto Von Warburg. This implies that mitochondria are poorly active in tumors [3]. However, an increasing amount of evidence demonstrates that, despite several cancers satisfying their energetic requirements using glycolysis, other tumors—in particular if drug resistant—heavily rely on OXPHOS to fuel their metabolism [4].

For many years, mitochondria have been considered only as the energy powerhouse of the cell. Nonetheless, in addition to their role in generating ATP, mitochondria are key signaling centers regulating cancer development and progression, including metabolic reprogramming in response to anticancer drugs. In fact, the mitochondrial oxidative decarboxylation of pyruvate, the fatty acid β-oxidation (FAO) and the glutaminolysis are the key fuel of the tricarboxylic acid (TCA) cycle that sustains production of ATP via OXPHOS. The mitochondrial intermediate metabolism interconnects amino acid, lipid and carbohydrate metabolism that are involved in both TCA anaplerotic fluxes, to obtain energy equivalents, and TCA cataplerotic fluxes towards the synthesis of building blocks such as proteins and nucleotides. Higher energetic mitochondrial metabolism, higher anaplerotic and cataplerotic fluxes are hallmarks of drug resistant cancers [5]. Indeed, this metabolic phenotype replenishes cancer cells either of ATP and building blocks, attenuating the damages of cytotoxic stresses, including chemotherapy. Moreover, blocking the pyruvate dehydrogenase complex, i.e., the influx of glucose-derived acetyl-CoA into TCA cycle and/or anaplerotic pathways (such as FAO, glutaminolysis, glutamate oxidative metabolism, arginine, proline, asparagine, aspartate and phenylalanine catabolism) [6], buffers production of the reactive oxide species (ROS) by electron transport chain (ETC) [7], maintaining them below a "danger threshold" and determining the production of low levels of ROS that train cancer cells to resistance to oxidative stress and chemotherapeutic drugs, by upregulating antioxidant mechanisms [8].

Beside a key role in energetic metabolism and ROS production, mitochondria regulate the apoptotic response upon chemotherapy, by decreasing the BCL2/BAX ratio, increasing the permeabilization of mitochondrial membrane, the opening of mitochondrial permeability transition pore and the release of cytochrome c, which activates the apoptosome and the caspase 9/3 axis [9]. Furthermore, mitochondrial DNA (mtDNA) is frequently mutated in tumors, spontaneously or upon the damage induced by chemotherapeutic drugs, such as cisplatin and gemcitabine [10]. Since mtDNA mainly encodes for mitochondrial translation machinery and ETC complexes, mutations in these key players of OXPHOS may produce the synthesis of complexes characterized by a defective reduction of electron shuttles (ubiquinone, cytochrome c), structural components (Fe-S cluster-, cytochrome-containing proteins) or O_2, determining the generation of radical species or ROS. This mitochondrial dysfunction promotes metabolic alterations, changes the ROS buffering and the balance between pro-apoptotic and anti-apoptotic signaling, contributing to drug resistance [11].

Genetic alterations of TCA cycle enzymes such as succinate dehydrogenase (SDH), also shared with complex II of ETC, fumarate hydratase (FH) or isocitrate dehydrogenase (IDH) lead to the accumulation of the upstream intermediates—succinate, fumarate and 2-hydroxyglutarate (2-HG), respectively. They are known as oncometabolites, because of their role in cancer growth, aggressiveness and progression [12]. This review will describe the current understanding of oncometabolite role in cancer aggressiveness, with a special emphasis on drug resistance. Next, we will focus on potential pharmacological strategies targeting the production of oncometabolites as potential tools improving the efficacy of anti-cancer treatments.

2. Mitochondrial Oncometabolites and Cancer Biology

Succinate, fumarate and 2-HG dysregulate a plethora of cellular processes associated with invasiveness and drug resistance, such as protein post-translational modifications, metabolic and epigenetic events, epithelial-to-mesenchymal transition (EMT), inhibition of α-ketoglutarate (α-KG)-dependent dioxygenase enzymes [12]. Since α-KG is part of TCA cycle, its modulation by the oncometabolites generated within the TCA cycle itself may represent a finely tuned feedback control on the cycle itself.

Succinate is generated from succinyl-CoA and oxidized into fumarate by SDH. Fumarate is the substrate for FH, an enzyme that catalyzes the reversible hydration/dehydration of fumarate to malate. SDH complex is built of four subunits (SDHA, SDHB, SDHC, SDHD). It is the only TCA enzyme that produces FADH2 [12,13]. Mutations in SDH have been reported in all subunits. In addition, some SDH-deficient tumors either have hypermethylation in the SDHC promoter, which phenotypically makes these tumors without a functioning SDH [14] or have hyper-expressed the tumor necrosis factor-associated protein (TRAP1) that inhibits SDH [15]. Moreover, down-regulation of SDH mRNA by miR-210, miR-31 and miR-37, post-translational modifications such as dephosphorylation by PTEN-like mitochondrial phosphatase-1, deacetylation of lysines consequent to the loss of sirtuin 3, competitive inhibition by itaconate, a TCA cycle side-metabolite produced by the decarboxylation of cis-aconitate during inflammation [16], result in the inhibition of SDH activity [17]. In all these cases succinate accumulates, as reported in paragangliomas, pheochromocytomas, neuroblastomas [18], gastrointestinal stromal cancer [19], colon [20], renal and ovarian cancers [21].

FH has isoforms with different cellular localization: one mitochondrial isoform participates in TCA cycle; one cytosolic isoform is involved in the metabolism of amino acids and fumarate [22]. When FH is mutated, as described for instance in renal cell cancer (RCC) and kidney renal papillary cell carcinoma (KIRP) [23], fumarate accumulates [13]. Importantly, RCC with mutant FH is one of the most aggressive forms of renal cancer, characterized by early metastasis and a poor clinical outcome [24]. Sporadic cases of deficient FH were also reported for paragangliomas, pheochromocytomas [25], neuroblastoma [26], uterine and skin leiomyoma [27], and endometrial cancer [28]. A similar metabolic phenotype with fumarate accumulation is described in nasopharyngeal carcinomas overexpressing the lymphoid-specific helicase, a chromatin remodeling ATPase that causes FH repression: this phenotype has been linked to increased migration and invasion [29].

Differently from succinate and fumarate, 2-HG is produced by an abnormal catalytic activity of IDH, a TCA enzyme that in physiological conditions catalyzes the decarboxylation of isocitrate into α-KG and CO_2, using NADP+ and Mg^{2+} as cofactors [30]. The reverse reaction produces isocitrate through the reductive carboxylation of α-KG, consuming NAD(P)H and CO_2: when this reaction is incomplete and does not involve CO_2, α-KG is reduced into 2-HG [31]. IDH enzymes are present in three isoforms, each with a different subcellular localization and co-substrates specificity: IDH1 is localized in peroxisomes and cytosol and uses NADP+/NADPH, the NADP+/NADPH-dependent IDH2 and the NAD+/NADH-dependent IDH3 are present in mitochondria. IDH1 reversibly interconverts α-KG into isocitrate as part of the reductive glutamine metabolism [32]. IDH2 is mainly involved in the oxidative metabolism of isocitrate in the TCA cycle, while IDH3 irreversibly oxidizes isocitrate to produce α-KG and NADH. Somatic point mutations in IDH1 and IDH2 genes have been found in glioma, glioblastoma multiforme (GBM) and acute myeloid leukemia (AML), prevalently concentrated in specific hot spots [30]. The IDH1 R132H/C/Q, IDH2 R140Q/W/L and R172K/M/G/T/S are the most common mutations conferring a new catalytic activity with overproduction of 2-HG [33].

Succinate, fumarate and 2-HG contribute to cancer growth with pleiotropic mechanisms, such as stabilization of the hypoxic inducible factor-1α (HIF-1α), epigenetic changes, apoptosis alteration, increased production of mitochondrial ROS (mtROS) and protein or chromatin "succinylation", all events that occur often concurrently and are interconnected [34].

The accumulation of succinate in tumors causes the so-called pseudohypoxia, a condition characterized by the stabilization of HIF-1α notwithstanding the normoxic environment. This pseudohypoxic phenotype promotes cell survival, proliferation, angiogenesis and drug resistance [35]. Succinate mediates HIF-1α stabilization by inhibiting the prolylhydroxylases (PHDs), which are responsible for hydroxylating HIF-1α and marking it for proteasomal degradation. The mechanism of PHDs inhibition by succinate was first demonstrated in HEK293 cells silenced for SDHD subunit that has increased succinate and lacked HIF-1α degradation [36]. The same results were obtained in the human colon cancer cell line HCT116, knocked-down for SDHB, where succinate accumulation and HIF-1α stabilization were accompanied by lower mitochondrial O_2 consumption rate and higher extracellular acidification, indicative of a metabolic shift toward glycolysis induced by HIF-1α [37]. Succinate may act also through succinate receptor SUCNR1, which stabilizes HIF-1α in non-small cell lung cancer by engaging the downstream mediators phosphatidylinositol 3-phosphate kinase (PI3K)/Akt that phosphorylate HIF-1α on serine [38]. Of note, SUCNR1 is highly expressed also in kidney cancer, where its signaling promotes angiogenesis, hematopoiesis and inflammation [39], and in tumor-associated macrophages (TAMs), where the binding of succinate favors the polarization toward a tumor-permissive M2-phenotype, facilitating cancer cell migration, invasion and metastasis [38]. Further, the increase in mtROS that is associated with SDH deficiency [40] may increase HIF-1α because ROS inactivate PHDs, thus preventing HIF-1α degradation [41,42]. In neuroblastoma, the increase of HIF-1α has also been caused by the inhibition of the ten-eleven translocation proteins (TETs) that antagonize DNA methylation in specific loci by oxidizing 5-methylcytosines. Both succinate and fumarate inhibited TETs and induced the simultaneous transcriptional increase of HIF-1α and HIF-2α. However not all hypoxia-responsive genes were upregulated [26], suggesting that differential circuitries—dependent and independent from mitochondrial oncometabolites—control the transcriptional activity of HIFs. In addition, 2-HG causes pseudohypoxia: in the presence of mutated IDH2, the high ratio between 2-HG and α-KG reduces the activity of PHDs, stabilizing HIF-1α [33].

As mentioned before, mitochondrial oncometabolites cause epigenetic changes in cancer cells, boosting oncogenesis and cancer progression. SDH deficient tumors are characterized by hypermethylation of histones and DNA cytosine [14,43], as a result of the succinate-mediated inhibition of histone lysine demethylases (KDMs) and TETs [26,44]. The hypermethylation changes the expression profile of specific genes, leading for instance to the activation of the EMT program, as demonstrated in pheochromocytomas and paragangliomas knocked-down for SDHB [45]. Moreover, fumarate inhibits TETs and KDMs, suppressing the anti-metastatic miR-200, up-regulating specific transcription factors, such as Twist and HIF-1α, that promote EMT. As proof of concept, the reintroduction of full-length Fh1 in mouse and human FH-deficient cells was sufficient to prevent the EMT signature, reducing vimentin and restoring E-cadherin expression [46]. In addition, epigenetic changes in FH deficient cells can contribute to defects in DNA Damage Response (DDR) and to the bypass of the cell cycle checkpoints activated after DNA damage, e.g., after irradiation. In vitro studies on RCC-derived cell lines showed that FH deficiency causes either the arrest in G1-phase or the more rapidly progress through mitosis after DNA damage. Fumarate accumulation enhances the bypass of G2-phase checkpoints, activates the error-prone non-homologous end-joining (NHEJ) repair system during cell mitosis, and favors the accumulation of ROS, known inducers of DNA damage, with the result of an increased genome instability [47]. The effects of fumarate in chromatin remodeling and DNA damage are not tumor specific, because the DNA hypermethylation observed in HepG2 cells exposed to millimolar concentrations of fumarate were comparable to the hypermethylation detected in FH deficient cells [48]. Of note, hypermethylation can be also caused by 2-HG that acts at the epigenetic level by competitively inhibiting TET2 and JMJD2A/lysine demethylase 4A [33].

FH plays a physiological role in controlling cell proliferation, independent on the effects on cell cycle and chromatin remodeling. This role is often altered in cancer cells, as a consequence of the activation of other pathways peculiar of transformed cells, such as the O-glycosylation (O-GlcNAc) pathway or the p21 Activated Kinase 4 (PAK4)-dependent activity. While in non-transformed cells, FH binds the Activation Transcription Factor 2 (ATF2) and enhances its transcriptional activity, favoring cell cycle arrest, in cancer cells, particularly in those tumors that display a high activity of O-GlcNAc transferase (OGT) such as pancreatic adenocarcinoma (PDAC) [49], the FH/ATF2-mediated events are impaired by the O-GlcNAc glycosylation of FH. This post-translational modification limits the interaction between FH and ATF2, maintaining high levels of cell proliferation [50]. Accordingly, PDAC patients with high OGT and O-GlcNAc-FH levels have a lower median survival [50]. Transforming growth factor β (TGFβ) is responsible for a second mechanism of fumarate-dependent inhibition of cell proliferation, disrupted in cancer cells. TGFβ signaling favors growth arrest by increasing the phosphorylation of FH on Thr90 by p38 mitogen activated kinase (MAPK). Such phosphorylation favors the interaction between FH and recombination signal binding protein for immunoglobulin kappa J region, also known as CSL, a downstream effector of Notch. The FH/CSL complex associates p53 and is recruited on the promoter of the p53-targeted gene p21/cyclin dependent kinase inhibitor 1A, which prevents cell cycle progression. PAK4, highly expressed in lung cancers, counteracts the anti-proliferative effect induced by TGFβ/FH/CSL cascade by phosphorylating FH on Ser46, an event that—contrarily to the phosphorylation on Thr90—impairs the interaction between FH and CSL, favoring tumor proliferation and metastasis. Conversely, the PAK4 inhibitor PF-3758309 favors the FH-CSL interaction in non-small cell lung cancer cells and enhances the anti-proliferative effect induced by TGFβ [51].

Multiple pathways regulating cell proliferation and/or inhibiting of apoptosis are controlled also by 2-HG [31]. In IDH1-R132Q knock-in mutant cells, 2-HG physically binds Cdc42, a small GTPase of Rho family involved in the regulation of cell cycle. By doing so, 2-HG blocks Cdc42 interaction with mixed lineage kinase 3 (MLK3), a component of the pro-apoptotic cascade MLK3/MKK4-7/JNK/Bim. Typically, 2-HG prevents the association between Cdc42 and MLK3, preventing apoptosis and favoring cancer cells proliferation and tumor mass expansion [52]. Moreover, it has been reported an important decrease of p53 in mouse embryonic fibroblasts and HCT116 cells carrying IDH1-R132Q/R132H mutations: the high levels of 2-HG stabilize HIF-2α, which activates the transcription of miR-380-5p. The latter triggers the degradation of p53 mRNA, favoring cell proliferation and tumorigenesis [30]. In agreement, the levels of p53 are negatively correlated with IDH1-R132H levels in human gliomas [30], supporting at clinical levels the molecular mechanism dependent on the 2-HG/HIF-2α/miR-380-5p axis described in vitro. A p53-independent mechanism by which 2-HG prevents apoptosis has been documented in AML cells engineered to express mutant IDH1-R132H, where 2-HG accumulates and inhibits the cytochrome c oxidase complex of the ETC. This metabolic shut down increases the activation of the anti-apoptotic BCL2 protein, promoting tumor growth and progression [33,53], likely by reducing mtROS.

A peculiar mechanism that links the production of TCA-derived oncometabolites to oncogenesis and tumor progression is proteins succinylation, a post-translational modification in which succinyl group is added to a lysine residue. After the attachment of succinate, the positive charge of lysine is negatively charged, leading to important changes in protein structure and function. Although hyper-succinylated proteins have been already associated with the tumors with SDH, FH and IDH deficiency, the impact of this post-translational modification in cancer cells is still matter of investigation [54]. The best studied protein regulated by succinylation is Kelch-like ECH-associated protein 1 (KEAP1), the endogenous inhibitor of the redox-sensitive transcription factor Nuclear Factor, Erythroid 2 Like 2 (NRF2). KEAP1 succinylation prevents its binding to NRF2, activating the NFR2-mediated transcriptional program, including several genes involved in the antioxidant response [55]. Interestingly, the hyper-succinylation of several mitochondrial proteins in SDH and IDH deficient cells may alter mitochondrial-dependent apoptosis and metabolism. For instance, hyper-succinylated proteins in mitochondria increase the association of the pro-survival BCL-2 protein to the mitochondrial membrane [56], a condition that confers resistance to apoptosis. An intriguing cross-talk occurs between the three enzymes of TCA cycle producing oncometabolites in glioma with mutated IDH1. Since 2-HG is a structural analogue of succinate and fumarate it may inhibit both SDH and FH, determining the concurrent accumulation of succinate and fumarate, the consequent hyper-succinylation of several proteins and the inhibition of apoptosis. In line with this data, the reduction of succinylation, obtained by overexpressing the desuccinylase SIRT5 in IDH1-R132C-harboring HT1080 cells, decreases BCL-2 accumulation and slows tumor growth [7,56]. Interestingly, protein succinylation and epigenetic changes are two events strictly interconnected in tumors with high levels of mitochondrial oncometabolites. Histones have about 30% lysine targets of succinylation. Notably, histone and chromatin succinylation have been correlated with an increased transcription of the succinylated gene [34], although the detailed mechanisms of how histone and non-histone protein succinylation affects tumorigenesis are still unexplored [19]. The main effects of oncometabolites on cancer biology are summarized in Figure 1.

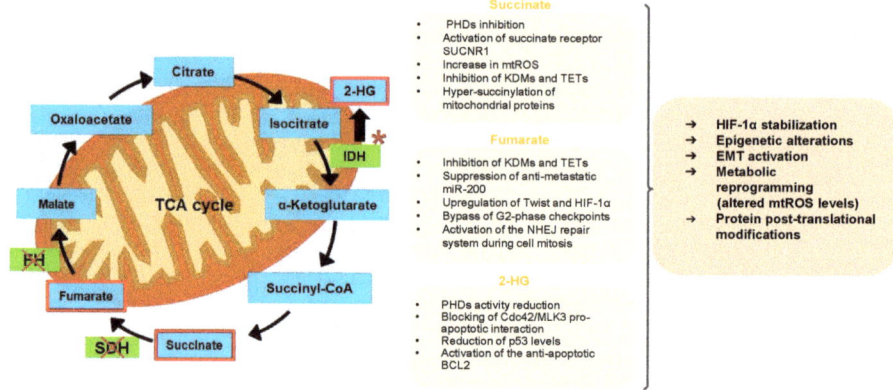

Figure 1. TCA cycle, main oncometabolites and effects on cancer biology. An altered tricarboxylic acid (TCA) cycle due to gain-of-function mutations (*) in isocitrate dehydrogenase (IDH) and loss-of-function mutations (X) in succinate dehydrogenase (SDH) and fumarate hydratase (FH), produces high levels of 2-hydroxyglutarate (2-HG), succinate and fumarate, respectively, that act as oncometabolites by pleiotropic mechanisms. PHDs: prolyl-hydroxylases; SUCNR1: succinate receptor 1; mtROS: mitochondrial reactive oxygen species; KDMs: histone lysine demethylases; TET: ten-eleven translocation proteins; HIF-1α: hypoxia-induced transcriptional factor; NHEJ: non-homologous end-joining; Cdc42: cell division control protein 42; MLK3: mixed lineage kinase 3; BCL2: B-cell lymphoma 2; EMT: epithelial mesenchymal transition.

3. Mitochondrial Oncometabolites and Drug Resistance

The first indirect indication linking mitochondria-derived oncometabolites and drug resistance is that tumors producing high amounts of oncometabolites are characterized by highly aggressive phenotype and poor prognosis. Indeed, SDH deficiency is found in about 5–10% of gastrointestinal stromal tumors, which affect younger patients, are resistant to tyrosine kinase inhibitors and have a higher recurrence rate after surgical resection [14]. A similar phenotype characterizes extra-adrenal paragangliomas with by SHD mutations that have early onset, high aggressiveness and poor prognosis [57]. A poor survival has also been observed in patients affected by KIRP with FH deficiency, where FH levels are positively correlated with overall survival. The poor prognosis in FH deficient tumors is explained by the down-regulation of the anti-metastatic miR-200a and miR-200b, and by the activation of the EMT program [46,48]. In line with these data, the analysis of kidney renal clear cell carcinoma (KIRC) TCGA database, showed that the levels of FH mRNA and protein negatively correlate with vimentin, positively correlate with E-cadherin and patients' survival, confirming the role of FH loss in tumor malignancy and patient poor outcome [46]. Moreover, fumarate accumulation is linked with endometrial cancer aggressiveness, via adenylosuccinate lyase (ADSL) and killer cell lectin-like receptor C3 (KLRC3): the knock-down of ADSL decreases KLRC3 that in turn reduces cell proliferation, migration and invasion. Fumarate recovers KLRC3 expression in ADSL-knocked down cells, counteracting these anti-tumor effects and contributing to cancer aggressiveness [28]. Accordingly, in GBM, a tumor where oncometabolites are often increased, the fumarate-dependent increase of KLRC3 has been correlated with radio-resistance and poor outcome [58]. FH deficiency also protects cancer cells from drugs targeting mitochondrial ETC and causing a metabolic catastrophe, as demonstrated in

FH-deficient UOK262 cells treated with ONC201 [59], an anti-GBM agent that decreases OXPHOS-mediated production of ATP [60].

In contrast with the finding suggesting that fumarate facilitates tumor aggressiveness and resistance, in HeLa cells the increase of fumarate and malate chemosensitizes to cisplatin, as demonstrated by slower cell proliferation and reduced tumor size in mice. However, in this work the increase of fumarate seemed a consequence of the decreased level of adenylate kinase 4, a key enzyme in regulating the high-energy phosphoryl transfer reactions, rather than a deficiency of FH [61]. This discrepancy leads to hypothesize that a TCA-independent increase of fumarate may have opposite effects than a TCA-dependent increase in terms of chemotherapy efficacy.

Succinate is linked to chemoresistance because it stabilizes HIF-1α, a transcription factor with a known role in drug resistance. First, as a consequence of the metabolic shift toward a more glycolytic and acidic TME, HIF-1α inactivates weak bases chemotherapeutic agents as anthracyclines. Moreover, it stimulates angiogenesis and EMT program, and increases several drug efflux transporters, such as P-glycoprotein, multidrug resistance-related protein 1 (MRP1) and breast cancer resistance protein [35]. Considering the plethora of chemotherapeutic drugs effluxed by these transporters, tumors with high levels of HIF-1α stabilized by succinate are characterized by a multidrug resistant phenotype. Lastly, the hyper-succinylation increases also NRF2 that protects tumors from the chemotherapy-induced oxidative damages by upregulating anti-oxidant enzymes, drug-inactivating enzymes and MRP1 [62].

IDH1/IDH2-mutated tumors are also resistant to a plethora of drugs. One of the most promising drugs for the treatment of refractory or relapsed AML is enasidenib/AG-221, a IDH2 inhibitor [60]. However, two mutations of IDH2 in the wild-type allele, specifically Q316E and I319M, induce resistance to enasidenib because they alter the binding site between the drug and the IDH2 dimer. The presence of these mutations in trans with the R140Q gain-of-function mutation on the second allele further enhances the resistance to enasidenib [63]. Some cases of resistance to IDH-targeting therapies, such as enasidenib/AG-221 for IDH2 or ivosidenib/AG-120 for IDH1, are caused by an isoform switch induced by the treatment that shifts the prevailing isoform between the cytoplasmic mutant IDH1 and the mitochondrial mutant IDH2. This switch has been reported in a four-case study, and in chondrosarcoma cells harboring the double mutations IDH1-R132G/IDH2-R172V and IDH1-R132H/IDH2-R172S. In these situations, the selective pressure caused by the treatment with a single IDH inhibitor confers a growth advantage to the subclones with prevalent activity of the IDH isoform not inhibited by the treatment [64]. This process is at the basis of the acquired resistance towards IDH-inhibitors and is common particularly in hematological cancers, where IDH1 and IDH2 mutations often co-exist. The use of the combined IDH1 and IDH2 inhibitors may likely prevent the onset of resistance due to the IDH isoform switch. However, this approach has the risks of undesired toxicity and unexpected drug-drug interaction.

IDH mutations confer the resistance also to other anti-cancer agents different from IDH inhibitors. In solid tumors like GBM, IDH1 mutations prevail and confer not only drug resistance but also radioresistance, because of the increased activity of DDR systems and the high activity of de novo and salvage pathways of nucleotide synthesis [65]. GBM cells carrying the R132H-IDH1 are specifically resistant to histone deacetylase inhibitors (HDACi), such as trichostatin A, vorinostat and valproic acid as a consequence of the 2-HG-induced transcriptional increase of NANOG [66], a key regulator of stemness and self-renewal properties of cancer cells. Mechanisms oncometabolites mediated drug resistance are summarized in Figure 2.

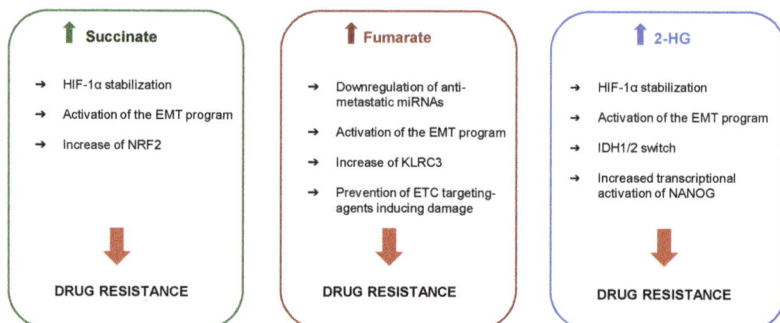

Figure 2. Effects of oncometabolites in drug resistance. The accumulation of oncometabolites such as succinate, fumarate and 2-hydroxyglutarate (2-HG) activates different mechanisms leading to drug resistance such as stabilization of hypoxia inducible factor-1α (HIF-1α), downregulation of anti-metastatic and oncosuppressor miRNAs, induction of epithelial-mesenchymal transition (EMT), overexpression of nuclear factor erythroid 2-related factor 2 (NRF2) and of the killer cell lectin like receptor C3 (KLRC3), prevention of the damages elicited by electron transport chain (ETC)-targeting agents, switch between isocitrate dehydrogenase (IDH) 1 and 2, activation of the stemness regulator NANOG.

4. Pharmacological Approaches to Reduce Mitochondrial Oncometabolites

On the one hand the metabolic re-arrangements of cancer cells with over-production of TCA-derived oncometabolites increase tumor aggressiveness; on the other hand, these tumors expose some metabolic vulnerabilities, offering new therapeutic opportunities to eradicate the cells over-producing oncometabolites (Table 1; Figure 3).

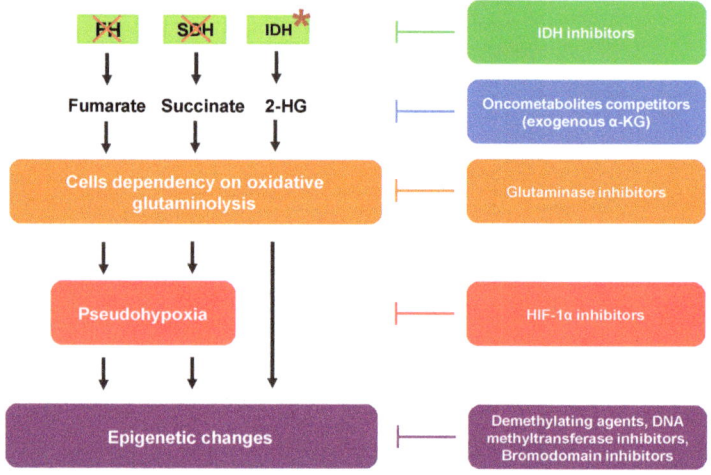

Figure 3. Overview of the main pharmacological strategies to prevent the synthesis and the effects of oncometabolites. Different pharmacological strategies are currently being investigated to counteract the action of oncometabolites. Some of them target the enzyme that produces the oncometabolites, as isocitrate dehydrogenase (IDH) inhibitors, while others target the downstream effects of oncometabolites, such as glutaminolysis, pseudohypoxia or epigenetic changes. Differently, other approaches aim at competing with the oncometabolites themselves, such as the administration of exogenous α-ketoglutarate (α-KG). (*) Gain-of-function mutations in isocitrate dehydrogenase (IDH); (X) loss-of-function mutations in succinate dehydrogenase (SDH) and fumarate hydratase (FH).

Since succinate and fumarate accumulation mainly derive from loss-of-function mutations in SDH and FH, a genetic correction reintroducing the deficient gene is still challenging and poorly feasible. Most attempts to counteract succinate and fumarate accumulation target the downstream pathways activated by these oncometabolites. Indeed, as shown in SDHB knocked-out cells, cells with deficient SDH become extremely dependent on the oxidative glutaminolysis to meet their energy requirement. Therein, they are selectively killed by the glutaminase 1 inhibitors compound 968 and CB-839 [37]. Similarly, also the bromodomain proteins inhibitor JQ1 displays a high selectivity against SDH deficient cells, because it down-regulates c-Myc which transcriptionally enhances glutaminolysis enzymes [37]. Targeting glutaminolysis or its controllers is therefore an effective strategy to eradicate succinate hyper-producing cells. Succinate accumulation caused by SDH deficiency inhibits pyruvate dehydrogenase and stabilizes HIF-1α, but these effects are counteracted by exogenous αKG. The latter appeared indeed an effective antitumor and antiangiogenic compound in SHD-deficient tumors [67–69]. Moreover, since HIF-1α is activated by succinate, the use of HIF-1α inhibitors has been proposed as an alternative and effective strategy to block the tumor progression driven by succinate [36]. The major limitations to the use of HIF-1α inhibitors in patients are the high side-effect toxicity, due to the inhibition of the physiological functions of HIF-1α, and the limited anti-tumor efficacy, likely because several downstream effectors of HIF-1α become independent drivers of oncogenesis and progression (https://clinicaltrials.gov/ct2/results/details?cond=Cancer&term=HIF), accessed on April 2021.

Differently from succinate and fumarate, the accumulation of 2-HG may be overcome by the inhibition of mutated IDH. The first drug introduced against IDH mutated AML, venetoclax, was not a direct inhibitor of IDH, but it inhibited the anti-apoptotic protein BCL-2, which is increased by 2-HG [33,53]. After venetoclax, several direct inhibitors of IDH have been tested in clinical trials to antagonize 2-HG, but only two of them—enasidenib/AG-221 and ivosidenib/AG-120—have been approved for the treatment of refractory AML [70]. Enasidenib is a small molecule inhibiting mutant IDH2, which is overexpressed in hematological cancers: it has high selectivity, good solubility and oral bioavailability [33]. Ivosidenib, also characterized by good oral bioavailability, shows a preferential inhibition on IDH1 and is evaluated for solid tumors including GBM [33]. Since in some cases the tumors display the shift between IDH1 and IDH2 mutant isoforms, making isoform-selective inhibitors progressively ineffective [64], dual IDH1/IDH2 inhibitors are under evaluation. One of the most promising dual inhibitors is vorasidenib, and has been proposed for the treatment of GBM since it is able to cross the blood brain barrier [71]. Importantly, the response to IDH inhibitors is affected by the type of mutations [72]. Indeed, it has been demonstrated that R132Q mutation alters the catalytic site structure in such a way that the IDH1 inhibitors ML309, AGI-5198 and GSK864 are less potent. By contrast they are instead more active against R132H-IDH1 or wild-type IDH1 expressing cells [72]. This aspect must be carefully considered in choosing the right inhibitor for the right mutant tumor.

Besides specific inhibitors, several miRNA-targeting agents are also considered since it has been clearly demonstrated that miR-181a had inhibitory effect on IDH1 and miR-183 on IDH2 [73,74]. However, despite the promising results obtained in vitro and in preclinical models, miRNA technology is still problematic in clinical use. Therefore, its efficacy in targeting IDH1/IDH2 activated tumors must be re-evaluated when technical issues concerning delivery, stability and specificity will be overcome.

Table 1. Main pharmacological approaches counteracting oncometabolites effects on cancer progression and drug resistance.

Targeted Oncometabolite	Mutated Gene	Drugs
Succinate	SDH	Compound 968 and CB-839 [37]
		JQ1 [37]
Fumarate	FH	Exogenous αKG [67–69]
		HIF-1α inhibitors [36]
		Venetoclax [33,53].
		Enasidenib/AG-221 [33,70]
		Ivosidenib/AG-120 [33,64] Vorasidenib [71]
		ML309 [72]
2-HG	IDH	AGI-5198 [72]
		GSK864 [72]
		Azacytidine [75,76]
		Decitabine [75,76]
		Temozolomide [77,78]

2-HG: 2-hydroxyglutarate; SDH: succinate dehydrogenase; FH: fumarate dehydratase; IDH: isocitrate dehydrogenase; αKG: α-ketoglutarate; HIF-1α: hypoxia-induced transcriptional factor.

Notably, IDH mutant tumors are characterized by hyper-methylation of DNA, as a result of the epigenetic changes induced by TCA-derived oncometabolites [12]. Hence, some demethylating agents are under investigation in IDH mutated tumors. For instance, the DNA methyltransferase inhibitors azacytidine and decitabine have showed clinical benefits in AML, including IDH mutated leukemias [75,76]. Interestingly, IDH1 and IDH2 mutated GBM, SDHB deficient pheochromocytoma and paraganglioma are more sensitive to temozolomide (TMZ), and IDH1/2 mutations are con-sidered a good prognostic factor. This is likely explained by the hypermethylation of the O6-methylguanine DNA methyltransferase promoter, one of the key antagonists of TMZ activity, in mutated tumors [77,78]. Consistently, the exposure of GBM cells to exogenous 2-HG slows down tumor progression and has a synergistic effect with chemotherapeutic agents inhibiting DNA demethylation, such as azacytidine and decitabine, or inducing DNA damage as daunorubicin [79]. This example shows that oncometabolites cannot be considered entirely under a negative light, because high levels of 2-HG may exert anti-tumor and chemosensitizing effects in IDH1/IDH2 mutated GBM.

It remains to be clarified, however, which factor between the level of oncometabolites or the oncogenic/oncosuppressor pathways altered by mutated TCA enzymes play the most prominent role in chemosensization or chemoresistance.

5. Conclusions

The involvement of mitochondria metabolism in cancer growth, progression and drug resistance has been established since a long time. However, many processes related to mitochondrial metabolic reprogramming and linked to drug resistance still need to be explored in depth. Among them, great attention has been recently paid to the mechanisms underlying aggressiveness and drug resistance associated with defects of SDH and FH, and hyper-activating mutations of IDH, all leading to the accumulation of mitochondrial oncometabolites. The generation of a pseudohypoxic phenotype, the epigenetic changes and the post-translational modification in specific proteins induced by the oncometabolites have been regarded as the main mechanism promoting cancer progression. The mechanisms behind the drug resistance displayed by tumors with high levels of succinate, fumarate and 2-HG are in part similar. For instance, oncometabolite-induced resistance often relies on the oncometabolite-driven activation of HIF1-α and EMT programs. Oncometabolites also specifically modulate oncogenic and/or oncosuppressor pathways, determining a complex crosstalk between different genetic alterations co-existing in the same tumors, contributing to aggressiveness and resistance.

To slow down tumor progression and improve drugs sensitivity, different therapeutic strategies targeting the mitochondria-derived oncometabolites have been experimented, and some of them reached phase I/II clinical trials. This is the situation of tumors with IDH1/IDH2 mutations that can be treated with small molecules acting as selective inhibitors, with good success in AML and GBM. Since the defects related to SDH and FH are prevalently due to loss of function, the direct targeting of these enzyme with specific activators or with genetic engineering is more difficult. A better strategy, although indirect, is interfering with the pathways activated by succinate and fumarate. Inhibitors of EMT program, which is downstream of all three TCA-derived oncometabolites—may be another approach limiting tumor aggressiveness, invasion and chemoresistance. In this perspective, epigenetic drugs such as demethylating agents and DNA methyltransferase inhibitors that have been demonstrated to block EMT program [80] are of particular interest. Indeed, IDH1 mutants GBM are resistant to HDACi [66]. The combination of the IDH1 inhibitors ivosidenib/AG-120 associated with other epigenetic drugs such as decitabine or azacytabine, may open new therapeutic possibilities for aggressive and chemorefractory tumors producing oncometabolites.

Another intriguing point is understanding the possible cross-talk between each oncometabolite produced within the tumor cell. If defective SDH and FH lead to the accumulation of succinate and fumarate, this derangement of TCA flux can slow down the upstream steps of the cycle. The accumulation of citrate and isocitrate may favor the generation of 2-HG, thus generating tumors with all three oncometabolites increased. Conversely, a hyperactive/mutated IDH subtracts α-KG from the TCA cycle, and this diversion can indirectly reduce the rate of downstream enzymes, thus limiting the production of succinate and fumarate in tumors with wild-type SDH and FH. Of course, the presence of defective forms of SDH and FH produces the accumulation of fumarate and succinate also in case of mutated IDH. Different combination strategies, depending on the relative amounts of 2-HG, fumarate and succinate, and on the activity of their downstream effectors, should be adopted in order to maximize the efficacy of anti-oncometabolite agents.

Since several genetic lesions within a tumor may co-exist, an in-depth genomic profiling of the TCA cycle genes may help identifying the TCA cycle genotypic profile and the best choice of treatment. The presence of different clones within the same tumors, harboring different mutations, further complicates the situation, because different areas within the tumor bulk may behave metabolically differently. To partially circumvent this issue, the coupling of high-throughput metabolomic analysis and high-resolution imaging analysis by MALDI-imaging techniques can map the intratumor areas with different levels of TCA cycle metabolism and identify the most prominent metabolic phenotype within the tumor mass. The simultaneous advancement in diagnostic techniques and oncometabolite-targeting agents will help the development of an "oncometabolite-based precision medicine" in the next future.

Indeed, despite the limited number of drugs targeting the mitochondria-derived oncometabolites currently available, the research in this field can open very interesting therapeutic opportunities. First tumors with mutations in TCA offer the possibility of targeting either the TCA cycle mutated enzymes or the downstream pathways controlled by the oncometabolite, leading the way to different combination therapies that can be exploited with anti-tumor, anti-metastatic or chemosensitizer purpose. Second, it is noteworthy that the agents targeting the production of mitochondrial derived oncometabolite are rather tumor-selective, because they hit isoforms of the TCA cycle enzymes detected in tumors, but not in non-transformed cells. Therefore, the pharmacological development of these drugs is particularly attractive, because it may lead to the realization of the first "metabolic targeted therapy" in the oncological field, conceived as a multi-target therapy peculiarly effective against tumors resistant to conventional treatments.

Author Contributions: Conceptualization, J.K. and C.R.; writing—original draft preparation D.P.A., M.G., G.O., M.P., G.R.; writing—review and editing, M.G., J.K. and C.R.; supervision, J.K. and C.R. All authors have read and agreed to the published version of the manuscript.

Funding: This research was funded by Associazione Italiana per la Ricerca sul Cancro (AIRC; grant IG21408).

Institutional Review Board Statement: Not applicable.

Informed Consent Statement: Not applicable.

Data Availability Statement: The data presented in this study are openly available in https://clinicaltrials.gov/ct2/results/details?cond=Cancer&term=HIF).

Conflicts of Interest: The authors declare no conflict of interest.

References

1. Zheng, H.C. The molecular mechanisms of chemoresistance in cancers. *Oncotarget* **2017**, *8*, 59950–59964. [CrossRef] [PubMed]
2. Bokil, A.; Sancho, P. Mitochondrial determinants of chemoresistance. *Cancer Drug Resist.* **2019**, 634–646. [CrossRef]
3. Potter, M.; Newport, E.; Morten, K.J. The Warburg effect: 80 years on. *Biochem. Soc. Trans.* **2016**, *44*, 1499–1505. [CrossRef]
4. Hirpara, J.; Eu, J.Q.; Tan, J.K.M.; Wong, A.L.; Clement, M.V.; Kong, L.R.; Ohi, N.; Tsunoda, T.; Qu, J.; Goh, B.C.; et al. Metabolic reprogramming of oncogene-addicted cancer cells to OXPHOS as a mechanism of drug resistance. *Redox Biol.* **2019**, *25*, 101076. [CrossRef]
5. Vyas, S.; Zaganjor, E.; Haigis, M.C. Mitochondria and cancer. *Cell* **2016**, *166*, 555–566. [CrossRef] [PubMed]
6. Woolbright, B.L.; Choudhary, D.; Mikhalyuk, A.; Trammel, C.; Shanmugam, S.; Abbott, E.; Pilbeam, C.C.; Taylor, J.A. The role of pyruvate dehydrogenase kinase-4 (PDK4) in bladder cancer and chemoresistance. *Mol. Cancer Ther.* **2018**, *17*, 2004–2012. [CrossRef] [PubMed]
7. Li, L.; Yu, A.Q. The functional role of peroxiredoxin 3 in reactive oxygen species, apoptosis, and chemoresistance of cancer cells. *J. Cancer Res. Clin. Oncol.* **2015**, *141*, 2071–2077. [CrossRef]
8. Alexa-Stratulat, T.; Pešić, M.; Gašparović, A.Č.; Trougakos, I.P.; Riganti, C. What sustains the multidrug resistance phenotype beyond ABC efflux transporters? Looking beyond the tip of the iceberg. *Drug Resist. Updat.* **2019**, *46*. [CrossRef]
9. Kapoor, I.; Bodo, J.; Hill, B.T.; Hsi, E.D.; Almasan, A. Targeting BCL-2 in B-cell malignancies and overcoming therapeutic resistance. *Cell Death Dis.* **2020**, *11*. [CrossRef]
10. Van Gisbergen, M.W.; Voets, A.M.; Starmans, M.H.; De Coo, I.F.; Yadak, R.; Hoffmann, R.F.; Boutros, P.C.; Smeets, H.J.; Dubois, L.; Lambin, P. How do changes in the mtDNA and mitochondrial dysfunction influence cancer and cancer therapy? Challenges, opportunities and models. *Mutat. Res. Rev. Mutat. Res.* **2015**, *764*, 16–30. [CrossRef]
11. Aminuddin, A.; Ng, P.Y.; Leong, C.O.; Chua, E.W. Mitochondrial DNA alterations may influence the cisplatin responsiveness of oral squamous cell carcinoma. *Sci. Rep.* **2020**, *10*, 1–17. [CrossRef] [PubMed]
12. Dando, I.; Pozza, E.D.; Ambrosini, G.; Torrens-Mas, M.; Butera, G.; Mullappilly, N.; Pacchiana, R.; Palmieri, M.; Donadelli, M. Oncometabolites in cancer aggressiveness and tumour repopulation. *Biol. Rev. Camb. Philos. Soc.* **2019**, *94*, 1530–1546. [CrossRef] [PubMed]
13. Aldera, A.P.; Govender, D. Gene of the month: SDH. *J. Clin. Pathol.* **2018**, *71*, 95–97. [CrossRef]
14. Neppala, P.; Banerjee, S.; Fanta, P.T.; Yerba, M.; Porras, K.A.; Burgoyne, A.M.; Sicklick, J.K. Current management of succinate dehydrogenase–deficient gastrointestinal stromal tumors. *Cancer Metastasis Rev.* **2019**, *38*, 525–535. [CrossRef] [PubMed]
15. Sciacovelli, M.; Guzzo, G.; Morello, V.; Frezza, C.; Zheng, L.; Nannini, N.; Calabrese, F.; Laudiero, G.; Esposito, F.; Landriscina, M.; et al. The mitochondrial chaperone TRAP1 promotes neoplastic growth by inhibiting succinate dehydrogenase. *Cell Metab.* **2013**, *17*, 988–999. [CrossRef]
16. Yu, H.E.; Wang, F.; Yu, F.; Zeng, Z.L.; Wang, Y.; Lu, Y.X.; Jin, Y.; Wang, D.S.; Qiu, M.Z.; Pu, H.Y.; et al. Suppression of fumarate hydratase activity increases the efficacy of cisplatin-mediated chemotherapy in gastric cancer. *Cell Death Dis.* **2019**, *10*. [CrossRef]
17. Dalla Pozza, E.; Dando, I.; Pacchiana, R.; Liboi, E.; Scupoli, M.T.; Donadelli, M.; Palmieri, M. Regulation of succinate dehydrogenase and role of succinate in cancer. *Semin. Cell Dev. Biol.* **2020**, *9*, 4–14. [CrossRef]
18. Hoekstra, A.S.; Bayley, J.P. The role of complex II in disease. *Biochim. Biophys. Acta Bioenerg.* **2013**, *1827*, 543–551. [CrossRef]
19. Zhao, Y.; Feng, F.; Guo, Q.H.; Wang, Y.P.; Zhao, R. Role of succinate dehydrogenase deficiency and oncometabolites in gastrointestinal stromal tumors. *World J. Gastroenterol.* **2020**, *26*, 5074–5089. [CrossRef]
20. Wang, H.; Chen, Y.; Wu, G. SDHB deficiency promotes TGFβ-mediated invasion and metastasis of colorectal cancer through transcriptional repression complex SNAIL1-SMAD3/4. *Transl. Oncol.* **2016**, *9*, 512–520. [CrossRef]
21. Hsu, C.C.; Tseng, L.M.; Lee, H.C. Role of mitochondrial dysfunction in cancer progression. *Exp. Biol. Med.* **2016**, *241*, 1281–1295. [CrossRef] [PubMed]
22. Schmidt, C.; Sciacovelli, M.; Frezza, C. Fumarate hydratase in cancer: A multifaceted tumour suppressor. *Semin. Cell Dev. Biol.* **2020**, *98*, 15–25. [CrossRef] [PubMed]
23. Tomlinson, I.P.M.; Alam, N.A.; Rowan, A.J.; Barclay, E.; Jaeger, E.E.M.; Kelsell, D.; Leigh, I.; Gorman, P.; Lamlum, H.; Rahman, S.; et al. Germline mutations in FH predispose to dominantly inherited uterine fibroids, skin leiomyomata and papillary renal cell cancer the multiple leiomyoma consortium. *Nat. Genet.* **2002**, *30*, 406–410. [CrossRef] [PubMed]
24. Schmidt, L.S.; Linehan, W.M. Hereditary leiomyomatosis and renal cell carcinoma. *Int. J. Nephrol. Renov. Dis.* **2014**, *7*, 253–260. [CrossRef] [PubMed]

25. Castro-Vega, L.J.; Buffet, A.; De Cubas, A.A.; Cascón, A.; Menara, M.; Khalifa, E.; Amar, L.; Azriel, S.; Bourdeau, I.; Chabre, O.; et al. Germline mutations in FH confer predisposition to malignant pheochromocytomas and paragangliomas. *Hum. Mol. Genet.* **2014**, *23*, 2440–2446. [CrossRef]
26. Laukka, T.; Mariani, C.J.; Ihantola, T.; Cao, J.Z.; Hokkanen, J.; Kaelin, W.G.; Godley, L.A.; Koivunen, P. Fumarate and succinate regulate expression of hypoxia-inducible genes via TET enzymes. *J. Biol. Chem.* **2016**, *291*, 4256–4265. [CrossRef]
27. Martinez-Mir, A.; Glaser, B.; Chuang, G.S.; Horev, L.; Waldman, A.; Engler, D.E.; Gordon, D.; Spelman, L.J.; Hatzibougias, I.; Green, J.; et al. Germline fumarate hydratase mutations in families with multiple cutaneous and uterine leiomyomata. *J. Invest. Dermatol.* **2003**, *121*, 741–744. [CrossRef]
28. Park, H.; Ohshima, K.; Nojima, S.; Tahara, S.; Kurashige, M.; Hori, Y.; Okuzaki, D.; Wada, N.; Ikeda, J.I.; Morii, E. Adenylosuccinate lyase enhances aggressiveness of endometrial cancer by increasing killer cell lectin-like receptor C3 expression by fumarate. *Lab. Investig.* **2018**, *98*, 449–461. [CrossRef]
29. He, X.; Yan, B.; Liu, S.; Jia, J.; Lai, W.; Xin, X.; Tang, C.E.; Luo, D.; Tan, T.; Jiang, Y.; et al. Chromatin remodeling factor LSH drives cancer progression by suppressing the activity of fumarate hydratase. *Cancer Res.* **2016**, *76*, 5743–5755. [CrossRef]
30. Jiang, B.; Zhao, W.; Shi, M.; Zhang, J.; Chen, A.; Ma, H.; Suleman, M.; Lin, F.; Zhou, L.; Wang, J.; et al. IDH1 Arg-132 mutant promotes tumor formation through down-regulating P53. *J. Biol. Chem.* **2018**, *293*, 9747–9758. [CrossRef]
31. Ježek, P. 2-Hydroxyglutarate in cancer cells. *Antioxid. Redox Signal.* **2020**, *33*, 903–926. [CrossRef]
32. Tinoco, G.; Wilky, B.A.; Paz-Mejia, A.; Rosenberg, A.; Trent, J.C. The biology and management of cartilaginous tumors: A role for targeting isocitrate dehydrogenase. *Am. Soc. Clin. Oncol. Educ. Book* **2015**, *35*, e648–e655. [CrossRef]
33. Amaya, M.L.; Pollyea, D.A. Targeting the IDH2 pathway in acute myeloid leukemia. *Clin. Cancer Res.* **2018**, *24*, 4931–4936. [CrossRef] [PubMed]
34. Smestad, J.; Erber, L.; Chen, Y.; Maher, L.J. Chromatin succinylation correlates with active gene expression and is perturbed by defective TCA cycle metabolism. *Iscience* **2018**, *2*, 63–75. [CrossRef] [PubMed]
35. Belisario, D.C.; Kopecka, J.; Pasino, M.; Akman, M.; Smaele, E.D.; Donadelli, M.; Riganti, C. Hypoxia dictates metabolic rewiring of tumors: Implications for chemoresistance. *Cells* **2020**, *9*, 2598. [CrossRef]
36. Selak, M.A.; Armour, S.M.; MacKenzie, E.D.; Boulahbel, H.; Watson, D.G.; Mansfield, K.D.; Pan, Y.; Simon, M.C.; Thompson, C.B.; Gottlieb, E. Succinate links TCA cycle dysfunction to oncogenesis by inhibiting HIF-α prolyl hydroxylase. *Cancer Cell* **2005**, *7*, 77–85. [CrossRef] [PubMed]
37. Kitazawa, S.; Ebara, S.; Ando, A.; Baba, Y.; Satomi, Y.; Soga, T.; Hara, T. Succinate dehydrogenase B-deficient cancer cells are highly sensitive to bromodomain and extra-terminal inhibitors. *Oncotarget* **2017**, *8*, 28922–28938. [CrossRef] [PubMed]
38. Wu, J.Y.; Huang, T.W.; Hsieh, Y.T.; Wang, Y.F.; Yen, C.C.; Lee, G.L.; Yeh, C.C.; Peng, Y.J.; Kuo, Y.Y.; Wen, H.T.; et al. Cancer-derived succinate promotes macrophage polarization and cancer metastasis via succinate receptor. *Mol. Cell* **2020**, *77*, 213–227.e5. [CrossRef] [PubMed]
39. Ristic, B.; Bhutia, Y.; Ganapathy, V. Cell-surface G-protein-coupled receptors for tumor-associated metabolites: A direct link to mitochondrial dysfunction in cancer. *Biochim. Biophys. Acta* **2017**, *1868*, 246–257. [CrossRef] [PubMed]
40. Mills, E.L.; Kelly, B.; Logan, A.; Costa, A.S.H.; Varma, M.; Bryant, C.E.; Tourlomousis, P.; Däbritz, J.H.M.; Gottlieb, E.; Latorre, I.; et al. Succinate dehydrogenase supports metabolic repurposing of mitochondria to drive inflammatory macrophages. *Cell* **2016**, *167*, 457–470.e13. [CrossRef] [PubMed]
41. Sena, L.A.; Chandel, N.S. Physiological roles of mitochondrial reactive oxygen species. *Mol. Cell* **2012**, *48*, 158–167. [CrossRef] [PubMed]
42. Ratcliffe, P.J. Oxygen sensing and hypoxia signalling pathways in animals: The implications of physiology for cancer. *J. Physiol.* **2013**, *591*, 2027–2042. [CrossRef]
43. Aggarwal, R.K.; Zou, Y.; Luchtel, R.A.; Pradhan, K.; Ashai, N.; Ramachandra, N.; Albanese, J.M.; Yang, J.-I.; Wang, X.; Aluri, S.; et al. Functional succinate dehydrogenase deficiency is a pathognomonic adverse feature of clear cell renal cancer. *bioRxiv* **2020**. [CrossRef]
44. Cervera, A.M.; Bayley, J.P.; Devilee, P.; McCreath, K.J. Inhibition of succinate dehydrogenase dysregulates histone modification in mammalian cells. *Mol. Cancer* **2009**, *8*, 89. [CrossRef] [PubMed]
45. Loriot, C.; Domingues, M.; Berger, A.; Menara, M.; Ruel, M.; Morin, A.; Castro-Vega, L.J.; Letouzé, É.; Martinelli, C.; Bemelmans, A.P.; et al. Deciphering the molecular basis of invasiveness in sdhbdeficient cells. *Oncotarget* **2015**, *6*, 32955–32965. [CrossRef] [PubMed]
46. Sciacovelli, M.; Frezza, C. Metabolic reprogramming and epithelial-to-mesenchymal transition in cancer. *FEBS J.* **2017**, *284*, 3132–3144. [CrossRef]
47. Johnson, T.I.; Costa, A.S.H.; Ferguson, A.N.; Frezza, C. Fumarate hydratase loss promotes mitotic entry in the presence of DNA damage after ionising radiation. *Cell Death Dis.* **2018**, *9*. [CrossRef] [PubMed]
48. Wentzel, J.F.; Lewies, A.; Bronkhorst, A.J.; Van Dyk, E.; Du Plessis, L.H.; Pretorius, P.J. Exposure to high levels of fumarate and succinate leads to apoptotic cytotoxicity and altered global DNA methylation profiles in vitro. *Biochimie* **2017**, *135*, 28–34. [CrossRef] [PubMed]
49. Ricciardiello, F.; Gang, Y.; Palorini, R.; Li, Q.; Giampà, M.; Zhao, F.; You, L.; La Ferla, B.; De Vitto, H.; Guan, W.; et al. Hexosamine pathway inhibition overcomes pancreatic cancer resistance to gemcitabine through unfolded protein response and EGFR-Akt pathway modulation. *Oncogene* **2020**, *39*, 4103–4117. [CrossRef]

50. Wang, T.; Yu, Q.; Li, J.; Hu, B.; Zhao, Q.; Ma, C.; Huang, W.; Zhuo, L.; Fang, H.; Liao, L.; et al. O-GlcNAcylation of fumarase maintains tumour growth under glucose deficiency. *Nat. Cell Biol.* **2017**, *19*, 833–843. [CrossRef]
51. Chen, T.; Wang, T.; Liang, W.; Zhao, Q.; Yu, Q.; Ma, C.M.; Zhuo, L.; Guo, D.; Zheng, K.; Zhou, C.; et al. PAK4 phosphorylates fumarase and blocks TGFβ-induced cell growth arrest in lung cancer cells. *Cancer Res.* **2019**, *79*, 1383–1397. [CrossRef]
52. Jiang, B.; Zhang, J.; Xia, J.; Zhao, W.; Wu, Y.; Shi, M.; Luo, L.; Zhou, H.; Chen, A.; Ma, H.; et al. IDH1 mutation promotes tumorigenesis by inhibiting JNK activation and apoptosis induced by serum starvation. *Cell Rep.* **2017**, *19*, 389–400. [CrossRef] [PubMed]
53. Chan, M.S.; Daniel, T.; Corces-Zimmerman, M.R.; Xavy, S.; Rastogi, S.; Hong, W.-J.; Zhao, F.; Medeiros, B.C.; Tyvoll, D.A.; Majeti, R. Isocitrate dehydrogenase 1 and 2 mutations induce BCL-2 dependence in acute myeloid leukemia. *Nat. Med.* **2015**, *21*, 178–184. [CrossRef] [PubMed]
54. Sreedhar, A.; Wiese, E.K.; Hitosugi, T. Enzymatic and metabolic regulation of lysine succinylation. *Genes Dis.* **2020**, *7*, 166–171. [CrossRef]
55. Kinch, L.; Grishin, N.V.; Brugarolas, J. Succination of keap1 and activation of Nrf2-dependent antioxidant pathways in FH-deficient papillary renal cell carcinoma type 2. *Cancer Cell* **2011**, *20*, 418–420. [CrossRef] [PubMed]
56. Li, F.; He, X.; Ye, D.; Lin, Y.; Yu, H.; Yao, C.; Huang, L.; Zhang, J.; Wang, F.; Xu, S.; et al. NADP(+)-IDH mutations promote hypersuccinylation that impairs mitochondria respiration and induces apoptosis resistance. *Mol. Cell* **2015**, *60*, 661–675. [CrossRef]
57. Timmers, H.J.; Gimenez-Roqueplo, A.P.; Mannelli, M.; Pacak, K. Clinical aspects of SDHx-related pheochromocytoma and paraganglioma. *Endocr. Relat. Cancer* **2009**, *16*, 391–400. [CrossRef] [PubMed]
58. Cheray, M.; Bessette, B.; Lacroix, A.; Mélin, C.; Jawhari, S.; Pinet, S.; Deluche, E.; Clavère, P.; Durand, K.; Sanchez-Prieto, R.; et al. KLRC3, a natural killer receptor gene, is a key factor involved in glioblastoma tumourigenesis and aggressiveness. *J. Cell Mol. Med.* **2017**, *21*, 244–253. [CrossRef] [PubMed]
59. Greer, Y.E.; Porat-Shliom, N.; Nagashima, K.; Stuelten, C.; Crooks, D.; Koparde, V.N.; Gilbert, S.F.; Islam, C.; Ubaldini, A.; Ji, Y.; et al. ONC201 kills breast cancer cells in vitro by targeting mitochondria. *Oncotarget* **2018**, *9*, 18454–18479. [CrossRef]
60. Pruss, M.; Dwucet, A.; Tanriover, M.; Hlavac, M.; Kast, R.E.; Debatin, K.M.; Wirtz, C.R.; Halatsch, M.E.; Siegelin, M.D.; Westhoff, M.A.; et al. Dual metabolic reprogramming by ONC201/TIC10 and 2-deoxyglucose induces energy depletion and synergistic anti-cancer activity in glioblastoma. *Br. J. Cancer* **2020**, *122*, 1146–1157. [CrossRef]
61. Fujisawa, K.; Terai, S.; Takami, T.; Yamamoto, N.; Yamasaki, T.; Matsumoto, T.; Yamaguchi, K.; Owada, Y.; Nishina, H.; Noma, T.; et al. Modulation of anti-cancer drug sensitivity through the regulation of mitochondrial activity by adenylate kinase 4. *J. Exp. Clin. Cancer Res.* **2016**, *35*, 1–15. [CrossRef]
62. Salaroglio, I.C.; Panada, E.; Moiso, E.; Buondonno, I.; Provero, P.; Rubinstein, M.; Kopecka, J.; Riganti, C. PERK induces resistance to cell death elicited by endoplasmic reticulum stress and chemotherapy. *Mol. Cancer* **2017**, *16*, 1–13. [CrossRef] [PubMed]
63. Intlekofer, A.M.; Shih, A.H.; Wang, B.; Nazir, A.; Ariën, S.; Albanese, S.K.; Patel, M.; Famulare, C.; Fabian, N.; Takemoto, N.; et al. Acquired resistance to IDH inhibition through trans or cis dimer-interface mutations. *Nature* **2018**, *559*, 125–129. [CrossRef]
64. Harding, J.J.; Lowery, M.A.; Shih, A.H.; Schvartzman, J.M.; Hou, S.; Famulare, C.; Patel, M.; Roshal, M.; Do, R.K.; Zehir, A.; et al. Isoform switching as a mechanism of acquired resistance to mutant isocitrate dehydrogenase inhibition. *Cancer Discov.* **2018**, *8*, 1540–1546. [CrossRef] [PubMed]
65. Garrett, M.; Sperry, J.; Braas, D.; Yan, W.; Le, T.M.; Mottahedeh, J.; Ludwig, K.; Eskin, A.; Qin, Y.; Levy, R.; et al. Metabolic characterization of isocitrate dehydrogenase (IDH) mutant and IDH wildtype gliomaspheres uncovers cell type-specific vulnerabilities. *Cancer Metab.* **2018**, *6*, 1–15. [CrossRef]
66. Kim, G.H.; Choi, S.Y.; Oh, T.I.; Kan, S.Y.; Kang, H.; Lee, S.; Oh, T.; Ko, H.M.; Lim, J.H. IDH1R132H causes resistance to HDAC inhibitors by increasing NANOG in glioblastoma cells. *Int. J. Mol. Sci.* **2019**, *20*, 2679. [CrossRef]
67. Brière, J.J.; Favier, J.; Bénit, P.; El Ghouzzi, V.; Lorenzato, A.; Rabier, D.; Di Renzo, M.F.; Gimenez-Roqueplo, A.P.; Rustin, P. Mitochondrial succinate is instrumental for HIF1α nuclear translocation in SDHA-mutant fibroblasts under normoxic conditions. *Hum. Mol. Genet.* **2005**, *14*, 3263–3269. [CrossRef]
68. Letouzé, E.; Martinelli, C.; Loriot, C.; Burnichon, N.; Abermil, N.; Ottolenghi, C.; Janin, M.; Menara, M.; Nguyen, A.T.; Benit, P.; et al. SDH mutations establish a hypermethylator phenotype in paraganglioma. *Cancer Cell* **2013**, *23*, 739–752. [CrossRef] [PubMed]
69. Matsumoto, K.; Obara, N.; Ema, M.; Horie, M.; Naka, A.; Takahashi, S.; Imagawa, S. Antitumor effects of 2-Oxoglutarate through inhibition of angiogenesis in a murine tumor model. *Cancer Sci.* **2009**, *100*, 1639–1647. [CrossRef]
70. Golub, D.; Iyengar, N.; Dogra, S.; Wong, T.; Bready, D.; Tang, K.; Modrek, A.S.; Placantonakis, D.G. Mutant isocitrate dehydrogenase inhibitors as targeted cancer therapeutics. *Front. Oncol.* **2019**, *9*. [CrossRef]
71. Konteatis, Z.; Artin, E.; Nicolay, B.; Straley, K.; Padyana, A.K.; Jin, L.; Chen, Y.; Narayaraswamy, R.; Tong, S.; Wang, F.; et al. Vorasidenib (AG-881): A first-in-class, brain-penetrant dual inhibitor of mutant IDH1 and 2 for treatment of glioma. *ACS Med. Chem. Lett.* **2020**, *11*, 101–107. [CrossRef] [PubMed]
72. Matteo, D.A.; Wells, G.; Luna, L.; Grunseth, A.; Zagnitko, O.; Scott, D.; Hoang, A.; Luthra, A.; Swairjo, M.; Schiffer, J.; et al. Inhibitor potency varies widely among tumor-relevant human isocitrate dehydrogenase 1 mutants. *Biochem. J.* **2019**, *475*, 3221–3238. [CrossRef] [PubMed]
73. Chu, B.; Wu, T.; Miao, L.; Mei, Y.; Wu, M. MiR-181a regulates lipid metabolism via IDH1. *Sci. Rep.* **2015**, *5*, 1–8. [CrossRef]

74. Tanaka, H.; Sasayama, T.; Tanaka, K.; Nakamizo, S.; Nishihara, M.; Mizukawa, K.; Kohta, M.; Koyama, J.; Miyake, S.; Taniguchi, M.; et al. MicroRNA-183 upregulates HIF-1α by targeting isocitrate dehydrogenase 2 (IDH2) in glioma cells. *J. Neurooncol.* **2013**, *111*, 273–283. [CrossRef]
75. Dombret, H.; Seymour, J.F.; Butrym, A.; Wierzbowska, A.; Selleslag, D.; Jang, J.H.; Kumar, R.; Cavenagh, J.; Schuh, A.C.; Candoni, A.; et al. International phase 3 study of azacitidine vs. conventional care regimens in older patients with newly diagnosed AML with >30% blasts. *Blood* **2015**, *126*, 291–299. [CrossRef]
76. Kantarjian, H.; Ravandi, F.; Wilson, W.; Estey, E. Decitabine in older adults with acute myeloid leukemia: Why was the dream broken? *J. Clin. Oncol.* **2013**, *31*, 1795–1796. [CrossRef]
77. Hadoux, J.; Favier, J.; Scoazec, J.-Y.; Leboulleux, S.; Ghuzlan, A.A.; Caramella, C.; Deandreis, D.; Borget, I.; Loriot, C.; Chougnet, C.; et al. SDHB mutations are associated with response to temozolomide in patients with metastatic pheochromocytoma or paraganglioma. *Int. J. Cancer* **2014**, *135*, 2711–2720. [CrossRef] [PubMed]
78. Songtao, Q.; Lei, Y.; Si, G.; Yanqing, D.; Huixia, H.; Xuelin, Z.; Lanxiao, W.; Fei, Y. IDH mutations predict longer survival and response to temozolomide in secondary glioblastoma. *Cancer Sci.* **2012**, *103*, 269–273. [CrossRef]
79. Su, R.; Lei, D.; Chenying, L.; Nachtergaele, S.; Wunderlich, M.; YQing, Y.; Deng, X.; Wang, Y.; Weng, X.; Hu, C.; et al. R-2HG exhibits anti-tumor activity by targeting FTO/M6 A/MYC/CEBPA signaling. *Cell* **2018**, *172*, 90–105.e23. [CrossRef]
80. Dong, B.; Qiu, Z.; Wu, Y. Tackle epithelial-mesenchymal transition with epigenetic drugs in cancer. *Front. Pharmacol.* **2020**, *11*, 596239. [CrossRef]

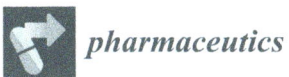

Review

Mitochondrial Targeting Involving Cholesterol-Rich Lipid Rafts in the Mechanism of Action of the Antitumor Ether Lipid and Alkylphospholipid Analog Edelfosine

Faustino Mollinedo * and Consuelo Gajate

Centro de Investigaciones Biológicas Margarita Salas, Consejo Superior de Investigaciones Científicas (CSIC), Laboratory of Cell Death and Cancer Therapy, Department of Molecular Biomedicine, C/Ramiro de Maeztu 9, E-28040 Madrid, Spain; cgajate@cib.csic.es
* Correspondence: fmollin@cib.csic.es

Citation: Mollinedo, F.; Gajate, C. Mitochondrial Targeting Involving Cholesterol-Rich Lipid Rafts in the Mechanism of Action of the Antitumor Ether Lipid and Alkylphospholipid Analog Edelfosine. *Pharmaceutics* **2021**, *13*, 763. https://doi.org/10.3390/pharmaceutics13050763

Academic Editor: Joanna Kopecka

Received: 12 April 2021
Accepted: 11 May 2021
Published: 20 May 2021

Publisher's Note: MDPI stays neutral with regard to jurisdictional claims in published maps and institutional affiliations.

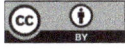

Copyright: © 2021 by the authors. Licensee MDPI, Basel, Switzerland. This article is an open access article distributed under the terms and conditions of the Creative Commons Attribution (CC BY) license (https://creativecommons.org/licenses/by/4.0/).

Abstract: The ether lipid edelfosine induces apoptosis selectively in tumor cells and is the prototypic molecule of a family of synthetic antitumor compounds collectively known as alkylphospholipid analogs. Cumulative evidence shows that edelfosine interacts with cholesterol-rich lipid rafts, endoplasmic reticulum (ER) and mitochondria. Edelfosine induces apoptosis in a number of hematological cancer cells by recruiting death receptors and downstream apoptotic signaling into lipid rafts, whereas it promotes apoptosis in solid tumor cells through an ER stress response. Edelfosine-induced apoptosis, mediated by lipid rafts and/or ER, requires the involvement of a mitochondrial-dependent step to eventually elicit cell death, leading to the loss of mitochondrial membrane potential, cytochrome c release and the triggering of cell death. The overexpression of Bcl-2 or Bcl-xL blocks edelfosine-induced apoptosis. Edelfosine induces the redistribution of lipid rafts from the plasma membrane to the mitochondria. The pro-apoptotic action of edelfosine on cancer cells is associated with the recruitment of F_1F_O–ATP synthase into cholesterol-rich lipid rafts. Specific inhibition of the F_O sector of the F_1F_O–ATP synthase, which contains the membrane-embedded c-subunit ring that constitutes the mitochondrial permeability transcription pore, hinders edelfosine-induced cell death. Taking together, the evidence shown here suggests that the ether lipid edelfosine could modulate cell death in cancer cells by direct interaction with mitochondria, and the reorganization of raft-located mitochondrial proteins that critically modulate cell death or survival. Here, we summarize and discuss the involvement of mitochondria in the antitumor action of the ether lipid edelfosine, pointing out the mitochondrial targeting of this drug as a major therapeutic approach, which can be extrapolated to other alkylphospholipid analogs. We also discuss the involvement of cholesterol transport and cholesterol-rich lipid rafts in the interactions between the organelles as well as in the role of mitochondria in the regulation of apoptosis in cancer cells and cancer therapy.

Keywords: mitochondria; cholesterol; lipid raft; mitochondrial permeability transition pore; alkylphospholipid analog; edelfosine

1. Introduction

The ether lipid edelfosine (1-*O*-octadecyl-2-*O*-methyl-*rac*-glycero-3-phosphocholine, ET-18-OCH$_3$) (Figure 1) is considered as the prototype of a family of synthetic antitumor drugs collectively known as alkylphospholipid analogs (APLs) or antitumor ether lipids (AELs) [1–3]. Among the distinct APLs, it is worth highlighting miltefosine, perifosine, erucylphosphocholine and erufosine, in addition to edelfosine (Figure 1). Miltefosine (hexadecyl 2-(trimethylazaniumyl)ethyl phosphate, also known as hexadecylphosphocholine) represents the minimal structural requirement for the antitumor activity of APLs and has become the first oral drug in the treatment of visceral leishmaniasis [4–6], being commercialized under the trademark name of Impavido®(oral solid human pharmaceutical product; Zentaris, Frankfurt, Germany). Miltefosine is also used in the clinic as a topical treatment for cutaneous metastases of breast cancer [7], and commercialized under the trademark name of Miltex® (topical liquid human pharmaceutical product; Baxter, Newbury, UK). Miltefosine is also used under the trademark of Miltefloran® for the treatment of canine leishmaniasis (oral liquid veterinary pharmaceutical product for dogs; Virbac, Carros, France) [8]. Perifosine (octadecyl-[1,1-dimethyl-piperidino-4-yl]phosphate), where the choline moiety of miltefosine is replaced by a heterocyclic piperidine group, shows a promising orally active antitumor APL [9,10] that is currently used in clinical trials [11–15]. Erucylphosphocholine ([13Z]-docos-13-en-1-yl 2-(trimethylammonio)ethyl phosphate, ErPC), an APL-derivative with a 22 carbon atom chain and a *cis*-13, 14 double bond, shows distinctive reduced hemolytic activity, thereby allowing intravenous injection, and holds promise for the treatment of human brain tumors [16–19]. The ErPC closely related congener erufosine (erucylphosphohomocholine, or erucylphospho-*N,N,N*-trimethylpropylammonium, ErPC3) [20,21], a member of the latest generation of APLs, can be applied intravenously and can cross the blood–brain barrier [22–25].

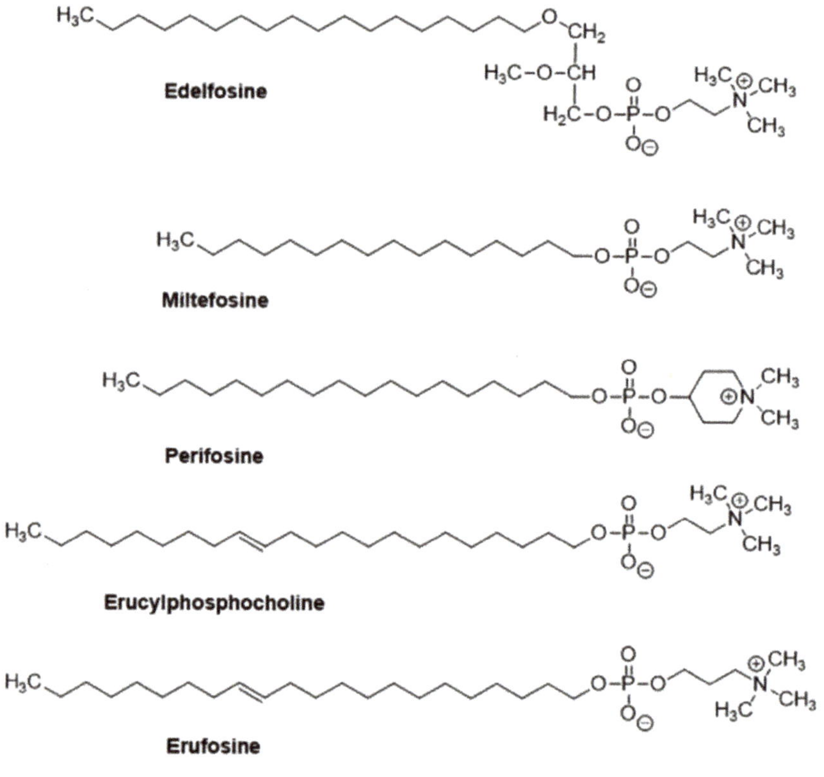

Figure 1. Chemical structures of some clinically relevant alkylphospholipid analogs.

However, edelfosine remains as the most active antitumor APL, and is the golden standard and prototype for other APLs and for studies on the mechanism of action of this family of compounds. Furthermore, our in vitro and in vivo results have revealed that edelfosine, orally administered, is the most potent APL in killing different *Leishmania spp.*, showing higher anti-*Leishmania* activity than miltefosine, and is less prone to generate drug resistance than miltefosine [26].

A major feature of the above APLs is that they target cell membranes, particularly lipid rafts, affecting several biochemical processes, ion transport and signaling pathways [1,2,27–30]. Edelfosine shows a high affinity for both model and cell membranes, but weak detergent activity [31]. A remarkable characteristic of the ether lipid edelfosine is its selectivity in inducing apoptosis in cancer cells, whereas non-transformed cells are spared [1,2,9,27,32]. This selectivity is due to the preferential drug uptake by cancer cells by a not fully understood mechanism [1,2,27,33–35]. Edelfosine targets the cell membrane and, depending on the cell type, leads to the onset of different types of cell death [36], ranging from apoptosis, which is predominantly triggered in most cancer cells [1,2,27,33–35], to necrosis/necroptosis [37,38], with mitochondria playing a key role in the irreversible onset of the cell death process [9,39,40].

2. The Alkylphospholipid Analog Edelfosine Induces Apoptosis Selectively in Cancer Cells

A direct antitumor action of edelfosine on cancer cells was already reported in the late 1970s and 1980s [41–44], but it was not until the 1990s and 2000s that the molecular mechanism underlying the antitumor activity of this drug started to be unveiled, showing that the induction of apoptosis by edelfosine was the main effect that explained the direct antitumor action of APLs [45,46]. Then, a number of findings in the Faustino Mollinedo's and Consuelo Gajate's laboratory, first in Valladolid (Spain) and then in Salamanca (Spain) in the late 1990s and early 2000s, respectively, demonstrated the selective pro-apoptotic effect of edelfosine on cancer cells, following the preferential drug uptake in tumor cells [32,33,47] and the reorganization of membrane lipid raft platforms [27,48]. These data provided the first evidence for a selective pro-apoptotic drug and for the involvement of lipid rafts in cancer chemotherapy. Edelfosine (Figure 1) is an oral drug showing potent antitumor activity against different kinds of tumors in cancer animal models [34,35,40,49], and lacks toxicity in rats after edelfosine oral treatment at pharmacological relevant doses, with no cardiotoxicity, hepatotoxicity or renal toxicity [50].

In general, apoptosis can be mainly induced either by an extrinsic pathway, mediated through the activation of death receptors, or by an intrinsic pathway or mitochondria-mediated process, which permeabilizes the outer mitochondrial membrane (OMM), leading to the release of cytochrome *c*, located in the mitochondrial intermembrane/intercristae spaces where it functions as an electron shuttle in the respiratory chain. Mitochondria-mediated apoptosis is characterized by mitochondrial outer membrane permeabilization (MOMP) and the subsequent release of mitochondrial cytochrome *c* into the cytoplasm to activate caspases. Once in the cytosol, cytochrome *c* binds the adaptor molecule APAF-1 (apoptosis protease-activating factor-1), causing it to oligomerize through a conformational change, and form a heptameric structure called the apoptosome complex, made up of cytochrome *c* and APAF-1. The apoptosome recruits and potentiates the activation of procaspase-9, which in turn cleaves and activates downstream effector caspases, such as caspase-3 and -7 [51]. MOMP is regulated by the Bcl-2 family of proteins [51].

3. Edelfosine Accumulates in Lipid Rafts and the Endoplasmic Reticulum of Cancer Cells, and the Generated Apoptotic Signals Converge on Mitochondria to Elicit Apoptosis

A major milestone in the study of the mechanism of action of APLs was achieved in 2001 when the apoptosis induced by the ether lipid edelfosine was first found to be mediated by lipid rafts [48]. Edelfosine accumulates in the lipid rafts of a wide array of hematological cancer cells [9,27,34,52–54], leading to apoptosis through the reorganization of these membrane domains, especially by promoting co-clustering of lipid rafts and Fas/CD95 death receptor signaling [9,27,34,53,54]. These seminal reports identified lipid rafts as a novel and promising target in cancer therapy [9,27,34,53–57], and paved the way for future studies in raft-targeted cancer therapy [29,30,56,58–63]. Edelfosine induced the clustering and recruitment of the Fas/CD95 death receptor, as well as other death receptors and downstream signaling molecules in lipid rafts, thus triggering apoptosis in a variety of cancer cells, including myeloid and lymphoid cancer cells [9,27,33,48]. This mechanism of action involved a raft-mediated activation of apoptosis via Fas/CD95, independently of its physiological FasL/CD95L ligand, which could be pharmacologically modulated, thus opening a new therapeutic approach in cancer therapy [1,27,34,35,53,59,64]. Interestingly, edelfosine prompted the recruitment of death receptors and downstream signaling molecules in lipid rafts, whereas Akt survival signaling was displaced from the rafts [30,65].

Yeast cells show different raft domains that contain transporters and proteins involved in the control of Na^+, K^+ and pH homeostasis, required for the proper function of yeast, and that modulate yeast growth and death [66]. The active transport of ions and nutrients in yeast relies on the existence of an electrochemical gradient of protons across the plasma membrane, and this electrochemical gradient is mainly generated in Saccharomyces cerevisiae by the H^+-ATPase gene *pma1*, an essential H^+ pump for yeast growth [67] and a resident raft protein [68]. We found that edelfosine treatment in S. cerevisiae displaced Pma1p from lipid rafts [69–71], and induced its internalization as well as of the plasma membrane arginine/H^+ symporter Can1p (arginine permease) and the uracil/H^+ symporter Fura4p (uracil permease), two nutrient H^+-symporters associated with yeast lipid rafts [66,72,73]. Our studies on the mechanism of action of edelfosine in S. cerevisase showed that the ether lipid displaces the essential proton pump Pma1p from the lipid rafts, inducing its internalization into the vacuole, the yeast equivalent to the mammalian endosome–lysosome system, and subsequent degradation, thus leading to altered pH homeostasis and cell death [69–71]. The displacement of Pma1p from the rafts following edelfosine treatment was preceded by the rapid movement of the yeast sterol ergosterol out of the plasma membrane and into the cell [69–71].

Taking together, edelfosine induces cell death through the reorganization of lipid rafts by modifying the balance of apoptotic versus survival signaling molecules in these membrane domains. Thus, the recruitment of apoptotic signaling molecules into lipid rafts and the displacement of survival molecules from these membrane domains is critical in the mechanism of action of this ether lipid.

Biophysical studies have shown that edelfosine has a high affinity for cholesterol, increases membrane thickness, and alters raft organization [74]. The high affinity of edelfosine for cholesterol is easily and visually explained on the basis of the complementarity of the molecular geometries of edelfosine and sterols in general [75]. The combination of "cone-shape" sterols and "inverted cone-shape" edelfosine leads to a more stable bilayer [75].

Studies on solid tumor cells, including pancreatic adenocarcinoma, lung adenocarcinoma, cervix epithelioid carcinoma and Ewing's sarcoma cells, have shown that edelfosine accumulated mainly in the endoplasmic reticulum (ER), triggering an ER stress response that eventually led to apoptosis [39,40,49,76]. Interestingly, edelfosine accumulated first in plasma membrane lipid rafts and subsequently in the ER of S. cerevisiae, used as a eukaryotic model organism [70].

However, although edelfosine has been found to accumulate in the membrane rafts [9,27,34,53,54] and the ER [40,49] of human tumor cells, as assessed by using radioactive edelfosine and fluorescent analogs of the ether lipid, all the apoptotic signals generated from either the plasma membrane rafts or the ER converge on the mitochondria to eventually trigger apoptosis (Figure 2). Thus, the overexpression of Bcl-2 or Bcl-x_L totally prevents the apoptotic response induced by edelfosine in cancer cells, either from a hematological or solid tumor origin [9,32,40,77]. These data highlight the critical role of mitochondria as a meeting and convergence point of different apoptotic signaling pathways, irreversibly leading to apoptosis.

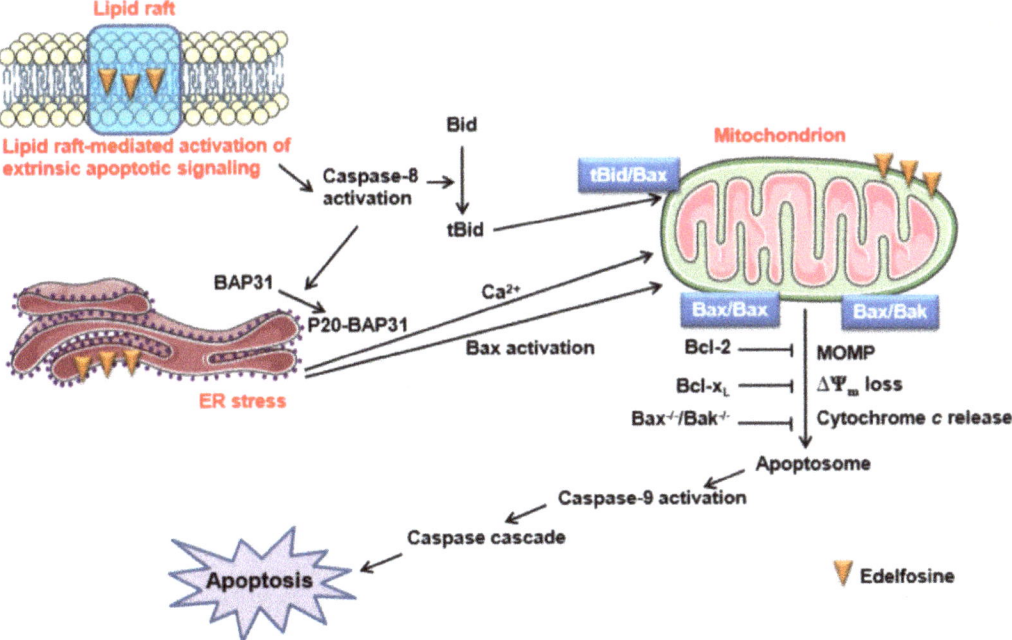

Figure 2. Schematic model of the involvement of plasma membrane lipid rafts, ER and mitochondria in edelfosine-induced apoptosis in cancer cells. Protection of mitochondria by Bcl-2 or Bcl-xL overexpression, or by Bax/Bak double knock-out (Bax$^{-/-}$/Bak$^{-/-}$), prevents cell death, indicating that the apoptotic signals derived from plasma membrane and ER converge on mitochondria. See text for details. MOMP, mitochondrial outer membrane permeabilization.

Edelfosine-induced apoptosis involved mitochondria as assessed by the disruption of the mitochondrial transmembrane potential ($\Delta\Psi_m$), measured using 3,3'-dihexyloxacarbocyanine iodide [DiOC6(3)] fluorescence, and the production of reactive oxygen species (ROS), detected using the conversion of dihydroethidium into ethidium, in both leukemic [47] and solid tumor cells [49]. Edelfosine also induced Bax activation, cytochrome c release, caspase-9 activation, and DNA fragmentation in both leukemic [9,47] and solid tumor cells [40,49], and Bcl-2 or Bcl-x$_L$ overexpression prevented the above-mentioned mitochondria-related responses [9,40,77].

4. Localization of Edelfosine in the Mitochondria of Cancer Cells Using Fluorescent Analogs

In 2004, we synthesized the first fluorescent edelfosine analog, which preserved pro-apoptotic activity comparable to that of the parent drug [27,78], as an excellent tool to unveil the mechanism of action of this drug. To this aim, we tried to synthesize a fluorescent edelfosine analog with a minimum modification of the chemical structure. Our previous structure–activity relationship studies at the time showed that some modifications preserved the apoptotic activity, including the presence of a double bond in the O-octadecyl chain at the C1 of edelfosine [32]. In this regard, a conjugated pentaene group appeared as a convenient candidate, considering that this fluorophore had led to the development of useful fluorescent probes for lipid membranes [79,80]. On these grounds, we reasoned that the replacement of the C18 aliphatic chain by a lipophilic fluorescent group of similar length could preserve the unique properties of this drug regarding its activity and selectivity. This led to the synthesis of the first fluorescent analog, containing the conjugated all-(E)-phenyltetraene blue-emitting chromophore, which was coined as PTE-ET [27] (Figure 3). This PTE-ET fluorescent analog, as well as the subsequently synthesized PTRI-ET (Figure 3), containing the all-(E)-phenyltrienyne blue-emitting chromophore, were the first fluorescent edelfosine analogs [27,70,78,81]. These fluorescent edelfosine analogs largely preserved the chemical structure of edelfosine (Figure 3), and shared analogous fluorescence traits with a poor fluorescence yield and photostability under intense near-UV laser excitation [28,78,81]. In order to improve the fluorescence yield and provide a more stable fluorescent signal, we synthesized a second generation of fluorescent analogs by adding a BODIPY (4,4-difluoro-4-bora-3a,4a-diaza-s-indacene; boron-dipyrromethene) fluorochrome attached to the alkyl chain of edelfosine, leading to the green-emitting Et-BDP-ET and Yn-BDP-ET fluorescent edelfosine analogs [28,81] (Figure 3). These two compounds had a higher fluorescence yield and resistance to photodegradation than the first generation fluorescent edelfosine analogs, and allowed a thorough analysis through confocal microscopy [28,81]. The use of all the above fluorescent edelfosine analogs, either first or second generation, allowed to localize edelfosine in the mitochondria of cancer cells (Figure 4) [81,82], in addition to the subcellular localizations of this drug in the ER [40,49,76] and lipid rafts [9,27,34,35] in solid tumor cells and hematological cancer cells, respectively. Interestingly, mitochondrial localization of edelfosine was also found in *Leishmania* parasites [82].

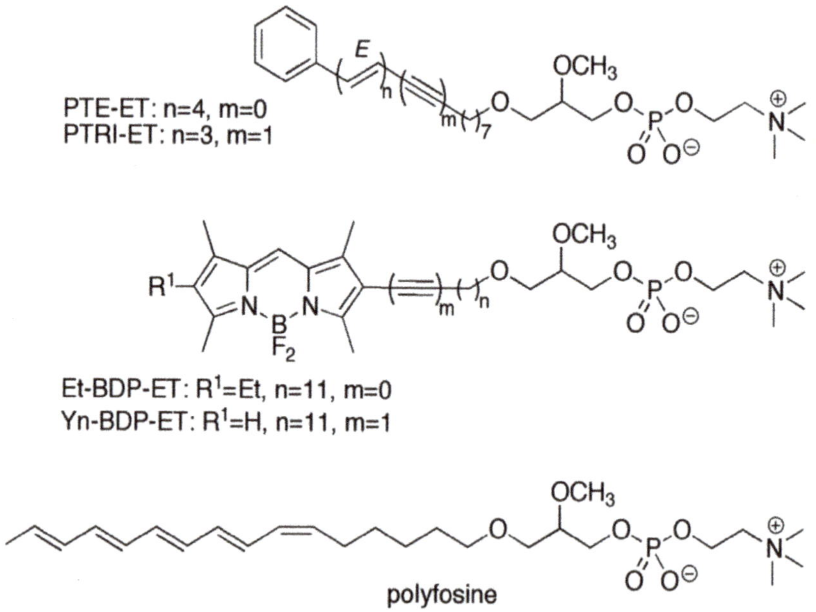

Figure 3. Chemical structures of fluorescent edelfosine analogs.

Polyene lipids (linear hydrocarbons containing a conjugated double-bond system) display a unique structural similarity to natural lipids, which results in minimal effects on the lipid properties. The above PTE-ET fluorescent analog could be included in this type of lipids. In this regard, polyfosine (Figure 3), a polyene fluorescent analog of edelfosine containing five conjugated double bonds, was also found to accumulate in the mitochondria and to induce morphological changes and apoptosis in COS7 cells [83].

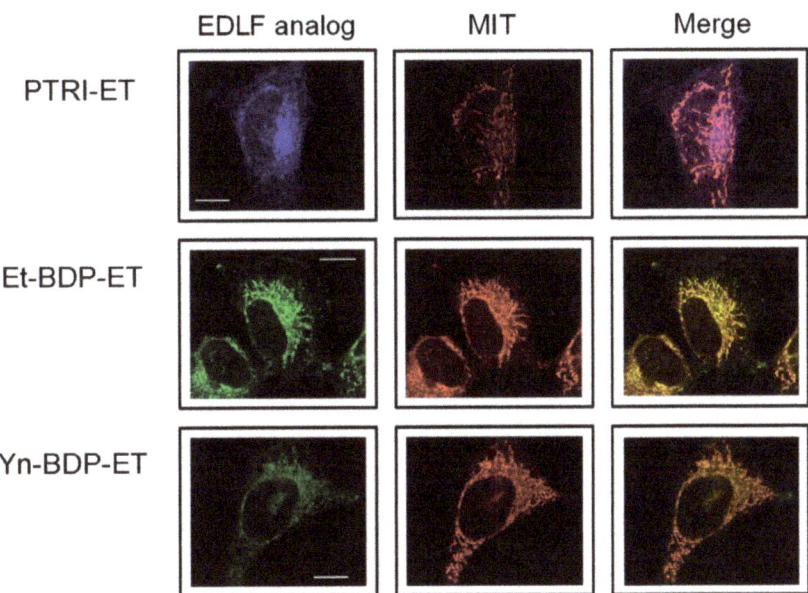

Figure 4. Colocalization of fluorescent edelfosine analogs and mitochondria in cancer cells. HeLa cells were incubated for 12 h with 10 μM of the indicated fluorescent edelfosine (EDLF) analogs (PTRI-ET, blue fluorescence; Et-BDP-ET, green fluorescence; Yn-BDP-ET, green fluorescence) to visualize edelfosine subcellular localization. Mitochondrial location was examined using MitoTracker Red probe (MIT, red fluorescence). Areas of colocalization between edelfosine analogs and mitochondria in the merge panels are purple (for PTRI-ET) or yellow (for Et-BDP-ET and Yn-BDP-ET). Bar, 10 μm. Image taken from [81], Springer Nature, 2011.

5. Cholesterol in Mitochondria

A major question raises from the above subcellular localization experiments. How does edelfosine accumulate in the mitochondrial membrane? We reason that a putative explanation for this accumulation could lie in the above-stated high affinity of edelfosine for cholesterol.

Lipids are not randomly distributed among biological membranes, but their relative content is characteristic for each organelle, affecting their shape, structure and function [84]. Lipids constitute approximately 50% of the mass of most cell membranes (e.g., plasma membrane), although this proportion is highly dependent on the type of membrane (e.g., mitochondrial inner membrane contains 75% protein as a result of the abundance of protein complexes involved in electron transport and oxidative phosphorylation). However, one must bear always in mind that there are many more lipid molecules than protein molecules in membranes because lipid molecules are small compared with proteins. On these grounds, it might be estimated the presence of about 50 lipid molecules for each protein molecule in the plasma membrane.

Among the distinct lipids, cholesterol (a major sterol component in animal cell membranes, making up about 30% of the lipid bilayer on average) has attracted much attention since its first isolation from gallstones in the eighteen century. The French doctor and chemist François-Paul Poulletier de la Salle (1719–1788) first identified cholesterol in gallstones in about 1758–1769, albeit his work was never published [85–87]. Later on, cholesterol was rediscovered in 1815 by the French chemist Michel Eugène Chevreul (1786–1889) who named it "cholesterine" [85–87].

Cholesterol is an essential building block of the plasma membrane, having diverse structural and functional roles [88,89], and playing pleiotropic actions in normal and cancer cells [30]. Cholesterol plays a unique and pivotal role among the different lipids in maintaining the structural integrity and regulating the fluidity of the mammalian cell membranes [90,91]. As compared to other lipids, cholesterol moves rapidly as a monomer across membranes and between membrane organelles on protein carriers [89]. However, cholesterol is not uniformly distributed within biological membranes and across different cellular compartments. Cholesterol has been suggested to be enriched in the cytosolic (inner) leaflet of the plasma membrane [92]. Recent imaging methods, using tunable orthogonal cholesterol sensors, have revealed a marked transbilayer asymmetry of plasma membrane cholesterol in mammalian cells, with the cholesterol concentration in the inner leaflet being ~12-fold lower than in the outer leaflet [93]. Cellular cholesterol, derived from low-density lipoprotein receptor-mediated endocytosis or synthesized de novo in the ER, is mainly (up to 90%) located in the plasma membrane, constituting 10–45% (mol%) of the total plasma membrane lipids [93–95]. Cholesterol plays major roles in the structural and functional modulation of integral membrane proteins [96], and in the formation of cholesterol-rich membrane domains, such as the so-called lipid or membrane rafts. Lipid rafts are membrane microdomains enriched in cholesterol and sphingolipids, involved in the lateral compartmentalization of molecules at the cell surface, and can coalesce to form membrane raft platforms [30,97].

Mitochondrial membranes are cholesterol-poor, particularly the inner mitochondrial membrane, as compared to other subcellular membranes in mammalian cells [98,99]. The relative proportion of phospholipid/cholesterol in the rat liver plasma membrane is 5.25, whereas this rate increases up to 58.3 in the rat liver mitochondria [98,99]. The sterol-to-protein ratio in mitochondria is low compared to other subcellular fractions (rat liver), as follows: mitochondria (0.003 mg sterol/mg protein); ER (0.014 mg sterol/mg protein); lysosomes (0.038 mg sterol/mg protein); Golgi (0.038 mg sterol/mg protein); and plasma membrane (0.128 mg sterol/mg protein) [98,99].

The mitochondria are made up of an OMM, an inner mitochondrial membrane (IMM), an inter-membrane space (IMS) in between, and the mitochondrial matrix enclosed by the IMM (Figure 5). The IMM shows a number of invaginations, called cristae, thus making the surface of the IMM significantly larger than that of the OMM. The whole machinery of oxidative phosphorylation, including the electron transport chain (ETC) complexes (complexes I–IV) as well as the F_1F_O–ATP synthase (complex V), resides in the IMM. The OMM separates the mitochondrion from the cytosol. The OMM forms a smooth lipid-rich surface with high membrane fluidity, whereas the IMM is highly folded and shows an elevated protein level and lower lipid content [98,99]. In this regard, cholesterol is enriched in the OMM compared to the IMM (0.04 mg sterol/mg protein in OMM versus <0.01 mg sterol/mg protein in IMM, rat liver) [98,99].

As stated above, cholesterol levels vary widely between different subcellular membranes (e.g., plasma membrane contains about 40-fold higher cholesterol levels than the ER and mitochondria [98,99]). Although cholesterol levels are particularly low in mitochondria, especially in the IMM [98,99], cholesterol must reach this subcellular compartment for the correct functioning of several major biological processes, including the synthesis of steroids, oxysterols and bile acids.

This variety in cholesterol content between different biological membranes is consistent with its putative major role in the regulation of the correct functioning of the distinct subcellular organelles. The low level of cholesterol in the mitochondria suggests that even small changes in its concentration, either through a general increase in sterol content or a particular clustering of cholesterol in certain membrane regions, could have a large impact on the biophysical and functional features of the membrane and organelle.

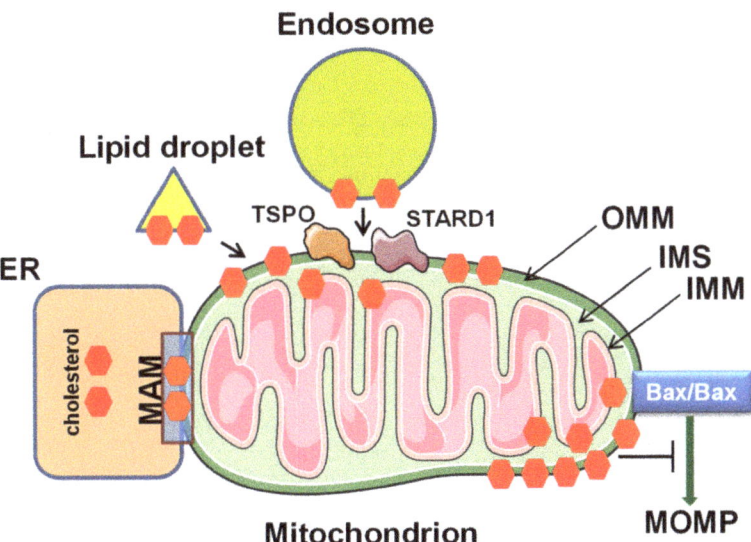

Figure 5. Import and transfer of cellular cholesterol into mitochondria. Cholesterol is transported to the mitochondria through vesicular and non-vesicular trafficking, involving the ER, lipid droplets, endosomes, TSPO and STARD1. Elevated mitochondrial cholesterol levels in cancer cells affect mitochondrial membrane and impair Bax/Bak oligomerization in OMM and subsequent MOMP formation, representing a mechanism of cell death resistance in tumor cells. See text for details. ER, endoplasmic reticulum. IMM, inner mitochondrial membrane. IMS, inter-membrane space. MAM, mitochondria-associated membrane. OMM, outer mitochondrial membrane. STARD1, steroidogenic acute regulatory protein-related lipid transfer domain containing protein 1. TSPO, translocator protein.

Cholesterol critically influences membrane fluidity, permeability, curvature and membrane protein interactions in biological cell membranes [30,60,100–102], affecting the cell surface distribution of membrane proteins, modulation of cellular signaling transmission and intracellular trafficking. A major feature of cholesterol is its ability to modulate the physicochemical properties of cellular membranes. Cholesterol orients in a phospholipid bilayer with its polar hydroxyl group towards the aqueous phase and the hydrophobic steroid ring oriented parallel to the hydrocarbon chains of the phospholipids, thus interacting with the membrane phospholipids and sphingolipids and being a critical contributor to lipid raft assembly [103].

6. Cholesterol Transport to Mitochondria

The insertion of cholesterol into the membrane lends rigidity and promotes the formation of protein-tethering platforms, such as lipid rafts [30,97]. In the mitochondria, cholesterol plays a number of major roles, some are as follows [104]: (a) a structural component of the OMM and IMM, providing the appropriate fluidity, curvature and biophysical properties; (b) a precursor of steroidogenesis, by which cholesterol is converted to biologically active steroid hormones, with the first biochemical reactions taking place in the mitochondrial matrix [105]; (c) the core of membrane platforms interacting with the ER, lysosomes and other vesicles or intracellular compartments; and (d) a tethering element for mitochondrial DNA.

Cholesterol is transported to the mitochondria through vesicular and non-vesicular trafficking. Some critical proteins and organelles/vesicles involved in mitochondrial cholesterol delivery to the mitochondria are schematically displayed in Figure 5, and indicated below.

STARD1 (30 kDa steroidogenic acute regulatory protein-related lipid transfer domain containing protein 1) acts at the OMM to mediate the import of cholesterol and transports cholesterol from the OMM to the IMM [106].

Translocator protein (18 kDa), TSPO (formerly known as the peripheral-type benzodiazepine receptor), is a ubiquitous mitochondrial protein, localized to the OMM, and involved in several biological functions, including mitochondrial cholesterol transport and steroid hormone biosynthesis [107,108]. TSPO is a five transmembrane domain protein found as a monomer, dimer and polymer, and is highly abundant in the OMM [107,108]. TSPO has been shown to interact with STARD1 and the voltage-dependent anion-selective channel 1 (VDAC1), the latter being the most abundant VDAC of the three isoforms VDAC1-3 [109,110]. TSPO is a high-affinity cholesterol-binding protein that oligomerizes to form a cholesterol transporting channel and prompts cholesterol transfer to the IMM [111,112]. TSPO has been shown to associate with different cytosolic and mitochondrial proteins as part of a large multiprotein complex involved in mitochondrial cholesterol transport [108,109].

Cholesterol transfer to the mitochondria is mediated by a series of direct interactions between the mitochondria and a series of intracellular organelles, such as ER, lipid droplets and endosomes (Figure 5). The mitochondria and the ER interact through the so-called mitochondria-associated membranes (MAMs) [113], which are involved in the transfer of cholesterol and other lipids between the ER and mitochondria [114]. Wide-field fluorescence microscopy combined with digital deconvolution has revealed that mitochondria form a largely interconnected dynamic network, and by expressing different fluorescent markers targeted to the mitochondria and ER, 5–20% of the mitochondrial surface was estimated to be in close apposition to (10–30 nm distance) or in association with the ER [115]. In fact, a large body of evidence demonstrates that mitochondria interact and communicate directly with the ER through MAMs to modulate several cellular responses [115–121].

Lipid droplets, originating from the ER, are dynamic structures able to interact with most other cellular organelles, are critical to buffer the levels of toxic lipid species [122,123] and are involved in lipid storage and mobilization [123]. Lipid droplets have been envisaged to interact directly with mitochondria to facilitate lipid transfer [124,125]. These lipid droplet–mitochondria interactions have been suggested to be mediated by SNAP-23 (23-kDa synaptosome-associated protein) [126], a protein that plays a major role in general membrane fusion processes, and serves as an important regulator of transport vesicle docking and fusion in all mammalian cells [127–130].

A major source of cholesterol is derived from the endocytosis of exogenous lipoproteins, transferring cholesterol from the lipoproteins and plasma membrane to the endosomes and multivesicular late endosomes [131–133]. The subsequent transport of cholesterol out of late endosomes requires the so-called Niemann-Pick type C1 (NPC1) and NCP2 proteins. Niemann-Pick disease type C (NP-C) is a rare neurodegenerative disorder of autosomal recessive inheritance, with an estimated incidence of 1 in 120,000–150,000 live births, and affects cholesterol trafficking [134,135]. NP-C is characterized by endosomal accumulation of unesterified cholesterol and glycolipids in various tissues, including the brain, leading to progressive central nervous system neurodegeneration and death [135]. This disease is caused by mutations of the *NPC1* (accounting for 95% of NP-C cases) or the *NPC2* gene (5% of NP-C cases). Currently, there is no cure for NP-C and patients usually die before adulthood (frequently in the second decade of life), but adult forms of NP-C are being increasingly recognized, having a more insidious onset and slower progression [136,137]. NP-C is characterized by impaired cholesterol efflux from late endosomes and lysosomes, and secondary accumulation of lipids due to mutations in the NPC1 or NPC2 proteins, which act in coordination to mediate the efflux of unesterified cholesterol from lysosomes or late endosomes. Human NPC1 encodes a 1278 amino acid (170–190 kDa) glycoprotein, found in late endosomes and lysosomal membranes, with 13 transmembrane domains, which binds both cholesterol and oxysterol [138]. NPC2 (18 kDa) is a soluble lysosomal glycoprotein containing 132 amino acids and is found in the lumen of late endosomes/lysosomes [139,140]. NPC1 binds cholesterol with nanomolar affinity, whereas NPC2 binds cholesterol with micromolar affinity [138,141]. In relation to this review, it is interesting to note that resistance to the ether lipid drug edelfosine represents the first phenotype caused by the deletion of the *NCR1* gene in *S. cerevisiae* [142], further supporting the strong relationship between the ether lipid edelfosine and cholesterol. *NCR1* is the *S. cerevisiae* homolog of the human *NCP1*, and the Ncr1p protein localizes to the vacuole [142]. Under normal circumstances, NPC2, as a soluble sterol transfer protein in the late endosome, transfers cholesterol from the internal vesicle to the membrane-bound NPC1, which mediates cholesterol egress from the late endosomes to the ER and plasma membrane. Putative transport from the late endosome to the mitochondria could be mediated through STARD3 (also known as metastatic lymph node 64 protein (MLN64)), a 50.5 kDa protein (containing 445 amino acids) that localizes in the membrane of late endosomes, and is involved in cholesterol transport [143,144]. However, the direct transport from endosomes to mitochondria or through an ER-mediated step is still a matter of controversy.

7. Mitochondrial Cholesterol in Cancer

Mitochondria are considered cholesterol-poor organelles, with estimates ranging from 0.5–3% of the content found in the plasma membrane [145]. However, increased mitochondrial cholesterol levels have been reported in a number of diseases or pathophysiological conditions, including some types of cancer, steatohepatitis, cardiac ischemia, aging and neurodegenerative diseases [146]. When it comes to neurodegenerative diseases, Alzheimer's disease and the lysosomal disorder NP-C call particular attention [147]. The functions of mitochondria are altered in all of the above conditions, and it is tempting to suggest the existence of an interplay between the abnormally increased mitochondrial cholesterol levels, mitochondria dysfunction and disease pathology [146,147]. The accumulation of intracellular cholesterol alters mitophagy and reduces the clearance of defective mitochondria in neurodegenerative diseases [148]. Regarding cancer, larger amounts of mitochondrial cholesterol have been found in solid tumors as compared to their normal counterparts, and this correlates with tumor growth and malignancy [149]. About 2- to 5-fold higher levels of mitochondrial cholesterol were found in the tumors from Buffalo rats containing transplanted Morris hepatomas, when compared to the content found in the mitochondria prepared from a host liver [150,151]. The mitochondrial cholesterol levels in H35 rat hepatoma cells and HepG2 human hepatoma cells were 3- to 10-fold higher than the corresponding cholesterol levels in normal rat and human liver mitochondria [152]. The high levels of mitochondrial cholesterol contribute to chemotherapy resistance [149,152].

As stated above, cholesterol level tends to be high in cancer cells, the meaning of which is currently controversial [30,153,154]. A number of studies have shown elevated mitochondrial cholesterol levels in cancer cells, being associated with chemotherapy resistance, low mitochondrial proton leak, and altered patterns of the Krebs cycle metabolism, which might affect the activity of certain mitochondrial enzymes [150–152,155,156]. An increased cholesterol level in the OMM, and its subsequent decrease in membrane fluidity, inhibits Bax oligomerization and activation (Figure 5), thus impairing MOMP and contributing to the resistance to apoptosis-inducing agents [149,157].

8. Mitochondrial Permeability Transition Pore (mPTP) and Regulation of Cell Death

Mitochondria are critical subcellular structures that control cellular life through energy production as well as cell death through the induction of apoptosis and necrosis. Different death signaling pathways converge on mitochondria, and the so-called mitochondrial permeability transition pore (mPTP) acts as a key nodal point in mediating cell death. Mitochondrial permeability transition is defined as the process whereby the IMM shows an increased permeability to solutes with a molecular mass of <1.5 kDa, thus resulting in the loss of the IMM potential, respiratory chain uncoupling, halt of mitochondrial ATP synthesis, mitochondrial swelling, OMM rupture, and eventually cell death [158–162]. The molecular identity of the mPTP is rather controversial, and different proteins have been suggested to be part of the mPTP complex or closely related to its function as regulators of mPTP activity. These proteins include the following: the adenine nucleotide translocator (ANT) [163], a 32 kDa protein located in the IMM responsible for the import of ADP into the mitochondrial matrix in exchange for ATP; VDAC1, the most abundant protein in the OMM with a molecular weight of ~32 kDa through which metabolites and nucleotides traverse the OMM [164]; the translocator protein (TSPO) (also known as the peripheral benzodiazepine receptor) [165], a 18 kDa transmembrane protein mainly found on the OMM [166], which is required for the mitochondrial cholesterol import that is essential for steroid hormone production [167]; the mitochondrial phosphate carrier (PiC) (also known as SLC25A3; solute carrier family 25, member 3), a ~40 kDa IMM solute carrier that is the primary transporter of inorganic phosphate (Pi) into the mitochondrial matrix [168]; and cyclophilin D (CypD), a 18.9 kDa matrix peptidyl-prolyl cis-trans isomerase that resides in the mitochondrial matrix, associates with the inner mitochondrial membrane during the mitochondrial membrane permeability transition [161], and interacts with and modulates F_1F_O–ATP synthase [169,170].

However, subsequent genetic studies showed the mPTP opening in the absence of ANT, VDAC, TSPO and PiC, suggesting that these proteins are not an integral component of the mPTP structure, but rather may play regulatory roles in pore formation [171–175].

The evidence accumulated in the last ten years has brought a new player to the scene that provides the key to the solution of the elusive and long-lasting enigma in mPTP biology. This new player is F_1F_O–ATP synthase, the ubiquitous and universal enzyme that provides cellular energy in the form of ATP by oxidative phosphorylation and photophosphorylation in animals, plants and microorganisms, thus leading to a dual and critical role of F_1F_O–ATP synthase in the regulation of cell life and death, playing major roles in energy generation and apoptosis regulation [176].

In mitochondria, oxidative phosphorylation has the following two critical parts: the ETC and chemiosmosis. The ETC includes a series of protein complexes (complex I, II, III and IV) bound to the IMM, through which electrons pass through in a series of redox reactions, leading to the translocation of protons from the mitochondrial matrix to the IMS, and thus forming an electrochemical gradient. This proton gradient increases the acidity in the IMS, generating an electrical difference with a positive charge outside and a negative charge inside. F_1F_O–ATP synthase (also known as complex V) uses the ETC-generated proton gradient across the IMM to form ATP through a chemiosmotic process. This enzyme is made up of two mechanical rotary motors, each driven by ATP hydrolysis or proton flux down the membrane potential of the protons. These two molecular motors, connected by a common rotor shaft, interconvert the chemical energy of ATP hydrolysis and proton electrochemical potential through mechanical rotation of the rotary shaft.

Mitochondrial F_1F_O–ATP synthase can undergo a Ca^{2+}-dependent transformation to form channels with properties matching those of the mPTP, as a key player in cell death [177]. The catalytic site of the F_1F_O–ATP synthase β subunit constitutes the Ca^{2+} trigger site, involved in the induction of a conformational change and transition of the F_1F_O–ATP synthase to a channel, behaving as an mPTP [177]. F_1F_O–ATP synthase is a complex enzyme with a molecular weight of >500 kDa, made up of two sectors, the inner membrane bound F_O region (indicating that it can be inhibited by the antibiotic oligomycin) and the matrix-exposed F_1 region, acting as rotary motors (Figure 6). The F1 sector (~380 kDa) is the hydrophilic water-soluble part of the complex, which acts as an ATP-driven motor and is composed of three copies of each of the subunits α and β (catalytic subunit), forming the catalytic head of the complex, and one each of the subunits γ, δ and ε, which constitute the central stalk of the complex. F_1 faces the mitochondrial matrix, and conformational changes in the F_1 subunits catalyze the formation of ATP from ADP and Pi. The F_O sector (~120 kDa) is hydrophobic and embedded in the IMM. F_O contains a proton corridor that is protonated and deprotonated repeatedly as H^+ ions flow down the gradient from the IMS to the matrix, causing rotation, which in turn alters the orientation and conformation of the F_1 subunits, thus driving ATP synthesis. F_O consists of several copies of subunit c

(8 to 10 copies in mammalian mitochondria) [178–180], which form a ring complex, and one copy each of the following subunits: b, the oligomycin sensitivity-conferring protein (OSCP); d and F6, which constitute the F_O peripheral stalk; f, the 6.8-kDa mitochondrial proteolipid (6.8PL), diabetes-associated protein in insulin-sensitive tissues (DAPIT); and g e, a and A6L, which act as F_O supernumerary subunits [180] (Figure 6). The c-ring is critical for the transport of protons through the F_O region [180]. The two F_O and F_1 sectors of the F_1F_O–ATP synthase complex push each other in the opposite direction [181], thus transforming a proton electrochemical potential into the synthesis of ATP from ADP and P_i. However, this complex can also act in the reverse direction, hydrolyzing ATP to pump protons and form an electrochemical potential. When the electrochemical potential of the protons is large enough to surpass the free energy of ATP hydrolysis, it drives the F_O sector to generate a rotary torque upon proton translocation through the c-ring to produce ATP synthesis in the F_1 sector. Conversely, when the electrochemical potential is small, the F_1 sector, acting as an F_1–ATPase (hydrolyzing ATP) induces F_O to rotate the c-ring in the reverse direction to pump protons against the electrochemical potential [181]. Thus, the proton electrochemical potential can drive the complex to synthesize ATP and, conversely, ATP hydrolysis (as an ATP-driven motor) can lead to the transfer of protons in the opposite way. Dimers of the F_1F_O–ATP synthase complex have been shown to be distributed along the inner folds of the mitochondrial cristae by high-resolution transmission electron microscopy [182,183]. This dimerization and localization of the F_1F_O–ATP synthase at the tips of the cristae induces a strong curvature to the membrane, leading to the characteristic folded morphology of the mitochondrial cristae [183,184]. The F_1F_O–ATP synthase would act as a sink of protons [182], generating a H^+ gradient higher at the cristae than in the rest of the intermembrane space. Compelling evidence has led to the novel concept that the IMM-embedded c-subunit ring of the membrane-spanning component F_O of the human mitochondrial ATP synthase complex, forms the mPTP [185–188], and this pore is also functional in the ATP synthase monomer, not requiring ATP synthase dimerization [189,190]. The purified reconstituted c-subunit ring of the F_1F_O–ATP synthase forms a voltage-sensitive channel, the persistent opening of which leads to the rapid and uncontrolled depolarization of the IMM in cells [187]. Depletion of the c-subunit hinders Ca^{2+}-induced IMM depolarization as well as Ca^{2+}- and ROS-induced cell death, whereas the overexpression of the c-subunit favors cell death [187]. Genetic manipulation of c-subunit expression levels by siRNA in HeLa cervical cancer cells affected the mPTP activity [185]. Knockdown of the c-subunits of the F_1F_O–ATP synthase reduced the mPTP opening in response to ionomycin or hydrogen peroxide and their overexpression enhanced the mPTP opening [185].

The current view of the mPTP includes a c-subunit channel embedded in the IMM (Figure 6). Mnatsakanyan and Jonas [190] have proposed a model of the F_1F_O–ATP synthase c-subunit channel, in which there are physiological reversible and pathological non-reversible openings of the c-subunit ring pore (Figure 6). It has been envisaged that the F_1 sector of the F_1F_O–ATP synthase can act as an inhibitor of the c-subunit ring pore and it can be reversibly tilted, through a conformational change, to release the close contact between the F_1 sector and the c-subunit pore in the F_O sector. This conformational change pulls away F_1 from the mouth of the c-subunit pore to open the channel from the matrix side (Figure 6). Under certain circumstances, including during long-lasting openings of the c-subunit channel, F_1 dissociates from F_O, thus leading to a permanent opening, mitochondria swelling, OMM rupture, and cell death. These conformational changes can be induced by the mPTP inducers CypD and Ca^{2+} through their binding to the OSCP and β subunit of the F_1F_O–ATP synthase, respectively, thus inducing a conformational change in the ATP synthase peripheral stalk subunits, promoting the removal of the F_1 sector from the top of the c-ring.

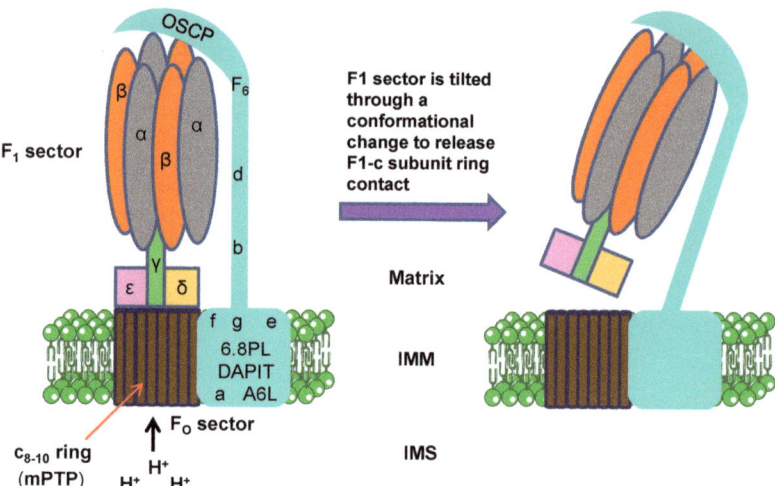

Figure 6. Organization of subunits in F_1F_O–ATP synthase in mammalian mitochondria and opening of the mPTP. OSCP, F6, d, and b constitute the F_O peripheral stalk. Under certain circumstances, the F_O peripheral stalk and F_1 sector are tilted to free the c-subunit ring channel from the side facing the matrix, thus opening the mPTP (see [190]). See text for details. IMM, inner mitochondrial membrane. IMS, inter-membrane space. mPTP, mitochondrial permeability transition pore.

The pro-apoptotic Bcl-2 family members Bax and Bak have been suggested to function as the OMM component of the mPTP in regulating cell death [191]. The mitochondria from Bax and Bak double-deleted mouse embryonic fibroblasts (MEFs) were resistant to Ca^{2+}-induced swelling, and displayed reduced OMM permeability and conductance as well as cell death [191]. In contrast, Bcl-2 (~26 kDa) and its homologue Bcl-x_L (~27 kDa), as well as other anti-apoptotic Bcl-2 family members, protect mitochondria by interacting with pro-apoptotic Bcl-2 members and hence prevent MOMP and subsequent apoptosis. The anti-apoptotic Bcl-2 members can also mediate the activity of the mPTP by direct interactions with regulatory components [192,193]. In addition, Bcl-x_L has been found to interact directly with the β-subunit of the F_1F_O–ATP synthase, regulating metabolic efficiency [194]. Thus, Bcl-x_L, once thought to be present exclusively on the OMM, is now accepted to be an F_1F_O–ATP synthase regulator in the IMM that stabilizes the inner membrane potential [194,195].

Oligomycin has been recognized as a potent inhibitor of the mitochondrial ATP synthase since the late 1950s and 1960s [196,197], with the F_O sector being responsible to confer oligomycin sensitivity [197,198]. In fact, the high-resolution (1.9 Å) crystal structure of oligomycin bound to the subunit c_{10} ring of the yeast mitochondrial ATP synthase has been reported [199].

OSCP is located on top of the catalytic F1 sector (Figure 6), connecting F_1 and the peripheral stalk, and ensuring the structural and functional coupling between F_O and F_1, which is disrupted by oligomycin [200].

The Bcl-2 family of proteins have the capacity to regulate the permeability of intracellular membranes to ions and proteins. The pro-apoptotic members of the Bcl-2 family (e.g., Bax and Bid) are able to form channels in the membranes and regulate preexisting channels, whereas the anti-apoptotic Bcl-2 members have the opposing effects on membrane channel formation [201].

9. Edelfosine Induces Indirect and Direct Effects on Mitochondria

The inhibitor of the mPTP cyclosporin A [202] inhibited [47,82], whereas Bcl-2 or Bcl-x_L overexpression totally prevented [9,40,47] edelfosine-induced apoptosis in cancer cells. These results, together with the edelfosine-induced mitochondrial-mediated changes depicted in Figure 2, provide strong evidence for the major role of mitochondria in the apoptotic response triggered by edelfosine in cancer cells.

The fact that edelfosine induces Bid cleavage, generating the 15 kDa cleaved form of truncated Bid (tBid), as well as BAP31 cleavage into the p20 fragment [39,40,49], further supports the involvement of mitochondria in the pro-apoptotic action of the ether lipid. Taken together, this suggests a complex interplay between the plasma membrane, ER and mitochondria in edelfosine action. Bid is a potent pro-apoptotic Bcl-2 family member which, upon proteolytic activation by caspases 8 or 10, translocates onto mitochondria and promotes the activation of Bax/Bak, thus contributing to cytochrome c release [203]. BAP31 is an integral membrane protein of the ER that modulates ER-mediated apoptosis through its caspase-8-mediated cleavage into a 20 kDa fragment. This p20–BAP31 fragment prompts the discharge of Ca^{2+} from the ER and its concomitant uptake into the mitochondria, thus directing pro-apoptotic signals between the ER and mitochondria [204]. Edelfosine induces all these changes, namely, caspase-8 and -10 activation, Bax activation, cytochrome c release, $\Delta\Psi_m$ loss, depletion of ER-stored Ca^{2+}, and the generation of the p20–BAP31 fragment, leading to cell death [9,27,28,39,40] (Figure 2). In addition, $bax^{-/-}$ $bak^{-/-}$ double-knockout SV-40-transformed MEFs were resistant to edelfosine [39], further supporting the involvement of mitochondria in the ether lipid-induced apoptosis response. These data strongly suggest the mitochondrial involvement in the pro-apoptotic effect of edelfosine, through signals generated from the death receptor-mediated extrinsic apoptotic signaling in membrane lipid rafts and from an ER stress response.

The accumulation of edelfosine in the mitochondria also raises the possibility that the ether lipid could have a direct effect on the mitochondria during the onset of apoptosis. In fact, we found that edelfosine accumulates in the mitochondria in cancer cells [81,82] and affects the mitochondria in a direct way [81,205]. Edelfosine induced swelling in isolated mitochondria from adult rat livers, indicating an increase in the mitochondrial membrane permeability [81,205]. This mitochondrial swelling was independent of ROS generation [81,205]. Furthermore, edelfosine was also found to inhibit mitochondrial respiration and decrease transmembrane electric potential on the isolated mitochondria [205]. These latter effects were also observed with the APL perifosine, together with its ability to induce mitochondrial permeability transition [205], suggesting that the above actions constitute a rather general feature of APLs. Interestingly, preincubation with the cholesterol-depleting agent methyl-β-cyclodextrin (MCD) [9,206], which disrupts membrane rafts, inhibited edelfosine-induced mitochondrial swelling in the isolated mitochondria [81], suggesting that the action of edelfosine on isolated mitochondria seems to be dependent on mitochondrial lipid rafts.

10. Edelfosine-Induced Apoptosis Involves F_1F_O–ATPase and Its Recruitment to Lipid Rafts

Oligomycin is a highly selective inhibitor of the membrane-embedded F_O sector (proton channel) of the F_1F_O–ATP synthase that binds to the rotating c-ring within the membrane and inhibits the enzyme complex [199,207,208]. We found that oligomycin prevented edelfosine-induced $\Delta\Psi_m$ dissipation and DNA degradation in cancer cells and *Leishmania* parasites [82], suggesting a major role of the F_O component of the F_1F_O–ATP synthase in the antitumor and anti-*Leishmania* activity of the ether lipid. In fact, recent data indicate that the accumulation of edelfosine in the kinetoplast-mitochondrion, leading to $\Delta\Psi_m$ loss and to the successive breakdown of mitochondrial and nuclear DNA, underlies the potent action of this alkylphosphocholine analog against *Leishmania* parasites [82]. Oligomycin also attenuated apoptosis and $\Delta\Psi_m$ loss induced by erufosine in glioblastoma cells [209]. Erufosine was found to interact with the 18 kDa translocator protein (TSPO), leading to the activation of the mitochondrial apoptosis cascade [20]. Furthermore, the *Saccharomyces cerevisiae ATP7Δ* mutant, with a deletion in the gene encoding for subunit d of the stator stalk of mitochondrial F_1F_O–ATP synthase, which is conserved in mammalian cells [210], was resistant to edelfosine [82]. This edelfosine-resistant phenotype could be reverted by transformation with the wild-type *ATP7* gene [82]. The above evidence strongly supports the involvement of F_1F_O–ATPase in the killing activity of edelfosine and in the onset of APL-induced apoptosis in general.

Edelfosine affects membrane lipid organization, making membranes more fluid [211,212]. On these grounds, edelfosine could be hypothesized to make the OMM more porous and permeable, thus favoring the leakage of H^+ ions. This would lead to the dissipation of the proton gradient, and therefore the F_1F_O–ATP synthase could run in reverse, that is, hydrolyzing ATP and alkalinizing the matrix by proton extrusion. Matrix alkalinization causes the mPTP opening [213], and then it could be envisaged that the F_1F_O–ATP synthase could promote the onset of cell death by this F_1F_O–ATP synthase-mediated increase in the matrix pH. This mechanism has been previously proposed for the inhibition of Bax-induced apoptosis by oligomycin in yeast and mammalian cells [214].

By proteomic analyses in lipid rafts, isolated from different hematological cancer cells through discontinuous sucrose gradient centrifugation [215,216], we found that edelfosine treatment in hematological cancer cells led to a dramatic recruitment of mitochondrial F_1F_O–ATP synthase to the rafts [82]. This remarkable F_1F_O–ATP synthase translocation into the rafts could suggest that the enzyme is either translocated to lipid rafts present at the cell surface or in the mitochondria. Several studies have reported the presence of raft-located F_1F_O–ATP synthase at the plasma membrane of different normal and tumor cells, having been proposed to act as a proton channel, a modulator of extracellular ATP level, or as a regulator of intracellular Ca^{2+} levels, involved in numerous biological processes, including cell migration and intracellular pH modulation [217–224].

11. Edelfosine Promotes Raft Translocation to Mitochondria and Presence of Raft-Like Domains in Mitochondria

The present evidence cannot discern between the translocation of F_1F_O–ATP synthase to lipid rafts at the cell surface or to raft domains present in the mitochondria. However, edelfosine has been shown to promote the redistribution of lipid rafts from the plasma membrane to the mitochondria, suggesting a raft-mediated plasma membrane–mitochondria link [81]. In this context, we have found a lipid raft-mediated connection between the extrinsic and intrinsic apoptotic pathways in human multiple myeloma MM144 cells [225].

The fact that edelfosine can interact with plasma membrane lipid rafts and mitochondria could led us to suggest that the ether lipid could be translocated from the plasma membrane to the mitochondria, where it would ultimately exert its pro-apoptotic activity promoting the accumulation of F_1F_O–ATP synthase into mitochondrial rafts, $\Delta\Psi_m$ dissipation, cytochrome *c* release, leading eventually to cell demise. Lipid rafts were mainly located at the plasma membrane in untreated HeLa cells, as assessed by the raft marker fluorescein isothiocyanate-cholera toxin B subunit that binds ganglioside GM1 [226], mainly found in these domains [227]. Mitochondria (stained with MitoTracker Red) were observed as a widespread network in the interior of the cell. Following edelfosine treatment, the membrane rafts were gradually internalized into the cell, and colocalized with mitochondria at the time of apoptosis onset, thus unveiling a link between plasma membrane rafts and mitochondria driven by edelfosine [81]. This suggests the presence of cholesterol-rich raft-like domains in mitochondria that could be involved in edelfosine-induced apoptosis. It is interesting to note that the GD3 raft component can proceed from the cell plasma membrane to the mitochondria via a microtubule-dependent mechanism, which could be regulated by CLIPR-59, a new CLIP-170-related protein involved in microtubule dynamics [228–230]. Although the presence of lipid rafts in mitochondria remains a controversial issue [231–234], there is increasing evidence favoring the presence of raft-like domains in theses organelles. Lipid raft-like domains enriched in ganglioside GD3 have been found in mitochondria and are involved in apoptosis regulation [229,232,235]. It is tempting to speculate that mitochondrial membrane rafts represent specific sites where certain critical biochemical processes, including apoptosis modulation, take place. Consistently, raft disruption prevented edelfosine-induced swelling in isolated mitochondria [81] as well as mitochondrial depolarization induced by GD3 or tBid [232]. Cholesterol levels in MAMs are higher than in the rest of the ER and they influence ER–mitochondria association [106,236,237], suggesting the importance of MAMs in providing cholesterol, and likely raft components, to the mitochondria membranes. The ganglioside GM1, abundant in lipid rafts, has been reported to accumulate in the glycosphingolipid-enriched domains of MAMs, linking ER stress to Ca^{2+}-dependent mitochondrial apoptosis [238]. The physical interaction between the ER and mitochondria [239] could underlie the localization of edelfosine in both the ER [40,49,76] and mitochondria [81,82] of cancer cells. This could explain how edelfosine-mediated ER stress, which releases ER-stored Ca^{2+}, requires mitochondria for the apoptotic outcome [40,49,76].

12. Conclusions

This review presents a compilation and discussion of the different pieces of evidence that support the involvement and critical role of mitochondria in the antitumor action of the ether lipid edelfosine, and likely other APLs. Edelfosine accumulates in the lipid rafts, ER and mitochondria in tumor cells. The close interplay between the lipid rafts, ER and mitochondria could explain the above physical localization of edelfosine within cancer cells. Lipid rafts could be the common hypothetical link and means of ether lipid transport between the different cellular loci. Figure 7 summarizes the pleiotropic effects exerted by edelfosine on several cellular functions as a result of the drug action in a number of biochemical processes occurring in lipid rafts, ER and mitochondria. The apoptotic signaling triggered by edelfosine following raft-mediated Fas/CD95 engagement and ER stress converge through the mitochondria to render an apoptotic outcome. Mitochondria behave as the critical subcellular master regulator of cell demise. Thus, protection of mitochondria with the overexpression of Bcl-2 or Bcl-x_L blocks the apoptotic signals triggered by Fas/CD95 or ER stress, and prevents cell death. The affinity of edelfosine for cholesterol, a major and essential constituent of membrane rafts, could explain the above interplay between the rafts, ER and mitochondria as well as the presence of the ether lipid in the above membrane domains and organelles. The higher cholesterol level in mitochondria from tumor cells as well as in the MAMs, connecting the ER and mitochondria, together with the presence of raft domains in the mitochondria could explain the presence of edelfosine in mitochondria. Interestingly, edelfosine induces the translocation of lipid rafts from the plasma membrane to the mitochondria, pointing out a link between the cell surface and mitochondria that could also involve the ER. Although a hypothetical translocation of lipid rafts from the plasma membrane to the mitochondria, through yet unknown mechanisms, could take place, an alternative and plausible explanation could involve edelfosine-induced changes in the mitochondrial membrane (e.g., through altered cholesterol levels or distribution) resulting in the formation of raft-like structures in the mitochondria. The presence of lipid rafts or raft-like domains in mitochondria is a controversial issue, but increasing evidence supports their existence. Furthermore, the higher level of cholesterol in the mitochondria of tumor cells might suggest that cancer cell mitochondria are rather enriched in cholesterol-rich rafts that could harbor proteins and biochemical processes critical for the modulation of cell fate. In this regard, it is interesting to note that F_1F_O–ATP synthase is located in lipid rafts and that the c-subunit ring of the F_O sector constitutes the mPTP. Thus, the evidence discussed here strongly suggests that lipid rafts play a key role in the regulation of cell survival or cell death. Edelfosine, which interacts with cholesterol and accumulates in lipid rafts, promotes cell death through reorganizing the lipid rafts and their composition. In this context, edelfosine induces the recruitment of F_1F_O–ATP synthase into membrane rafts, and oligomycin, the potent inhibitor of the F_O sector, blocks edelfosine-induced apoptosis. These data support a major role for F_1F_O–ATP synthase in the modulation of cell death. A plausible mechanism for the pro-apoptotic effect of edelfosine in tumor cells could involve the lipid raft-mediated translocation of edelfosine from the plasma membrane to the mitochondria, where it will ultimately exert its cytotoxic activity promoting the accumulation of F_1F_O–ATP synthase in mitochondrial rafts, thus leading to $\Delta\Psi_m$ dissipation, cytochrome c release, and eventually cell demise. The localization of edelfosine in the ER and mitochondria is in close agreement with the interaction between the ER and mitochondria, and suggests that this ether lipid could be studied as an interesting molecule to yield a further insight into these organelle interactions. This ether lipid could be used as a tool to understand the physiological and pharmacological relevance of ER–mitochondria junctions. Membrane targeting by the APL edelfosine might unveil a fascinating network of communication between the plasma membrane and organelle membranes to control cell death, as well as new insights into the role of novel membrane domains within mitochondria. These studies should help to understand membrane trafficking to mitochondria, and the link between lipid rafts and mitochondria, thus opening new avenues for novel therapeutic approaches in cancer therapy and other biomedical applications where cell death should be critically controlled. The results discussed in this review highlight the importance of cholesterol and lipid rafts in the control of cell death by mitochondria as well as in mitochondrial targeting in cancer therapy.

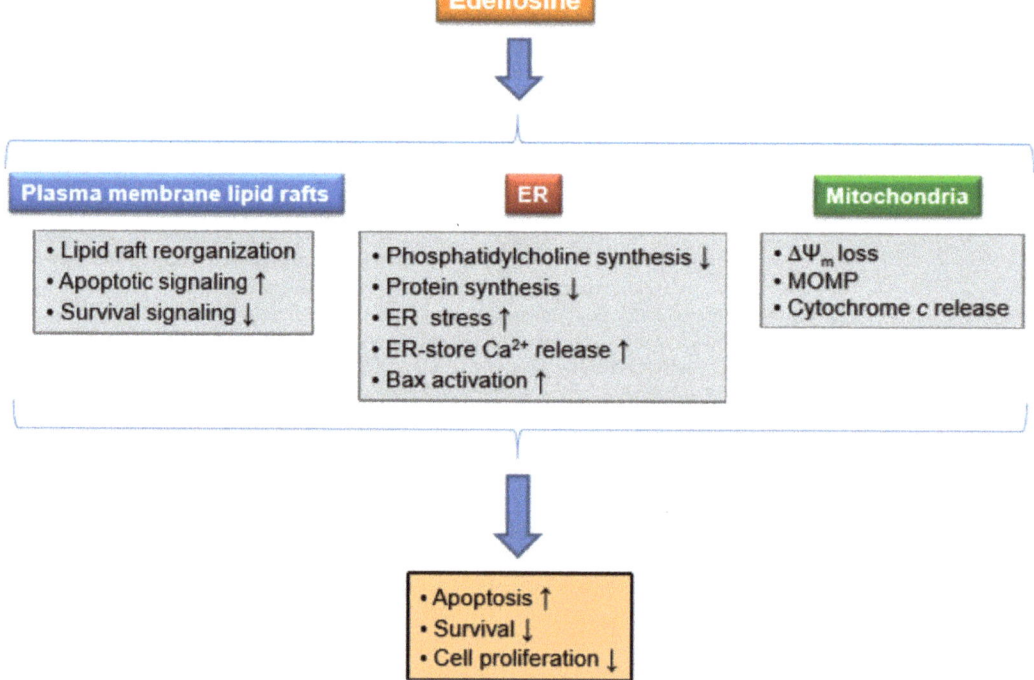

Figure 7. Major effects of edelfosine on lipid rafts, ER and mitochondria, and the subsequent consequences on cellular functions related to cell fate. This scheme represents several biochemical processes and cellular functions affected by edelfosine in cancer cells as discussed in the text and references therein.

Author Contributions: The manuscript was written through the contributions of all authors. All authors have read and agreed to the published version of the manuscript.

Funding: This work was funded by the Spanish Ministry of Science, Innovation and Universities (SAF2017-89672-R grant).

Institutional Review Board Statement: Not applicable.

Informed Consent Statement: Not applicable.

Data Availability Statement: Not applicable.

Conflicts of Interest: The authors declare no conflict of interest.

Abbreviations

AELs	antitumor ether lipids
ANT	adenine nucleotide translocator
APAF-1	apoptosis protease-activating factor-1
APLs	alkylphospholipid analogs
BODIPY	4,4-difluoro-4-bora-3a,4a-diaza-s-indacene; boron-dipyrromethene
CypD	cyclophilin D
$\Delta\Psi_m$	mitochondrial transmembrane potential
DiOC6(3)	3,3′-dihexyloxacarbocyanine iodide
ER	endoplasmic reticulum
ET-18-OCH$_3$	1-O-octadecyl-2-O-methyl-rac-glycero-3-phosphocholine (edelfosine)
ETC	electron transport chain
IMM	inner mitochondrial membrane
IMS	inter-membrane space
MAMs	mitochondria-associated membranes
MCD	methyl-β-cyclodextrin
MEFs	mouse embryonic fibroblasts
MLN64	metastatic lymph node 64 protein
MOMP	mitochondrial outer membrane permeabilization
mPTP	mitochondrial permeability transition pore
NP-C	Niemann-Pick disease type C
NPC1	Niemann-Pick type C1 protein
OMM	outer mitochondrial membrane
OSCP	oligomycin sensitivity-conferring protein
PiC	mitochondrial phosphate carrier (PiC)
ROS	reactive oxygen species
SLC25A3	solute carrier family 25, member 3
SNAP-23	23-kDa synaptosome associated protein
STARD1	steroidogenic acute regulatory protein-related lipid transfer domain containing protein 1
STARD3	steroidogenic acute regulatory protein-related lipid transfer domain containing protein 3
tBid	truncated Bid
TSPO	translocator protein
VDAC1	voltage-dependent anion-selective channel 1

References

1. Gajate, C.; Mollinedo, F. Biological activities, mechanisms of action and biomedical prospect of the antitumor ether phospholipid ET-18-OCH$_3$ (Edelfosine), a proapoptotic agent in tumor cells. *Curr. Drug Metab.* **2002**, *3*, 491–525. [CrossRef] [PubMed]
2. Mollinedo, F.; Gajate, C.; Martin-Santamaria, S.; Gago, F. ET-18-OCH$_3$ (edelfosine): A selective antitumour lipid targeting apoptosis through intracellular activation of Fas/CD95 death receptor. *Curr. Med. Chem.* **2004**, *11*, 3163–3184. [CrossRef]
3. Mollinedo, F. Editorial: Antitumor alkylphospholipid analogs: A promising and growing family of synthetic cell membrane-targeting molecules for cancer treatment. *Anticancer Agents Med. Chem.* **2014**, *14*, 495–498. [CrossRef]
4. Sundar, S.; Jha, T.K.; Thakur, C.P.; Bhattacharya, S.K.; Rai, M. Oral miltefosine for the treatment of Indian visceral leishmaniasis. *Trans. R. Soc. Trop. Med. Hyg.* **2006**, *100* (Suppl. S1), S26–S33. [CrossRef] [PubMed]
5. Sundar, S.; Jha, T.K.; Thakur, C.P.; Engel, J.; Sindermann, H.; Fischer, C.; Junge, K.; Bryceson, A.; Berman, J. Oral miltefosine for Indian visceral leishmaniasis. *N. Engl. J. Med.* **2002**, *347*, 1739–1746. [CrossRef]
6. Dorlo, T.P.; Balasegaram, M.; Beijnen, J.H.; de Vries, P.J. Miltefosine: A review of its pharmacology and therapeutic efficacy in the treatment of leishmaniasis. *J. Antimicrob. Chemother.* **2012**, *67*, 2576–2597. [CrossRef]
7. Smorenburg, C.H.; Seynaeve, C.; Bontenbal, M.; Planting, A.S.; Sindermann, H.; Verweij, J. Phase II study of miltefosine 6% solution as topical treatment of skin metastases in breast cancer patients. *Anticancer Drugs* **2000**, *11*, 825–828. [CrossRef]

8. Dos Santos Nogueira, F.; Avino, V.C.; Galvis-Ovallos, F.; Pereira-Chioccola, V.L.; Moreira, M.A.B.; Romariz, A.; Molla, L.M.; Menz, I. Use of miltefosine to treat canine visceral leishmaniasis caused by *Leishmania infantum* in Brazil. *Parasit Vectors* **2019**, *12*, 79. [CrossRef] [PubMed]
9. Gajate, C.; Mollinedo, F. Edelfosine and perifosine induce selective apoptosis in multiple myeloma by recruitment of death receptors and downstream signaling molecules into lipid rafts. *Blood* **2007**, *109*, 711–719. [CrossRef] [PubMed]
10. Richardson, P.G.; Eng, C.; Kolesar, J.; Hideshima, T.; Anderson, K.C. Perifosine, an oral, anti-cancer agent and inhibitor of the Akt pathway: Mechanistic actions, pharmacodynamics, pharmacokinetics, and clinical activity. *Expert Opin. Drug Metab. Toxicol.* **2012**, *8*, 623–633. [CrossRef] [PubMed]
11. Hasegawa, K.; Kagabu, M.; Mizuno, M.; Oda, K.; Aoki, D.; Mabuchi, S.; Kamiura, S.; Yamaguchi, S.; Aoki, Y.; Saito, T.; et al. Phase II basket trial of perifosine monotherapy for recurrent gynecologic cancer with or without PIK3CA mutations. *Invest. New Drugs* **2017**, *35*, 800–812. [CrossRef] [PubMed]
12. Becher, O.J.; Millard, N.E.; Modak, S.; Kushner, B.H.; Haque, S.; Spasojevic, I.; Trippett, T.M.; Gilheeney, S.W.; Khakoo, Y.; Lyden, D.C.; et al. A phase I study of single-agent perifosine for recurrent or refractory pediatric CNS and solid tumors. *PLoS ONE* **2017**, *12*, e0178593. [CrossRef] [PubMed]
13. Kaley, T.J.; Panageas, K.S.; Mellinghoff, I.K.; Nolan, C.; Gavrilovic, I.T.; DeAngelis, L.M.; Abrey, L.E.; Holland, E.C.; Lassman, A.B. Phase II trial of an AKT inhibitor (perifosine) for recurrent glioblastoma. *J. Neurooncol.* **2019**, *144*, 403–407. [CrossRef]
14. Richardson, P.G.; Nagler, A.; Ben-Yehuda, D.; Badros, A.; Hari, P.N.; Hajek, R.; Spicka, I.; Kaya, H.; LeBlanc, R.; Yoon, S.-S.; et al. Randomized, placebo-controlled, phase 3 study of perifosine combined with bortezomib and dexamethasone in patients with relapsed, refractory multiple myeloma previously treated with bortezomib. *eJHaem* **2020**, *1*, 94–102. [CrossRef]
15. Kaley, T.J.; Panageas, K.S.; Pentsova, E.I.; Mellinghoff, I.K.; Nolan, C.; Gavrilovic, I.; DeAngelis, L.M.; Abrey, L.E.; Holland, E.C.; Omuro, A.; et al. Phase I clinical trial of temsirolimus and perifosine for recurrent glioblastoma. *Ann. Clin. Transl. Neurol.* **2020**, *7*, 429–436. [CrossRef]
16. Erdlenbruch, B.; Jendrossek, V.; Kugler, W.; Eibl, H.; Lakomek, M. Increased delivery of erucylphosphocholine to C6 gliomas by chemical opening of the blood-brain barrier using intracarotid pentylglycerol in rats. *Cancer Chemother. Pharmacol.* **2002**, *50*, 299–304. [CrossRef] [PubMed]
17. Erdlenbruch, B.; Jendrossek, V.; Marx, M.; Hunold, A.; Eibl, H.; Lakomek, M. Antitumor effects of erucylphosphocholine on brain tumor cells in vitro and in vivo. *Anticancer Res.* **1998**, *18*, 2551–2557.
18. Jendrossek, V.; Kugler, W.; Erdlenbruch, B.; Eibl, H.; Lang, F.; Lakomek, M. Erucylphosphocholine-induced apoptosis in chemoresistant glioblastoma cell lines: Involvement of caspase activation and mitochondrial alterations. *Anticancer Res.* **2001**, *21*, 3389–3396.
19. Jendrossek, V.; Muller, I.; Eibl, H.; Belka, C. Intracellular mediators of erucylphosphocholine-induced apoptosis. *Oncogene* **2003**, *22*, 2621–2631. [CrossRef]
20. Veenman, L.; Gavish, M.; Kugler, W. Apoptosis induction by erucylphosphohomocholine via the 18 kDa mitochondrial translocator protein: Implications for cancer treatment. *Anticancer Agents Med. Chem.* **2014**, *14*, 559–577. [CrossRef] [PubMed]
21. Chometon, G.; Cappuccini, F.; Raducanu, A.; Aumailley, M.; Jendrossek, V. The membrane-targeted alkylphosphocholine erufosine interferes with survival signals from the extracellular matrix. *Anticancer Agents Med. Chem.* **2014**, *14*, 578–591. [CrossRef]
22. Henke, G.; Lindner, L.H.; Vogeser, M.; Eibl, H.J.; Worner, J.; Muller, A.C.; Bamberg, M.; Wachholz, K.; Belka, C.; Jendrossek, V. Pharmacokinetics and biodistribution of Erufosine in nude mice—Implications for combination with radiotherapy. *Radiat. Oncol.* **2009**, *4*, 46. [CrossRef] [PubMed]
23. Henke, G.; Meier, V.; Lindner, L.H.; Eibl, H.; Bamberg, M.; Belka, C.; Budach, W.; Jendrossek, V. Effects of ionizing radiation in combination with Erufosine on T98G glioblastoma xenograft tumours: A study in NMRI nu/nu mice. *Radiat. Oncol.* **2012**, *7*, 172. [CrossRef] [PubMed]
24. Ansari, S.S.; Sharma, A.K.; Soni, H.; Ali, D.M.; Tews, B.; Konig, R.; Eibl, H.; Berger, M.R. Induction of ER and mitochondrial stress by the alkylphosphocholine erufosine in oral squamous cell carcinoma cells. *Cell Death Dis.* **2018**, *9*, 296. [CrossRef] [PubMed]
25. Tzoneva, R.; Stoyanova, T.; Petrich, A.; Popova, D.; Uzunova, V.; Momchilova, A.; Chiantia, S. Effect of erufosine on membrane lipid order in breast cancer cell models. *Biomolecules* **2020**, *10*, 802. [CrossRef] [PubMed]
26. Varela-M, R.E.; Villa-Pulgarin, J.A.; Yepes, E.; Muller, I.; Modolell, M.; Munoz, D.L.; Robledo, S.M.; Muskus, C.E.; Lopez-Aban, J.; Muro, A.; et al. In vitro and in vivo efficacy of ether lipid edelfosine against *Leishmania* spp. and SbV-resistant parasites. *PLoS Negl. Trop. Dis.* **2012**, *6*, e1612. [CrossRef] [PubMed]
27. Gajate, C.; Del Canto-Janez, E.; Acuna, A.U.; Amat-Guerri, F.; Geijo, E.; Santos-Beneit, A.M.; Veldman, R.J.; Mollinedo, F. Intracellular triggering of Fas aggregation and recruitment of apoptotic molecules into Fas-enriched rafts in selective tumor cell apoptosis. *J. Exp. Med.* **2004**, *200*, 353–365. [CrossRef] [PubMed]
28. Gajate, C.; Mollinedo, F. Lipid rafts, endoplasmic reticulum and mitochondria in the antitumor action of the alkylphospholipid analog edelfosine. *Anticancer Agents Med. Chem.* **2014**, *14*, 509–527. [CrossRef]
29. Jaffres, P.A.; Gajate, C.; Bouchet, A.M.; Couthon-Gourves, H.; Chantome, A.; Potier-Cartereau, M.; Besson, P.; Bougnoux, P.; Mollinedo, F.; Vandier, C. Alkyl ether lipids, ion channels and lipid raft reorganization in cancer therapy. *Pharmacol. Ther.* **2016**, *165*, 114–131. [CrossRef]

30. Mollinedo, F.; Gajate, C. Lipid rafts as signaling hubs in cancer cell survival/death and invasion: Implications in tumor progression and therapy. *J. Lipid Res.* **2020**, *61*, 611–635. [CrossRef]
31. Busto, J.V.; Sot, J.; Goni, F.M.; Mollinedo, F.; Alonso, A. Surface-active properties of the antitumour ether lipid 1-O-octadecyl-2-O-methyl-rac-glycero-3-phosphocholine (edelfosine). *Biochim. Biophys. Acta* **2007**, *1768*, 1855–1860. [CrossRef] [PubMed]
32. Mollinedo, F.; Fernandez-Luna, J.L.; Gajate, C.; Martin-Martin, B.; Benito, A.; Martinez-Dalmau, R.; Modolell, M. Selective induction of apoptosis in cancer cells by the ether lipid ET-18-OCH$_3$ (Edelfosine): Molecular structure requirements, cellular uptake, and protection by Bcl-2 and Bcl-X$_L$. *Cancer Res.* **1997**, *57*, 1320–1328. [PubMed]
33. Gajate, C.; Fonteriz, R.I.; Cabaner, C.; Alvarez-Noves, G.; Alvarez-Rodriguez, Y.; Modolell, M.; Mollinedo, F. Intracellular triggering of Fas, independently of FasL, as a new mechanism of antitumor ether lipid-induced apoptosis. *Int. J. Cancer* **2000**, *85*, 674–682. [CrossRef]
34. Mollinedo, F.; de la Iglesia-Vicente, J.; Gajate, C.; Estella-Hermoso de Mendoza, A.; Villa-Pulgarin, J.A.; Campanero, M.A.; Blanco-Prieto, M.J. Lipid raft-targeted therapy in multiple myeloma. *Oncogene* **2010**, *29*, 3748–3757. [CrossRef]
35. Mollinedo, F.; de la Iglesia-Vicente, J.; Gajate, C.; Estella-Hermoso de Mendoza, A.; Villa-Pulgarin, J.A.; de Frias, M.; Roue, G.; Gil, J.; Colomer, D.; Campanero, M.A.; et al. In vitro and in vivo selective antitumor activity of Edelfosine against mantle cell lymphoma and chronic lymphocytic leukemia involving lipid rafts. *Clin. Cancer Res.* **2010**, *16*, 2046–2054. [CrossRef]
36. Melo-Lima, S.; Gajate, C.; Mollinedo, F. Triggers and signaling cross-talk controlling cell death commitment. *Cell Cycle* **2015**, *14*, 465–466. [CrossRef] [PubMed]
37. Melo-Lima, S.; Celeste Lopes, M.; Mollinedo, F. Necroptosis is associated with low procaspase-8 and active RIPK1 and -3 in human glioma cells. *Oncoscience* **2014**, *1*, 649–664. [CrossRef] [PubMed]
38. Melo-Lima, S.; Lopes, M.C.; Mollinedo, F. ERK1/2 acts as a switch between necrotic and apoptotic cell death in ether phospholipid edelfosine-treated glioblastoma cells. *Pharmacol. Res.* **2015**, *95*, 2–11. [CrossRef] [PubMed]
39. Nieto-Miguel, T.; Fonteriz, R.I.; Vay, L.; Gajate, C.; Lopez-Hernandez, S.; Mollinedo, F. Endoplasmic reticulum stress in the proapoptotic action of edelfosine in solid tumor cells. *Cancer Res.* **2007**, *67*, 10368–10378. [CrossRef] [PubMed]
40. Gajate, C.; Matos-da-Silva, M.; Dakir, E.L.; Fonteriz, R.I.; Alvarez, J.; Mollinedo, F. Antitumor alkyl-lysophospholipid analog edelfosine induces apoptosis in pancreatic cancer by targeting endoplasmic reticulum. *Oncogene* **2012**, *31*, 2627–2639. [CrossRef]
41. Andreesen, R.; Modolell, M.; Weltzien, H.U.; Eibl, H.; Common, H.H.; Lohr, G.W.; Munder, P.G. Selective destruction of human leukemic cells by alkyl-lysophospholipids. *Cancer Res.* **1978**, *38*, 3894–3899. [PubMed]
42. Modolell, M.; Andreesen, R.; Pahlke, W.; Brugger, U.; Munder, P.G. Disturbance of phospholipid metabolism during the selective destruction of tumor cells induced by alkyl-lysophospholipids. *Cancer Res.* **1979**, *39*, 4681–4686. [PubMed]
43. Andreesen, R.; Modolell, M.; Oepke, G.H.; Common, H.; Lohr, G.W.; Munder, P.G. Studies on various parameters influencing leukemic cell destruction by alkyl-lysophospholipids. *Anticancer Res.* **1982**, *2*, 95–100. [PubMed]
44. Scholar, E.M. Inhibition of the growth of human lung cancer cells by alkyl-lysophospholipid analogs. *Cancer Lett.* **1986**, *33*, 199–204. [CrossRef]
45. Mollinedo, F.; Martinez-Dalmau, R.; Modolell, M. Early and selective induction of apoptosis in human leukemic cells by the alkyl-lysophospholipid ET-18-OCH$_3$. *Biochem. Biophys. Res. Commun.* **1993**, *192*, 603–609. [CrossRef]
46. Diomede, L.; Colotta, F.; Piovani, B.; Re, F.; Modest, E.J.; Salmona, M. Induction of apoptosis in human leukemic cells by the ether lipid 1-octadecyl-2-methyl-*rac*-glycero-3-phosphocholine. A possible basis for its selective action. *Int. J. Cancer* **1993**, *53*, 124–130. [CrossRef]
47. Gajate, C.; Santos-Beneit, A.M.; Macho, A.; Lazaro, M.; Hernandez-De Rojas, A.; Modolell, M.; Munoz, E.; Mollinedo, F. Involvement of mitochondria and caspase-3 in ET-18-OCH$_3$-induced apoptosis of human leukemic cells. *Int. J. Cancer* **2000**, *86*, 208–218. [CrossRef]
48. Gajate, C.; Mollinedo, F. The antitumor ether lipid ET-18-OCH$_3$ induces apoptosis through translocation and capping of Fas/CD95 into membrane rafts in human leukemic cells. *Blood* **2001**, *98*, 3860–3863. [CrossRef]
49. Bonilla, X.; Dakir el, H.; Mollinedo, F.; Gajate, C. Endoplasmic reticulum targeting in Ewing's sarcoma by the alkylphospholipid analog edelfosine. *Oncotarget* **2015**, *6*, 14596–14613. [CrossRef]
50. Mollinedo, F.; Gajate, C.; Morales, A.I.; del Canto-Janez, E.; Justies, N.; Collia, F.; Rivas, J.V.; Modolell, M.; Iglesias, A. Novel anti-inflammatory action of edelfosine lacking toxicity with protective effect in experimental colitis. *J. Pharmacol. Exp. Ther.* **2009**, *329*, 439–449. [CrossRef]
51. Lopez, J.; Tait, S.W. Mitochondrial apoptosis: Killing cancer using the enemy within. *Br. J. Cancer* **2015**, *112*, 957–962. [CrossRef] [PubMed]
52. Van der Luit, A.H.; Budde, M.; Ruurs, P.; Verheij, M.; van Blitterswijk, W.J. Alkyl-lysophospholipid accumulates in lipid rafts and induces apoptosis via raft-dependent endocytosis and inhibition of phosphatidylcholine synthesis. *J. Biol. Chem.* **2002**, *277*, 39541–39547. [CrossRef]
53. Mollinedo, F.; Gajate, C. Fas/CD95 death receptor and lipid rafts: New targets for apoptosis-directed cancer therapy. *Drug Resist. Updat.* **2006**, *9*, 51–73. [CrossRef]
54. Gajate, C.; Gonzalez-Camacho, F.; Mollinedo, F. Involvement of raft aggregates enriched in Fas/CD95 death-inducing signaling complex in the antileukemic action of edelfosine in Jurkat cells. *PLoS ONE* **2009**, *4*, e5044. [CrossRef] [PubMed]
55. Reis-Sobreiro, M.; Gajate, C.; Mollinedo, F. Involvement of mitochondria and recruitment of Fas/CD95 signaling in lipid rafts in resveratrol-mediated antimyeloma and antileukemia actions. *Oncogene* **2009**, *28*, 3221–3234. [CrossRef] [PubMed]

56. Mollinedo, F.; Gajate, C. Lipid rafts and clusters of apoptotic signaling molecule-enriched rafts in cancer therapy. *Future Oncol.* **2010**, *6*, 811–821. [CrossRef]
57. Mollinedo, F.; Gajate, C. Lipid rafts, death receptors and CASMERs: New insights for cancer therapy. *Future Oncol.* **2010**, *6*, 491–494. [CrossRef]
58. Mollinedo, F. Death receptors in multiple myeloma and therapeutic opportunities. In *Myeloma Therapy. Pursuing the Plasma Cell*; Lonial, S., Ed.; Humana Press: Totowa, NJ, USA, 2008; pp. 393–419.
59. Gajate, C.; Mollinedo, F. Lipid rafts and Fas/CD95 signaling in cancer chemotherapy. *Recent Pat. Anticancer Drug Discov.* **2011**, *6*, 274–283. [CrossRef]
60. Gajate, C.; Mollinedo, F. Lipid rafts and raft-mediated supramolecular entities in the regulation of CD95 death receptor apoptotic signaling. *Apoptosis* **2015**, *20*, 584–606. [CrossRef]
61. Gajate, C.; Mollinedo, F. Lipid raft-mediated Fas/CD95 apoptotic signaling in leukemic cells and normal leukocytes and therapeutic implications. *J. Leukoc. Biol.* **2015**, *98*, 739–759. [CrossRef]
62. Mollinedo, F.; Gajate, C. Lipid rafts as major platforms for signaling regulation in cancer. *Adv. Biol. Regul.* **2015**, *57*, 130–146. [CrossRef] [PubMed]
63. Mollinedo, F.; Gajate, C. Fas/CD95, Lipid rafts, and cancer. In *TRAIL, Fas Ligand, TNF and TLR3 in Cancer*; Micheau, O., Ed.; Springer International Publishing AG: Cham, Switzerland, 2017; pp. 187–227.
64. Mollinedo, F.; Gajate, C. FasL-independent activation of Fas. In *Fas Signaling*; Wajant, H., Ed.; Landes Bioscience and Springer Science: Georgetown, TX, USA, 2006; pp. 13–27.
65. Reis-Sobreiro, M.; Roue, G.; Moros, A.; Gajate, C.; de la Iglesia-Vicente, J.; Colomer, D.; Mollinedo, F. Lipid raft-mediated Akt signaling as a therapeutic target in mantle cell lymphoma. *Blood Cancer J.* **2013**, *3*, e118. [CrossRef] [PubMed]
66. Mollinedo, F. Lipid raft involvement in yeast cell growth and death. *Front. Oncol.* **2012**, *2*, 140. [CrossRef] [PubMed]
67. Serrano, R.; Kielland-Brandt, M.C.; Fink, G.R. Yeast plasma membrane ATPase is essential for growth and has homology with ($Na^+ + K^+$)-, K^+- and Ca^{2+}-ATPases. *Nature* **1986**, *319*, 689–693. [CrossRef]
68. Bagnat, M.; Chang, A.; Simons, K. Plasma membrane proton ATPase Pma1p requires raft association for surface delivery in yeast. *Mol. Biol. Cell* **2001**, *12*, 4129–4138. [CrossRef]
69. Zaremberg, V.; Gajate, C.; Cacharro, L.M.; Mollinedo, F.; McMaster, C.R. Cytotoxicity of an anti-cancer lysophospholipid through selective modification of lipid raft composition. *J. Biol. Chem.* **2005**, *280*, 38047–38058. [CrossRef]
70. Cuesta-Marban, A.; Botet, J.; Czyz, O.; Cacharro, L.M.; Gajate, C.; Hornillos, V.; Delgado, J.; Zhang, H.; Amat-Guerri, F.; Acuna, A.U.; et al. Drug uptake, lipid rafts, and vesicle trafficking modulate resistance to an anticancer lysophosphatidylcholine analogue in yeast. *J. Biol. Chem.* **2013**, *288*, 8405–8418. [CrossRef] [PubMed]
71. Czyz, O.; Bitew, T.; Cuesta-Marban, A.; McMaster, C.R.; Mollinedo, F.; Zaremberg, V. Alteration of plasma membrane organization by an anticancer lysophosphatidylcholine analogue induces intracellular acidification and internalization of plasma membrane transporters in yeast. *J. Biol. Chem.* **2013**, *288*, 8419–8432. [CrossRef]
72. Malinska, K.; Malinsky, J.; Opekarova, M.; Tanner, W. Visualization of protein compartmentation within the plasma membrane of living yeast cells. *Mol. Biol. Cell* **2003**, *14*, 4427–4436. [CrossRef]
73. Hearn, J.D.; Lester, R.L.; Dickson, R.C. The uracil transporter Fur4p associates with lipid rafts. *J. Biol. Chem.* **2003**, *278*, 3679–3686. [CrossRef]
74. Ausili, A.; Martinez-Valera, P.; Torrecillas, A.; Gomez-Murcia, V.; de Godos, A.M.; Corbalan-Garcia, S.; Teruel, J.A.; Gomez Fernandez, J.C. Anticancer agent edelfosine exhibits a high affinity for cholesterol and disorganizes liquid-ordered membrane structures. *Langmuir* **2018**, *34*, 8333–8346. [CrossRef]
75. Busto, J.V.; del Canto-Jañez, E.; Goñi, F.M.; Mollinedo, F.; Alonso, A. Combination of the anti-tumour cell ether lipid edelfosine with sterols abolishes haemolytic side effects of the drug. *J. Chem. Biol.* **2008**, *1*, 89–94. [CrossRef] [PubMed]
76. Nieto-Miguel, T.; Gajate, C.; Mollinedo, F. Differential targets and subcellular localization of antitumor alkyl-lysophospholipid in leukemic versus solid tumor Cells. *J. Biol. Chem.* **2006**, *281*, 14833–14840. [CrossRef] [PubMed]
77. Zhang, H.; Gajate, C.; Yu, L.P.; Fang, Y.X.; Mollinedo, F. Mitochondrial-derived ROS in edelfosine-induced apoptosis in yeasts and tumor cells. *Acta Pharmacol. Sin.* **2007**, *28*, 888–894. [CrossRef]
78. Quesada, E.; Delgado, J.; Gajate, C.; Mollinedo, F.; Acuna, A.U.; Amat-Guerri, F. Fluorescent phenylpolyene analogues of the ether phospholipid edelfosine for the selective labeling of cancer cells. *J. Med. Chem.* **2004**, *47*, 5333–5335. [CrossRef] [PubMed]
79. Mateo, C.R.; Souto, A.A.; Amat-Guerri, F.; Acuna, A.U. New fluorescent octadecapentaenoic acids as probes of lipid membranes and protein-lipid interactions. *Biophys. J.* **1996**, *71*, 2177–2191. [CrossRef]
80. Quesada, E.; Acuna, A.U.; Amat-Guerri, F. New Transmembrane Polyene Bolaamphiphiles as Fluorescent Probes in Lipid Bilayers. *Angew. Chem. Int. Ed. Engl.* **2001**, *40*, 2095–2097. [CrossRef]
81. Mollinedo, F.; Fernandez, M.; Hornillos, V.; Delgado, J.; Amat-Guerri, F.; Acuna, A.U.; Nieto-Miguel, T.; Villa-Pulgarin, J.A.; Gonzalez-Garcia, C.; Cena, V.; et al. Involvement of lipid rafts in the localization and dysfunction effect of the antitumor ether phospholipid edelfosine in mitochondria. *Cell Death Dis.* **2011**, *2*, e158. [CrossRef] [PubMed]
82. Villa-Pulgarin, J.A.; Gajate, C.; Botet, J.; Jimenez, A.; Justies, N.; Varela, M.R.; Cuesta-Marban, A.; Muller, I.; Modolell, M.; Revuelta, J.L.; et al. Mitochondria and lipid raft-located F_OF_1-ATP synthase as major therapeutic targets in the antileishmanial and anticancer activities of ether lipid edelfosine. *PLoS Negl. Trop. Dis.* **2017**, *11*, e0005805. [CrossRef]

83. Kuerschner, L.; Richter, D.; Hannibal-Bach, H.K.; Gaebler, A.; Shevchenko, A.; Ejsing, C.S.; Thiele, C. Exogenous ether lipids predominantly target mitochondria. *PLoS ONE* **2012**, *7*, e31342. [CrossRef]
84. Dowhan, W. Molecular basis for membrane phospholipid diversity: Why are there so many lipids? *Annu. Rev. Biochem.* **1997**, *66*, 199–232. [CrossRef]
85. Olson, R.E. Discovery of the lipoproteins, their role in fat transport and their significance as risk factors. *J. Nutr.* **1998**, *128*, 439S–443S. [CrossRef]
86. Kuijpers, P. History in medicine: The story of cholesterol, lipids and cardiology. *J. Cradiol. Pract.* **2021**, *19*, 1–5.
87. Walusinski, O. Charcot and cholesterin. *Eur. Neurol.* **2019**, *81*, 309–318. [CrossRef] [PubMed]
88. Maxfield, F.R.; Tabas, I. Role of cholesterol and lipid organization in disease. *Nature* **2005**, *438*, 612–621. [CrossRef] [PubMed]
89. Maxfield, F.R.; van Meer, G. Cholesterol, the central lipid of mammalian cells. *Curr. Opin. Cell Biol.* **2010**, *22*, 422–429. [CrossRef] [PubMed]
90. Chapman, D. Phase transitions and fluidity characteristics of lipids and cell membranes. *Q. Rev. Biophys.* **1975**, *8*, 185–235. [CrossRef] [PubMed]
91. Jaipuria, G.; Ukmar-Godec, T.; Zweckstetter, M. Challenges and approaches to understand cholesterol-binding impact on membrane protein function: An NMR view. *Cell Mol. Life Sci.* **2018**, *75*, 2137–2151. [CrossRef]
92. Mondal, M.; Mesmin, B.; Mukherjee, S.; Maxfield, F.R. Sterols are mainly in the cytoplasmic leaflet of the plasma membrane and the endocytic recycling compartment in CHO cells. *Mol. Biol. Cell* **2009**, *20*, 581–588. [CrossRef]
93. Liu, S.L.; Sheng, R.; Jung, J.H.; Wang, L.; Stec, E.; O'Connor, M.J.; Song, S.; Bikkavilli, R.K.; Winn, R.A.; Lee, D.; et al. Orthogonal lipid sensors identify transbilayer asymmetry of plasma membrane cholesterol. *Nat. Chem. Biol.* **2017**, *13*, 268–274. [CrossRef]
94. Lange, Y.; Swaisgood, M.H.; Ramos, B.V.; Steck, T.L. Plasma membranes contain half the phospholipid and 90% of the cholesterol and sphingomyelin in cultured human fibroblasts. *J. Biol. Chem.* **1989**, *264*, 3786–3793. [CrossRef]
95. Das, A.; Brown, M.S.; Anderson, D.D.; Goldstein, J.L.; Radhakrishnan, A. Three pools of plasma membrane cholesterol and their relation to cholesterol homeostasis. *eLife* **2014**, *3*, e02882. [CrossRef]
96. Fantini, J.; Barrantes, F.J. How cholesterol interacts with membrane proteins: An exploration of cholesterol-binding sites including CRAC, CARC, and tilted domains. *Front. Physiol.* **2013**, *4*, 31. [CrossRef] [PubMed]
97. Lingwood, D.; Simons, K. Lipid rafts as a membrane-organizing principle. *Science* **2010**, *327*, 46–50. [CrossRef] [PubMed]
98. Daum, G.; Vance, J.E. Import of lipids into mitochondria. *Prog. Lipid Res.* **1997**, *36*, 103–130. [CrossRef]
99. Horvath, S.E.; Daum, G. Lipids of mitochondria. *Prog Lipid Res.* **2013**, *52*, 590–614. [CrossRef]
100. Simons, K.; Vaz, W.L. Model systems, lipid rafts, and cell membranes. *Annu. Rev. Biophys. Biomol. Struct.* **2004**, *33*, 269–295. [CrossRef]
101. Subczynski, W.K.; Pasenkiewicz-Gierula, M.; Widomska, J.; Mainali, L.; Raguz, M. High Cholesterol/Low Cholesterol: Effects in biological membranes: A review. *Cell Biochem. Biophys.* **2017**, *75*, 369–385. [CrossRef]
102. Zakany, F.; Kovacs, T.; Panyi, G.; Varga, Z. Direct and indirect cholesterol effects on membrane proteins with special focus on potassium channels. *Biochim. Biophys. Acta Mol. Cell Biol. Lipids* **2020**, *1865*, 158706. [CrossRef]
103. Ohvo-Rekila, H.; Ramstedt, B.; Leppimaki, P.; Slotte, J.P. Cholesterol interactions with phospholipids in membranes. *Prog. Lipid Res.* **2002**, *41*, 66–97. [CrossRef]
104. Desai, R.; Campanella, M. Exploring mitochondrial cholesterol signalling for therapeutic intervention in neurological conditions. *Br. J. Pharmacol.* **2019**, *176*, 4284–4292. [CrossRef]
105. Miller, W.L.; Bose, H.S. Early steps in steroidogenesis: Intracellular cholesterol trafficking. *J. Lipid Res.* **2011**, *52*, 2111–2135. [CrossRef] [PubMed]
106. Elustondo, P.; Martin, L.A.; Karten, B. Mitochondrial cholesterol import. *Biochim. Biophys. Acta Mol. Cell Biol. Lipids* **2017**, *1862*, 90–101. [CrossRef] [PubMed]
107. Li, F.; Liu, J.; Liu, N.; Kuhn, L.A.; Garavito, R.M.; Ferguson-Miller, S. Translocator protein 18 kDa (TSPO): An old protein with new functions? *Biochemistry* **2016**, *55*, 2821–2831. [CrossRef] [PubMed]
108. Papadopoulos, V.; Fan, J.; Zirkin, B. Translocator protein (18 kDa): An update on its function in steroidogenesis. *J. Neuroendocrinol.* **2018**, *30*, e12500. [CrossRef]
109. Liu, J.; Rone, M.B.; Papadopoulos, V. Protein-protein interactions mediate mitochondrial cholesterol transport and steroid biosynthesis. *J. Biol. Chem.* **2006**, *281*, 38879–38893. [CrossRef]
110. Shoshan-Barmatz, V.; Pittala, S.; Mizrachi, D. VDAC1 and the TSPO: Expression, interactions, and associated functions in health and disease states. *Int. J. Mol. Sci.* **2019**, *20*, 3348. [CrossRef]
111. Delavoie, F.; Li, H.; Hardwick, M.; Robert, J.C.; Giatzakis, C.; Peranzi, G.; Yao, Z.X.; Maccario, J.; Lacapere, J.J.; Papadopoulos, V. In vivo and in vitro peripheral-type benzodiazepine receptor polymerization: Functional significance in drug ligand and cholesterol binding. *Biochemistry* **2003**, *42*, 4506–4519. [CrossRef]
112. Fantini, J.; Di Scala, C.; Evans, L.S.; Williamson, P.T.; Barrantes, F.J. A mirror code for protein-cholesterol interactions in the two leaflets of biological membranes. *Sci. Rep.* **2016**, *6*, 21907. [CrossRef]
113. Vance, J.E. Phospholipid synthesis in a membrane fraction associated with mitochondria. *J. Biol. Chem.* **1990**, *265*, 7248–7256. [CrossRef]
114. Flis, V.V.; Daum, G. Lipid transport between the endoplasmic reticulum and mitochondria. *Cold Spring Harb. Perspect. Biol.* **2013**, *5*, a013235. [CrossRef]

115. Rizzuto, R.; Pinton, P.; Carrington, W.; Fay, F.S.; Fogarty, K.E.; Lifshitz, L.M.; Tuft, R.A.; Pozzan, T. Close contacts with the endoplasmic reticulum as determinants of mitochondrial Ca^{2+} responses. *Science* **1998**, *280*, 1763–1766. [CrossRef]
116. Csordas, G.; Renken, C.; Varnai, P.; Walter, L.; Weaver, D.; Buttle, K.F.; Balla, T.; Mannella, C.A.; Hajnoczky, G. Structural and functional features and significance of the physical linkage between ER and mitochondria. *J. Cell Biol.* **2006**, *174*, 915–921. [CrossRef] [PubMed]
117. Rowland, A.A.; Voeltz, G.K. Endoplasmic reticulum-mitochondria contacts: Function of the junction. *Nat. Rev. Mol. Cell Biol.* **2012**, *13*, 607–625. [CrossRef] [PubMed]
118. Helle, S.C.; Kanfer, G.; Kolar, K.; Lang, A.; Michel, A.H.; Kornmann, B. Organization and function of membrane contact sites. *Biochim. Biophys. Acta* **2013**, *1833*, 2526–2541. [CrossRef]
119. Van Vliet, A.R.; Verfaillie, T.; Agostinis, P. New functions of mitochondria associated membranes in cellular signaling. *Biochim. Biophys. Acta* **2014**, *1843*, 2253–2262. [CrossRef] [PubMed]
120. Annunziata, I.; Sano, R.; d'Azzo, A. Mitochondria-associated ER membranes (MAMs) and lysosomal storage diseases. *Cell Death Dis.* **2018**, *9*, 328. [CrossRef] [PubMed]
121. Lee, S.; Min, K.T. The interface between ER and mitochondria: Molecular compositions and functions. *Mol. Cells* **2018**, *41*, 1000–1007. [PubMed]
122. Barbosa, A.D.; Siniossoglou, S. Function of lipid droplet-organelle interactions in lipid homeostasis. *Biochim. Biophys. Acta Mol. Cell Res.* **2017**, *1864*, 1459–1468. [CrossRef]
123. Olzmann, J.A.; Carvalho, P. Dynamics and functions of lipid droplets. *Nat. Rev. Mol. Cell Biol.* **2019**, *20*, 137–155. [CrossRef]
124. Murphy, S.; Martin, S.; Parton, R.G. Lipid droplet-organelle interactions; sharing the fats. *Biochim. Biophys. Acta* **2009**, *1791*, 441–447. [CrossRef] [PubMed]
125. Lin, Y.; Hou, X.; Shen, W.J.; Hanssen, R.; Khor, V.K.; Cortez, Y.; Roseman, A.N.; Azhar, S.; Kraemer, F.B. SNARE-mediated cholesterol movement to mitochondria supports steroidogenesis in rodent cells. *Mol. Endocrinol.* **2016**, *30*, 234–247. [CrossRef] [PubMed]
126. Jagerstrom, S.; Polesie, S.; Wickstrom, Y.; Johansson, B.R.; Schroder, H.D.; Hojlund, K.; Bostrom, P. Lipid droplets interact with mitochondria using SNAP23. *Cell Biol. Int.* **2009**, *33*, 934–940. [CrossRef] [PubMed]
127. Ravichandran, V.; Chawla, A.; Roche, P.A. Identification of a novel syntaxin- and synaptobrevin/VAMP-binding protein, SNAP-23, expressed in non-neuronal tissues. *J. Biol. Chem.* **1996**, *271*, 13300–13303. [CrossRef]
128. Mollinedo, F.; Lazo, P.A. Identification of two isoforms of the vesicle-membrane fusion protein SNAP-23 in human neutrophils and HL-60 cells. *Biochem. Biophys. Res. Commun.* **1997**, *231*, 808–812. [CrossRef]
129. Martin-Martin, B.; Nabokina, S.M.; Blasi, J.; Lazo, P.A.; Mollinedo, F. Involvement of SNAP-23 and syntaxin 6 in human neutrophil exocytosis. *Blood* **2000**, *96*, 2574–2583. [CrossRef] [PubMed]
130. Mollinedo, F.; Calafat, J.; Janssen, H.; Martin-Martin, B.; Canchado, J.; Nabokina, S.M.; Gajate, C. Combinatorial SNARE complexes modulate the secretion of cytoplasmic granules in human neutrophils. *J. Immunol.* **2006**, *177*, 2831–2841. [CrossRef]
131. Bissig, C.; Gruenberg, J. Lipid sorting and multivesicular endosome biogenesis. *Cold Spring Harb. Perspect. Biol.* **2013**, *5*, a016816. [CrossRef]
132. Luo, J.; Jiang, L.; Yang, H.; Song, B.L. Routes and mechanisms of post-endosomal cholesterol trafficking: A story that never ends. *Traffic* **2017**, *18*, 209–217. [CrossRef]
133. Ouweneel, A.B.; Thomas, M.J.; Sorci-Thomas, M.G. The ins and outs of lipid rafts: Functions in intracellular cholesterol homeostasis, microparticles, and cell membranes. *J. Lipid Res.* **2020**, *61*, 676–686. [CrossRef]
134. Vanier, M.T.; Millat, G. Niemann-Pick disease type C. *Clin. Genet.* **2003**, *64*, 269–281. [CrossRef] [PubMed]
135. Chang, T.Y.; Reid, P.C.; Sugii, S.; Ohgami, N.; Cruz, J.C.; Chang, C.C. Niemann-Pick type C disease and intracellular cholesterol trafficking. *J. Biol. Chem.* **2005**, *280*, 20917–20920. [CrossRef]
136. Sevin, M.; Lesca, G.; Baumann, N.; Millat, G.; Lyon-Caen, O.; Vanier, M.T.; Sedel, F. The adult form of Niemann-Pick disease type C. *Brain* **2007**, *130*, 120–133. [CrossRef] [PubMed]
137. Piroth, T.; Boelmans, K.; Amtage, F.; Rijntjes, M.; Wierciochin, A.; Musacchio, T.; Weiller, C.; Volkmann, J.; Klebe, S. Adult-onset niemann-pick disease type C: Rapid treatment initiation advised but early diagnosis remains difficult. *Front. Neurol.* **2017**, *8*, 108. [CrossRef] [PubMed]
138. Infante, R.E.; Abi-Mosleh, L.; Radhakrishnan, A.; Dale, J.D.; Brown, M.S.; Goldstein, J.L. Purified NPC1 protein. I. Binding of cholesterol and oxysterols to a 1278-amino acid membrane protein. *J. Biol. Chem.* **2008**, *283*, 1052–1063. [CrossRef] [PubMed]
139. Naureckiene, S.; Sleat, D.E.; Lackland, H.; Fensom, A.; Vanier, M.T.; Wattiaux, R.; Jadot, M.; Lobel, P. Identification of HE1 as the second gene of Niemann-Pick C disease. *Science* **2000**, *290*, 2298–2301. [CrossRef] [PubMed]
140. Storch, J.; Xu, Z. Niemann-Pick C2 (NPC2) and intracellular cholesterol trafficking. *Biochim. Biophys. Acta* **2009**, *1791*, 671–678. [CrossRef]
141. Cheruku, S.R.; Xu, Z.; Dutia, R.; Lobel, P.; Storch, J. Mechanism of cholesterol transfer from the Niemann-Pick type C2 protein to model membranes supports a role in lysosomal cholesterol transport. *J. Biol. Chem.* **2006**, *281*, 31594–31604. [CrossRef]
142. Berger, A.C.; Hanson, P.K.; Wylie Nichols, J.; Corbett, A.H. A yeast model system for functional analysis of the Niemann-Pick type C protein 1 homolog, Ncr1p. *Traffic* **2005**, *6*, 907–917. [CrossRef]

143. Zhang, M.; Liu, P.; Dwyer, N.K.; Christenson, L.K.; Fujimoto, T.; Martinez, F.; Comly, M.; Hanover, J.A.; Blanchette-Mackie, E.J.; Strauss, J.F., 3rd. MLN64 mediates mobilization of lysosomal cholesterol to steroidogenic mitochondria. *J. Biol. Chem.* **2002**, *277*, 33300–33310. [CrossRef]
144. Bose, H.S.; Whittal, R.M.; Ran, Y.; Bose, M.; Baker, B.Y.; Miller, W.L. StAR-like activity and molten globule behavior of StARD6, a male germ-line protein. *Biochemistry* **2008**, *47*, 2277–2288. [CrossRef]
145. Soccio, R.E.; Breslow, J.L. Intracellular cholesterol transport. *Arterioscler. Thromb Vasc. Biol.* **2004**, *24*, 1150–1160. [CrossRef] [PubMed]
146. Martin, L.A.; Kennedy, B.E.; Karten, B. Mitochondrial cholesterol: Mechanisms of import and effects on mitochondrial function. *J. Bioenerg. Biomembr.* **2016**, *48*, 137–151. [CrossRef] [PubMed]
147. Arenas, F.; Garcia-Ruiz, C.; Fernandez-Checa, J.C. Intracellular Cholesterol Trafficking and Impact in Neurodegeneration. *Front. Mol. Neurosci.* **2017**, *10*, 382. [CrossRef]
148. Roca-Agujetas, V.; Barbero-Camps, E.; de Dios, C.; Podlesniy, P.; Abadin, X.; Morales, A.; Mari, M.; Trullas, R.; Colell, A. Cholesterol alters mitophagy by impairing optineurin recruitment and lysosomal clearance in Alzheimer's disease. *Mol. Neurodegener.* **2021**, *16*, 15. [CrossRef] [PubMed]
149. Ribas, V.; Garcia-Ruiz, C.; Fernandez-Checa, J.C. Mitochondria, cholesterol and cancer cell metabolism. *Clin. Transl. Med.* **2016**, *5*, 22. [CrossRef] [PubMed]
150. Feo, F.; Canuto, R.A.; Garcea, R.; Gabriel, L. Effect of cholesterol content on some physical and functional properties of mitochondria isolated from adult rat liver, fetal liver, cholesterol-enriched liver and hepatomas AH-130, 3924A and 5123. *Biochim. Biophys. Acta* **1975**, *413*, 116–134. [CrossRef]
151. Crain, R.C.; Clark, R.W.; Harvey, B.E. Role of lipid transfer proteins in the abnormal lipid content of Morris hepatoma mitochondria and microsomes. *Cancer Res.* **1983**, *43*, 3197–3202.
152. Montero, J.; Morales, A.; Llacuna, L.; Lluis, J.M.; Terrones, O.; Basanez, G.; Antonsson, B.; Prieto, J.; Garcia-Ruiz, C.; Colell, A.; et al. Mitochondrial cholesterol contributes to chemotherapy resistance in hepatocellular carcinoma. *Cancer Res.* **2008**, *68*, 5246–5256. [CrossRef]
153. Krycer, J.R.; Brown, A.J. Cholesterol accumulation in prostate cancer: A classic observation from a modern perspective. *Biochim. Biophys. Acta* **2013**, *1835*, 219–229. [CrossRef]
154. Kuzu, O.F.; Noory, M.A.; Robertson, G.P. The role of cholesterol in cancer. *Cancer Res.* **2016**, *76*, 2063–2070. [CrossRef] [PubMed]
155. Parlo, R.A.; Coleman, P.S. Enhanced rate of citrate export from cholesterol-rich hepatoma mitochondria. The truncated Krebs cycle and other metabolic ramifications of mitochondrial membrane cholesterol. *J. Biol. Chem.* **1984**, *259*, 9997–10003. [CrossRef]
156. Baggetto, L.G.; Clottes, E.; Vial, C. Low mitochondrial proton leak due to high membrane cholesterol content and cytosolic creatine kinase as two features of the deviant bioenergetics of Ehrlich and AS30-D tumor cells. *Cancer Res.* **1992**, *52*, 4935–4941.
157. Lucken-Ardjomande, S.; Montessuit, S.; Martinou, J.C. Bax activation and stress-induced apoptosis delayed by the accumulation of cholesterol in mitochondrial membranes. *Cell Death Differ.* **2008**, *15*, 484–493. [CrossRef] [PubMed]
158. Zoratti, M.; Szabo, I. The mitochondrial permeability transition. *Biochim. Biophys. Acta* **1995**, *1241*, 139–176. [CrossRef]
159. Halestrap, A.P.; McStay, G.P.; Clarke, S.J. The permeability transition pore complex: Another view. *Biochimie* **2002**, *84*, 153–166. [CrossRef]
160. Halestrap, A.P. What is the mitochondrial permeability transition pore? *J. Mol. Cell Cardiol.* **2009**, *46*, 821–831. [CrossRef]
161. Rao, V.K.; Carlson, E.A.; Yan, S.S. Mitochondrial permeability transition pore is a potential drug target for neurodegeneration. *Biochim. Biophys. Acta* **2014**, *1842*, 1267–1272. [CrossRef]
162. Kwong, J.Q.; Molkentin, J.D. Physiological and pathological roles of the mitochondrial permeability transition pore in the heart. *Cell Metab.* **2015**, *21*, 206–214. [CrossRef]
163. Halestrap, A.P.; Brenner, C. The adenine nucleotide translocase: A central component of the mitochondrial permeability transition pore and key player in cell death. *Curr. Med. Chem.* **2003**, *10*, 1507–1525. [CrossRef] [PubMed]
164. Camara, A.K.S.; Zhou, Y.; Wen, P.C.; Tajkhorshid, E.; Kwok, W.M. Mitochondrial VDAC1: A key gatekeeper as potential therapeutic target. *Front. Physiol.* **2017**, *8*, 460. [CrossRef] [PubMed]
165. Papadopoulos, V.; Baraldi, M.; Guilarte, T.R.; Knudsen, T.B.; Lacapere, J.J.; Lindemann, P.; Norenberg, M.D.; Nutt, D.; Weizman, A.; Zhang, M.R.; et al. Translocator protein (18kDa): New nomenclature for the peripheral-type benzodiazepine receptor based on its structure and molecular function. *Trends Pharmacol. Sci.* **2006**, *27*, 402–409. [CrossRef] [PubMed]
166. Si Chaib, Z.; Marchetto, A.; Dishnica, K.; Carloni, P.; Giorgetti, A.; Rossetti, G. Impact of cholesterol on the stability of monomeric and dimeric forms of the translocator protein TSPO: A molecular simulation study. *Molecules* **2020**, *25*, 4299. [CrossRef] [PubMed]
167. Selvaraj, V.; Stocco, D.M.; Tu, L.N. Minireview: Translocator protein (TSPO) and steroidogenesis: A reappraisal. *Mol. Endocrinol.* **2015**, *29*, 490–501. [CrossRef] [PubMed]
168. Rochette, L.; Meloux, A.; Zeller, M.; Malka, G.; Cottin, Y.; Vergely, C. Mitochondrial SLC25 carriers: Novel targets for cancer therapy. *Molecules* **2020**, *25*, 2417. [CrossRef]
169. Giorgio, V.; Bisetto, E.; Soriano, M.E.; Dabbeni-Sala, F.; Basso, E.; Petronilli, V.; Forte, M.A.; Bernardi, P.; Lippe, G. Cyclophilin D modulates mitochondrial F_0F_1-ATP synthase by interacting with the lateral stalk of the complex. *J. Biol. Chem.* **2009**, *284*, 33982–33988. [CrossRef]
170. Beutner, G.; Alanzalon, R.E.; Porter, G.A., Jr. Cyclophilin D regulates the dynamic assembly of mitochondrial ATP synthase into synthasomes. *Sci. Rep.* **2017**, *7*, 14488. [CrossRef] [PubMed]

171. Kokoszka, J.E.; Waymire, K.G.; Levy, S.E.; Sligh, J.E.; Cai, J.; Jones, D.P.; MacGregor, G.R.; Wallace, D.C. The ADP/ATP translocator is not essential for the mitochondrial permeability transition pore. *Nature* **2004**, *427*, 461–465. [CrossRef]
172. Krauskopf, A.; Eriksson, O.; Craigen, W.J.; Forte, M.A.; Bernardi, P. Properties of the permeability transition in VDAC1(-/-) mitochondria. *Biochim. Biophys. Acta* **2006**, *1757*, 590–595. [CrossRef]
173. Baines, C.P.; Kaiser, R.A.; Sheiko, T.; Craigen, W.J.; Molkentin, J.D. Voltage-dependent anion channels are dispensable for mitochondrial-dependent cell death. *Nat. Cell Biol.* **2007**, *9*, 550–555. [CrossRef]
174. Sileikyte, J.; Blachly-Dyson, E.; Sewell, R.; Carpi, A.; Menabo, R.; Di Lisa, F.; Ricchelli, F.; Bernardi, P.; Forte, M. Regulation of the mitochondrial permeability transition pore by the outer membrane does not involve the peripheral benzodiazepine receptor (Translocator Protein of 18 kDa (TSPO)). *J. Biol. Chem.* **2014**, *289*, 13769–13781. [CrossRef] [PubMed]
175. Gutierrez-Aguilar, M.; Douglas, D.L.; Gibson, A.K.; Domeier, T.L.; Molkentin, J.D.; Baines, C.P. Genetic manipulation of the cardiac mitochondrial phosphate carrier does not affect permeability transition. *J. Mol. Cell Cardiol.* **2014**, *72*, 316–325. [CrossRef] [PubMed]
176. Nath, S. A novel conceptual model for the dual role of FOF1-ATP synthase in cell life and cell death. *Biomol. Concepts* **2020**, *11*, 143–152. [CrossRef] [PubMed]
177. Giorgio, V.; Burchell, V.; Schiavone, M.; Bassot, C.; Minervini, G.; Petronilli, V.; Argenton, F.; Forte, M.; Tosatto, S.; Lippe, G.; et al. Ca^{2+} binding to F-ATP synthase beta subunit triggers the mitochondrial permeability transition. *EMBO Rep.* **2017**, *18*, 1065–1076. [CrossRef]
178. Watt, I.N.; Montgomery, M.G.; Runswick, M.J.; Leslie, A.G.; Walker, J.E. Bioenergetic cost of making an adenosine triphosphate molecule in animal mitochondria. *Proc. Natl. Acad. Sci. USA* **2010**, *107*, 16823–16827. [CrossRef] [PubMed]
179. He, J.; Ford, H.C.; Carroll, J.; Douglas, C.; Gonzales, E.; Ding, S.; Fearnley, I.M.; Walker, J.E. Assembly of the membrane domain of ATP synthase in human mitochondria. *Proc. Natl. Acad. Sci. USA* **2018**, *115*, 2988–2993. [CrossRef] [PubMed]
180. Song, J.; Pfanner, N.; Becker, T. Assembling the mitochondrial ATP synthase. *Proc. Natl. Acad. Sci. USA* **2018**, *115*, 2850–2852. [CrossRef]
181. Okuno, D.; Iino, R.; Noji, H. Rotation and structure of FoF1-ATP synthase. *J. Biochem.* **2011**, *149*, 655–664. [CrossRef]
182. Davies, K.M.; Strauss, M.; Daum, B.; Kief, J.H.; Osiewacz, H.D.; Rycovska, A.; Zickermann, V.; Kuhlbrandt, W. Macromolecular organization of ATP synthase and complex I in whole mitochondria. *Proc. Natl. Acad. Sci. USA* **2011**, *108*, 14121–14126. [CrossRef]
183. Strauss, M.; Hofhaus, G.; Schroder, R.R.; Kuhlbrandt, W. Dimer ribbons of ATP synthase shape the inner mitochondrial membrane. *EMBO J.* **2008**, *27*, 1154–1160. [CrossRef]
184. Paumard, P.; Vaillier, J.; Coulary, B.; Schaeffer, J.; Soubannier, V.; Mueller, D.M.; Brethes, D.; di Rago, J.P.; Velours, J. The ATP synthase is involved in generating mitochondrial cristae morphology. *EMBO J.* **2002**, *21*, 221–230. [CrossRef]
185. Bonora, M.; Bononi, A.; De Marchi, E.; Giorgi, C.; Lebiedzinska, M.; Marchi, S.; Patergnani, S.; Rimessi, A.; Suski, J.M.; Wojtala, A.; et al. Role of the c subunit of the FO ATP synthase in mitochondrial permeability transition. *Cell Cycle* **2013**, *12*, 674–683. [CrossRef] [PubMed]
186. Azarashvili, T.; Odinokova, I.; Bakunts, A.; Ternovsky, V.; Krestinina, O.; Tyynela, J.; Saris, N.E. Potential role of subunit c of F0F1-ATPase and subunit c of storage body in the mitochondrial permeability transition. Effect of the phosphorylation status of subunit c on pore opening. *Cell Calcium* **2014**, *55*, 69–77. [CrossRef] [PubMed]
187. Alavian, K.N.; Beutner, G.; Lazrove, E.; Sacchetti, S.; Park, H.A.; Licznerski, P.; Li, H.; Nabili, P.; Hockensmith, K.; Graham, M.; et al. An uncoupling channel within the c-subunit ring of the F_1F_O ATP synthase is the mitochondrial permeability transition pore. *Proc. Natl. Acad. Sci. USA* **2014**, *111*, 10580–10585. [CrossRef] [PubMed]
188. Neginskaya, M.A.; Solesio, M.E.; Berezhnaya, E.V.; Amodeo, G.F.; Mnatsakanyan, N.; Jonas, E.A.; Pavlov, E.V. ATP synthase C-subunit-deficient mitochondria have a small cyclosporine A-sensitive channel, but lack the permeability transition pore. *Cell Rep.* **2019**, *26*, 11–17.e12. [CrossRef]
189. Mnatsakanyan, N.; Llaguno, M.C.; Yang, Y.; Yan, Y.; Weber, J.; Sigworth, F.J.; Jonas, E.A. A mitochondrial megachannel resides in monomeric F1FO ATP synthase. *Nat. Commun.* **2019**, *10*, 5823. [CrossRef] [PubMed]
190. Mnatsakanyan, N.; Jonas, E.A. ATP synthase c-subunit ring as the channel of mitochondrial permeability transition: Regulator of metabolism in development and degeneration. *J. Mol. Cell Cardiol.* **2020**, *144*, 109–118. [CrossRef] [PubMed]
191. Karch, J.; Kwong, J.Q.; Burr, A.R.; Sargent, M.A.; Elrod, J.W.; Peixoto, P.M.; Martinez-Caballero, S.; Osinska, H.; Cheng, E.H.; Robbins, J.; et al. Bax and Bak function as the outer membrane component of the mitochondrial permeability pore in regulating necrotic cell death in mice. *eLife* **2013**, *2*, e00772. [CrossRef]
192. Naumova, N.; Sachl, R. Regulation of cell death by mitochondrial transport systems of calcium and Bcl-2 proteins. *Membranes* **2020**, *10*, 299. [CrossRef]
193. Lamb, H.M. Double agents of cell death: Novel emerging functions of apoptotic regulators. *FEBS J.* **2020**, *287*, 2647–2663. [CrossRef]
194. Alavian, K.N.; Li, H.; Collis, L.; Bonanni, L.; Zeng, L.; Sacchetti, S.; Lazrove, E.; Nabili, P.; Flaherty, B.; Graham, M.; et al. Bcl-xL regulates metabolic efficiency of neurons through interaction with the mitochondrial F1FO ATP synthase. *Nat. Cell Biol.* **2011**, *13*, 1224–1233. [CrossRef]
195. Chen, Y.B.; Aon, M.A.; Hsu, Y.T.; Soane, L.; Teng, X.; McCaffery, J.M.; Cheng, W.C.; Qi, B.; Li, H.; Alavian, K.N.; et al. Bcl-xL regulates mitochondrial energetics by stabilizing the inner membrane potential. *J. Cell Biol.* **2011**, *195*, 263–276. [CrossRef] [PubMed]

196. Lardy, H.A.; Johnson, D.; Mc, M.W. Antibiotics as tools for metabolic studies. I. A survey of toxic antibiotics in respiratory, phosphorylative and glycolytic systems. *Arch. Biochem. Biophys.* **1958**, *78*, 587–597. [CrossRef]
197. Racker, E. A mitochondrial factor conferring oligomycin sensitivity on soluble mitochondrial ATPase. *Biochem. Biophys. Res. Commun.* **1963**, *10*, 435–439. [CrossRef]
198. Kagawa, Y.; Racker, E. Partial resolution of the enzymes catalyzing oxidative phosphorylation. 8. Properties of a factor conferring oligomycin sensitivity on mitochondrial adenosine triphosphatase. *J. Biol. Chem.* **1966**, *241*, 2461–2466. [CrossRef]
199. Symersky, J.; Osowski, D.; Walters, D.E.; Mueller, D.M. Oligomycin frames a common drug-binding site in the ATP synthase. *Proc. Natl. Acad. Sci. USA* **2012**, *109*, 13961–13965. [CrossRef] [PubMed]
200. Antoniel, M.; Giorgio, V.; Fogolari, F.; Glick, G.D.; Bernardi, P.; Lippe, G. The oligomycin-sensitivity conferring protein of mitochondrial ATP synthase: Emerging new roles in mitochondrial pathophysiology. *Int. J. Mol. Sci.* **2014**, *15*, 7513–7536. [CrossRef] [PubMed]
201. Sharpe, J.C.; Arnoult, D.; Youle, R.J. Control of mitochondrial permeability by Bcl-2 family members. *Biochim. Biophys. Acta* **2004**, *1644*, 107–113. [CrossRef]
202. Di Lisa, F.; Bernardi, P. Mitochondrial function as a determinant of recovery or death in cell response to injury. *Mol. Cell Biochem.* **1998**, *184*, 379–391. [CrossRef]
203. Kuwana, T.; Bouchier-Hayes, L.; Chipuk, J.E.; Bonzon, C.; Sullivan, B.A.; Green, D.R.; Newmeyer, D.D. BH3 domains of BH3-only proteins differentially regulate Bax-mediated mitochondrial membrane permeabilization both directly and indirectly. *Mol. Cell* **2005**, *17*, 525–535. [CrossRef] [PubMed]
204. Breckenridge, D.G.; Stojanovic, M.; Marcellus, R.C.; Shore, G.C. Caspase cleavage product of BAP31 induces mitochondrial fission through endoplasmic reticulum calcium signals, enhancing cytochrome c release to the cytosol. *J. Cell Biol.* **2003**, *160*, 1115–1127. [CrossRef]
205. Burgeiro, A.; Pereira, C.V.; Carvalho, F.S.; Pereira, G.C.; Mollinedo, F.; Oliveira, P.J. Edelfosine and perifosine disrupt hepatic mitochondrial oxidative phosphorylation and induce the permeability transition. *Mitochondrion* **2013**, *13*, 25–35. [CrossRef] [PubMed]
206. Christian, A.E.; Haynes, M.P.; Phillips, M.C.; Rothblat, G.H. Use of cyclodextrins for manipulating cellular cholesterol content. *J. Lipid Res.* **1997**, *38*, 2264–2272. [CrossRef]
207. Pagliarani, A.; Nesci, S.; Ventrella, V. Novel Drugs Targeting the c-Ring of the F_1F_O-ATP Synthase. *Mini Rev. Med. Chem.* **2016**, *16*, 815–824. [CrossRef] [PubMed]
208. Srivastava, A.P.; Luo, M.; Zhou, W.; Symersky, J.; Bai, D.; Chambers, M.G.; Faraldo-Gomez, J.D.; Liao, M.; Mueller, D.M. High-resolution cryo-EM analysis of the yeast ATP synthase in a lipid membrane. *Science* **2018**, *360*, 6389. [CrossRef]
209. Veenman, L.; Alten, J.; Linnemannstons, K.; Shandalov, Y.; Zeno, S.; Lakomek, M.; Gavish, M.; Kugler, W. Potential involvement of F0F1-ATP(synth)ase and reactive oxygen species in apoptosis induction by the antineoplastic agent erucylphosphohomocholine in glioblastoma cell lines: A mechanism for induction of apoptosis via the 18 kDa mitochondrial translocator protein. *Apoptosis* **2010**, *15*, 753–768. [PubMed]
210. Norais, N.; Prome, D.; Velours, J. ATP synthase of yeast mitochondria. Characterization of subunit d and sequence analysis of the structural gene ATP7. *J. Biol. Chem.* **1991**, *266*, 16541–16549. [CrossRef]
211. Ausili, A.; Torrecillas, A.; Aranda, F.J.; Mollinedo, F.; Gajate, C.; Corbalan-Garcia, S.; de Godos, A.; Gomez-Fernandez, J.C. Edelfosine is incorporated into rafts and alters their organization. *J. Phys. Chem. B* **2008**, *112*, 11643–11654. [CrossRef] [PubMed]
212. Castro, B.M.; Fedorov, A.; Hornillos, V.; Delgado, J.; Acuna, A.U.; Mollinedo, F.; Prieto, M. Edelfosine and miltefosine effects on lipid raft properties: Membrane biophysics in cell death by antitumor lipids. *J. Phys. Chem. B* **2013**, *117*, 7929–7940. [CrossRef]
213. Bernardi, P.; Vassanelli, S.; Veronese, P.; Colonna, R.; Szabo, I.; Zoratti, M. Modulation of the mitochondrial permeability transition pore. Effect of protons and divalent cations. *J. Biol. Chem.* **1992**, *267*, 2934–2939. [CrossRef]
214. Matsuyama, S.; Xu, Q.; Velours, J.; Reed, J.C. The Mitochondrial F_0F_1-ATPase proton pump is required for function of the proapoptotic protein Bax in yeast and mammalian cells. *Mol. Cell* **1998**, *1*, 327–336. [CrossRef]
215. Gajate, C.; Mollinedo, F. Isolation of lipid rafts through discontinuous sucrose gradient centrifugation and Fas/CD95 death receptor localization in raft fractions. *Methods Mol. Biol.* **2017**, *1557*, 125–138. [PubMed]
216. Gajate, C.; Mollinedo, F. Lipid raft isolation by sucrose gradient centrifugation and visualization of raft-located proteins by fluorescence microscopy: The use of combined techniques to assess Fas/CD95 location in rafts during apoptosis triggering. *Methods Mol. Biol.* **2021**, *2187*, 147–186. [PubMed]
217. Das, B.; Mondragon, M.O.; Sadeghian, M.; Hatcher, V.B.; Norin, A.J. A novel ligand in lymphocyte-mediated cytotoxicity: Expression of the beta subunit of H+ transporting ATP synthase on the surface of tumor cell lines. *J. Exp. Med.* **1994**, *180*, 273–281. [CrossRef] [PubMed]
218. Bae, T.J.; Kim, M.S.; Kim, J.W.; Kim, B.W.; Choo, H.J.; Lee, J.W.; Kim, K.B.; Lee, C.S.; Kim, J.H.; Chang, S.Y.; et al. Lipid raft proteome reveals ATP synthase complex in the cell surface. *Proteomics* **2004**, *4*, 3536–3548. [CrossRef]
219. Ma, Z.; Cao, M.; Liu, Y.; He, Y.; Wang, Y.; Yang, C.; Wang, W.; Du, Y.; Zhou, M.; Gao, F. Mitochondrial F1Fo-ATP synthase translocates to cell surface in hepatocytes and has high activity in tumor-like acidic and hypoxic environment. *Acta Biochim. Biophys. Sin.* **2010**, *42*, 530–537. [CrossRef]

220. Kim, B.W.; Lee, C.S.; Yi, J.S.; Lee, J.H.; Lee, J.W.; Choo, H.J.; Jung, S.Y.; Kim, M.S.; Lee, S.W.; Lee, M.S.; et al. Lipid raft proteome reveals that oxidative phosphorylation system is associated with the plasma membrane. *Expert Rev. Proteom.* **2010**, *7*, 849–866. [CrossRef]
221. Kawai, Y.; Kaidoh, M.; Yokoyama, Y.; Ohhashi, T. Cell surface F1/FO ATP synthase contributes to interstitial flow-mediated development of the acidic microenvironment in tumor tissues. *Am. J. Physiol. Cell Physiol.* **2013**, *305*, C1139–C1150. [CrossRef]
222. Wang, W.J.; Shi, X.X.; Liu, Y.W.; He, Y.Q.; Wang, Y.Z.; Yang, C.X.; Gao, F. The mechanism underlying the effects of the cell surface ATP synthase on the regulation of intracellular acidification during acidosis. *J. Cell Biochem.* **2013**, *114*, 1695–1703. [CrossRef]
223. Allen-Worthington, K.; Xie, J.; Brown, J.L.; Edmunson, A.M.; Dowling, A.; Navratil, A.M.; Scavelli, K.; Yoon, H.; Kim, D.G.; Bynoe, M.S.; et al. The F_0F_1 ATP synthase complex localizes to membrane rafts in gonadotrope cells. *Mol. Endocrinol.* **2016**, *30*, 996–1011. [CrossRef]
224. Zhu, B.; Feng, Z.; Guo, Y.; Zhang, T.; Mai, A.; Kang, Z.; Weijen, T.; Wang, D.; Yin, D.; Zhu, D.; et al. F0F1 ATP synthase regulates extracellular calcium influx in human neutrophils by interacting with Cav2.3 and modulates neutrophil accumulation in the lipopolysaccharide-challenged lung. *Cell Commun. Signal.* **2020**, *18*, 19. [CrossRef] [PubMed]
225. Gajate, C.; Gonzalez-Camacho, F.; Mollinedo, F. Lipid raft connection between extrinsic and intrinsic apoptotic pathways. *Biochem. Biophys. Res. Commun.* **2009**, *380*, 780–784. [CrossRef] [PubMed]
226. Schon, A.; Freire, E. Thermodynamics of intersubunit interactions in cholera toxin upon binding to the oligosaccharide portion of its cell surface receptor, ganglioside GM1. *Biochemistry* **1989**, *28*, 5019–5024. [CrossRef] [PubMed]
227. Harder, T.; Scheiffele, P.; Verkade, P.; Simons, K. Lipid domain structure of the plasma membrane revealed by patching of membrane components. *J. Cell Biol.* **1998**, *141*, 929–942. [CrossRef] [PubMed]
228. Sorice, M.; Matarrese, P.; Manganelli, V.; Tinari, A.; Giammarioli, A.M.; Mattei, V.; Misasi, R.; Garofalo, T.; Malorni, W. Role of GD3-CLIPR-59 association in lymphoblastoid T cell apoptosis triggered by CD95/Fas. *PLoS ONE* **2010**, *5*, e8567. [CrossRef]
229. Sorice, M.; Garofalo, T.; Misasi, R.; Manganelli, V.; Vona, R.; Malorni, W. Ganglioside GD3 as a raft component in cell death regulation. *Anticancer Agents Med. Chem.* **2012**, *12*, 376–382. [CrossRef]
230. Sorice, M.; Mattei, V.; Matarrese, P.; Garofalo, T.; Tinari, A.; Gambardella, L.; Ciarlo, L.; Manganelli, V.; Tasciotti, V.; Misasi, R.; et al. Dynamics of mitochondrial raft-like microdomains in cell life and death. *Commun. Integr. Biol.* **2012**, *5*, 217–219. [CrossRef]
231. Ciarlo, L.; Manganelli, V.; Garofalo, T.; Matarrese, P.; Tinari, A.; Misasi, R.; Malorni, W.; Sorice, M. Association of fission proteins with mitochondrial raft-like domains. *Cell Death Differ.* **2010**, *17*, 1047–1058. [CrossRef]
232. Garofalo, T.; Giammarioli, A.M.; Misasi, R.; Tinari, A.; Manganelli, V.; Gambardella, L.; Pavan, A.; Malorni, W.; Sorice, M. Lipid microdomains contribute to apoptosis-associated modifications of mitochondria in T cells. *Cell Death Differ.* **2005**, *12*, 1378–1389. [CrossRef]
233. Sorice, M.; Manganelli, V.; Matarrese, P.; Tinari, A.; Misasi, R.; Malorni, W.; Garofalo, T. Cardiolipin-enriched raft-like microdomains are essential activating platforms for apoptotic signals on mitochondria. *FEBS Lett.* **2009**, *583*, 2447–2450. [CrossRef]
234. Zheng, Y.Z.; Berg, K.B.; Foster, L.J. Mitochondria do not contain lipid rafts, and lipid rafts do not contain mitochondrial proteins. *J. Lipid Res.* **2009**, *50*, 988–998. [CrossRef] [PubMed]
235. Garofalo, T.; Manganelli, V.; Grasso, M.; Mattei, V.; Ferri, A.; Misasi, R.; Sorice, M. Role of mitochondrial raft-like microdomains in the regulation of cell apoptosis. *Apoptosis* **2015**, *20*, 621–634. [CrossRef]
236. Fujimoto, M.; Hayashi, T.; Su, T.P. The role of cholesterol in the association of endoplasmic reticulum membranes with mitochondria. *Biochem. Biophys. Res. Commun.* **2012**, *417*, 635–639. [CrossRef] [PubMed]
237. Area-Gomez, E.; Del Carmen Lara Castillo, M.; Tambini, M.D.; Guardia-Laguarta, C.; de Groof, A.J.; Madra, M.; Ikenouchi, J.; Umeda, M.; Bird, T.D.; Sturley, S.L.; et al. Upregulated function of mitochondria-associated ER membranes in Alzheimer disease. *EMBO J.* **2012**, *31*, 4106–4123. [CrossRef]
238. Sano, R.; Annunziata, I.; Patterson, A.; Moshiach, S.; Gomero, E.; Opferman, J.; Forte, M.; d'Azzo, A. GM1-ganglioside accumulation at the mitochondria-associated ER membranes links ER stress to Ca(2+)-dependent mitochondrial apoptosis. *Mol. Cell* **2009**, *36*, 500–511. [CrossRef]
239. De Brito, O.M.; Scorrano, L. Mitofusin 2 tethers endoplasmic reticulum to mitochondria. *Nature* **2008**, *456*, 605–610. [CrossRef] [PubMed]

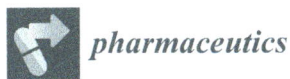

Article

Oxoglutarate Carrier Inhibition Reduced Melanoma Growth and Invasion by Reducing ATP Production

Jae-Seon Lee [1], Jiwon Choi [2], Seon-Hyeong Lee [1], Joon Hee Kang [1], Ji Sun Ha [1], Hee Yeon Kim [1], Hyonchol Jang [1], Jong In Yook [2] and Soo-Youl Kim [1],*

1. Division of Cancer Biology, Research Institute, National Cancer Center, Goyang, Gyeonggi-do 10408, Korea; ljs891109@gmail.com (J.-S.L.); shlee1987@gmail.com (S.-H.L.); wnsl2820@gmail.com (J.H.K.); jsha9595@gmail.com (J.S.H.); 74790@ncc.re.kr (H.Y.K.); hjang@ncc.re.kr (H.J.)
2. Department of Oral Pathology, Oral Cancer Research Institute, Yonsei University College of Dentistry, Seoul 03722, Korea; edccjw3235@yuhs.ac (J.C.); jiyook@yuhs.ac (J.I.Y.)
* Correspondence: kimsooyoul@gmail.com; Tel.: +82-31-920-2221; Fax: +82-31-920-2278

Received: 20 October 2020; Accepted: 20 November 2020; Published: 23 November 2020

Abstract: Recent findings indicate that (a) mitochondria in proliferating cancer cells are functional, (b) cancer cells use more oxygen than normal cells for oxidative phosphorylation, and (c) cancer cells critically rely on cytosolic NADH transported into mitochondria via the malate-aspartate shuttle (MAS) for ATP production. In a spontaneous lung cancer model, tumor growth was reduced by 50% in heterozygous oxoglutarate carrier (OGC) knock-out mice compared with wild-type counterparts. To determine the mechanism through which OGC promotes tumor growth, the effects of the OGC inhibitor N-phenylmaleimide (NPM) on mitochondrial activity, oxygen consumption, and ATP production were evaluated in melanoma cell lines. NPM suppressed oxygen consumption and decreased ATP production in melanoma cells in a dose-dependent manner. NPM also reduced the proliferation of melanoma cells. To test the effects of NPM on tumor growth and metastasis in vivo, NPM was administered in a human melanoma xenograft model. NPM reduced tumor growth by approximately 50% and reduced melanoma invasion by 70% at a dose of 20 mg/kg. Therefore, blocking OGC activity may be a useful approach for cancer therapy.

Keywords: oxoglutarate carrier; malate-aspartate shuttle; cancer metabolism; ATP production

1. Introduction

Recently, we reported that up to 80% of the total ATP production in melanoma and lung cancer cells [1], and about 40% of the ATP production in pancreatic cancer cells [2,3], depends on cytosolic NADH and the malate-aspartate shuttle (MAS). The MAS transfers cytosolic NADH into mitochondria for ATP production through oxidative phosphorylation (OxPhos) in the mitochondrial membrane [1]. The MAS consists of four metabolic enzymes, glutamic-oxaloacetic transaminase (GOT) 1 and 2 and malate dehydrogenase (MDH) 1 and 2, and two antiporters, oxoglutarate carrier (OGC, oxoglutarate/malate antiporter, *SLC25A11*) and mitochondrial aspartate-glutamate carrier (AGC1) (Figure 1A) [1,4]. Knock-down of OGC reduced ATP production by 80% and inhibited the growth of lung and melanoma cancer cells by over 90% [1]. ATP depletion by more than 50% induces cell cycle arrest and cell death in a time-dependent manner in cancer cells [5–8]. Furthermore, in in vivo experiments, heterozygous OGC knock-out mice showed 50% less spontaneous tumor development in the *KRAS*^{LA2} lung cancer model [1]. Blocking OGC may selectively inhibit cancer growth by reducing ATP production in cancer cells because cancer cells rely on the MAS for ATP generation while normal cells do not [1,2].

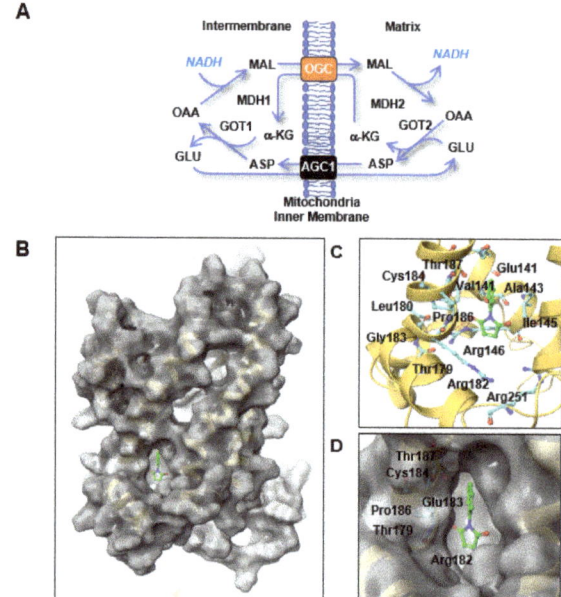

Figure 1. Important binding interactions for the docked conformations of NPM using the OGC homology model. (**A**) The MAS for NADH transport into the mitochondrial matrix. NPM, N-phenylmaleimide; OGC, oxoglutarate carrier; AGC1, aspartate-glutamate carrier isoform 1; OAA, oxaloacetate; α-KG, α-ketoglutarate. (**B**) The binding site in the OGC model is shown as a light orange ribbon; NPM is shown in green in a stick-ball structure. (**C**) Detailed interactions between NPM and OGC are shown with a stick model, and residues involved in the interaction with NPM are presented in the stick-ball style colored by atom type (C, cyan; N, blue; O, red). H-bonds are indicated by red dashed lines. (**D**) Close-up left-hand view of the predicted binding of NPM to OGC. The ligand is depicted in the stick-ball style. Figures were drawn in Maestro (Schrödinger, LLC, New York, NY, USA, 2020).

A specific mitochondrial transport system for 2-oxoglutarate was first proposed by Dr. Chappell in 1967 [9], and the biochemical properties of this system, including its structure and activity, were recently reviewed by Dr. Fiermonte [10]. OGC has a similar structure to that of mitochondrial ADP/ATP carriers, although a three-dimensional (3D) study of the OGC structure by X-ray crystallography failed [10]. Inhibitors of OGC were therefore developed based on the starting compounds of the biochemical reaction instead of the OGC structure. Most OGC inhibitors are derived from substrate analogues such as succinate, butylmalonate, and phthalonate [11,12], which do not bind to the translocation site but do block transport. OGC contains three cysteine residues at positions 184, 221, and 224 that can create S-S bridges with sulfhydryl reagents [13]. Dr. Palmieri's group found that both mercurials and maleimides integrated specifically with Cys184 [13]. This binding was associated with inhibition of the OGC active conformation. The degree of OGC inhibition by N-phenylmaleimide (NPM) binding to OGC was enhanced in the presence of OGC substrates [13]. This suggests that a substrate-induced conformational change in OGC increases the reactivity of Cys184 to sulfhydryl reagents such as NPM [13]. NPM inhibited OGC transport activity with a 50% inhibitory concentration (IC_{50}) of 1.25 mmol/min/g [13], and NPM analogues inhibited the proliferation of H460 cancer cells with IC_{50} values of 0.84–9 μM using in vitro assay system using reconstituted liposome with purified OGC [14].

In this study, we investigated whether OGC inhibition with NPM inhibited cancer growth by reducing ATP production. Although NPM itself is known to have some off-target effects, this study demonstrates the potential therapeutic efficacy of OGC inhibitors.

2. Materials and Methods

2.1. Cell Culture

Tumor spheres (TS) generated from the UACC-62 and B16F10 melanoma cell lines were used in this study. UACC-62 cells were obtained from the US National Cancer Institute (NCI; Bethesda, MD, USA) (MTA 1-2702-09) and B16F10 cells (CRL-6475) were obtained from the American Type Culture Collection (ATCC; Manassas, VA, USA). For TS culture, cells were cultured in TS complete media, which was composed of Dulbecco's modified Eagle's medium/F12 (SH30023.01, Hyclone, Logan, UT, USA), B27 supplement (17504044, Thermo Fisher Scientific, Waltham, MA, USA), 20 ng/mL basic fibroblast growth factor (F0291, Sigma-Aldrich, St. Louis, MO, USA), and 20 ng/mL epidermal growth factor (E9644, Sigma-Aldrich, St. Louis, MO, USA).

2.2. Homology Modeling and Molecular Docking

To obtain a homology model of OGC, we used the nuclear magnetic resonance (NMR)-based structure of mitochondrial uncoupling protein 2 (UCP2; Protein Data Bank (PDB) ID, 2LCK) as a template structure. The sequence alignment and homology modeling procedure were executed using Prime (Schrödinger, New York, NY, USA, 2020) [15]. The overall quality of the modeled structure was assessed using a Ramachandran plot. The active binding sites of OGC were identified using the modeled protein structure in the SiteMap program of the Schrödinger software [16]. To examine the binding interactions of the protein–ligand complexes, molecular docking studies were performed using the Glide software (Schrödinger, New York, NY, USA), which uses an optimized potential for liquid simulations (OPLS)-2005 force field, and refinement was carried out as per the recommendations of the Schrödinger Protein Preparation Wizard. LigPrep (Schrödinger, New York, NY, USA) was used to generate 3D structures of the ligands. The active grid was generated using the Receptor grid application in the Glide module. On a defined receptor grid, flexible docking was performed using the standard precision mode of Glide [17]. The best docking pose for a compound was selected based on the best-scoring conformations from Glide, the binding patterns, and visual inspection.

2.3. Sulforhodamine B Assay (SRB): Cell Growth Assay

Cancer cells were counted, and approximately 2×10^4 cells per well were seeded in 96-well cell culture plates (Corning Inc., Corning, NY, USA). After incubation at 37 °C in a humidified atmosphere with 5% CO_2 for 72 h, cells were treated with the indicated concentrations of NPM. The assay was performed following to the previously established method [2].

2.4. Measurement of the NADH/NAD^+ Ratio and ATP Levels

To quantify NADH/NAD in cell lines, the Ultra-GloTM Recombinant Luciferase assay kit (Promega, #G9071) was used according to the manufacturer's instructions. Briefly, the cyclic enzyme included in the kit converts NAD^+ to NADH, which subsequently activates a reductase that converts pro-luciferin to luciferin. The samples were subsequently detected with Ultra-GloTM r-Luciferase. To this end, the cells were seeded into a 96-well culture plate at a density of 10^4 cells/well and incubated for 24 h, then treated with NPM for 72 h. Subsequently, 50 µL of NAD/NADH-GloTM Detection Reagent and an equal volume of sample were incubated at room temperature for 30 min. To measure ATP levels in cell lines, the cell titer-Glo 2.0 assay (Promega, #G9241) was used according to the manufacturer's instructions. The cells were seeded into a 96-well culture plate at a density of 10^5 cells/well and incubated for 24 h and treated with NPM for 72 h. A volume of CellTiter-Glo® 2.0 Reagent equal to the volume of ATP standard present in each well was added. The mixed contents were incubated at room temperature for 10 min and luminescence was measured.

2.5. Measurement of Apoptosis

Tumor cells were incubated with or without NPM. The cells were collected, washed with cold PBS, centrifuged at 1400 rpm for 3 min, and resuspended in binding buffer from a kit (556547, BD Biosciences, San Jose, CA, USA) at a density of 1×10^6 cells/mL. Cells (1×10^5 cells in a 100 µL volume) were transferred to a 5 mL culture tube, and 5 µL each of annexin V-FITC and propidium iodide (PI) were added. The cells were gently vortexed and incubated for 15 min at room temperature in the dark. A total of 400 µL of binding buffer was added to each tube, and the samples were analyzed by flow cytometry (FACSCalibur BD Biosciences, San Jose, CA, USA).

2.6. Measurement of Mitochondrial Membrane Potential ($\Delta\psi m$)

Mitochondrial membrane potential (MMP) was assessed by measuring the mean fluorescence intensity of tetramethylrodamine ester (TMRE) loaded cells. TMRE (87917, Sigma-Aldrich, St. Louis, MO, USA) is a fluorescence probe that specifically accumulates within mitochondria in an MMP-dependent manner. Cells were plated in a 100 mm plate and treated as indicted. Twenty minutes prior to the end of each treatment, 100 nM TMRE was added to the culture medium. Cells were washed two times with ice-cold PBS. Cells were collected immediately for flow cytometric analysis (FACSCalibur, BD Biosciences, San Jose, CA, USA) of fluorescence intensity using the 585 nm (FL-2) channel.

2.7. Immunohistochemistry

Immunohistochemistry was performed on a Ventana Discovery XT automated staining instrument (Ventana Medical Systems, Tucson, AZ, USA) followed by the established method [2]. Staining was performed with a Ki-67 antibody (ab15580; Abcam, Cambridge, UK) and KI-67 positive cells were quantified using ImageJ software (64-bit Java 1.8.0_112).

2.8. XF Cell Mito Stress Analysis

Cells were treated with the indicated drugs for 24 h. For determination of the oxygen consumption rate (OCR), cells were incubated in XF base medium supplemented with 10 mM glucose, 1 mM sodium pyruvate, and 2 mM of L-glutamine, and were equilibrated in a non-CO_2 incubator for 1 h before starting the assay. The samples were incubated for 3 min and then data were acquired for 3 min using the XFe96 extracellular flux analyzer (Seahorse Bioscience, North Billerica, MA, USA). Oligomycin (0.75 µM), carbonyl cyanide-4-(trifluoromethoxy) phenylhydrazone (FCCP; 1 µM), and rotenone/antimycin A (0.5 µM) (103015-100, Agilent Technologies, Santa Clara, CA, USA) were injected at the indicated time points. Finally, the OCR was normalized to the cell number, as determined by CCK-8 assay.

2.9. CCK-8 Assay

Cancer cells were counted, and approximately 5×10^3 cells per well were seeded in 96-well cell culture plates (Corning Inc., Corning, NY, USA). After incubation at 37 °C in a humidified atmosphere with 5% CO_2 for 72 h, cells were treated with the indicated concentrations of NPM. At the end of XF Cell Mito Stress Analysis, 10 µL of CCK-8 reagent (ALX-850-039, Enzo Life Sciences, Farmingdale, NY, USA) was added to each well, and the optical density (OD) at 450 nm was measured using a multifunction microplate reader (Infinite M200 Pro, Tecan, Männedorf, Switzerland) after incubation for 1 h at 37 °C.

2.10. Invasion Assay

The upper compartments of 8 mm Transwells (6.5 mm diameter; Coastar Corp., Cambridge, MA, USA) were precoated with Matrigel (1 mg/mL). Cells (10^5 cells) were suspended in DMEM and placed in the upper compartments of the Transwells, and the lower compartments were filled with DMEM supplemented with 3% FBS. After 24 h, the filters were washed with PBS and fixed with methanol. Migrated cells on the filter membrane were stained using a Diff-Quik staining kit (38721, Sysmex,

Kobe, Japan). Each assay was conducted at least three times, and three random fields under 20× magnification were analyzed for each filter membrane.

2.11. Preclinical Xenograft Model

Balb/c-nu mice (Orient, Seoul, Korea) were between 6 and 8 weeks of age before tumor induction. This study was reviewed and approved by the Institutional Animal Care and Use Committee (IACUC) of the National Cancer Center Research Institute, which is an Association for Assessment and Accreditation of Laboratory Animal Care (AAALAC) International-accredited facility that abides by the Institute of Laboratory Animal Resources guidelines (protocol NCC-19-195). Mice were inoculated with UACC-62 cells (1×10^7) in 100 µL PBS subcutaneously using a 1 mL syringe. After 1 week, the mice were divided into two groups, a control group treated with vehicle and an NPM-treated group (n = 5 mice/group). Vehicle (5% dimethyl sulfoxide (DMSO) and 10% Kolliphor in PBS; 100 µL) and NPM (20 mg/kg) were administered orally once per day, 5 days/week, for 3 weeks. The primary tumor size was measured every week using calipers. The tumor volume was calculated using the formula $V = (A \times B^2)/2$, where V is the volume (mm^3), A is the long diameter, and B is the short diameter.

2.12. Syngeneic Lung Tumor Metastasis Model

This study was reviewed and approved by the IACUC of the National Cancer Center Research Institute (protocol NCC-20-557). To determine the effect of NPM on tumor metastasis in vivo, the formation of lung metastases was assessed in C57BL/6 mice injected intravenously with B16F10 cells (1×10^5) via the tail vein. Three weeks after injection of B16F10 cells, the mice were sacrificed by CO_2 asphyxiation, images of the lungs were captured, and the lung metastases were counted. Tissue specimens from each group were fixed in formalin and embedded in paraffin for histologic examination. Metastatic lesions were quantified using ImageJ software (64-bit Java 1.8.0_112).

2.13. hERG K^+ Channel Binding Assay

E-4031 (M5060, Sigma-Aldrich, St. Louis, MO, USA) compound was used as a positive control. Membrane containing the hERG channel was mixed with the tracer for 4 h. The fluorescence intensity in the presence of NPT (excitation at 530 nm, emission at 590 nm) was measured by Synergy Neo (Biotek, Winooski, VT, USA) using the hERG Fluorescence Polarization Assay kit (PV5365, Thermo Fisher Scientific) and compared with the fluorescence intensity of the DMSO solvent control. The hERG assay was performed by a licensed contract research organization, Daegu-Gyeongbuk Medical Innovation Foundation (Daegu, Korea).

2.14. Statistical Analysis

Statistical analysis was performed using the Student's t-test as appropriate. Tumor growth and tumor weight was analyzed statistically by two-way analysis of variance (ANOVA) tests using GraphPad PRISM 5 (GraphPad Software, San Diego, CA, USA).

3. Results

3.1. Molecular Docking of NPM to OGC

Tumor spheres (TSs) were generated from the UACC-62 and B16F10 melanoma cell lines and used in this study to mimic a 3D culture system. The OGC inhibitor NPT was used to test whether OGC inhibition could block the MAS, reduce ATP production, and inhibit cancer growth [13]. Unlike healthy cells, cancer cells utilize the MAS to transfer NADH from the cytosol to mitochondria. The MAS is composed of two antiporters, OGC and AGC1, as well as GOT1 and 2 and MDH1 and 2 (Figure 1A). Although OGC has a similar structure to that of mitochondrial ADP/ATP carriers (PDB ID: 1OKC), there is no crystal structure for the human OGC in the PDB database. By sequence similarity searching, the crystal structure of mouse mitochondrial uncoupling protein 2 (UCP2; PDB ID: 2LCK) was found to be most similar to the sequence of human OGC protein [18]. To obtain homology structure model of human OGC, we used the crystal structure of mouse UCP2 as a template. The Cys184 residue of mitochondrial OGC was found to be more accessible to sulfhydryl reagents when substrate and residues previously defined to be essential for substrate binding were added to the model [13]. Thus, we considered the binding site around Cys184 as the specific target site for the sulfhydryl reagent NPM. Grid-based docking of NPM around Cys184 in the OGC homology model produced a configuration in which the hydroxy group of NPM forms hydrogen bonds with Arg146 of the binding site (Figure 1B). As illustrated, the N-phenyl ring docked into a hydrophobic cavity formed by residues Val141, Ile145, Leu180, and Pro186 (Figure 1C,D). These residues involved in the interaction of OGC with NPM are likely essential for transport function and conformational changes. In particular, Arg146, which is involved in the salt-bridge network, is likely to play a major role in opening and closing the matrix gate to alter the conformational state of the carrier.

3.2. The Effect of NPM on Mitochondrial Activity and ATP Production in Cancer Cells

Recently, we showed that knock-down of OGC reduced ATP production by up to 80%, with a concomitant reduction in mitochondrial activity [1]. To test whether NPM reduces ATP production by inhibiting OGC and therefore inhibiting mitochondrial activity, the OCR and ATP production were analyzed using Seahorse analyzer after NPM treatment (Figure 2). NPM treatment for 24 h reduced the OCR by about 20% and 33% in UACC-62 and B16F10 cells, respectively (Figure 2A). ATP production was also reduced by 28% and 24% in UACC-62 and B16F10 cells compared with nontreated control cells (Figure 2A). NPM treatment for 72 h reduced the OCR by approximately 50% and 60% in UACC-62 and B16F10 cells, respectively, which correlated with an approximately 52% and 57% reduction in ATP production compared with control UACC-62 and B16F10 cells (Figure 2A). These results suggest that cancer cells rely on OxPhos, which consumes oxygen to produce ATP using NADH from the cytosol, which is in turn transferred into mitochondria by OGC. To test whether the reduction in OCR by NPM is related to a decrease in OxPhos, mitochondrial membrane potential was measured by tetramethylrhodamine-ethylester (TMRE) staining (Figure 2B). Mitochondrial membrane potential was decreased by NPM treatment, which showed a dose and time dependence between 24 and 48 h at 10 μM (Figure 2B). NPM treatment at 10 μM for 48 h decreased mitochondrial activity to about 10% of the control in UACC-62 and B16F10 cells (Figure 2B). This implies that OGC inhibition reduces NADH flux into mitochondria from the cytosol, which reduces ATP production by OxPhos. To test whether NPM inhibits OGC, we analyzed the OCR and ATP production after treatment with 20 μM NPM for 24 h in OGC knock-down B16F10 cells (Figure 2C). OGC knock-down alone decreased the OCR and the ATP production, but there was no additional effect of NPM in OGC knock-down cells (Figure 2C). Therefore, NPM reduces ATP production by inhibiting OGC in melanoma cells.

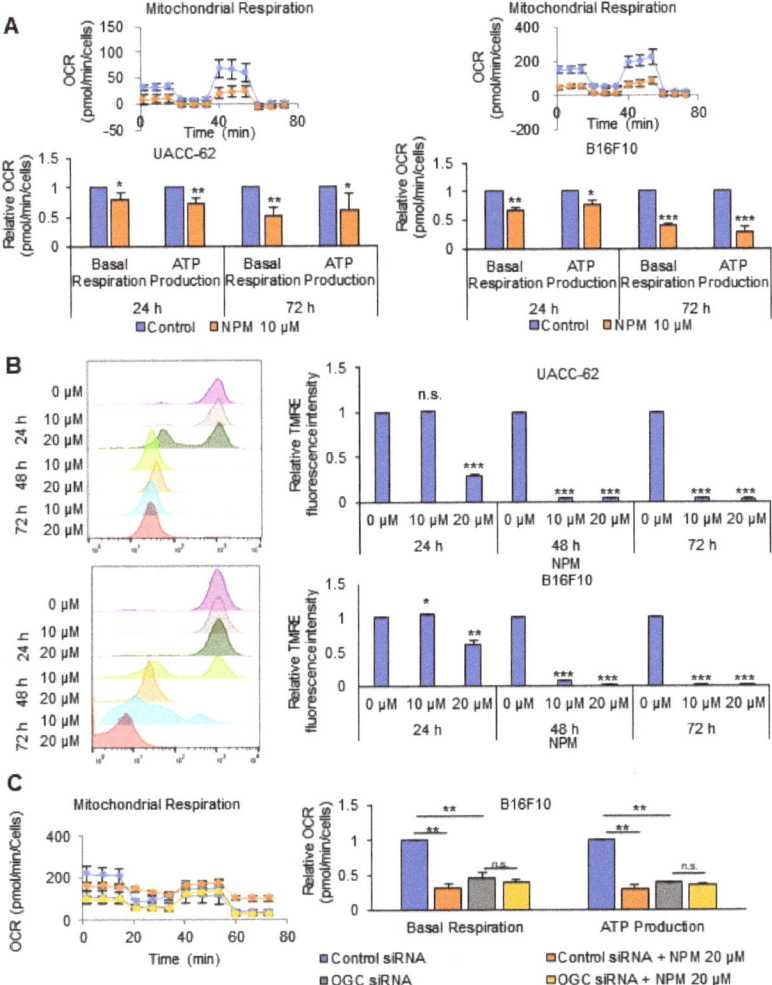

Figure 2. NPM reduced ATP production by decreasing the OCR and the mitochondrial membrane potential. (**A**) OCR was measured in UACC-62 and B16F10 cells treated with 10 µM of NPM for 24 h and 72 h using a Seahorse XFe96 analyzer. (**B**) The mitochondrial membrane potential was determined by tetramethylrodamine ester (TMRE) staining in UACC-62 and B16F10 cells treated with 10 or 20 µM of NPM for the indicated times. (**C**) The OCR and ATP production were analyzed by Seahorse XF analyzer after treatment of wild-type or OGC knock-down B16F10 cells with 20 µM of NPM for 24 h. Data represent the mean and standard deviation of three independent experiments. * $p < 0.05$, ** $p < 0.01$, and *** $p < 0.001$ compared with the vehicle control.

3.3. The Inhibitory Effect of NPM Treatment on Proliferation of Tumor Spheres

To test whether NPM can regulate cancer growth through OGC inhibition, cell proliferation was measured by Cell Counting Kit-8 (CCK-8) assay, a sensitive colorimetric assay for the determination of cell viability. Treatment with 20 µM NPM decreased TS proliferation to about 70% and 55% of the control in UACC-62 and B16F10 cells, respectively (Figure 3A). NPM is known as an OGC inhibitor, which transfers malate from the cytosol to mitochondria. The transferred malate is converted to oxaloacetate by MDH2, resulting in NADH production. Therefore, we tested whether NPM reduced the NADH and ATP level. NADH and ATP were reduced dose-dependently by NPM treatment for 72 h. The 20 µM of NPM decreased the NADH level to 12% and 4% of the level in control UACC-62 and B16F10 cells, respectively (Figure 3B). Additionally, 20 µM of NPM decreased the ATP level to 23% and 4% of the level in control UACC-62 and B16F10 cells, respectively (Figure 3C). This implies that OGC inhibition stalls the MAS and reduces NADH production by MDH2 by decreasing the amount of malate in mitochondria. To test whether the decrease in ATP was due to cell death resulting from NPM treatment, an annexin V and propidium iodide (PI) staining assay was performed with B16F10 cells treated with 10 or 20 µM NPM for 72 h (Figure 3D). There was no increase in cell death after NPM treatment for 72 h, which suggests that the ATP reduction is not due to an increase in apoptosis.

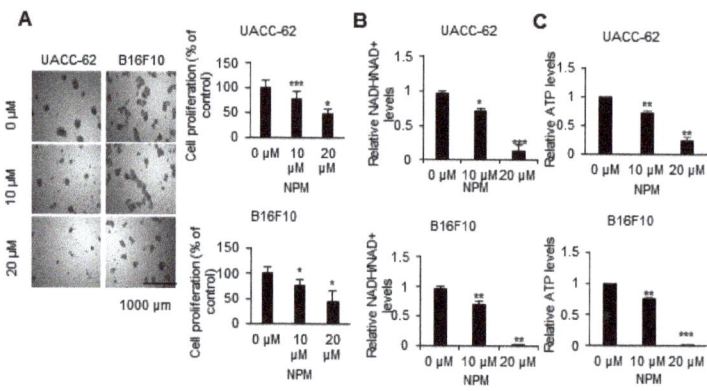

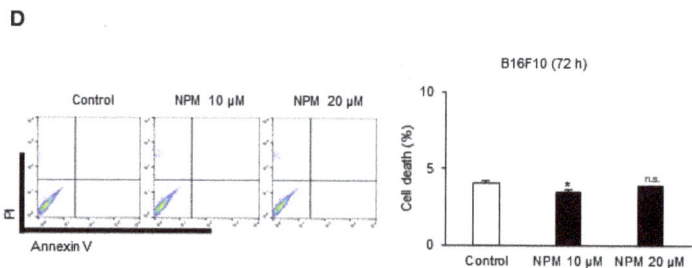

Figure 3. Cancer cell proliferation was regulated by NPM. (**A**) Cancer cell proliferation was determined by SRB assay in UACC-62 and B16F10 TSs treated with the indicated concentration of NPM for 72 h. (**B**) The NADH/NAD+ ratio was measured in UACC-62 and B16F10 cells treated with the indicated concentration of NPM for 72 h. (**C**) The ATP level was measured using luminescent ATP assay kit in UACC-62 and B16F10 cells following to the treatment of NPM for 72 h. (**D**) Cell death was determined by annexin V and propidium iodide (PI) staining in B16F10 cells treated with 10 and 20 µM NPM for 72 h. Data represent the mean and standard deviation of three independent experiments. * $p < 0.05$, ** $p < 0.01$, and *** $p < 0.001$ compared with the vehicle control.

3.4. Antiproliferative Effect of NPM in a Human Melanoma Xenograft Model

We observed an antiproliferative effect of NPM in cancer cells, as shown in Figure 3. To test whether NPM has anticancer effects on melanoma in vivo, NPM was administered in a mouse xenograft model using the human UACC-62 cell line (Figure 4). The maximum tolerated dose of NPM was determined to be 60 mg/kg/day (PO: per os, oral treatment) (Supplementary Figure S1). Three weeks of treatment with NPM reduced the UACC-62 tumor volume to about 50% of the control group (Figure 4A,C). Tumors were collected at the end of the in vivo experiment and tumors were weighed. The tumor mass in the NPM treatment group was reduced by 63% compared with the control group (Figure 4B). Immunohistochemical staining for Ki67, a marker of proliferation, was strongly reduced by NPM treatment. NPM treatment reduced the percentage of Ki67-positive cells by 67% compared with the control (Figure 4D).

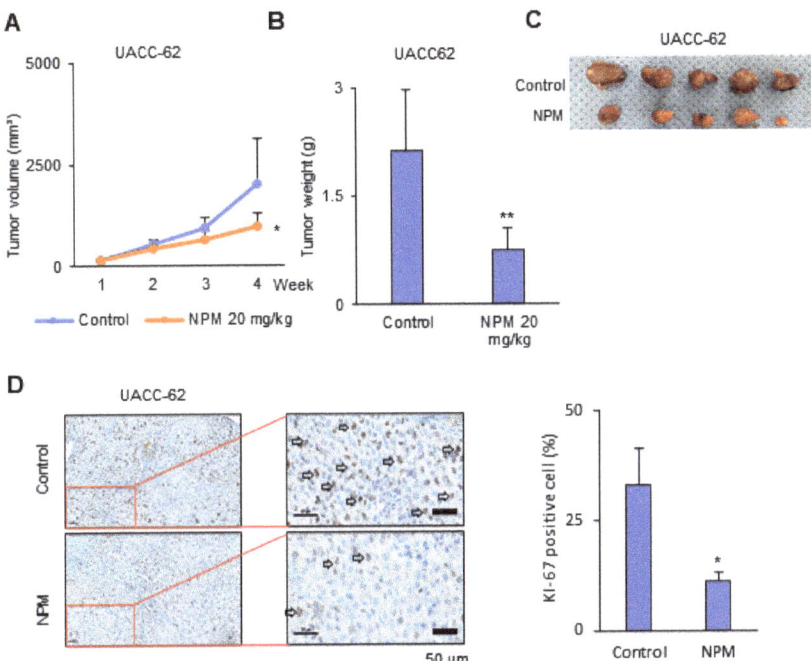

Figure 4. Tumor growth in a melanoma xenograft model was inhibited by NPM treatment. (**A**) The graph represents the tumor growth, as measured using calipers. (**B**) The weight of subcutaneous UACC-62 tumors from mice with or without NPM treatment. (**C**) Representative images of the removed tumors. (**D**) Immunohistochemical analysis of Ki-67 in UACC-62 xenografts from mice with or without NPM treatment. Quantification was measured by positive cell counting using Image J. Data represent the mean and standard deviation of three independent experiments. * $p < 0.05$ and ** $p < 0.01$ compared with the vehicle control. KI-67 positive cell was checked by arrow.

3.5. Antimetastasis Effect of NPM in a Human Melanoma Xenograft Model

One feature of malignant melanoma is invasiveness. A previous study demonstrated that an increase in the ATP production could promote cell migration and invasion in human cancer [19]. We tested whether NPM reduces cell invasion using an in vitro Transwell invasion assay. NPM treatment significantly reduced cell invasion in a dose-dependent manner in B16F10 and UACC-62 cells (Figure 5A). We next analyzed the melanoma metastasis in vivo by inoculating C57BL/6 mice intravenously with B16F10 cells (Figure 5B). Lungs were collected at the end of the study, and hematoxylin and eosin (H&E) staining was performed (Figure 5C). The number of metastatic lung nodules and the total area of the metastases were determined using ImageJ. NPT reduced the number of metastatic lung nodules and the total area of lung metastasis by 70% (Figure 5D,E).

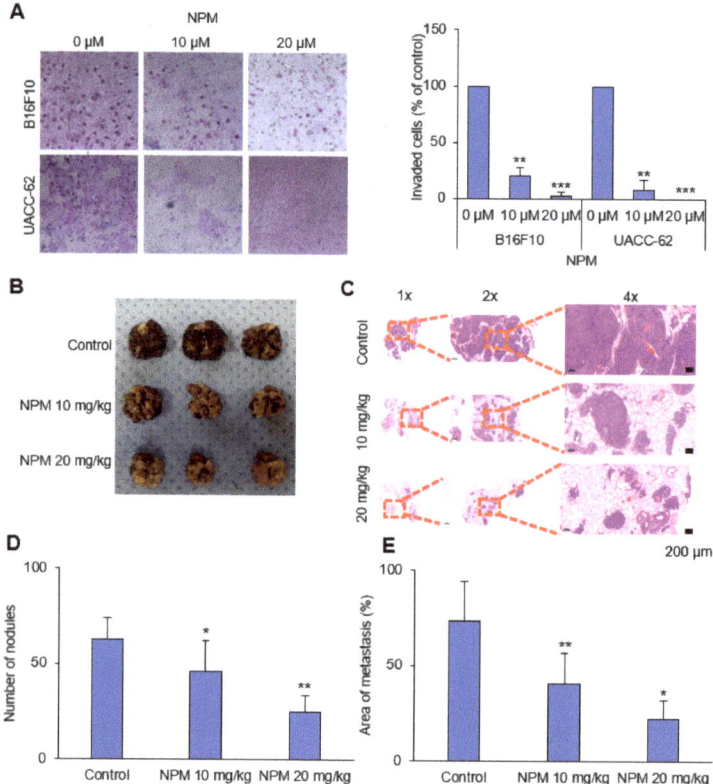

Figure 5. NPM reduces lung metastasis of B16F10 melanoma cells in immunocompetent mice. (**A**) Invasion assay performed with B16F10 and UACC-62 cell lines following NPM treatment for 16 h. Representative images of the invasion assay using B16F10 and UACC-62 cells (left). The numbers of invasive B16F10 and UACC-62 cells were measured using ImageJ (right). (**B**) Representative photographs of formalin-fixed lungs. (**C**) Metastatic lesions were observed with hematoxylin and eosin (H&E) staining. (**D**) Statistical analysis of the number of metastatic nodules. (**E**) Statistical analysis of the total metastatic area using ImageJ. Data represent the mean and standard deviation of three independent experiments. * $p < 0.05$, ** $p < 0.01$, and *** $p < 0.001$ compared with the vehicle control.

4. Discussion

In in vitro experiments with cultured melanoma tumor spheres, NPM suppressed mitochondrial activity, oxygen consumption, and ATP production in a dose-dependent manner by inhibiting OGC, resulting in decreased melanoma cell proliferation. NPM also reduced melanoma cell invasion by over 70% in a human melanoma metastasis model. Therefore, blocking OGC activity with NPM may be a useful approach for inhibiting cancer growth.

However, there are reports of the inhibitory effects of NPM on pyruvate transport, telomerase activity, and Bak protein activity. It is known that pyruvate transport may be inhibited by thiol-blocking reagents such as iodoacetate and NPM [20]. However, in cancer cells, pyruvate transport into mitochondria is limited because cancer cells have higher expression of lactate dehydrogenase (LDHA), which catalyzes pyruvate to lactate, compared with normal cells [21]. Furthermore, cancer cells do not rely on the tricarboxylic acid (TCA) cycle to produce NADH, while normal cells depend completely on the TCA cycle for NADH production [2]. Therefore, the decrease in ATP production observed in response to NPM likely does not occur through inhibition of pyruvate transport. Indeed, OCR and ATP production were measured in B16F10 cells treated with the indicated concentration of pyruvate inhibitor UK-5099 for 24 h. The analysis showed no decrease of these parameters. (Supplementary Figure S2). NPM is also known to inhibit telomerase activity, which plays a key role in maintaining telomerase length [22]. In in vitro assays, NPM inhibited telomerase activity. However, the IC_{50} of NPM for inhibition of telomerase activity was approximately 2 µM, at which concentration there was no telomerase inhibition in cancer cells [22]. This implies that the cytotoxicity of NPM is unrelated to inhibition of telomerase activity. Finally, NPM has been reported to induce apoptosis through Bak oligomerization in Jurkat cells at a concentration of 0.5 µM [23]. However, we did not observe apoptosis by FACS analysis of melanoma cell lines treated with 20 µM NPM for 72 h.

Maleimide is formed with a -C(O)NHC(O)- functional group from the reaction of maleic acid and imide. NPM is a derivative of maleimide in which the NH group of maleimide is replaced with the aryl group of phenyl. NPM can cause skin and eye irritation and showed acute toxicity, with a 50% lethal dose (LD_{50}) of 78 mg/kg in mice when administered orally (https://www.cdc.gov/niosh-rtecs/ON5ACA30.html). In this study, we did not observe any death or weight loss in mice treated with 20 mg/kg NPM. Although NPM is considered a nonspecific cytotoxic agent, NPM also did not show any cardiotoxicity by hERG assay (Supplementary Figure S3). The hERG channel inhibition assay is a highly sensitive assay that will identify compounds exhibiting cardiotoxicity related to hERG inhibition in vivo. The IC_{50} value of NPM in that assay was 78.75 µM, which indicates that it shows no hERG channel inhibition.

OGC with NPM significantly reduced ATP production in melanoma cells by decreasing NADH production. Treatment of mice with NPM reduced tumor growth and tumor invasion by 60% and 80%, respectively, in a human melanoma xenograft model. These data suggest that OGC inhibition combined with cytotoxic anticancer therapy may have synergistic effects on tumor growth.

5. Conclusions

Biochemical data from this study using the chemical inhibitor NPM and previous studies using OGC knock-out cells [1] together suggest that proliferating cancer cells rely on the MAS system to transport cytosolic NADH into the mitochondria, where it is then used to generate ATP through OxPhos. This study suggests that OGC, as a major regulatory component of the MAS, is a promising molecular target to inhibit cancer growth and invasion by inhibition of cancer metabolism. Therefore, more efforts should be devoted to developing OGC inhibitors for cancer therapy.

Supplementary Materials: The following are available online at http://www.mdpi.com/1999-4923/12/11/1128/s1. Supplementary Figure S1: The maximum tolerated dose (MTD) was determined in order to examine the acute toxicity of NPM in animals. Supplementary Figure S2: The cell mito stress test was performed to examine the effect of UK-5099 as mitochondria pyruvate carrier inhibitor. Figure S3: The binding of NPM to the hERG K$^+$ channel was evaluated as a measure of cardiac toxicity.

Author Contributions: Conceptualization: S.-Y.K.; validation: J.-S.L., J.C., S.-H.L., and H.Y.K.; methodology and formal analysis: J.-S.L., J.C., S.-H.L., and H.Y.K.; investigation and resources: J.-S.L., S.-H.L., J.H.K., J.S.H., and H.Y.K.; data curation: J.-S.L., J.C., and H.Y.K.; writing—original draft preparation: S.-Y.K.; writing—review and editing: H.J. and J.I.Y.; data visualization: J.-S.L., J.C., and S.-Y.K.; project administration: S.-Y.K.; funding acquisition: S.-Y.K. All authors have read and agreed to the published version of the manuscript.

Funding: This research was supported by the Bio & Medical Technology Development Program of the National Research Foundation (NRF) funded by the Ministry of Science & ICT in Korea (2019M3A9G110434521) to SK.

Acknowledgments: This work was supported by the Flow Cytometry Core Facility of the National Cancer Center of Korea.

Conflicts of Interest: The authors declare no conflict of interest.

References

1. Lee, J.S.; Lee, H.; Lee, S.; Kang, J.H.; Lee, S.H.; Kim, S.G.; Cho, E.S.; Kim, N.H.; Yook, J.I.; Kim, S.Y. Loss of SLC25A11 causes suppression of NSCLC and melanoma tumor formation. *EBioMedicine* **2019**, *40*, 184–197. [CrossRef]
2. Lee, J.S.; Oh, S.J.; Choi, H.J.; Kang, J.H.; Lee, S.H.; Ha, J.S.; Woo, S.M.; Jang, H.; Lee, H.; Kim, S.Y. ATP Production Relies on Fatty Acid Oxidation Rather than Glycolysis in Pancreatic Ductal Adenocarcinoma. *Cancers* **2020**, *12*, 2477. [CrossRef]
3. Kim, S.Y. Cancer Energy Metabolism: Shutting Power off Cancer Factory. *Biomol. Ther. (Seoul)* **2018**, *26*, 39–44. [CrossRef] [PubMed]
4. Greenhouse, W.V.; Lehninger, A.L. Occurrence of the malate-aspartate shuttle in various tumor types. *Cancer Res.* **1976**, *36*, 1392–1396. [PubMed]
5. Kang, J.H.; Lee, S.H.; Hong, D.; Lee, J.S.; Ahn, H.S.; Ahn, J.H.; Seong, T.W.; Lee, C.H.; Jang, H.; Hong, K.M.; et al. Aldehyde dehydrogenase is used by cancer cells for energy metabolism. *Exp. Mol. Med.* **2016**, *48*, e272. [CrossRef] [PubMed]
6. Kang, J.H.; Lee, S.H.; Lee, J.S.; Nam, B.; Seong, T.W.; Son, J.; Jang, H.; Hong, K.M.; Lee, C.; Kim, S.Y. Aldehyde dehydrogenase inhibition combined with phenformin treatment reversed NSCLC through ATP depletion. *Oncotarget* **2016**, *7*, 49397–49410. [CrossRef] [PubMed]
7. Lee, J.S.; Kim, S.H.; Lee, S.; Kang, J.H.; Lee, S.H.; Cheong, J.H.; Kim, S.Y. Gastric cancer depends on aldehyde dehydrogenase 3A1 for fatty acid oxidation. *Sci. Rep.* **2019**, *9*, 16313. [CrossRef]
8. Lee, S.; Lee, J.S.; Seo, J.; Lee, S.H.; Kang, J.H.; Song, J.; Kim, S.Y. Targeting Mitochondrial Oxidative Phosphorylation Abrogated Irinotecan Resistance in NSCLC. *Sci. Rep.* **2018**, *8*, 15707. [CrossRef]
9. Robinson, B.H.; Chappell, J.B. The inhibition of malate, tricarboxylate and oxoglutarate entry into mitochondria by 2-n-butylmalonate. *Biochem. Biophys. Res. Commun.* **1967**, *28*, 249–255. [CrossRef]
10. Monne, M.; Miniero, D.V.; Iacobazzi, V.; Bisaccia, F.; Fiermonte, G. The mitochondrial oxoglutarate carrier: From identification to mechanism. *J. Bioenerg. Biomembr.* **2013**, *45*, 1–13. [CrossRef]
11. Stipani, I.; Natuzzi, D.; Daddabbo, L.; Ritieni, A.; Randazzo, G.; Palmieri, F. Photoaffinity labeling of the mitochondrial oxoglutarate carrier by azido-phthalonate. *Biochim. Biophys. Acta* **1995**, *1234*, 149–154. [CrossRef] [PubMed]
12. Meijer, A.J.; von Woerkom, G.M.; Eggelte, T.A. Phthalonic acid, an inhibitor of alpha-oxoglutarate transport in mitochondria. *Biochim. Biophys. Acta* **1976**, *430*, 53–61. [CrossRef] [PubMed]
13. Capobianco, L.; Bisaccia, F.; Mazzeo, M.; Palmieri, F. The mitochondrial oxoglutarate carrier: Sulfhydryl reagents bind to cysteine-184, and this interaction is enhanced by substrate binding. *Biochemistry* **1996**, *35*, 8974–8980. [CrossRef] [PubMed]
14. Ferri, N.; Beccalli, E.M.; Contini, A.; Corsini, A.; Antonino, M.; Radice, T.; Pratesi, G.; Tinelli, S.; Zunino, F.; Gelmi, M.L. Antiproliferative effects on human tumor cells and rat aortic smooth muscular cells of 2,3-heteroarylmaleimides and heterofused imides. *Bioorg. Med. Chem.* **2008**, *16*, 1691–1701. [CrossRef] [PubMed]
15. Jacobson, M.P.; Pincus, D.L.; Rapp, C.S.; Day, T.J.; Honig, B.; Shaw, D.E.; Friesner, R.A. A hierarchical approach to all-atom protein loop prediction. *Proteins* **2004**, *55*, 351–367. [CrossRef] [PubMed]
16. Halgren, T.A. Identifying and characterizing binding sites and assessing druggability. *J. Chem. Inf. Model.* **2009**, *49*, 377–389. [CrossRef]
17. Friesner, R.A.; Banks, J.L.; Murphy, R.B.; Halgren, T.A.; Klicic, J.J.; Mainz, D.T.; Repasky, M.P.; Knoll, E.H.; Shelley, M.; Perry, J.K.; et al. Glide: A new approach for rapid, accurate docking and scoring. 1. Method and assessment of docking accuracy. *J. Med. Chem.* **2004**, *47*, 1739–1749. [CrossRef]
18. Berardi, M.J.; Shih, W.M.; Harrison, S.C.; Chou, J.J. Mitochondrial uncoupling protein 2 structure determined by NMR molecular fragment searching. *Nature* **2011**, *476*, 109–113. [CrossRef]
19. Yang, H.; Geng, Y.H.; Wang, P.; Yang, H.; Zhou, Y.T.; Zhang, H.Q.; He, H.Y.; Fang, W.G.; Tian, X.X. Extracellular ATP promotes breast cancer invasion and chemoresistance via SOX9 signaling. *Oncogene* **2020**, *39*, 5795–5810. [CrossRef]
20. Thomas, A.P.; Halestrap, A.P. Identification of the protein responsible for pyruvate transport into rat liver and heart mitochondria by specific labelling with [3H]N-phenylmaleimide. *Biochem. J.* **1981**, *196*, 471–479. [CrossRef]

21. Feng, Y.; Xiong, Y.; Qiao, T.; Li, X.; Jia, L.; Han, Y. Lactate dehydrogenase A: A key player in carcinogenesis and potential target in cancer therapy. *Cancer Med.* **2018**, *7*, 6124–6136. [CrossRef] [PubMed]
22. Huang, P.R.; Yeh, Y.M.; Pao, C.C.; Chen, C.Y.; Wang, T.C. N-(1-Pyrenyl) maleimide inhibits telomerase activity in a cell free system and induces apoptosis in Jurkat cells. *Mol. Biol. Rep.* **2012**, *39*, 8899–8905. [CrossRef] [PubMed]
23. Huang, P.R.; Hung, S.C.; Pao, C.C.; Wang, T.C. N-(1-pyrenyl) maleimide induces bak oligomerization and mitochondrial dysfunction in Jurkat Cells. *Biomed. Res. Int.* **2015**, *2015*, 798489. [CrossRef] [PubMed]

Publisher's Note: MDPI stays neutral with regard to jurisdictional claims in published maps and institutional affiliations.

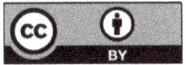

© 2020 by the authors. Licensee MDPI, Basel, Switzerland. This article is an open access article distributed under the terms and conditions of the Creative Commons Attribution (CC BY) license (http://creativecommons.org/licenses/by/4.0/).

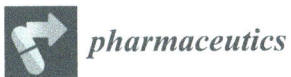

Article

Plumbagin Elicits Cell-Specific Cytotoxic Effects and Metabolic Responses in Melanoma Cells

Haoran Zhang [1,2], Aijun Zhang [1,3], Anisha A. Gupte [1,4] and Dale J. Hamilton [1,4,*]

1 Center for Bioenergetics, Houston Methodist Research Institute, Houston, TX 77030, USA; hzhang@houstonmethodist.org (H.Z.); azhang@houstonmethodist.org (A.Z.); aagupte@houstonmethodist.org (A.A.G.)
2 Department of Dermatology, Xiangya Hospital, Central South University, Changsha 410008, China
3 Molecular Biology Research in Medicine, Houston Methodist Research Institute, Weill Cornell Medicine Affiliate, Houston, TX 77030, USA
4 Department of Medicine, Houston Methodist, Weill Cornell Medicine Affiliate, Houston, TX 77030, USA
* Correspondence: djhamilton@houstonmethodist.org; Tel.: +1-(713)-441-4483

Abstract: Melanoma is one of the most malignant skin cancers that require comprehensive therapies, including chemotherapy. A plant-derived drug, plumbagin (PLB), exhibits an anticancer property in several cancers. We compared the cytotoxic and metabolic roles of PLB in A375 and SK-MEL-28 cells, each with different aggressiveness. In our results, they were observed to have distinctive mitochondrial respiratory functions. The primary reactive oxygen species (ROS) source of A375 can be robustly attenuated by cell membrane permeabilization. A375 cell viability and proliferation, migration, and apoptosis induction are more sensitive to PLB treatment. PLB induced metabolic alternations in SK-MEL-28 cells, which included increasing mitochondrial oxidative phosphorylation (OXPHOS), mitochondrial ATP production, and mitochondrial mass. Decreasing mitochondrial OXPHOS and total ATP production with elevated mitochondrial membrane potential (MMP) were observed in PLB-induced A375 cells. PLB also induced ROS production and increased proton leak and non-mitochondria respiration in both cells. This study reveals the relationship between metabolism and cytotoxic effects of PLB in melanoma. PLB displays stronger cytotoxic effects on A375 cells, which exhibit lower respiratory function than SK-MEL-28 cells with higher respiratory function, and triggers cell-specific metabolic changes in accordance with its cytotoxic effects. These findings indicate that PLB might serve as a promising anticancer drug, targeting metabolism.

Keywords: melanoma; plumbagin; cytotoxic effect; metabolism; mitochondria; reactive oxygen species

1. Introduction

Cutaneous melanoma, mainly caused by exposure to ultraviolet light, is the most dangerous skin cancer. It accounts for 1% of skin cancer diagnoses but results in 90% of deaths from all skin cancers [1]. Surgery is generally considered a typical treatment for localized melanoma. Multidisciplinary approaches, including chemotherapy, immunotherapy, and radiation therapy, are performed in advanced cases to improve the prognosis since advanced melanomas display high aggressiveness and a metastatic characteristic [2]. With current evidence-based treatment, cutaneous melanoma with lymph node and distant metastasis is reported to have 66.2% and 27.3% five-year survival rates, respectively, in the United States compared with up to 99% survival for localized melanoma [3]. Accordingly, it is necessary to explore novel treatments in the management of melanomas with different aggressiveness. A375 and SK-MEL-28 are two human melanoma cell lines with the BRAF mutation at V600E; they were selected as representative models according to the Melanoma Aggressiveness Score (MAGS). A375 has a higher MAGS than SK-MEL-28 because of the great differences in cell proliferation, migration, invasion, cell-doubling time, and other aggressive phenotypes [4].

Several natural phytochemical compounds with high anticancer potential are promising drugs in cancer therapy, including the treatment of melanoma [5–7]. Plumbagin (PLB), a naphthoquinone derivative mainly extracted from the plant, exhibits anticancer potential in different cancers, including inhibition of invasion and metastasis, induction of autophagy and apoptosis, and alteration of the cell cycle [8–11]. PLB is also considered a potent suppressor of cellular glutathione and an inducer of ROS [9,12]. Furthermore, PLB shows an anticancer effect on breast cancer depending on NQ01 activity [13], an inhibiting effect on mitochondrial electron transport, and an Nrf-2-mediated antioxidative response in several cancer cell lines [14]. It indicates the latent role of PLB on energy metabolism and mitochondrial bioenergetics. PLB has been proven to have anti-invasion and anti-metastasis effects via MAPK pathways [15] and the effect of triggering mitochondrial apoptosis by ROS and c-Jun N-terminal kinase pathways in melanoma cells [12].

However, little is known about the metabolic effect of PLB on human melanoma cells with different aggressiveness. This study aims to investigate the phenotypic alteration of cancer progression and energy metabolic changes in melanoma cell lines with different aggressiveness by applying the PLB treatment in vitro.

2. Materials and Methods

2.1. Chemicals and Reagents

Plumbagin from Plumbago indica (P7262), superoxide dismutase (SOD, S8409), L-glutamic acid (49449), L-malic (M1000), adenosine 5′-diphosphate monopotassium salt dihydrate (A5285), pyruvate (P2256), succinate (S2378), digitonin (D5628), oligomycin (O4876), carbonyl cyanide-4-(trifluoromethoxy) phenylhydrazone (FCCP, C2920), rotenone (R8875), antimycin A (A8674), L-glutamine solution (200mM, 59202C), D-(+)-glucose (G7021), H_2O_2 solution, 323381), and propidium iodide (PI, 11348639001) were purchased from Sigma (St. Louis, MO, USA). Dulbecco's modified Eagle's medium (DMEM, 30-2002), Eagle's minimum essential medium (EMEM, 30-2003), dermal cell basal medium (PCS-200-030), and the Adult Melanocyte Growth Kit (PCS-200-042) were obtained from American Type Culture Collection (ATCC, Manassas, VA, USA). Sodium pyruvate solution (1136-070) was obtained from Gibco (Grand Island, NY, USA). Horseradish peroxidase (A22188), Amplex UltraRed (AmR, A36006), MitoTracker Green dye (M7514), and Hoechst 33,258 (H3569) were purchased from Invitrogen (Foster City, CA, USA). Total OXPHOS human WB antibody cocktail (MS601) was purchased from Abcam (Cambridge, UK). GAPDH rabbit antibody (2118) was purchased from Cell Signaling Technology (Danvers, MA, USA). Goat anti-rabbit IgG-HRP (sc-2004) and goat anti-mouse IgG-HRP (sc-2005) were obtained from Santa Cruz BioTechnology (Dallas, TX, USA); 4–20% protein gels (456-1096) were purchased from BioRad (Hercules, CA, USA). A nonradioactive cell proliferation MTS assay (G6521) was purchased from Promega (Madison, WI, USA). XF DMEM base medium (102353-100), a Seahorse XF cell Mito Stress Test kit (103015-100), and a Seahorse XF Real-Time ATP Rate Assay kit (103592-100) were obtained from Agilent (Santa Clara, CA, USA). A MiR05 kit (60101-01) was purchased from Oroboros (Innsbruck, Austria). Annexin V-FITC (556419) and 10X Annexin V binding buffer (556454) were purchased from BD Biosciences (San Jose, CA, USA).

2.2. Cell Culture

Human melanoma cell lines A375 (ATCC-CRL-1619), with higher aggressiveness, SK-MEL-28 (ATCC-HTB-72), with lower aggressiveness, and normal human primary epidermal melanocytes (HEMa, ATCC-PCS-200-013) were purchased from ATCC. A375 cells were cultured in DMEM and SK-MEL-28 cells were cultured in EMEM; both kinds of the medium were supplemented with 10% fetal bovine serum, 100 IU/mL penicillin, and 100 μg/mL streptomycin. HEMa cells were cultured in dermal cell basal medium supplemented with an Adult Melanocyte Growth Kit. Cells were maintained at 37 °C in a humidified incubator with 5% CO_2. A 0.25% (w/v) trypsin-0.53mM EDTA solution was used to detach and collect the cells for subculturing or further experiments.

2.3. Dose–Response Curve Analysis

PLB was dissolved in DMSO at a series of stock concentrations and 1:1000 diluted to specific concentrations for cell treatments. The control group had the same volume of DMSO added during the treatment. A375 and SK-MEL-28 cells were seeded in a 96-well plate at the density of 1×10^4 cells/well, A375 cells were treated with DMSO and PLB with concentrations of 1, 2, 2.5, 3, 3.5, 4, 6 µM, while DMSO and 1, 2, 4, 6, 7, 8, and 10 µM PLB were added to the SK-MEL-28 wells four times to repeat for each condition. HEMa cells were seeded at 5×10^4 and treated with DMSO and 1, 2, 4, 6, 7, 8 µM PLB to test its cytotoxic effect on normal cells. An MTS assay was applied to assess the number of viable cells after 48 h incubation with different concentrations of PLB. Briefly, 20 ul of MTS solution was added to each well with 100 µL of renewed medium. After 2 h incubation at 37 °C in a humidified, 5% CO_2 atmosphere, the absorbance was measured at 490 nm using a microplate reader (BioTek Instruments, Winooski, VT, USA). The IC50 values were calculated by GraphPad Prism 8.1.0 (GraphPad Software Inc., San Diego, CA, USA).

A375 and SK-MEL-28 cells were seeded at the density of 6×10^4 and 4×10^4 cells/well, respectively, in the 12-well plate and treated with DMSO and 1 and 3 µM PLB. Each condition was repeated twice. Trypan blue was used to determine viable cells. The cell numbers were counted at the same time each day within the following 4 days.

2.4. Determination of Cell Migration

Cell migration was measured by the wound-healing method. After two cell lines reaching confluence in 6-well culture plates, sterile P-1000 pipette tips were used to make artificial parallel scratches on the cell layer, and the floating cells were washed twice with PBS, which was finally replaced with complete culture medium containing DMSO or 1 or 3 µM PLB. The distance of migration was photographed with a microscope at different time points and quantified with ImageJ software (US National Institutes of Health, Bethesda, MA, USA), and the migration inhibition rate was calculated by the formula below:

$$migration\ inhibition\ rate = \frac{distance\ of\ PLB - distance\ of\ DMSO}{distance\ of\ initial\ scratch}$$

2.5. Apoptosis Analysis

The percentage of apoptotic A375 and SK-MEL-28 was quantified by Annexin V-FITC/PI double-staining. Briefly, cells were pretreated with varying doses of PLB (control, 1 and 3 µM) for 48 h. Harvested cells were resuspended in 100 µL 1X binding buffer and labeled for 15 min with 5 µL Annexin V-FITC and 1 µL of the 50 µg/mL PI at room temperature in the dark. A positive control group was conducted by heating cells at 55 °C for 16 min. The green (FITC) and red (PE-Texas Red) fluorescence were evaluated by flow cytometric analysis (FACSAria™ II, BD Biosciences, San Jose, CA, USA).

2.6. Seahorse Real-Time Cell Metabolic Analysis

Two melanoma cell lines were seeded in seahorse XF96 cell culture microplates at the density of 20,000 per well the day before the experiment. After 24 h of incubation, cells were rinsed and replaced with 180 µL of XF DMEM base medium supplemented with 1 mM pyruvate, 2 mM glutamine, and 25 mM glucose for A375 or 5.56 mM glucose for SK-MEL-28, with pH adjusted to 7.4, and incubated in a 37 °C, non-CO_2 incubator for at least 1 h. The cellular oxygen consumption rate (OCR) and the extracellular acidification rate (ECAR) were measured by the Seahorse XF96e extracellular flux analyzer (Agilent, Santa Clara, CA, USA), during which the Seahorse XF cell Mito Stress Test Kit, consisting of oligomycin (Oligo), FCCP, and a mixture of ROT and AA, was added in turn to reach 1, 2, 0.5, and 0.5 µM final concentration; specifically, DMSO and 1, 3, and 6 µM PLB were injected acutely prior to the Oligo in control and PLB treatment groups. The ATP assay with acute injection consisted of DMSO or 1, 3, or 6 µM PLB, 1 µM Oligo, and the combination of 0.5 µM ROT and 0.5 µM AA. Each sample was run in triplicates at least. An Agilent

Seahorse XF Mito Stress Test Report Generator (Agilent, Santa Clara, CA, USA) was applied to data analysis.

2.7. High-Resolution Respirometry and ROS Production Analysis

Cells were exposed to the DMSO or PLB treatment the day prior to the experiment, then harvested and resuspended with complete culture medium or MiR05 buffer at pH 7.4. The oxygen consumption and H_2O_2 production rates were measured with a high-resolution Oroboros respirometer (Oroboros Instruments Corp., Innsbruck, Austria). After calibration with H_2O_2 solution, each of the two chambers of the Oroboros machine was filled with 2 mL of the cell suspension along with SOD (2 µL, 5 kU/mL), HRP (4 µL, 500 U/mL), and AmR (2 µL, 10 mM). After 5 to 10 min stabilization, the oxygen consumption rate (OCR) and the H_2O_2 production rate were monitored dynamically by series of injections with substrates and inhibitors, the order of which was as the following: L-glutamate (10 µL, 2 M), malate (5 µL, 0.8 M), ADP (10 µL, 0.5 M), pyruvate (5 µL, 2 M), succinate (5 µL, 1 M), digitonin (3 µL, 8.1 mM), Oligo (3 µL, 5 mM), an inhibitor of ATPase synthetase, FCCP (3 µL, 1 mM), an oxidative phosphorylation (OXPHOS) uncoupler, ROT (1 µL, 1 mM), a complex I inhibitor, and AA (1 µL, 5 mM), a complex III inhibitor. Data were normalized by cell number and analyzed by DatLab 4 software (OROBOROS Instruments Corp., Innsbruck, Austria).

2.8. Mitochondria Mass Assessment

A MitoTracker Green probe that was able to diffuse across the cell membrane and accumulate in active mitochondria was used to assess mitochondria mass. Hoechst and PI were used to distinguish live from dead cells. In short, cells were seeded in a 4-well chamber slide at a density of 5×10^4 (A375) or 2×10^4 (SK-MEL-28) with DMSO or 1 µM PLB treatment. After 24 h incubation, cells were labeled with 50 nM MitoTracker Green dye and 2 µg/mL Hoechst in PBS at 37 °C for 25 min, protected from light. After washing with PBS, cells were covered and sealed on the slide. Fluorescence imaging was performed using a fluorescence microscope (Eclipse Ti, Nikon, Tokyo, Japan), and the intensity of fluorescence was quantified by ImageJ software (version 1.53e, National Institutes of Health, Bethesda, MD, USA).

2.9. Measurement of Mitochondria Membrane Potential

JC-1 dye, a kind of mitochondria membrane potential probe, was applied to measure the polarization changes due to the PLB treatment. After pretreated with DMSO or 1 or 3 µM PLB for 48 h, A375 and SK-MEL-28 cells were collected and resuspended with PBS consisting of 2 µM JC-1 dye. FCCP and JC-1 dye, both with 2 µM working concentration, were applied successively to the positive control cells. All the samples were incubated in the dark at room temperature for 15 min. To assess the attached cells with treatment for 24 h, cells were processed as we described in the Mitochondria Mass Assessment section and stained with 2 µM JC-1 dye and 2 µg/mL Hoechst, with 15-min incubation in a cell culture incubator at 37 °C. Thereafter, cells were washed once with PBS before measurement. Stained cells were examined through flow cytometry and a fluorescence microscope in FITC (green) and PE Texas-Red (red) channels.

2.10. Western Blotting

Proteins were extracted from DMSO and 1 and 3 µM PLB pretreated melanoma cells by RIPA buffer with protease inhibitor. After measuring the protein concentration, an equal volume of protein samples with equal concentration were loaded to 4–20% protein gels and transferred onto polyvinylidene difluoride membranes. The membranes were then blocked with 5% fatty-acid-free milk and incubated with total OXPHOS human WB antibodies (1:500) at 4 °C overnight. Next, the membranes were incubated with corresponding secondary antibodies (1:2000) for 1.5 h. The chemiluminescence bands were detected by ECL Western blotting substrate. To normalize the expression of the target protein, we stripped the membrane and incubated it with the GAPDH antibody. Following the steps we described above, the control bands were obtained. The expression of target proteins was measured by ImageJ software.

2.11. Statistical Data Analysis

The data were analyzed by GraphPad Prism 8 and displayed as mean ± standard deviation. To compare the data between the two groups, a *t*-test was used. Analysis of variance (ANOVA) was performed in the comparison of more than two groups, followed by Tukey's test for posthoc analysis. $p < 0.05$ was considered statistically significant.

3. Results

3.1. A375 and SK-MEL-28 Melanoma Cells Display Comparative Mitochondria Respiratory Phenotypes

SK-MEL-28 cells displayed a stronger mitochondrial oxygen consumption rate (OCR) with the injection of different substrates and blockers compared to the A375 cells (Figure 1a–c). After using digitonin to permeabilize the cell membrane in the Oroboros machine, the basal mitochondria OCR increased in both A375 and SK-MEL-28 cells since the substrates of the mitochondrial complex I (Cx I) and complex II (Cx II), including L-glutamate, L-malic, pyruvate, and succinate, along with adenosine diphosphate (ADP), entered the cells and were oxidized by mitochondria in the mitochondria respiration buffer (MiR05; Figure 1a,b). Oligomycin (Oligo), an inhibitor of adenosine triphosphate (ATP) synthase, blocks the proton channel of complex V (Cx V). The comparative mitochondrial proton leak in SK-MEL-28 cells was higher than in A375 cells, as determined by assessing the difference of the OCR between oligomycin and antimycin A (AA) (Figure 1c). ATP-linked respiration, the value of digitonin (Digi) minus the value of Oligo, was higher in SK-MEL-28 cells (Figure 1d). FCCP, a mitochondrial OXPHOS uncoupler that facilitates the proton transfer across the mitochondrial inner membrane by bypassing the F0 subunit of the Cx V pathway, increased the OCR to the maximum in both cells. The maximum mitochondrial respiration in A375 cells was inferior to SK-MEL-28 cells (Figure 1e). The respiratory control ratio (RCR) is defined as the ratio of ADP-stimulated respiration (State 3) to leak respiration when ATP production is shut off by Oligo (State 4 oligo). The RCR of A375 cells was higher than SK-MEL-28 cells (Figure 1f), indicating a high capacity for substrate oxidation [16].

3.2. H_2O_2 Production Rates Vary in A375 and SK-MEL-28 Cells

AmR fluorescence was recorded concurrently with OCR, as above (Figure 2a,b). A375 cells displayed a higher H_2O_2 production rate than SK-MEL-28 cells at the baseline without the addition of digitonin. Surprisingly, the H_2O_2 production rate dropped significantly, with no response to the addition of any blockers to A375 cells after cell membrane permeabilization occurred with the injection of digitonin. By contrast, digitonin has no effect on the H_2O_2 production rate in SK-MEL-28 cells, which were unresponsive to the blockers (Figure 2a,b).

3.3. H_2O_2 Production Triggered Differentially by PLB in A375 and SK-MEL-28

Melanoma cells were pretreated with DMSO and 0.5 and 1 µM PLB and subsequently injected into the chambers of Oroboros. Before digitonin application, PLB induced H_2O_2 production in both intact A375 and SK-MEL-28 cells. The increased H_2O_2 production rate in the DMSO group and PLB groups declined in A375 cells permeabilized with digitonin (Figure 2c). Conversely, the rate in permeabilized SK-MEL-28 cells slightly increased and was amplified by PLB treatment (Figure 2d).

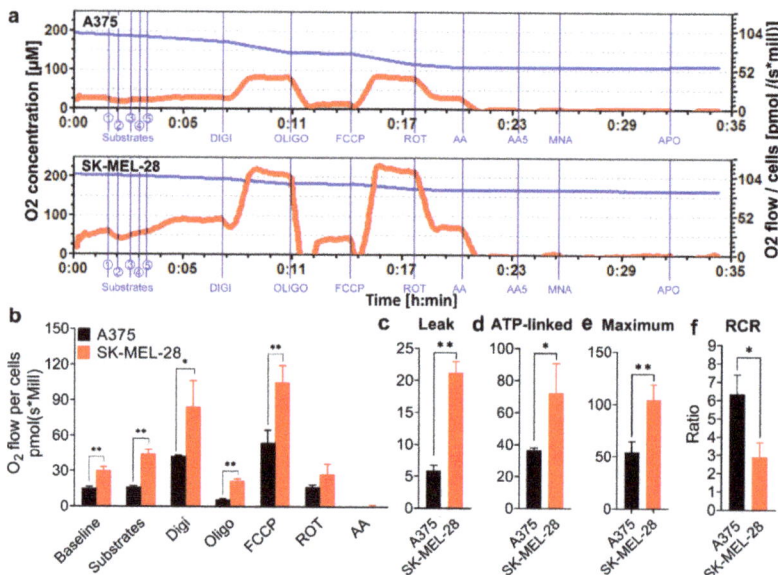

Figure 1. Comparative mitochondria phenotypes in melanoma cell lines. A375 and SK-MEL-28 cells were counted and placed in the Oroboros respiratory chambers, with sequential injections of Cx I and Cx II substrates (① L-glutamate; ② L-malic; ③ ADP; ④ pyruvate; ⑤ succinate), Digi (8.1 mM), Oligo (5 mM), FCCP (1 mM), ROT (1 mM), and AA (5 mM). (**a**) The O_2 concentration (blue line) and OCR for per million A375 and SK-MEL-28 cells (red line) were monitored in real-time. (**b**) The stable OCR values for per million A375 and SK-MEL-28 cells, measured by Oroboros, are displayed in the bar graph (n = 3). The data accessed from Oroboros was further calculated. The results are shown as (**c**) proton leak, (**d**) ATP-linked respiration, (**e**) maximum respiration, and (**f**) RCR, which means the State 3 over State 4 oligo. Results are expressed as mean ± SD. * $p < 0.05$, ** $p < 0.01$. Cx I, complex I; Cx II, complex II; ADP, adenosine diphosphate; Digi, digitonin; Oligo, oligomycin; FCCP, carbonyl cyanide-4-(trifluoromethoxy) phenylhydrazone; ROT, rotenone; AA, antimycin A; OCR, oxygen consumption rate; ATP, adenosine triphosphate; RCR, respiratory control ratio; SD, standard deviation.

3.4. Inhibitory Effects of PLB on Cell Viability and Proliferation Are Robust in A375 Cells

Metabolically active cells were able to react with the MTS assay, a number of which were positively related to the absorbance value detected by the microplate reader. The dose–response curves were displayed in Figure 3a. Based on this, the 50% inhibitory concentration (IC50) of PLB was calculated. The results revealed that PLB inhibited cell viability and proliferation in A375 cells (IC50 = 2.790 μM) more effectively than in SK-MEL-28 cells (IC50 = 3.872 μM). PLB has no cytotoxic effect on normal melanocytes (HEMa). On the contrary, we found an increasing survival rate of HEMa cells with PLB treatment, even in high concentrations, compared with the DMSO group (Figure S1). Moreover, time and dose–response of the PLB treatment were also determined by cell number counting. In the control group, A375 cells displayed a stronger exponential growth pattern than SK-MEL-28 cells over time. The growth of A375 cells was significantly inhibited by 1 μM PLB, and the inhibition effect was even stronger in the 3 μM PLB group (Figure 3b). However, PLB's inhibitory effect on SK-MEL-28 was not as strong compared with that on A375 cells with the 1 and 3 μM PLB treatments (Figure 3c).

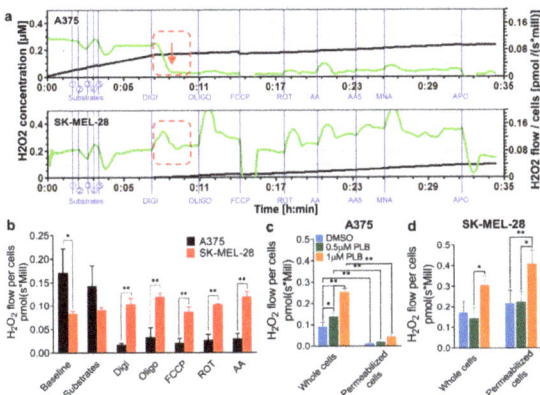

Figure 2. H_2O_2 production rate for whole and permeabilized melanoma cells at basal and PLB induced levels. A375 and SK-MEL-28 cells were counted and placed in the Oroboros respiratory chambers, with sequential injections of Cx I and Cx II substrates (① L-glutamate; ② L-malic; ③ ADP; ④ pyruvate; ⑤ succinate), Digi (8.1 mM), Oligo (5 mM), FCCP (1 mM), ROT (1 mM), and AA (5 mM). H_2O_2 signals were detected by Amplex UltraRed. (**a**) The H_2O_2 level (black line) and H_2O_2 flow for per million A375 and SK-MEL-28 cells (green line) were monitored in real-time. The red dashed box, along with a red arrow, highlights the H_2O_2 production drop in A375 cells compared to SK-MEL-28 cells. (**b**) The stable H_2O_2 flow values for per million A375 and SK-MEL-28 cells are displayed in the bar graph. ($n = 3$) The H_2O_2 production rates for whole and permeabilized (**c**) A375 cells and (**d**) SK-MEL-28 cells with DMSO and 1 and 3 μM PLB treatments are represented as the H_2O_2 flow before and after digitonin is applied ($n = 3$). Results are expressed as mean ± SD. * $p < 0.05$, ** $p < 0.01$. DMSO, dimethyl sulfoxide; PLB, plumbagin.

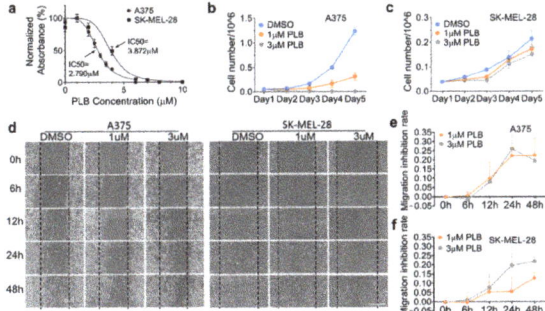

Figure 3. Differential inhibition effects of PLB on cell viability and migration in A375 and SK-MEL-28. (**a**) A375 and SK-MEL-28 cells were seeded in the 96-well plate at the density of 1×10^4 cells/well and treated with PLB (DMSO and 1, 2, 2.5, 3, 3.5, 4, and 6 μM PLB for A375 cells; DMSO and 1, 2, 4, 6, 7, 8, and 10 μM PLB for SK-MEL-28 cells) for two days. Viable cell numbers were measured by MTS assay. The IC50 of A375 and SK-MEL-28 cells were 2.790 and 3.872 μM, respectively ($n = 3$). (**b**) A375 cells and (**c**) SK-MEL-28 cells treated with DMSO and 1 and 3 μM PLB were counted for 5 days ($n = 2$). (**d**) Two cell lines were seeded in a 6-well plate, and the migration status was displayed by different treatments (DMSO and 1 and 3 μM PLB) and time points (0, 6, 12, 24, and 48 h). The migration inhibition rates in the 1 and 3 μM PLB groups were compared with the DMSO group. Scale bar = 0.1 mm. (**e**) Migration inhibition rate of A375 cells. (**f**) Migration inhibition rate of SK-MEL-28 cells ($n = 3$). Results are expressed as mean ± SD. MTS, nonradioactive cell proliferation assay; IC50, 50% inhibitory concentration.

3.5. Inhibitory Effects of PLB on A375 and SK-MEL-28 Cell Migration

The migration results of two melanoma cell lines with DMSO or 1 or 3 µM PLB treatment, monitored by microscopy at different time points (0, 6, 12, 24, and 48 h), are exhibited in Figure 3d. The inhibition of migration is defined as the difference of cell migration distance between DMSO and PLB groups, which is divided by the width of scratch at the beginning for each condition, respectively. In A375 cells, PLB had a relatively parallel inhibitory effect at concentrations of 1 and 3 µM (Figure 3e), while only a 21.8% inhibition of migration was seen in SK-MEL-28 cells with the 3 µM treatment. A low concentration of PLB treatment in SK-MEL-28 cells was unable to induce a similar suppression effect as in A375 cells (Figure 3f).

3.6. PLB-Induced Apoptosis in A375 But Not SK-MEL-28 Cells

According to the cells without staining, we drew the gate for flow cytometric analysis to differentiate the positive group from the negative group. Both late apoptosis or necrosis and early apoptosis were obviously induced in the 3 µM PLB group compared with the DMSO and 1 µM PLB groups in A375 cells. There was no significant difference between the DSMO group and the 1 µM group in A375 cells (Figure 4a,b). Neither 1 nor 3 µM PLB had any visible and statistical apoptotic effect on SK-MEL-28 cells (Figure 4a,c).

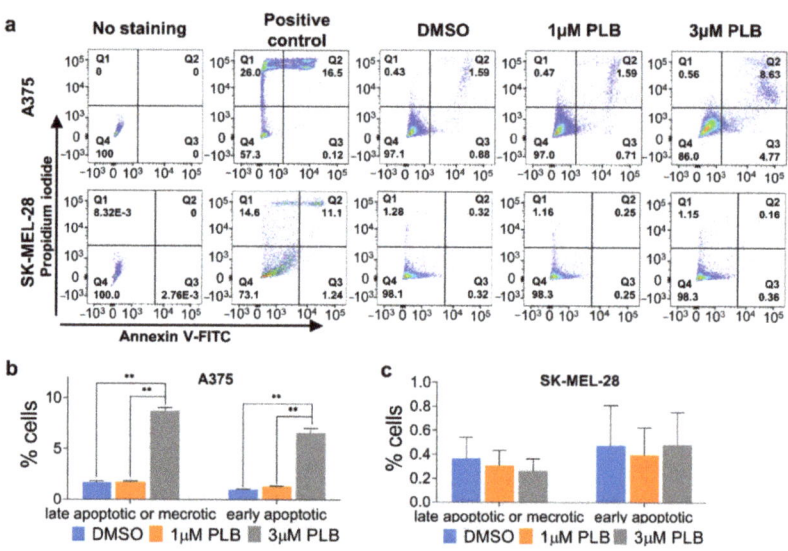

Figure 4. Differential effects of PLB on inducing A375 and SK-MEL-28 apoptosis. A375 and SK-MEL-28 cells pretreated with DMSO and 1 and 3 µM PLB were stained with Annexin V-FITC and PI. Cells heated at 55 °C for 16 min were the positive controls. (**a**) Cells with fluorescence were detected by flow cytometry. (**b**) The percentage of late apoptotic or necrotic and early apoptotic A375 cells in DMSO and 1 and 3 µM PLB groups. (**c**) The percentage of late apoptotic or necrotic and early apoptotic SK-MEL-28 cells in DMSO and 1 and 3 µM PLB groups. Results are expressed as mean ± SD (n = 3). ** $p < 0.01$. PI, propidium iodide.

3.7. Distinct Mitochondrial Responses to PLB Treatment in A375 and SK-MEL-28 Cells

The injection of PLB (DMSO and 1, 3, and 6 µM) triggered dose-dependent increases of the basal OCR and proton leak in both melanoma cell lines (Figure 5a–c). The maximum respiratory rate in SK-MEL-28 cells directly increased with the increasing PLB doses. On the contrary, the maximum respiration decreased in the high concentration group (3, 6 µM PLB) in A375 cells (Figure 5d). Furthermore, the percentage of spare respiratory capacity

PLB increases the respiratory rate in SK-MEL-28 cells mainly by inducing mitochondrial respiration, yet no obvious response was found in the mitostress energy map of A375 cells. Nevertheless, the increase of proton leak and decrease of maximum respiration, as well as spared respiration in A375 cells with PLB treatment, implies the negative effects of PLB in A375 cells. In SK-MEL-28 cells, the effects are positive despite the increase of proton leak because of the increased maximum respiration and stabilized spared respiration. The spared respiration, also called reserve respiration, is decreased by oxidative stress, the depletion of which, if exceeding the threshold of the basal respiration, can cause cell death [27,28]. Furthermore, we surprisingly found that mitochondria-independent respiration was stimulated by PLB in both cells. Nonmitochondrial respiration is generated from several pathways, including NADPH oxidases and lipoxygenases [27]. An elevated ROS level is also responsible for nonrespiration [29]. In our study, we first evaluated the innate abilities for ROS (H_2O_2) production, which are higher in A375 cells. Interestingly, after permeabilization, the ROS production rate declined sharply in A375 cells and increased a little bit in SK-MEL-28 cells. The results reveal that the major source of ROS in A375 cells may be outside the mitochondria, not mainly from the electron transport chain. Then, we confirmed that PLB induced ROS production, which is consistent with previous cancer research [9–11]. The reduction of ROS production due to cell permeabilization was enhanced by PLB in A375 cells. We can speculate that some oxidative enzymes, for example, the NADPH enzyme [30], may be involved in PLB-induced ROS production in A375 cells. ROS production in SK-MEL-28 cells is more dependent on mitochondrial respiration.

Our study demonstrates that PLB reduced ATP synthesis in A375 cells from both mitochondria and glycolysis, whereas mitochondrial ATP production in SK-MEL-28 cells was accelerated by PLB in a dose-dependent manner, which implies a degree of consistency with the results above. However, the expression of ATP5A basically remains stable, with or without PLB, in the two cell lines. As we described above, PLB-treated A375 cells display attenuated mitochondrial respiration; hence, more heat is generated, caused by leak-related respiration compared with ATP production [31]. Therefore, mitochondrial ATP production does not depend on the expression of ATP5A. Interestingly, we observed that MMP in A375 cells exceedingly increases with a lethal dose (3 µM) of PLB treatment. No significant MMP change was recorded in the SK-MEL-28 cells. Previous studies suggest a negative correlation between MMP and ATP production [32]. Consistently, the increase in MMP, accompanying diminished ATP production in A375 cells, is also proven in our experiments. Such an increase is reported in apoptosis and cancer [33,34]. The NDUFB8 subunit, located in the transmembrane domain of mitochondrial Cx I, functions as the proton pump to elevate MMP [35]. In our Western blotting results, the expression of NDUFB8 significantly increased in A375 cells under the 3 µM PLB treatment, which can be another explanation for the increased MMP. In addition, mitochondrial intensity is strengthened by PLB in SK-MEL-28 cells and unchanged in A375 cells. The results indicate an increased mitochondrial mass [31,36] and provide support for enhanced mitochondrial OXPHOS and bioenergetic capacity in the PLB-treated SK-MEL-28 cells we discussed above [29,37]. Based on our data and other research, PLB may also cause mitochondrial biogenesis to increase or mitophagy to decrease [38].

This investigation of melanoma cells, with different levels of aggressiveness and metabolic phenotypes, documents differential cytotoxic and metabolic responses when exposed to plumbagin. The study provides initial evidence that plumbagin, acting as a REDOX altering agent, might be utilized as an adjunct to melanoma therapy. Further studies on the anticancer characteristic of PLB could focus on specific molecular pathways, related gene expressions, and drug combination therapies.

Supplementary Materials: The following are available online at https://www.mdpi.com/article/10.3390/pharmaceutics13050706/s1, Figure S1: Survival rate in HEMa cells with PLB treatment.

Author Contributions: Conceptualization, H.Z., A.Z. and D.J.H.; methodology, H.Z. and A.Z.; software, A.Z.; validation, H.Z. and A.Z.; formal analysis, H.Z. and A.Z.; investigation, H.Z.; resources,

A.Z. and D.J.H.; data curation, H.Z. and A.Z.; writing—original draft preparation, H.Z.; writing—review and editing, A.Z., A.A.G. and D.J.H.; visualization, A.A.G. and D.J.H.; supervision, A.A.G. and D.J.H.; project administration, A.A.G.; funding acquisition, D.J.H. All authors have read and agreed to the published version of the manuscript.

Funding: This research received intramural and philanthropic funding.

Institutional Review Board Statement: Not applicable.

Informed Consent Statement: Not applicable.

Data Availability Statement: Data are contained within the article.

Acknowledgments: We thank Henry Pownall, our scientific advisor, for his mentorship of H.Z. and critical reading of the manuscript.

Conflicts of Interest: The authors declare no conflict of interest.

References

1. Siegel, R.L.; Miller, K.D.; Jemal, A. Cancer statistics, 2020. *CA Cancer J. Clin.* **2020**, *70*, 7–30. [CrossRef] [PubMed]
2. Heistein, J.B.; Acharya, U. Malignant Melanoma. In *StatPearls*; StatPearls Publishing: Treasure Island, FL, USA, 2020; bookshelf ID: NBK470409. Available online: https://www.ncbi.nlm.nih.gov/books/NBK430685/ (accessed on 11 May 2021).
3. Surveillance, Epidemiology, and End Results. (SEER) Program (www.seer.cancer.gov) SEER*Stat Database: Melanoma of the Skin. SEER 5-Year Relative Survival Rates, SEER 18 Areas (2010–2016). National Cancer Institute, DCCPS, Surveillance Research Program, Released December 2019. Underlying Mortality Data Provided by NCHS. Available online: https://seer.cancer.gov/statfacts/html/melan.html (accessed on 31 January 2021).
4. Rossi, S.; Cordella, M.; Tabolacci, C.; Nassa, G.; D'Arcangelo, D.; Senatore, C.; Pagnotto, P.; Magliozzi, R.; Salvati, A.; Weisz, A.; et al. TNF-alpha and metalloproteases as key players in melanoma cells aggressiveness. *J. Exp. Clin. Cancer Res.* **2018**, *37*, 326. [CrossRef] [PubMed]
5. Yoo, T.K.; Kim, J.S.; Hyun, T.K. Polyphenolic Composition and Anti-Melanoma Activity of White Forsythia (Abeliophyllum distichum Nakai) Organ Extracts. *Plants* **2020**, *9*, 757. [CrossRef] [PubMed]
6. Juszczak, A.M.; Czarnomysy, R.; Strawa, J.W.; Zovko Koncic, M.; Bielawski, K.; Tomczyk, M. In Vitro Anticancer Potential of Jasione montana and Its Main Components against Human Amelanotic Melanoma Cells. *Int. J. Mol. Sci.* **2021**, *22*, 3345. [CrossRef]
7. Nawrot-Hadzik, I.; Choromanska, A.; Abel, R.; Preissner, R.; Saczko, J.; Matkowski, A.; Hadzik, J. Cytotoxic Effect of Vanicosides A and B from Reynoutria sachalinensis Against Melanotic and Amelanotic Melanoma Cell Lines and in silico Evaluation for Inhibition of BRAFV600E and MEK1. *Int. J. Mol. Sci.* **2020**, *21*, 4611. [CrossRef] [PubMed]
8. Jamal, M.S.; Parveen, S.; Beg, M.A.; Suhail, M.; Chaudhary, A.G.; Damanhouri, G.A.; Abuzenadah, A.M.; Rehan, M. Anticancer compound plumbagin and its molecular targets: A structural insight into the inhibitory mechanisms using computational approaches. *PLoS ONE* **2014**, *9*, e87309. [CrossRef] [PubMed]
9. Yin, Z.; Zhang, J.; Chen, L.; Guo, Q.; Yang, B.; Zhang, W.; Kang, W. Anticancer Effects and Mechanisms of Action of Plumbagin: Review of Research Advances. *BioMed Res. Int.* **2020**, *2020*, 6940953. [CrossRef]
10. Zhang, R.; Wang, Z.; You, W.; Zhou, F.; Guo, Z.; Qian, K.; Xiao, Y.; Wang, X. Suppressive effects of plumbagin on the growth of human bladder cancer cells via PI3K/AKT/mTOR signaling pathways and EMT. *Cancer Cell Int.* **2020**, *20*, 520. [CrossRef]
11. Xue, D.; Pan, S.-T.; Zhou, X.; Ye, F.; Zhou, Q.; Shi, F.; He, F.; Yu, H.; Qiu, J. Plumbagin Enhances the Anticancer Efficacy of Cisplatin by Increasing Intracellular ROS in Human Tongue Squamous Cell Carcinoma. *Oxidative Med. Cell. Longev.* **2020**, *2020*, 1–21. [CrossRef]
12. Wang, C.C.; Chiang, Y.M.; Sung, S.C.; Hsu, Y.L.; Chang, J.K.; Kuo, P.L. Plumbagin induces cell cycle arrest and apoptosis through reactive oxygen species/c-Jun N-terminal kinase pathways in human melanoma A375.S2 cells. *Cancer Lett.* **2008**, *259*, 82–98. [CrossRef]
13. Pradubyat, N.; Sakunrangsit, N.; Mutirangura, A.; Ketchart, W. NADPH: Quinone oxidoreductase 1 (NQO1) mediated anti-cancer effects of plumbagin in endocrine resistant MCF7 breast cancer cells. *Phytomedicine* **2020**, *66*, 153133. [CrossRef]
14. Kapur, A.; Beres, T.; Rathi, K.; Nayak, A.P.; Czarnecki, A.; Felder, M.; Gillette, A.; Ericksen, S.S.; Sampene, E.; Skala, M.C.; et al. Oxidative stress via inhibition of the mitochondrial electron transport and Nrf-2-mediated anti-oxidative response regulate the cytotoxic activity of plumbagin. *Sci. Rep.* **2018**, *8*, 1073. [CrossRef]
15. Alem, F.Z.; Bejaoui, M.; Villareal, M.O.; Rhourri-Frih, B.; Isoda, H. Elucidation of the effect of plumbagin on the metastatic potential of B16F10 murine melanoma cells via MAPK signalling pathway. *Exp. Dermatol.* **2020**, *29*, 427–435. [CrossRef]
16. Brand, M.D.; Nicholls, D.G. Assessing mitochondrial dysfunction in cells. *Biochem. J.* **2011**, *435*, 297–312. [CrossRef]
17. Pasquali, S.; Hadjinicolaou, A.V.; Chiarion Sileni, V.; Rossi, C.R.; Mocellin, S. Systemic treatments for metastatic cutaneous melanoma. *Cochrane Database Syst. Rev.* **2018**, *2*, CD011123. [CrossRef]
18. Kuske, M.; Westphal, D.; Wehner, R.; Schmitz, M.; Beissert, S.; Praetorius, C.; Meier, F. Immunomodulatory effects of BRAF and MEK inhibitors: Implications for Melanoma therapy. *Pharmacol. Res.* **2018**, *136*, 151–159. [CrossRef]
19. Arslanbaeva, L.R.; Santoro, M.M. Adaptive redox homeostasis in cutaneous melanoma. *Redox Biol.* **2020**, *37*, 101753. [CrossRef]

20. Haq, R.; Shoag, J.; Andreu-Perez, P.; Yokoyama, S.; Edelman, H.; Rowe, G.C.; Frederick, D.T.; Hurley, A.D.; Nellore, A.; Kung, A.L.; et al. Oncogenic BRAF regulates oxidative metabolism via PGC1alpha and MITF. *Cancer Cell* **2013**, *23*, 302–315. [CrossRef]
21. Frederick, M.; Skinner, H.D.; Kazi, S.A.; Sikora, A.G.; Sandulache, V.C. High expression of oxidative phosphorylation genes predicts improved survival in squamous cell carcinomas of the head and neck and lung. *Sci. Rep.* **2020**, *10*, 6380. [CrossRef]
22. Vayalil, P.K. Mitochondrial oncobioenergetics of prostate tumorigenesis. *Oncol. Lett.* **2019**, *18*, 4367–4376. [CrossRef]
23. Elgendy, M.; Ciro, M.; Hosseini, A.; Weiszmann, J.; Mazzarella, L.; Ferrari, E.; Cazzoli, R.; Curigliano, G.; DeCensi, A.; Bonanni, B.; et al. Combination of Hypoglycemia and Metformin Impairs Tumor Metabolic Plasticity and Growth by Modulating the PP2A-GSK3beta-MCL-1 Axis. *Cancer Cell* **2019**, *35*, 798–815.e5. [CrossRef] [PubMed]
24. Di Biase, S.; Lee, C.; Brandhorst, S.; Manes, B.; Buono, R.; Cheng, C.W.; Cacciottolo, M.; Martin-Montalvo, A.; de Cabo, R.; Wei, M.; et al. Fasting-Mimicking Diet Reduces HO-1 to Promote T Cell-Mediated Tumor Cytotoxicity. *Cancer Cell* **2016**, *30*, 136–146. [CrossRef] [PubMed]
25. Zaal, E.A.; Berkers, C.R. The Influence of Metabolism on Drug Response in Cancer. *Front. Oncol.* **2018**, *8*, 500. [CrossRef] [PubMed]
26. Delgado-Goni, T.; Miniotis, M.F.; Wantuch, S.; Parkes, H.G.; Marais, R.; Workman, P.; Leach, M.O.; Beloueche-Babari, M. The BRAF Inhibitor Vemurafenib Activates Mitochondrial Metabolism and Inhibits Hyperpolarized Pyruvate-Lactate Exchange in BRAF-Mutant Human Melanoma Cells. *Mol. Cancer Ther.* **2016**, *15*, 2987–2999. [CrossRef] [PubMed]
27. Chacko, B.K.; Kramer, P.A.; Ravi, S.; Benavides, G.A.; Mitchell, T.; Dranka, B.P.; Ferrick, D.; Singal, A.K.; Ballinger, S.W.; Bailey, S.M.; et al. The Bioenergetic Health Index: A new concept in mitochondrial translational research. *Clin. Sci.* **2014**, *127*, 367–373. [CrossRef] [PubMed]
28. Dranka, B.P.; Hill, B.G.; Darley-Usmar, V.M. Mitochondrial reserve capacity in endothelial cells: The impact of nitric oxide and reactive oxygen species. *Free Radic. Biol. Med.* **2010**, *48*, 905–914. [CrossRef] [PubMed]
29. Hill, B.G.; Benavides, G.A.; Lancaster, J.R., Jr.; Ballinger, S.; Dell'Italia, L.; Jianhua, Z.; Darley-Usmar, V.M. Integration of cellular bioenergetics with mitochondrial quality control and autophagy. *Biol. Chem.* **2012**, *393*, 1485–1512. [CrossRef]
30. Gillette, M.U.; Wang, T.A. Brain circadian oscillators and redox regulation in mammals. *Antioxid. Redox Signal.* **2014**, *20*, 2955–2965. [CrossRef]
31. Cottet-Rousselle, C.; Ronot, X.; Leverve, X.; Mayol, J.F. Cytometric assessment of mitochondria using fluorescent probes. *Cytom. Part A* **2011**, *79*, 405–425. [CrossRef]
32. Logan, A.; Pell, V.R.; Shaffer, K.J.; Evans, C.; Stanley, N.J.; Robb, E.L.; Prime, T.A.; Chouchani, E.T.; Cocheme, H.M.; Fearnley, I.M.; et al. Assessing the Mitochondrial Membrane Potential in Cells and In Vivo using Targeted Click Chemistry and Mass Spectrometry. *Cell Metab.* **2016**, *23*, 379–385. [CrossRef]
33. Smith, R.A.; Hartley, R.C.; Cocheme, H.M.; Murphy, M.P. Mitochondrial pharmacology. *Trends Pharmacol. Sci.* **2012**, *33*, 341–352. [CrossRef]
34. Wallace, D.C.; Fan, W.; Procaccio, V. Mitochondrial energetics and therapeutics. *Annu. Rev. Pathol.* **2010**, *5*, 297–348. [CrossRef]
35. Protasoni, M.; Zeviani, M. Mitochondrial Structure and Bioenergetics in Normal and Disease Conditions. *Int. J. Mol. Sci.* **2021**, *22*, 586. [CrossRef]
36. Xiao, B.; Deng, X.; Zhou, W.; Tan, E.K. Flow Cytometry-Based Assessment of Mitophagy Using MitoTracker. *Front. Cell. Neurosci.* **2016**, *10*, 76. [CrossRef]
37. Yao, C.H.; Wang, R.; Wang, Y.; Kung, C.P.; Weber, J.D.; Patti, G.J. Mitochondrial fusion supports increased oxidative phosphorylation during cell proliferation. *eLife* **2019**, *8*. [CrossRef]
38. Valentin-Vega, Y.A.; Maclean, K.H.; Tait-Mulder, J.; Milasta, S.; Steeves, M.; Dorsey, F.C.; Cleveland, J.L.; Green, D.R.; Kastan, M.B. Mitochondrial dysfunction in ataxia-telangiectasia. *Blood* **2012**, *119*, 1490–1500. [CrossRef]

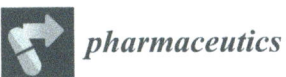

Article

Effect of Diphenyleneiodonium Chloride on Intracellular Reactive Oxygen Species Metabolism with Emphasis on NADPH Oxidase and Mitochondria in Two Therapeutically Relevant Human Cell Types

Sergejs Zavadskis [1], Adelheid Weidinger [1], Dominik Hanetseder [1], Asmita Banerjee [1], Cornelia Schneider [1], Susanne Wolbank [1], Darja Marolt Presen [1] and Andrey V. Kozlov [1,2,*]

[1] Ludwig Boltzmann Institute for Experimental and Clinical Traumatology in the AUVA Trauma Research Center, Austrian Cluster for Tissue Regeneration, A-1200 Vienna, Austria; sergejs.zavadskis@trauma.lbg.ac.at (S.Z.); adelheid.weidinger@trauma.lbg.ac.at (A.W.); dominik.hanetseder@trauma.lbg.ac.at (D.H.); asmita.banerjee@trauma.lbg.ac.at (A.B.); cornelia.schneider@trauma.lbg.ac.at (C.S.); susanne.wolbank@trauma.lbg.ac.at (S.W.); darja.marolt@trauma.lbg.ac.at (D.M.P.)

[2] Laboratory of Navigational Redox Lipidomics, Department of Human Pathology, IM Seche-Nov Moscow State Medical University, 119146 Moscow, Russia

* Correspondence: andrey.kozlov@trauma.lbg.ac.at; Tel.: +43-(0)-593-9341-980

Abstract: Reactive oxygen species (ROS) have recently been recognized as important signal transducers, particularly regulating proliferation and differentiation of cells. Diphenyleneiodonium (DPI) is known as an inhibitor of the nicotinamide adenine dinucleotide phosphate oxidase (NOX) and is also affecting mitochondrial function. The aim of this study was to investigate the effect of DPI on ROS metabolism and mitochondrial function in human amniotic membrane mesenchymal stromal cells (hAMSCs), human bone marrow mesenchymal stromal cells (hBMSCs), hBMSCs induced into osteoblast-like cells, and osteosarcoma cell line MG-63. Our data suggested a combination of a membrane potential sensitive fluorescent dye, tetramethylrhodamine methyl ester (TMRM), and a ROS-sensitive dye, CM-H2DCFDA, combined with a pretreatment with mitochondria-targeted ROS scavenger MitoTEMPO as a good tool to examine effects of DPI. We observed critical differences in ROS metabolism between hAMSCs, hBMSCs, osteoblast-like cells, and MG-63 cells, which were linked to energy metabolism. In cell types using predominantly glycolysis as the energy source, such as hAMSCs, DPI predominantly interacted with NOX, and it was not toxic for the cells. In hBMSCs, the ROS turnover was influenced by NOX activity rather than by the mitochondria. In cells with aerobic metabolism, such as MG 63, the mitochondria became an additional target for DPI, and these cells were prone to the toxic effects of DPI. In summary, our data suggest that undifferentiated cells rather than differentiated parenchymal cells should be considered as potential targets for DPI.

Keywords: diphenyleneiodonium; reactive oxygen species; mitochondria; NADPH-oxidase; differentiation; proliferation

1. Introduction

Diphenyleneiodonium (DPI) is known as a strong inhibitor of the nicotinamide adenine dinucleotide phosphate oxidase (NOX) and also interferes with mitochondrial function. NOX and the mitochondria are two major sources of reactive oxygen species (ROS) in the cell [1,2]. Beside their well-known role as inducers of oxidative stress, ROS have recently also been recognized as important signal transducers, regulating numerous physiological and pathophysiological processes [3]. Consequently, pharmacological treatments targeting ROS have come into focus as possible therapeutic strategies. In this context, DPI has already been tested as a potential drug for several diseases. For example, DPI has been shown to prevent the degeneration of neurons in Parkinson's disease [4] and show neuroprotective effects after focal cerebral ischemia [5,6]. Another study showed that ultra-low doses of DPI may be a therapeutic agent for the treatment of colitis and colitis-associated colorectal cancer [7]. Furthermore, it has been shown that the activation of NOX may represent a stimulus for cell-cycle activation and that DPI and apocynin inhibit this process in cardiac cells [8]. DPI has also been reported to induce a chemo-quiescence phenotype that potently inhibited the propagation of cancer stem-like cells. This action of DPI was associated with the inhibition of mitochondrial respiration [9]. The interaction of DPI in cancer stem-like cells attracted our attention. Several studies have shown that the inhibition of mitochondrial respiration can increase the production of mitochondrial ROS, which, in turn, can interact with NOX and vice versa (reviewed in [1,10]). Therefore, it can be assumed that DPI could influence different sources of intracellular ROS and orchestrate ROS-dependent processes of cellular metabolism in different cell types.

Human amniotic membrane mesenchymal stromal cells (hAMSCs), as well as bone marrow-derived mesenchymal stromal cells (hBMSCs), are two types of therapeutically relevant stromal cells [11]. However, hAMSCs reside in entirely different niches than hBMSCs and have different functions in vivo. While hBMSCs are multipotent cells [12], hAMSCs are known to express pluripotency markers, such as stage-specific embryonic antigen (SSEA)-3 and SSEA-4 [13]. Of note, considering the ontogenetic development, hAMSCs develop well before the formation of the three germ layers, whereas hBMSCs derive later in embryonic development from the mesodermal lineage [14].

hBMSCs constitute promising therapeutic cells for tissue regeneration, due to their secretory properties and/or their capacity to differentiate [15,16]. It has been shown that the cells change energy metabolism from glycolysis to mitochondrial energy conversion during the process of osteogenic differentiation [17,18].

The aim of this study was to investigate the effects of different DPI concentrations on the ROS metabolism and mitochondrial membrane potential of hAMSCs, undifferentiated hBMSCs, and their osteogenic-induced progeny, as well the osteosarcoma-derived cells (MG63) commonly used for osteoblastic models.

2. Materials and Methods

2.1. Chemicals and Materials

T75/T175 CELLSTAR® cell culture flasks were purchased from Greiner Bio-One (Kremsmünster, Austria), and 24-well plates were supplied by Corning Inc. (New York, NY, USA). Reagents were obtained from Merck/Sigma-Aldrich (Darmstadt, Germany) unless otherwise noted.

2.2. Preparation of Human Amniotic Membrane and Isolation of Human Amniotic Membrane Mesenchymal Stromal Cells

Human placentas were obtained from caesarian sections of term pregnancies with the patient's full informed consent (Ethikkommission des Landes Oberösterreich, No. 200, 12. 05. 2005) of approval and processed as described previously [19,20]. In brief, placentas were washed repeatedly with cold (4 °C) PBS solution (Szabo-Scandic, Vienna, Austria) before the amniotic membrane (AM) was carefully peeled off and separated from the chorion. The membrane was again washed repeatedly with cold PBS to remove blood remnants and then transferred to a 150 mm cell culture dish (Thermo Fisher Scientific, Waltham, MA, USA). The membranes were submerged in culture medium Dulbecco's Modified Eagle's Medium high-glucose, (DMEM-HG) supplemented with 10% fetal calf serum, (FCS), 1% L-glutamine, and 1% Pen/Strep) and cultured at 37 °C, 5% CO_2 in a humidified atmosphere (CO_2 incubator by Binder, Tuttlingen, Germany), until cell isolation on the following day.

For the isolation of hAMSCs, the membranes were washed twice with cold PBS and then dissected into pieces of about 2×3 cm² each. Subsequently, the pieces were transferred to T75 cell culture flasks and incubated in 1-mg/mL collagenase solution (collagenase type I, CLS1, 280 U/mg, Worthington Biochemical Corporation, Lakewood, NJ, USA) at 37 °C and continuous shaking for 2 h. Afterwards, an equal volume of cold PBS was added, and the cell suspension was filtered through 100 and 22-µm cell strainers (Thermo Fisher Scientific, Waltham, MA, USA and Karlsruhe, Germany). The suspension was then centrifuged for 9 min at $400 \times g$ and 4 °C, and the cell pellet was resuspended in DMEM HG medium supplemented with 10% FCS, 1% L-glutamine, 1% Pen/Strep, 1 ng/mL basic fibroblast growth factor (bFGF, Peprotech, Rocky Hill, CT, USA), and 15 mM HEPES. Cells were seeded in T175 cell culture flasks (2.5×10^6 cells/flask) and expanded for one passage. They were harvested at 70% confluency and cryopreserved at −80 °C.

After thawing, hAMSC were expanded in expansion medium (DMEM low-glucose, 10% FCS, 1% L-glutamine, 1% Pen/Strep, and 1 ng/mL bFGF (Peprotech, Rocky Hill, CT, USA) with 15 mM HEPES, passage 1) for 72 h and then split to 24-well plates for a pilot laser scan microscopy (LSM) analysis and a T75 flask, where they were further cultured in proliferation medium (DMEM/F-12, 10% FCS, 1% L-glutamine, 1% Pen/Strep, and 1 ng/mL bFGF (Peprotech, Rocky Hill, CT, USA) passage 2) for 72 h. The cells were split and cultivated in proliferation medium every 72 h, and passages 3 and 4 were used in the experiments.

2.3. Isolation of Human Bone Marrow-Derived Mesenchymal Stromal Cells

Human bone marrow mononuclear cells (hBMSCs) were purchased from Lonza (Basel, Switzerland), seeded on T75 tissue culture flasks and expanded in hBMSC culture medium consisting of DMEM- HG supplemented with 10% FCS, 1% Pen/Strep, 2 mM L-glutamine, and 1 ng/mL bFGF (Peprotech, Rocky Hill, CT, USA). Nonadherent bone marrow cells were removed during media changes. hBMSCs were routinely split upon reaching approx. 75% confluency. Trilineage differentiation potential and expression of mesenchymal surface antigens were confirmed (data not shown), and hBMSCs of passages 3, 4, and 5 were used in experiments.

2.4. Experimental Design

The effects of DPI on the mitochondrial membrane potential and cellular ROS levels were examined in undifferentiated hAMSCs, undifferentiated hBMSCs, and in hBMSCs after osteogenic induction for 14 days (osteoblast-like cells) in DMEM-HG supplemented with 10% FCS, 1% Pen/Strep, 2 mM L-glutamine, 10 nM dexamethasone, 50 µM ascorbic acid-2-phosphate, and 10 mM ß-glycerophosphate. Additionally, mitochondrial respiratory parameters were monitored in MG-63 cells (Merck, Sigma-Aldrich, St. Louis, MO, USA). Prior to the start of the experiments, the cells were synchronized by FCS starvation for 24 h. Synchronization was not performed on MG-63 cells.

2.5. Mitochondrial Respiration

Permeabilization of the cytoplasmic membrane of MG-63 cells was achieved by exposing the cells to 12 µM digitonin for 10 min. Permeabilized MG-63 cells were treated with different concentrations of DPI (0.625 µM, 1.25 µM, 2.5 µM, 5 µM, 10 µM, and 100 µM) and 0.5% dimethyl sulfoxide (DMSO) as the control. The concentration of MitoTEMPO (20 µM) was chosen based on the prior publication, where it was used to prevent oxidative damage caused by excessive mitochondrial ROS production [21]. MG-63 cells were seeded with a density of 10,000 cells/cm^2 in T175 flasks in DMEM-HG, supplemented with 10% FCS and 1% L-glutamine, ("cell culture medium"). After 3 days' incubation at 37 °C, 5% CO_2, and humidified atmosphere, the cells reached a confluency of 75%. The cells were detached with 2 mL trypsin/ ethylene diamine tetraacetic acid (EDTA) solution (10× concentration, 25% trypsin/EDTA and 75% PBS), centrifuged ($218 \times g$, 5 min), and counted with a hemocytometer (Neubauer type, Marienfeld, Lauda-Königshofen, Germany).

For the initial dose dependency, the cells were incubated for 30 min with different concentrations of DPI (0.625 µM, 1.25 µM, 2.5 µM, 5 µM, 10 µM, and 100 µM) directly in the measurement chambers of the high-resolution respirometer (Oroboros Instruments,

Innsbruck, Austria). A time point of 30 min was selected to test the direct effects of DPI. Delayed effects, possibly mediated by other intracellular processes, were examined in human primary cells only with laser scan microscopy (LSM; see below).

Permeabilized MG-63 were preincubated in cell culture flasks with 20 µM MitoTEMPO for 15 min and, after washing with PBS, treated with DPI for 30 min. Then, the cells were detached with trypsin/EDTA (10 × concentration, 25% trypsin/75% PBS), centrifuged (218× g, 5 min), counted with a hemocytometer (Neubauer type, Lauda-Königshofen, Germany), and examined with high-resolution respirometry (Oroboros Instruments, Innsbruck, Austria).

2.6. Mitochondrial Membrane Potential and Cellular ROS Measurement

Undifferentiated hBMSCs, hBMSCs after osteogenic induction, hAMSCs, and MG-63 cells were seeded in 24-well plates at a density of 10,000 cells/cm^2 in 1 mL culture medium/well. The cells were cultured for 48 h until 70–80% confluency was reached and synchronized for 24 h by FCS starvation. Then, the cells were pretreated for 15 min in a cell culture medium supplemented with 20 µM MitoTEMPO or 0.05% DMSO (control). The medium was then changed to a proliferation medium supplemented with 10 µM DPI, 100 µM DPI, or 0.05% DMSO (control), and the cells were incubated for various times, ranging from 30 min or longer, up to 96 h. At the end of incubation, the cells were stained with fluorescent probes in Hank's balanced salt solution according to the manufacturer's instructions. Fluorescent dye tetramethylrhodamine methyl ester (TMRM, 50 nM, 30 min, 37 °C, ex/em 543/565–583 nm; Promokine, Heidelberg, Germany) was used to evaluate mitochondrial membrane potential, fluorescent dye CM-H2DCFDA (5-(and-6)-chloromethyl-2′,7′-dichlorodihydrofluorescein diacetate, acetyl ester, 10 µM, 30 min, 37 °C, ex/em 488/505–550 nm; Thermo Fischer, Waltham, MA, USA) was used for the detection of cellular ROS, and fluorescent dye CM-H2XRos, 5 µM, 30 min, 37 °C, ex/em 543/ 596–617 nm; Thermo Fischer, Waltham, MA, USA) was used for the detection of mitochondrial ROS. LSM imaging was performed with an inverted confocal microscope (LSM 510, Zeiss, Oberkochen, Germany) and 10× objective. Image analysis was performed with ZEN 2009 (version 6.0.303; Carl Zeiss, Oberkochen, Germany) based on the region of interest selection consisting of multiple cells. The mean fluorescence magnitude obtained from single cells was determined after setting threshold at 2/255 in order to subtract the background signal.

2.7. Measurement of Mitochondrial Respiration

Mitochondrial respiratory parameters were monitored using high-resolution respirometry (Oxygraph-2k, Oroboros Instruments, Innsbruck, Austria). MG-63 cells (2 × 10^6/mL) were incubated in a buffer containing 115 mM KCl, 5 mM KH$_2$PO$_4$, 20 mM Tris-HCl, 0.5 mM EDTA, and 5 mg/mL fatty acid-free bovine serum albumin (pH 7.4, 37 °C). To assess Complex I- and Complex II-linked respiration, cells were permeabilized with digitonin (12 µM). State 2 respiration of Complex I was stimulated by the addition of 5 mM glutamate/5 mM malate. Transition to State 3 respiration was induced by the addition of adenosine diphosphate (ADP, 1 mM). Complex II-linked State 3 respiration was then stimulated with 10 mM succinate after the addition of Complex I inhibitor rotenone (1 µM). Maximum respiratory capacity was measured by the titration of carbonyl cyanide-4-(trifluoromethoxy)phenylhydrazone (FCCP) in steps of 0.5 µM. Respiration rates were obtained by calculating the negative time derivative of the measured oxygen concentration and subtraction of non-mitochondrial oxygen consumption (myxothiazol 10 µM).

2.8. Statistical Analysis

Prior to statistical analysis, the data was transformed to fraction of the control group, with the respective control group mean taken as 100%. The outliers were identified with the robust regression and outlier removal (ROUT) method (5% threshold), and ordinary ANOVA was performed on the whole dataset, with additional multiple comparisons of individual means against the mean of a control group using Fisher's Least Significant

Difference (LSD) test as the post-hoc test. All evaluations were performed using Graph-Pad Prism (GraphPad Software, San Diego, CA, USA, Version 8.0.1). For laser scanning microscopy experiments, the number of independent samples (n) is indicated as number of analyzed regions of interest, which comprise multiple adjacent cells with nonpathological morphology. For the measurement of mitochondrial respiration, the n number represents experiments with cells seeded on independent days. Data are presented as mean + SD. The significance level was set at 0.05 and is indicated as * $p < 0.05$, ** $p < 0.01$, *** $p < 0.001$, and **** $p < 0.0001$ compared to the control.

3. Results

The interaction between DPI and the mitochondria was first examined in permeabilized osteosarcoma cell line MG-63 to define the conditions for experiments with primary human cells, which were available in limited portions (Figure 1). Permeabilization allowed the testing of specific segments of the respiratory chain under conditions of substrate saturation (glutamate/malate or succinate). After 30 min of treatment, mitochondrial respiration with glutamate/malate (substrates of complex I) decreased with increasing DPI concentrations (0.625–100 M), reaching its minimum at approx. 5 µM DPI (Figure 1a). However, already at 0.625 µM DPI, we observed a strong inhibition of State 3 respiration linked to ATP synthesis. The recorded MG-63 mitochondrial respiration dataset is available in supplementary material (Figure S1). We showed that, although DPI inhibits the electron flow through Complex I, the total capacity of the respiratory chain determined in the presence of succinate and FCCP did not change in all ranges of DPI concentrations (Figure S1b).

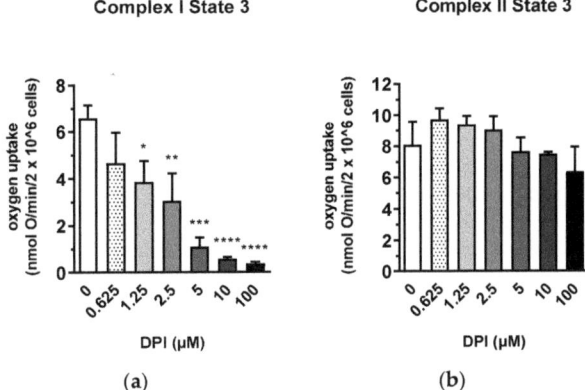

Figure 1. Inhibitory effect of diphenyleneiodonium chloride (DPI) on Complex I mitochondrial function in permeabilized MG-63 cells. (**a**) Effects of different concentrations of DPI on Complex I-linked State 3. * $p < 0.05$, ** $p < 0.01$, *** $p < 0.001$, and **** $p < 0.0001$ compared to the control. (**b**) Effects of different concentrations of DPI on Complex II-linked State 3. Data is represented as means + SD (error bars) (n = 3). One-way ANOVA followed by multiple comparison post-hoc Fisher's LSD test.

In contrast, an increase in the rate of respiration was observed with succinate (a substrate of Complex II) after the treatment with DPI up to 10 µM and slightly dropped only upon treatment with 100 µM DPI (Figure 1b). We considered that the insufficiency of Complex I in MG-63 cells is compensated by Complex II in a wide range of DPI concentrations. Thus, for the following experiments, we selected 10 µM DPI as the concentration where the inhibition of Complex I can be fully compensated by electron flow via Complex II and 100 µM DPI as the critical concentration where mitochondrial dysfunction was expected to occur.

The experiments with permeabilized MG-63 cells were performed under conditions of substrate saturation (glutamate/malate and succinate). That is not necessarily the case in living cells, where insufficient levels of intracellular succinate may induce a decrease in membrane potential if the electron transfer through Complex I is inhibited by DPI. To test this assumption, we determined the mitochondrial membrane potential in nonpermeabilized MG-63 cells in the presence of 10 and 100 µM DPI (Figure 2). We observed that 10 µM DPI did not influence the membrane potential, while 100 µM DPI significantly decreased the membrane potential (Figure 2a) and substantially elevated the levels of cellular ROS (Figure 2b).

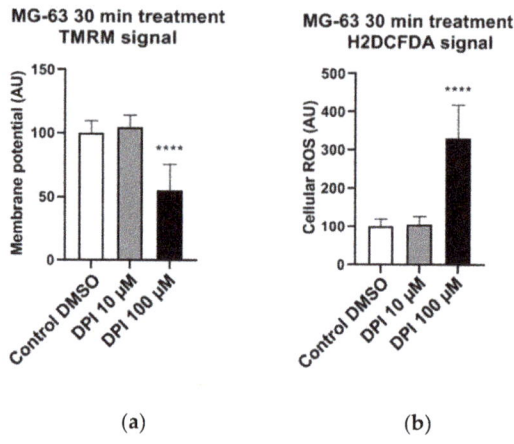

Figure 2. Effects of 30 min 10 µM and 100 µM diphenyleneiodonium chloride (DPI) in nonpermeabilized MG-63 cells, inducing a drop in mitochondrial membrane potential and a burst of reactive oxygen species (ROS) production on higher concentrations. The data is displayed in arbitrary units (AU). (**a**) Effects of 10 µM and 100 µM DPI on mitochondrial membrane potential. (**b**) Effects of 10 µM and 100 µM DPI on cellular ROS levels. Data is represented as means + SD (error bars) ($n = 24$; each point was obtained by analyzing 2–4 single cells. **** $p < 0.0001$; one-way ANOVA followed by multiple comparison post-hoc Fisher's LSD test.).

Cellular ROS may come from different sources, including mitochondria. To examine whether the observed increase in cytoplasmic ROS originated from the mitochondria, we stained cells with a mitochondria-specific ROS-sensitive fluorescent probe and treated the cells for 30 min with 100 µM DPI (Figure 3). We observed that the ROS-sensitive fluorescent probe accumulated in the intact mitochondria of the control group (Figure 3a), whereas, in response to the DPI treatment, the fluorescent probe was released in the cytoplasm (Figure 3b), thus suggesting a mitochondrial origin of the ROS. Additionally, we stained the cells with CM-H2XRos together with a nuclear dye (NucSpot® 650), and we did not find staining by CM-H2XRos in the nuclei of the control cells (Figure S2). To further prove the mitochondrial origin of cytoplasmic ROS, we tested whether the increase in ROS can be reduced by mitochondria-targeted antioxidant MitoTEMPO. If an excessive generation of ROS contributes to mitochondrial dysfunction, the treatment with MitoTEMPO should prevent a drop in membrane potential as well. Indeed, the LSM analysis showed that the treatment of MG-63 with MitoTEMPO abolished the increase in cytoplasmic ROS levels in DPI-treated cells and prevented the drop in the mitochondrial membrane potential (Figure 4a). The experiment performed with permeabilized cells with an excess of substrate MitoTEMPO did not affect the mitochondrial respiration recorded in the presence of 100 µM DPI (Figure 4b).

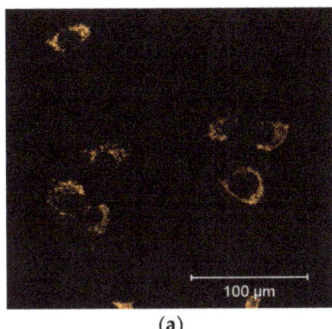 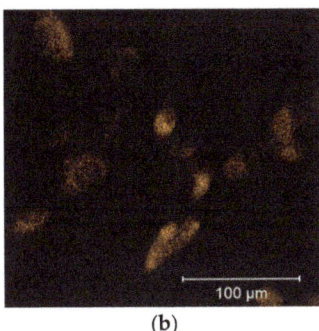

(a) (b)

Figure 3. Release of the mitochondrial ROS-sensitive CM-H2XRos fluorescent probe to the cytoplasm is induced by a 100 μM diphenyleneiodonium chloride (DPI) treatment of MG-63 cells. (**a**) Control group treated with 0.5% vol. DMSO. (**b**) Group exposed to a 100 μM DPI concentration. The images were taken with a Zeiss LSM 510 microscope, 10× objective, 5 μM CM-H2XRos probe concentration.

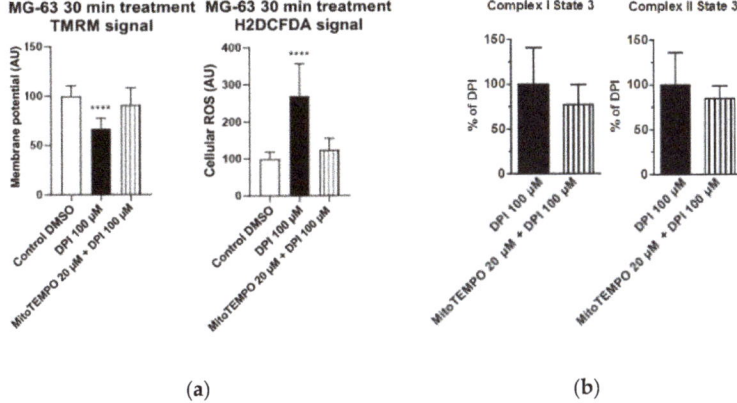

(a) (b)

Figure 4. Effects of 20 μM MitoTEMPO pretreatment on MG-63 cells exposed to 100 μM DPI. (**a**) Mitochondrial membrane potential and cellular ROS levels estimated with laser scan microscopy (LSM). MitoTEMPO is capable of preventing a decrease of the mitochondrial membrane potential and excessive generation of ROS. The images were taken with a Zeiss LSM 510 microscope, 10x objective, 50 nM tetramethylrhodamine methyl ester (TMRM) and 10 μMH2DCFDA probe concentration. Data is represented as means + SD (error bars) (n = 24; each point was obtained by analyzing 2–4 single cells. **** $p < 0.0001$; one-way ANOVA followed by multiple comparison post-hoc Fisher's LSD test. (**b**) Cellular respiration measurements of Complex I and Complex II State 3 MitoTEMPO does not cause recovery of mitochondrial respiration. Means + SD, n = 4.

Figure 4 demonstrates our observations made with LSM and high resolution respirometry; the full cellular respirometry datasets are available in Figure S3. The data presented above suggest that the generation of cellular ROS and membrane potential are driven by the succinate-mediated pathway, which is in line with a recent finding that, in human mesenchymal stem cells, succinate plays an important role in maintaining stem cell functions [22]. Furthermore, the data presented above show that the LSM analysis using a combination of TMRM and H2DCFDA probes to analyze the changes in membrane potential induced by DPI or another drug is sufficient for a general estimation of the cellular bioenergetic status and ROS metabolism. The levels of cytoplasmic ROS represent an important feature of ROS metabolism, particularly for ROS signaling [3,23]. To examine whether the permeabilization used for the detection of mitochondrial respiration influences the measurements with fluorescent probes, we repeated the experiments with permeabilized cells (Figure S4). Permeabilization increased the susceptibility of cells to 100 µM DPI, reducing strongly the amount of attached cells (Figure S5). The remaining cells had the same membrane potential as the control cells and cells treated with 10 µM DPI in contrast to nonpermeabilized cells, which showed a decrease of the membrane potential in response to 100 µM DPI (Figure 2a). We assume that this difference is due to a drastic increase in the intracellular glucose levels, which additionally stimulated the electron flow through the respiratory chain. There was no difference in ROS levels in response to DPI treatments in nonpermeabilized (Figure 2b) and permeabilized cells (Figure S4b).

Determination of mitochondrial respiration in permeabilized cells showed that the inhibition of Complex I by DPI can be compensated by the electron supply from the succinate to Complex II. However, these measurements were performed under conditions of excessive succinate availability from the medium. Nevertheless, the intracellular amounts of succinate may not be sufficient to compensate the inhibition of Complex I. To prove this, we inhibited Complex I with rotenone and determined its effects on the mitochondrial membrane potential and cellular ROS levels with and without DPI.

Interestingly, a low concentration of DPI combined with rotenone caused mitochondrial membrane hyperpolarization (Figure S6a), similar to our observations with the effects of DPI and rotenone in mitochondrial respiration measurements (Figure 1b). The cellular ROS levels were not affected in the 10 µM DPI treatment group and strongly increased in the 100 µM DPI group, similarly to the experiment results without rotenone (Figure 2b). This suggests that the increase of cellular ROS levels is not due to the reverse electron flow from the succinate.

Therefore, in the following set of experiments, we used these parameters to estimate the bioenergetics status and ROS metabolism in hAMSCs and undifferentiated hBMSCs, as well as their osteogenic-induced progeny, osteoblast-like cells.

3.1. 30-Minute Time Point

3.1.1. hAMSC

No statistically significant changes in mitochondrial membrane potential (Figure 5a) and cellular ROS levels (Figure 5b) were observed in hAMSC after the treatments with DPI (10 µM and 100 µM), suggesting the overall robustness of hAMSC in response towards all presented treatments.

3.1.2. hBMSC

In hBMSC, a combined treatment with 20 µM MitoTEMPO and 100 µM DPI substantially reduced the membrane potential in hBMSCs, whereas no significant differences were observed with the single MitoTEMPO and DPI treatment groups, even with the 100 µMDPI treatment (Figure 6a).

The treatments of hBMSCs with 10 µM and 100 µM DPI significantly reduced the cellular ROS levels (Figure 6b). An additional treatment with 20 µM MitoTEMPO did not affect the ROS levels compared to 10 µM DPI alone (Figure 6b). Taken together, the ROS level reduction in response to DPI and the absence of a MitoTEMPO effect implies that predominant target of DPI is NOX, not the mitochondria.

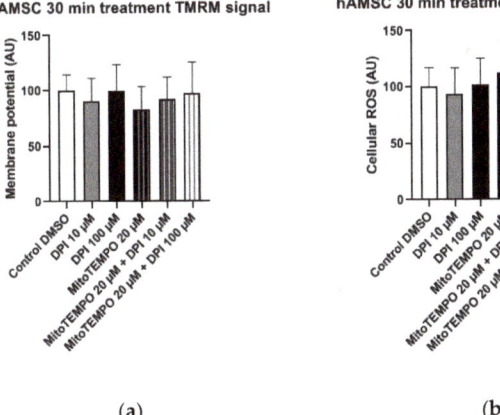

Figure 5. Mitochondrial membrane potential and cellular ROS levels 30 min after the treatment of human amniotic membrane mesenchymal stromal cells (hAMSCs) with diphenyleneiodonium chloride (DPI) and MitoTEMPO. (**a**) Changes in the mitochondrial membrane potential are not present. (**b**) Changes of the cellular ROS levels are not present. Data is represented as means + SD (error bars) ($n = 24$; each point was obtained by analyzing 2–4 single cells. $p > 0.05$; one-way ANOVA followed by multiple comparison post-hoc Fisher's LSD test. There was no significant differences.

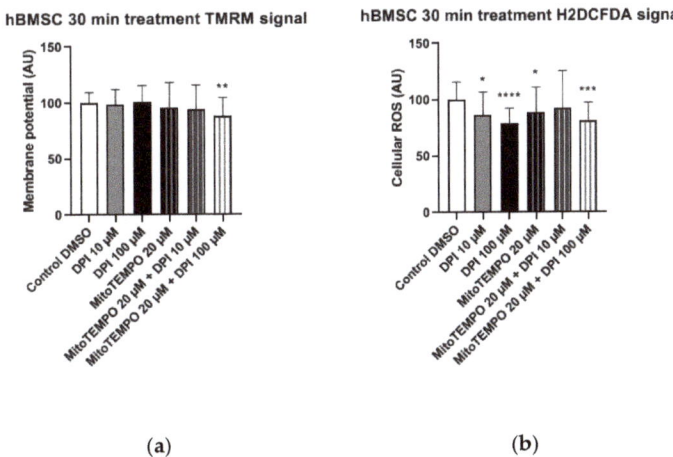

Figure 6. Mitochondrial membrane potential and cellular ROS levels 30 min after the treatment of hBMSCs with diphenyleneiodonium chloride (DPI) and MitoTEMPO. (**a**) Changes in the mitochondrial membrane potential. (**b**) Changes of the cellular ROS levels. Data is represented as means + SD (error bars) ($n = 36$; each point was obtained by analyzing 2–4 single cells. * $p < 0.05$, ** $p < 0.01$, *** $p < 0.001$, and **** $p < 0.0001$; one-way ANOVA followed by multiple comparison post-hoc Fisher's LSD test.

3.1.3. Osteoblast-Like Cells

In osteoblast-like cells, all treatments resulted in significantly reduced mitochondrial membrane potential compared to the control group (Figure 7a). Furthermore, treatments with 10 μM and 100 μM DPI significantly reduced the cellular ROS levels compared to the control group (Figure 7b). This reveals that, similarly to undifferentiated hBMSCs, DPI showed inhibitory properties in predifferentiated cells. The treatment with 20 μM

MitoTEMPO caused an increase of ROS compared to the control group, whereas the combined treatments exhibited no differences in the control group in these cells (Figure 7b).

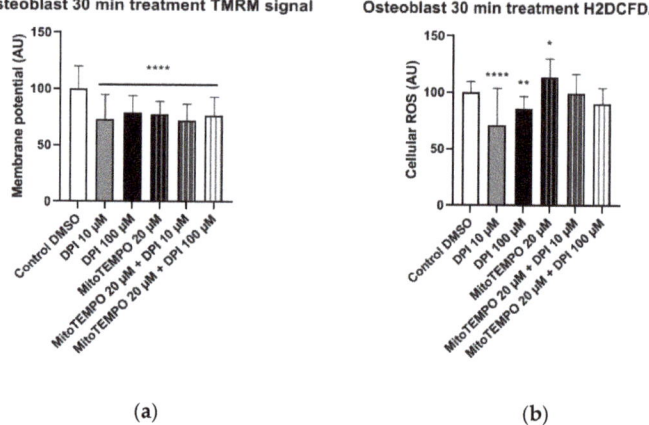

(a)   (b)

Figure 7. Mitochondrial membrane potential and cellular ROS levels 30 min after treatment of osteogenic-induced hBMSCs (osteoblast-like cells) with diphenyleneiodonium chloride (DPI) and MitoTEMPO. (**a**) Changes in the mitochondrial membrane potential. (**b**) Changes of the cellular ROS levels due to nicotinamide adenine dinucleotide phosphate oxidase (NOX) inhibition at high and low concentrations of DPI. Data is represented as means + SD (error bars) ($n = 24$; each point was obtained by analyzing 2–4 single cells. * $p < 0.05$, ** $p < 0.01$, and **** $p < 0.0001$; one-way ANOVA followed by multiple comparison post-hoc Fisher's LSD test.

3.2. Three-Hour Time Point

3.2.1. hAMSCs

In hAMSCs, we observed a significant increase in the mitochondrial membrane potential in the combined treatment groups with 20 μM MitoTEMPO and either 10 μM or 100 μMDPI (Figure 8a). A similar trend of increased mitochondrial membrane potential was observed in the 100 μM DPI group, but the difference to the control group was not statistically significant (Figure 8a). The treatment of hAMSCs with 100 μM DPI and combined treatments of hAMSCs with 20 μM MitoTEMPO and 10 μMor 100 μM DPI resulted in significantly decreased cellular ROS levels compared to the control group (Figure 8b). This could imply a presence of crosstalk between the mitochondria and NOX in hAMSCs, as the decrease in ROS levels was accompanied by an increase in the mitochondrial membrane potential. Paradoxically, the treatment with 20 μM MitoTEMPO caused a significant increase in cellular ROS levels compared to the control group (Figure 8b).

3.2.2. hBMSCs

In hBMSCs, no statistically significant changes in the mitochondrial membrane potential were observed in any of the treatment groups compared to the control group (Figure 9a). The treatment of hBMSCs with 100 μM DPI and combined treatments with 20 μM MitoTEMPO and 10 μM or 100 μM DPI led to significant increases in the cellular ROS levels compared to the control group (Figure 9b). This suggests the onset of DPI effects on the mitochondria, which were not prevented but, rather, exacerbated in a combined treatment with MitoTEMPO and 100 μM DPI compared to the treatment with 100 μM DPI alone (Figure 9b).

We observed a relatively big variance in the 100 μM DPI plus 20 μM MitoTEMPO groups (Figures 8 and 9). We assume the following reasons for that. In our experiments, the primary cells first underwent synchronization for 24 h. This implies that, 30 min after treatments, the cells were still synchronized; however, by three h, a portion of the cells already responded to the treatments changing their metabolic states, and another portion still did not. Eventually, all cells reached a steady state by 24 h. We presume that this is the reason for the higher variations at the three-h time point, including the combined treatment group with 100 μM DPI plus 20 μM MitoTEMPO.

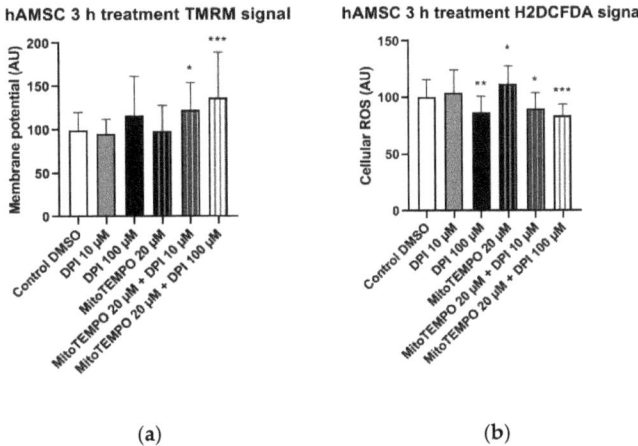

(a) (b)

Figure 8. Mitochondrial membrane potential and cellular ROS levels 3 h after the treatment of hAMSCs with diphenyleneiodonium chloride (DPI) and MitoTEMPO. (a) Changes in mitochondrial membrane potential. (b) Changes of cellular ROS levels; high concentrations of DPI induce an increase of the ROS via the mitochondrial effects. Data is represented as means + SD (error bars) ($n = 23$; each point was obtained by analyzing 2–4 single cells. * $p < 0.05$, ** $p < 0.01$, and *** $p < 0.001$; one-way ANOVA followed by multiple comparison post-hoc Fisher's LSD test.

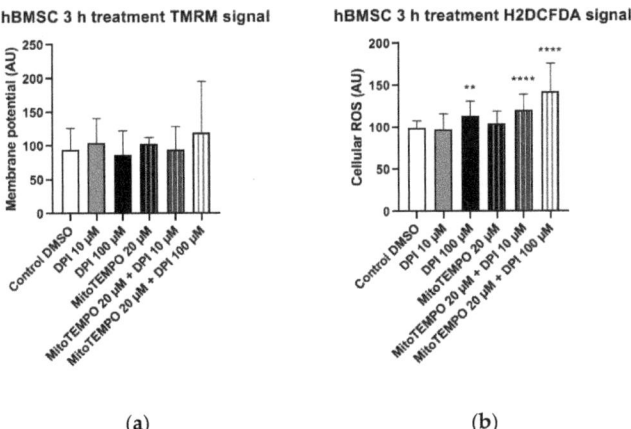

(a) (b)

Figure 9. Mitochondrial membrane potential and cellular ROS levels 3 h after treatment of hBMSCs with diphenyleneiodonium chloride (DPI) and MitoTEMPO. (a) Changes in the mitochondrial membrane potential. (b) Changes of cellular ROS levels; the increase is caused by the mitochondrial effects of DPI. Data is represented as means + SD (error bars) ($n = 36$; each point was obtained by analyzing 2–4 single cells. ** $p < 0.01$, and **** $p < 0.0001$; one-way ANOVA followed by multiple comparison post-hoc Fisher's LSD test.

3.2.3. Osteoblast-Like Cells

In osteoblast-like cells, no statistically significant differences in mitochondrial membrane potential changes were observed in any of the treatment groups compared to the control group (Figure 10a). However, the treatment with 20 μM MitoTEMPO, as well as the combined treatment with 20 μM MitoTEMPO and 10 μM DPI caused a statistically significant increase in the cellular ROS levels compared to the control group (Figure 10b).

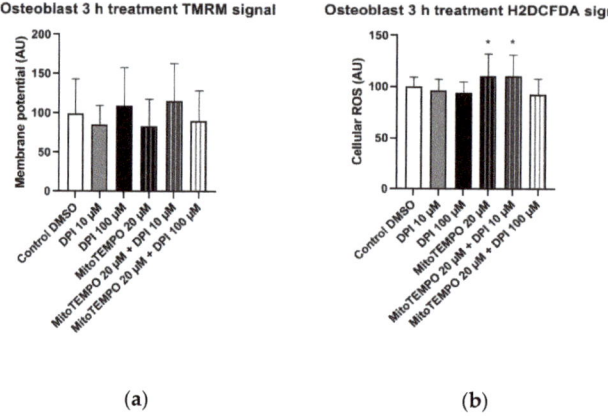

(a) (b)

Figure 10. Mitochondrial membrane potential and cellular ROS levels 3 h after the treatment of osteogenic-induced hBMSCs (osteoblast-like cells) with diphenyleneiodonium chloride (DPI) and MitoTEMPO. (a) Changes in the mitochondrial membrane potential. (b) Changes of the cellular ROS levels. Data is represented as means + SD (error bars) (n = 24; each point was obtained by analyzing 2–4 single cells; cells used in these experiments were obtained from the differentiating passage 2 hBMSCs. * $p < 0.05$; one-way ANOVA followed by multiple comparison post-hoc Fisher's LSD test.

3.3. 24-Hour Time Point
3.3.1. hAMSCs

In hAMSCs, a significant decrease in the mitochondrial membrane potential was observed after the treatment with 100 μM DPI and the combined treatment with 20 μM MitoTEMPO and 100 μM DPI (Figure 11a), which showed a direct inhibitory effect on the mitochondria. However, an increase in the mitochondrial membrane potential was observed after the combined treatment with 20 μM MitoTEMPO and 10 μM DPI (Figure 11a). The treatment with 100 μM DPI and combined treatment with 20 μM MitoTEMPO and 100 μM DPI induced a significant increase in the cellular ROS levels compared to the control group (Figure 11b). Thus, the 20 μM MitoTEMPO and 100 μM DPI treatment group exhibited a simultaneous decrease in mitochondrial membrane potential with an increase in the cellular ROS, suggesting a direct inhibitory effect of high concentrations of DPI on the mitochondria.

3.3.2. hBMSCs

In hBMSCs, both the mitochondrial membrane potential (Figure 12a) and cellular ROS levels (Figure 12b) showed a strong increase after the treatment with 10 μM DPI and the combined treatment with 20 μM MitoTEMPO and 10 μM DPI. However, no viable cells could be observed after the 24-h treatment with either 100 μM DPI alone or in combination with 20 μM MitoTEMPO (Figure 12). Additionally, morphological changes of the hBMSC shape compared to the control group were observed after the 10 μM DPI treatment (Figure 13). The cells appeared in a compacted form, building up round structures while exhibiting elevated mitochondrial membrane potential (Figure 12).

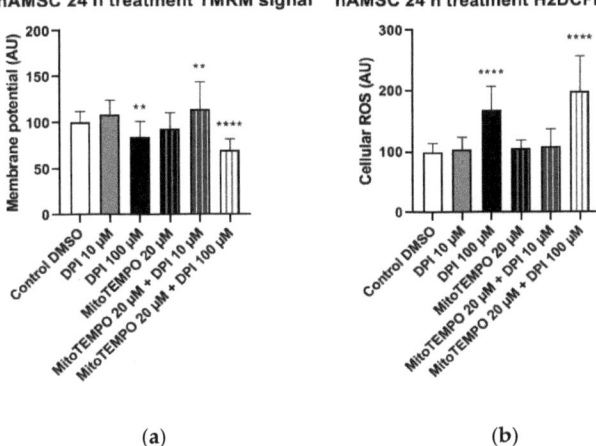

(a) (b)

Figure 11. Mitochondrial membrane potential and cellular ROS levels 24 h after the treatment of hAMSCs with diphenyleneiodonium chloride (DPI) and MitoTEMPO. (**a**) Changes in the mitochondrial membrane potential. (**b**) Changes of the cellular ROS levels, an increase caused by a high DPI. Data is represented as means + SD (error bars) (n = 23; each point was obtained by analyzing 2–4 single cells. ** $p < 0.01$, and **** $p < 0.0001$; one-way ANOVA followed by multiple comparison post-hoc Fisher's LSD test.

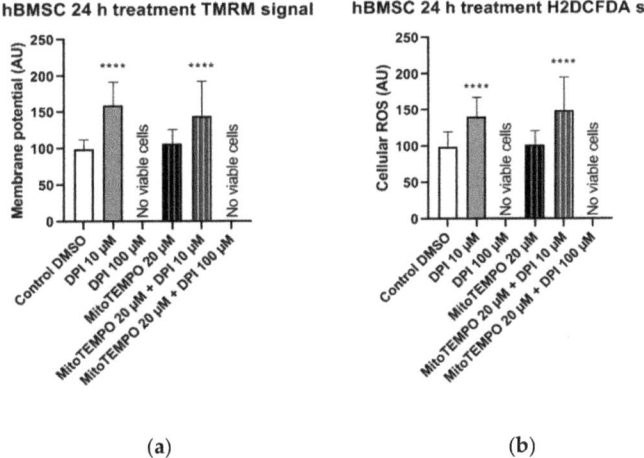

(a) (b)

Figure 12. Mitochondrial membrane potential and cellular ROS levels 24 h after the treatment of hBMSCs with diphenyleneiodonium chloride (DPI) and MitoTEMPO. (**a**) Changes in the mitochondrial membrane potential. (**b**) Changes of the cellular ROS levels. Data is represented as means + SD (error bars) (n = 36; each point was obtained by analyzing 2–4 single cells. **** $p < 0.0001$; one-way ANOVA followed by multiple comparison post-hoc Fisher's LSD test.

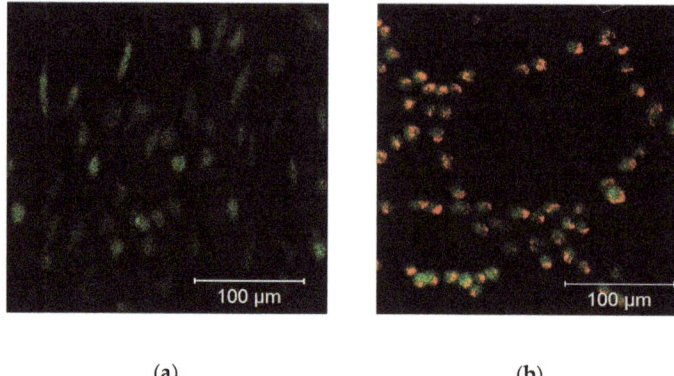

(a) (b)

Figure 13. Morphological changes of the hBMSCs (passage 3) in response to the 10 µM DPI 24-h treatment, mitochondrial membrane potential-sensitive TMRM probe, and cellular ROS-sensitive H2DCFDA probe. (**a**) Control group treated with 0.5% vol. DMSO. (**b**) Group treated with 10 µM DPI. The images were taken with a Zeiss LSM 510 microscope, 10× objective, 50 nM TMRM (red signal) or 10 µM (green signal) H2DCFDA probe concentration.

This suggests that a treatment with low DPI concentrations affects the mitochondrial activity of hBMSCs. Similar changes in the morphology were observed in after the treatment with 20 µM MitoTEMPO (data not shown). Taking into consideration the 3-h time point results, our data imply that, in hBMSCs, at a certain point after the DPI treatments, the scales are tipped from ROS reduction by 10 µM DPI via NOX inhibition (30-min time point) to ROS production by mitochondria (3 h and 24 h). However, hBMSCs treated with 100 µM DPI showed an increase of cellular ROS levels after 3 h, which eventually led to death after 24 h.

3.3.3. Osteoblast-Like Cells

In osteoblast-like cells, single and combined treatments with 10 µM DPI and 20 µM MitoTEMPO resulted in cell survival but no statistically significant alterations in mitochondrial membrane potential compared to the control group (Figure 14a). In contrast, a statistically significant increase in cellular ROS levels was detected after the combined treatment with 20 µM MitoTEMPO and 10 µM DPI (Figure 13b). Overall, this implies an increased robustness of osteoblast-like cells compared to their undifferentiated hBMSC counterparts, since no ROS increase was found after the treatment with 10 µM DPI after 24 h. However, similarly to hBMSCs, no viable osteoblast-like cells were detected after the single or combined treatments with 100 µM DPI and 20 µM MitoTEMPO (Figure 14). To better visualize the similarities within the cell types examined in this study, we applied a Ward's cluster analysis (Figure S7). We analyzed a total of 10 predictors of all H2DCFDA and TMRM groups. Cells connected closer to 0 on the x-axis were more similar to each other, e.g., BMSC 3 h and hAMSC at 24 h were more similar than the ROS at 24 h and BMSC at 24 h.

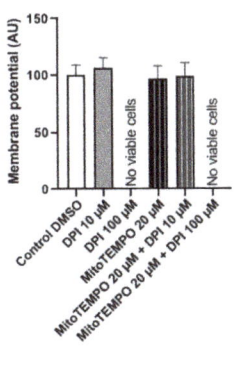
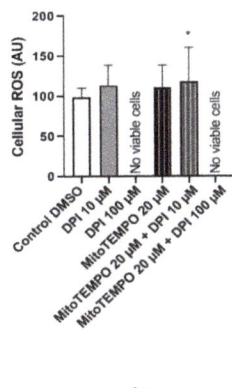

(a) (b)

Figure 14. Mitochondrial membrane potential and cellular ROS levels 24 h after the treatment of osteogenic-induced hBMSCs (osteoblast-like cells) with diphenyleneiodonium chloride (DPI) and MitoTEMPO. (**a**) Changes in the mitochondrial membrane potential. (**b**) Changes of the cellular ROS levels. Data is represented as means + SD (error bars) (n = 24; each point was obtained by analyzing 2–4 single cells; the cells used in these experiments were obtained from the differentiating passage 2 hBMSCs. * $p < 0.05$; one-way ANOVA followed by multiple comparison post-hoc Fisher's LSD test.

4. Discussion

The main findings of this study highlight the differences in ROS turnover between MG-63 cells, hAMSCs, hBMSCs, and hBMSCs differentiated towards osteogenic lineage in vitro. The treatment with 100 µM DPI induced the inhibition of mitochondrial Complex I-linked respiration in MG-63 cells (Figures 1 and 2), accompanied by a burst of mitochondrial ROS production, followed by the translocation of ROS into the cytoplasm (Figure 3). This translocation was accompanied by a decrease in mitochondrial membrane potential. Assuming that excessive ROS generation by the mitochondria may be the reason for the decreased membrane potential, we pretreated cells with mitochondria targeted ROS scavenger MitoTEMPO. Indeed, a drop in membrane potential was prevented by this antioxidant in MG-63 cells. In contrast to MG-63 cells, in hAMSCs, hBMSCs, and osteoblast-like cells derived from hBMSCs, 100 µM DPI did not induce excessive ROS production.

We examined and confirmed the potency of DPI to inhibit mitochondrial respiratory Complex I even at concentrations of 0.625 µM in MG-63 cells, while the Complex II activity remained unaffected. This suggests the presence of a compensatory mechanism, which may explain the lack of acute response towards the 10 µM DPI treatment. Indeed, 10 µM of DPI nearly fully inhibited Complex I but did not influence the membrane potential determined by the membrane potential sensitive fluorescent dye TMRM. In contrast, 100 µM DPI, which already partially affected Complex II (Figure 1) induced a drop in the mitochondrial membrane potential and elevated the ROS levels (Figure 4). Here, we should note that, in the experiments with mitochondrial respiration, the cells were permeabilized and had access to saturating substrate concentrations from the culture medium. In contrast, in the nonpermeabilized cells, the concentrations of substrate can limit the mitochondrial function, and, consequently, the effects of the DPI treatment can be stronger. Furthermore, our experiments with the MG-63 cells suggested that the determination of the mitochondrial membrane potential and the levels of cytoplasmic ROS with fluorescent probes, in combination with the effects of the mitochondria-targeted antioxidant MitoTEMPO, may bring key information about the ROS metabolism in various cell types. We considered that both NOX and mitochondria can contribute to the cellular pool of ROS and affect the mitochondrial function. In this sense, the application of MitoTEMPO allowed us to dissect the specific contribution of mitochondrial ROS. This strategy was applied for hAMSCs, hBMSCs, and differentiated hBMSCs.

Compared to MG-63 cells, hAMSCs of the reflected amniotic region are characterized by low mitochondrial activity [24] and possibly rely mostly on glycolytic pathways. This implies that hAMSC ROS metabolism is more likely to be influenced by NADPH oxidase (NOX) activity rather than the mitochondria. The 30-min treatments with DPI alone or in combination with MitoTEMPO did not result in any alterations in the hAMSC mitochondrial membrane potential and cellular ROS levels compared to the controls (Figure 5). After the three-h treatment, we observed a decrease in cellular ROS in groups treated with high concentrations of DPI, accompanied by an increase in the mitochondrial membrane potential. This effect was slightly more pronounced in the presence of MitoTEMPO. However, after 24 h of exposure to 100 μM DPI alone or in combination with MitoTEMPO, we observed an increase in cellular ROS, accompanied by a decrease in mitochondrial membrane potential. Together, these data suggest that the ROS metabolic pathways in hAMSCs are predominantly determined by NOX rather than by mitochondrial ROS, and high concentrations of DPI did not reduce substantially the numbers of cells by 24 h.

In experiments with hBMSCs, after 30 min, most single and combined treatments with DPI and MitoTEMPO reduced the levels of cytoplasmic ROS. An accompanying decrease of the mitochondrial membrane potential was found only in the combined treatment group with 20 μM MitoTEMPO and 100 μM DPI (Figure 6); 10 μM and 100 μM DPI did not affect the membrane potential but decreased the levels of cytoplasmic ROS. As the highest effects were observed with 100 μM DPI either with or without MitoTEMPO, our data suggests the involvement of NOX inhibition, similar to what we observed in hAMSCs after three h. After three h, the treatment of hBMSCs with 100 μM DPI either alone or in combination with MitoTEMPO elevated the cytoplasmic ROS production, an effect similar to what was observed at 24 h with the hAMSCs. However, the three-h treatment with DPI did not influence membrane potential. Surprisingly, we also observed an increase in the levels of cellular ROS upon the combined treatment with both 10 μM DPI and MitoTEMPO. We cannot explain this phenomenon; however, it demonstrates that MitoTEMPO does not exert a protective effect in these cells. After 24 h of hBMSC treatment with 100 μM DPI either alone or in combination with MitoTEMPO, more than 90% of the cells were dead (Figure 12). This shows that 100 μM DPI is toxic for hBMSCs, although it was not toxic for hAMSCs. Interestingly, the hBMSCs treated with 10 μM DPI exhibited an increase in both cellular ROS and mitochondrial membrane potential, accompanied by drastic changes in the morphology (Figure 13). These changes indirectly suggested that 10 μM DPI might affect the intracellular signaling processes potentially associated with cellular differentiation.

Consequently, our results show that the ROS turnover in hBMSCs is initially more influenced by NOX activity rather than by the mitochondria, with the mitochondria-related effects beginning to contribute after 3 h. Taken together, in both the hAMSCs as well as the hBMSCs, the initial response to the DPI treatment was mediated by NOX, while the mitochondrial response occurred after 24 h in hAMSCs and 3 h in hBMSCs.

We next examined the osteoblast-like cells differentiated from hBMSCs 30 min after DPI treatment (Figure 7). We observed a decrease in the cytoplasmic ROS levels in response to either 10 μM or 100 μM DPI. This response was not accompanied by an increase in the membrane potential. After three h, we did not see any changes in osteoblast-like cell membrane potentials, but we did observe a slight elevation of the cytoplasmic ROS by 20 μM MitoTEMPO alone or in combination with DPI (Figure 10). We do not have a reasonable explanation for this fact, perhaps other than the NOX or mitochondria source of ROS appears at this time point. After 24 h, there were no vital osteoblast-like cells upon the treatment with 100 μM DPI, similar with the hBMSCs (Figure 14). The mitochondrial membrane potential was not affected in all groups that survived the treatment; the levels of cellular ROS were increased only in the 20 μM MitoTEMPO combined with 10 μM DPI group. While the mode of action of MitoTEMPO as an antioxidant is well-defined in immortalized cell lines, here, we observed an opposite effect. This poses an open question regarding the other possible effects of MitoTEMPO in primary cells.

Our results suggest that the ROS metabolism in osteogenic predifferentiated hBMSCs is more dependent on mitochondrial ROS than on not differentiated BMSCs. This is in-line with the previous findings that undifferentiated cells are more dependent on the anerobic energy metabolism [25]. Consequently, DPI affects undifferentiated cells predominantly by inhibiting NOX, while, in predifferentiated cells, the mitochondrial effects of DPI become more pronounced. Consequently, our approach for the simultaneous determination of the mitochondrial membrane potential and cytoplasmic ROS can distinguish specific differences in the ROS metabolism in different types of mesenchymal stromal cells at different phases of their proliferation and differentiation. A Ward's cluster analysis (supplementary material, Figure S3) could further enhance the understanding of cell similarities after different treatments (with DPI) at different stages of differentiation.

5. Conclusions

Our study demonstrates critical differences in ROS metabolism between the osteoblastoma cell line (MG-63), osteoblast-like cells induced from hBMSCs, and undifferentiated hBMSCs and hAMSCs. These differences were uncovered by the examination of the cell responses to treatments with DPI and MitoTEMPO. Our data suggest that the mechanism of ROS generation and the levels of intracellular ROS predominantly depend on the type of energy metabolism used by the cell. Thus, in cell types with glycolysis, DPI predominantly interacts with NOX, while the mitochondria remain unaffected. In contrast, in cells with aerobic energy metabolism, the mitochondria become an additional target for DPI. As a result, cells relying more on aerobic metabolism such as MG-63 or osteoblast-like cells are more sensitive to the toxic effects of DPI, while cells predominantly living from glycolysis, such as hAMSCs, are more resistant to the toxic effects of DPI. In summary, our data suggest that undifferentiated cells rather than differentiated parenchymal cells should be considered as potential targets for DPI.

Supplementary Materials: The following are available online at https://www.mdpi.com/1999-4923/13/1/10/s1: Figure S1. Effects of diphenyleneiodonium chloride (DPI) on the mitochondrial function in MG-63 cells, Figure S2. MG-63 cell nuclear and mitochondrial ROS staining in the control cells, Figure S3. Combined effects of diphenyleneiodonium (DPI) and MitoTEMPO in permeabilized, Figure S4. Mitochondrial membrane potential and cellular ROS levels in permeabilized MG-63 cells, Figure S5. Response of permeabilized and nonpermeabilized MG-63 cells to 100 μM DPI, Figure S6. Mitochondrial membrane potential and cellular ROS levels in MG-63 cells exposed to DPI and 5 μM rotenone, Figure S7. Hierarchical cluster analysis of the hAMSCs, hBMSCs, and osteoblast similarity dendrogram.

Author Contributions: Conceptualization, A.V.K. and A.W.; methodology, S.Z. and D.H.; validation, S.Z., D.H., D.M.P., A.B., and C.S.; formal analysis, S.Z.; investigation, S.Z. and A.W.; resources, A.V.K.; data curation and writing—original draft preparation, A.V.K., A.W., and S.Z.; writing—review and editing, D.H., S.Z., A.B., C.S., S.W., and D.M.P.; supervision, A.V.K., A.W., and S.W.; project administration, A.V.K. and A.W.; and funding acquisition, A.V.K. and D.M.P. All authors have read and agreed to the published version of the manuscript.

Funding: This research was partially funded by FFG grant #FFG 854180, FFG Industrienahe Dissertation grant #867803, and the project Rejuvenate Bone funding from the European Union's Horizon 2020 Research and Innovation Program under the Marie Sklodowska-Curie grant agreement No. 657716.

Institutional Review Board Statement: Ethical review and approval were waived for this study, because the decision was made by the governmental ethic committee (Ethikkommission des Landes Oberösterreich, No. 200, 12. 05. 2005).

Informed Consent Statement: Human placentae from caesarean sections were collected with informed consent of the patients and approval of the local ethical commission (Ethikkommission des Landes Oberösterreich, 21 May 2014), in accordance to the Declaration of Helsinki.

Data Availability Statement: Data available on request due to ethical reasons.

Acknowledgments: The authors thank Sergiu Dumitrescu for providing the hAMSCs and the protocol for their isolation, as well as for stimulating discussions of the results, Markus Moik for assistance with the cultivation of the MG-63 cells, and Simone Hennerbichler-Lugscheider (Blutzentrale Linz) for her support.

Conflicts of Interest: The authors declare no conflict of interest.

References

1. Dikalov, S. Cross talk between mitochondria and NADPH oxidases. *Free Radic. Biol. Med.* **2011**, *51*, 1289–1301. [CrossRef]
2. Daiber, A. Redox signaling (cross-talk) from and to mitochondria involves mitochondrial pores and reactive oxygen species. *Biochim. Biophys. Acta (BBA)-Bioenerg.* **2010**, *1797*, 897–906. [CrossRef] [PubMed]
3. Weidinger, A.; Kozlov, A.V. Biological activities of reactive oxygen and nitrogen species: Oxidative stress versus signal transduction. *Biomolecules* **2015**, *5*, 472–484. [CrossRef] [PubMed]
4. Wang, Q.; Qian, L.; Chen, S.H.; Chu, C.H.; Wilson, B.; Oyarzabal, E.; Ali, S.; Robinson, B.; Rao, D.; Hong, J.S. Post-treatment with an ultra-low dose of NADPH oxidase inhibitor diphenyleneiodonium attenuates disease progression in multiple Parkinson's disease models. *Brain* **2015**, *138*, 1247–1262. [CrossRef] [PubMed]
5. Nagel, S.; Genius, J.; Heiland, S.; Horstmann, S.; Gardner, H.; Wagner, S. Diphenyleneiodonium and dimethylsulfoxide for treatment of reperfusion injury in cerebral ischemia of the rat. *Brain Res.* **2007**, *1132*, 210–217. [CrossRef] [PubMed]
6. Nagel, S.; Hadley, G.; Pfleger, K.; Grond-Ginsbach, C.; Buchan, A.M.; Wagner, S.; Papadakis, M. Suppression of the inflammatory response by diphenyleneiodonium after transient focal cerebral ischemia. *J. Neurochem.* **2012**, *123*, 98–107. [CrossRef] [PubMed]
7. Kuai, Y.; Liu, H.; Liu, D.; Liu, Y.; Sun, Y.; Xie, J.; Sun, J.; Fang, Y.; Pan, H.; Han, W. An ultralow dose of the NADPH oxidase inhibitor diphenyleneiodonium (DPI) is an economical and effective therapeutic agent for the treatment of colitis-associated colorectal cancer. *Theranostics* **2020**, *10*, 6743–6757. [CrossRef] [PubMed]
8. Buggisch, M.; Ateghang, B.; Ruhe, C.; Strobel, C.; Lange, S.; Wartenberg, M.; Sauer, H. Stimulation of ES-cell-derived cardiomyogenesis and neonatal cardiac cell proliferation by reactive oxygen species and NADPH oxidase. *J. Cell Sci.* **2007**, *120*, 885–894. [CrossRef]
9. Ozsvari, B.; Bonuccelli, G.; Sanchez-Alvarez, R.; Foster, R.; Sotgia, F.; Lisanti, M.P. Targeting flavin-containing enzymes eliminates cancer stem cells (CSCs), by inhibiting mitochondrial respiration: Vitamin B2 (Riboflavin) in cancer therapy. *Aging (Albany. NY)* **2017**, *9*, 2610–2628. [CrossRef]
10. Daiber, A.; Di Lisa, F.; Oelze, M.; Kröller-Schön, S.; Steven, S.; Schulz, E.; Münzel, T. Crosstalk of mitochondria with NADPH oxidase via reactive oxygen and nitrogen species signalling and its role for vascular function. *Br. J. Pharmacol.* **2017**, *174*, 1670–1689. [CrossRef]
11. Silini, A.R.; Cargnoni, A.; Magatti, M.; Pianta, S.; Parolini, O. The long path of human placenta, and its derivatives, in regenerative medicine. *Front. Bioeng. Biotechnol.* **2015**, *3*, 162. [CrossRef] [PubMed]
12. Caplan, A.I. Mesenchymal stem cells. *J. Orthop. Res.* **1991**, *9*, 641–650. [CrossRef] [PubMed]
13. Kim, J.; Kang, H.M.; Kim, H.; Kim, M.R.; Kwon, H.C.; Gye, M.C.; Kang, S.G.; Yang, H.S.; You, J. Ex vivo characteristics of human amniotic membrane-derived stem cells. *Cloning Stem Cells* **2007**, *9*, 581–594. [CrossRef] [PubMed]
14. Sadler, T. *Langman's Medical Embryology*, 9th ed.; Lippincott Williams & Wilkins: Philadelphia, PA, USA, 2004; ISBN 9780781743105.
15. Caplan, A.I.; Dennis, J.E. Mesenchymal stem cells as trophic mediators. *J. Cell. Biochem.* **2006**, *98*, 1076–1084. [CrossRef] [PubMed]
16. Zupan, J.; Tang, D.; Oreffo, R.O.C.; Redl, H.; Marolt Presen, D. Bone-Marrow-Derived Mesenchymal Stromal Cells: From Basic Biology to Applications in Bone Tissue Engineering and Bone Regeneration. In *Cell Engineering and Regeneration*; Springer International Publishing: Berlin/Heidelberg, Germany, 2020; pp. 1–55.
17. Chen, C.-T.; Shih, Y.-R.V.; Kuo, T.K.; Lee, O.K.; Wei, Y.-H. Coordinated Changes of Mitochondrial Biogenesis and Antioxidant Enzymes During Osteogenic Differentiation of Human Mesenchymal Stem Cells. *Stem Cells* **2008**, *26*, 960–968. [CrossRef] [PubMed]
18. Chen, C.T.; Hsu, S.H.; Wei, Y.H. Upregulation of mitochondrial function and antioxidant defense in the differentiation of stem cells. *Biochim. Biophys. Acta (BBA)-Gen. Subj.* **2010**, *1800*, 257–263. [CrossRef] [PubMed]
19. Banerjee, A.; Weidinger, A.; Hofer, M.; Steinborn, R.; Lindenmair, A.; Hennerbichler-Lugscheider, S.; Eibl, J.; Redl, H.; Kozlov, A.V.; Wolbank, S. Different metabolic activity in placental and reflected regions of the human amniotic membrane. *Placenta* **2015**, *36*, 1329–1332. [CrossRef]
20. Hennerbichler, S.; Reichl, B.; Pleiner, D.; Gabriel, C.; Eibl, J.; Redl, H. The influence of various storage conditions on cell viability in amniotic membrane. *Cell Tissue Bank.* **2007**, *8*, 1–8. [CrossRef]
21. Chang, H.W.; Wang, H.R.; Tang, J.Y.; Wang, Y.Y.; Farooqi, A.A.; Yen, C.Y.; Yuan, S.S.F.; Huang, H.W. Manoalide preferentially provides antiproliferation of oral cancer cells by oxidative stress-mediated apoptosis and dna damage. *Cancers* **2019**, *11*, 1303. [CrossRef]
22. Ko, S.H.; Choi, G.E.; Oh, J.Y.; Lee, H.J.; Kim, J.S.; Chae, C.W.; Choi, D.; Han, H.J. Succinate promotes stem cell migration through the GPR91-dependent regulation of DRP1-mediated mitochondrial fission. *Sci. Rep.* **2017**, *7*. [CrossRef]
23. Kozlov, A.V.; Lancaster, J.R.; Meszaros, A.T.; Weidinger, A. Mitochondria-meditated pathways of organ failure upon inflammation. *Redox Biol.* **2017**, *13*, 170–181. [CrossRef] [PubMed]

24. Banerjee, A.; Lindenmair, A.; Hennerbichler, S.; Steindorf, P.; Steinborn, R.; Kozlov, A.V.; Redl, H.; Wolbank, S.; Weidinger, A. Cellular and Site-Specific Mitochondrial Characterization of Vital Human Amniotic Membrane. *Cell Transpl.* **2018**, *27*, 3–11. [CrossRef] [PubMed]
25. Ito, K.; Suda, T. Metabolic requirements for the maintenance of self-renewing stem cells. *Nat. Rev. Mol. Cell Biol.* **2014**, *15*, 243–256. [CrossRef] [PubMed]

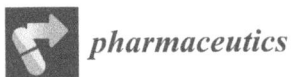

Article

Chimeric Drug Design with a Noncharged Carrier for Mitochondrial Delivery

Consuelo Ripoll [1], Pilar Herrero-Foncubierta [1,2], Virginia Puente-Muñoz [1,†], M. Carmen Gonzalez-Garcia [1], Delia Miguel [1], Sandra Resa [2], Jose M. Paredes [1], Maria J. Ruedas-Rama [1], Emilio Garcia-Fernandez [1], Mar Roldan [3], Susana Rocha [4], Herlinde De Keersmaecker [4], Johan Hofkens [4], Miguel Martin [3,‡], Juan M. Cuerva [2] and Angel Orte [1,*]

1 Departamento de Fisicoquimica, Unidad de Excelencia de Química Aplicada a Biomedicina y Medioambiente, Facultad de Farmacia, Universidad de Granada, Campus Cartuja, 18071 Granada, Spain; consueloripoll@ugr.es (C.R.); pilarhf@ugr.es (P.H-F.); vpuente@ugr.es (V.P.-M.); mcarmeng@ugr.es (M.C.G.-G.); dmalvarez@ugr.es (D.M.); jmparedes@ugr.es (J.M.P.); mjruedas@ugr.es (M.J.R.-R); emiliogf@ugr.es (E.G.-F)
2 Departamento de Quimica Organica, Unidad de Excelencia de Química Aplicada a Biomedicina y Medioambiente, Facultad de Ciencias, Universidad de Granada, Campus Fuentenueva, 18071 Granada, Spain; sra@ugr.es (S.R.); jmcuerva@ugr.es (J.M.C.)
3 GENYO, Pfizer-University of Granada-Junta de Andalucía Centre for Genomics and Oncological Research. Avda. Ilustracion 114. PTS, 18016 Granada, Spain; miguelmartin@ugr.es (M.M.); mar.roldan@genyo.es (M.R.)
4 Department of Chemistry, K. U. Leuven, Celestijnenlaan 200F, B-3001 Heverlee, Belgium; susana.rocha@kuleuven.be (S.R.); herlinde.dekeersmaecker@kuleuven.be (H.D.K.); johan.hofkens@kuleuven.be (J.H.)
* Correspondence: angelort@ugr.es; Tel.: +34-9-5824-3825
† Current address: Interdisciplinary Institute for Neuroscience, UMR 5297, Centre National de la Recherche Scientifique, F-33076 Bordeaux, France; and Interdisciplinary Institute for Neuroscience, University of Bordeaux, F-33076 Bordeaux, France.
‡ Current address: Departamento de Bioquimica y Biologia Molecular I, Facultad de Ciencias, Universidad de Granada, Campus Fuentenueva, 18071 Granada, Spain.

Abstract: Recently, it was proposed that the thiophene ring is capable of promoting mitochondrial accumulation when linked to fluorescent markers. As a noncharged group, thiophene presents several advantages from a synthetic point of view, making it easier to incorporate such a side moiety into different molecules. Herein, we confirm the general applicability of the thiophene group as a mitochondrial carrier for drugs and fluorescent markers based on a new concept of nonprotonable, noncharged transporter. We implemented this concept in a medicinal chemistry application by developing an antitumor, metabolic chimeric drug based on the pyruvate dehydrogenase kinase (PDHK) inhibitor dichloroacetate (DCA). The promising features of the thiophene moiety as a noncharged carrier for targeting mitochondria may represent a starting point for the design of new metabolism-targeting drugs.

Keywords: antitumor agents; fluorescence lifetime imaging; medicinal chemistry; metabolic drug; mitochondrial carrier

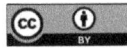

1. Introduction

Mitochondria are essential organelles for cellular metabolism; therefore, understanding their function is critical for biologists and biochemists [1]. Importantly, cellular metabolism, through mitochondrial activity, plays a central role in many physiological alterations and diseases. Alterations in mitochondrial metabolism play a crucial role in cancer [2,3]. The anabolic pathways derived from the mitochondrial oxidative metabolism, such as tricarboxylic acid cycle (TCA)-derived biosynthetic reactions, are significantly essential to sustain high proliferative rates in many cancer types [4]. Nevertheless, other cancer cells display an apparent independence on mitochondrial oxidative metabolism, thus fundamentally relying on cytosolic biosynthetic pathways derived from glycolytic intermediates [5–7]. Within this context, targeting the mitochondria for either visualization or sensing depends on the existence of different carriers capable of delivering the intended compound inside this organelle [8,9].

Mitochondrial visualization using fluorescent probes has been extensively studied and has yielded high- and super-resolution images of this organelle [10–12]. Moreover, fluorescent sensors that target mitochondria have been used to determine real-time chemical and physiological information [13–16], and specific drug delivery to this organelle has been accomplished to enhance drug activity [17–19]. The working mechanism of existing carriers is based on two different properties of the mitochondrial membrane: the negative membrane potential and selective use of the mitochondrial protein import machinery [20]. The latter implies the use of characteristic oligopeptide sequences that must be included in the probe [21]. The former depends on the incorporation of a lipophilic cation, usually a phosphonium, ammonium or pyridinium salt, in the structure of the fluorophore or drug [22–25]. In fact, one of the most commonly employed mitochondrial delivery carriers is the triphenylphosphonium cation (TPP), a bulky, positively charged group [25]. Recently, it has been shown that increasing the lipophilic volume of the carrier using methylated phenyl radicals in TPPs further enhances mitochondrial accumulation [18,26]. Cationic dyes [27,28] and delocalized lipophilic cations [29] are also known to efficiently gather in such organelle. Nevertheless, although this strategy is widely used, it has some drawbacks. The first of them is related to the inherent synthetic difficulties associated with salts, which hamper the use of standard purification/synthetic procedures in an organic chemistry lab, therefore implying that these ionic functionalities must be introduced in the last synthetic steps. Thus for example, liquid-liquid extraction with organic solvents, a general procedure to isolate most of the drugs, is based on that some reagents, solvents or by-products are ideally displaced to the water phase, in which cationic species would be also soluble preventing this type of purification. Likewise, the most used chromatographic techniques do not allow the separation of this kind of compounds due to its ionic nature. All of these limit the structures to which these mitochondria carriers can be coupled. The second important drawback is related to alterations that lipophilic cations cause to the mitochondrial function. Several authors have pointed out that these structures are able to reduce mitochondrial membrane potential ($\Delta\Psi_m$). During diverse stimulations or fixation with chemical agents, these dyes can easily leak out due to decrease in $\Delta\Psi_m$, and cannot work effectively [14,30]. Moreover, deleterious effects over the electron transport chain and mitochondrial respiration have been reported to be caused by cationic dyes, normally used to measure $\Delta\Psi_m$ [28], and mitochondria staining fluorescent probes [31].

Development of a nonprotonable, noncharged and simple mitochondrial carrier could represent a new paradigm applicable not only to fluorescent probes but also to the selective transport of therapeutic drugs to mitochondria, as highlighted by Xu and Xu in a recent review on mitochondria-targeting fluorescent sensors [32]. From a synthetic point of view, drug modification with noncharged carriers clearly represents an improvement over traditional approaches in terms of the simplicity of chemical reactions, purification steps, and subsequent characterization by spectroscopic techniques. Bearing this in mind, we aimed to develop very simple noncharged mitochondrial carriers that are practically unknown. The working hypothesis is that species with a partial positive charge are directly generated and trapped in the interior of the mitochondrial matrix from suitable nonprotonable, noncharged species. Mitochondria are rich in reactive oxygen species (ROS) [33], and basic electron pairs can be oxidized in such environments. A neutral carrier could be transformed into a partially charged carrier by oxidation of a basic electron pair in its structure, fostering accumulation inside the organelle. In our hypothesis, a neutral carrier diffuses into the cytoplasm and enters the mitochondrial membrane, becoming trapped in the mitochondrial matrix by an oxidation reaction (Scheme 1). During the progress of our research, a similar mechanism to this proposal was reported by Reshetnikov and colleagues [17] based on the oxidation of ferrocene to ferrocenium cations, and by Abelha et al. [34], who employed oxidation of the TPP moiety. Another potential candidate for oxidation-driven mitochondrial accumulation is pyridine, a very stable aromatic substrate with a basic pair that can be oxidized to yield well-known pyridine oxides [35,36]. Unfortunately, the basicity of such an electron pair is high enough for interaction with acidic lysosomes, preventing entry into the mitochondria. Hence, we focused our attention on the electron pair of thiophene, which is essentially not basic under physiological conditions. However, thiophenes can be oxidized by oxygen-based oxidants [37], e.g., H_2O_2, as well as by cytochrome P450 in vivo [38,39], to yield thiophene oxides, dioxides and epoxides. Indeed, thiophene carriers exhibit enhanced mitochondrial accumulation when linked to acridone fluorescent markers, especially when designed for fluorescence lifetime imaging microscopy (FLIM) [40]. In this previous work, although N-(3-hydroxypropyl)-4-methoxy-acridone accumulated in the cell nucleus, since acridone dyes are excellent DNA binding agents [41], the addition of a terminal thiophene ring resulted in the preferential delivery of the fluorescent dye to the mitochondria instead of the nuclei [40]. Importantly, mitochondrial delivery of a noncharged, thiophene-containing acridone dye cannot be predicted by current quantitative structure-activity relation (QSAR) algorithms [42]. Therefore, confirmation of the general applicability of thiophene as a mitochondrial carrier is still lacking.

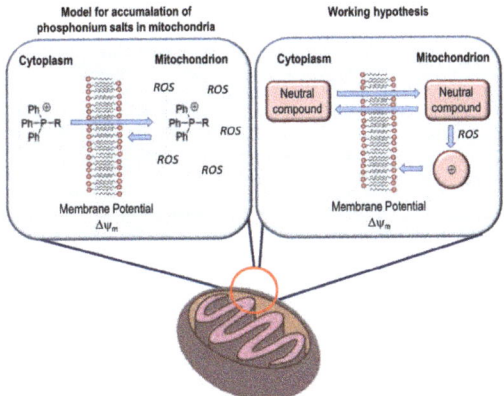

Scheme 1. Comparison of traditional mitochondrial carriers (**left**) and our hypothesized noncharged carriers oxidized inside the mitochondria (**right**).

Herein, we tested this new neutral mitochondrial carrier in a medicinal chemistry application by designing a thiophene-containing chimeric drug with potential anticancer activity after confirming the power of the thiophene ring to achieve mitochondrial delivery. One of the key targets in the regulation of cancer metabolism is pyruvate dehydrogenase complex (PDHC) [43], which catalyzes the key reaction to activate the TCA cycle. PDHC exhibits anomalously low activity in proliferative tumors that are resistant to conventional chemotherapies. This low pyruvate dehydrogenase (PDH) activity is caused by hyperactive pyruvate dehydrogenase kinase (PDHK), which phosphorylates PDH. In this context, therapies aiming to reactivate PDH would have an important impact, as they may decrease cellular metabolism to normal levels, circumventing the adaptive measures of tumor cells. With this in mind, mitochondrial accumulation of a PDHK inhibitor may lead to enhanced efficacy of metabolic treatment. Dichloroacetate (DCA) is a known PDHK inhibitor that has been tested in clinical trials, although its effectiveness has been questioned primarily because of the adverse side effects and toxicity due to the high doses needed to achieve antitumor activity [44]. Hence, we designed a very simple chimera of this PDHK inhibitor by merging DCA with a thiophene ring via an acetyl linker (Thio-DCA, Chart 1), and tested its efficacy against four different breast cancer cell lines that had shown resistance to DCA treatment, MDA-MB-468, MDA-MB-231, SKBR3, and MCF7, each with different metabolic features. It is relevant to work with all these cell lines due to their different cellular and molecular features and responses to chemotherapies and treatments [45].

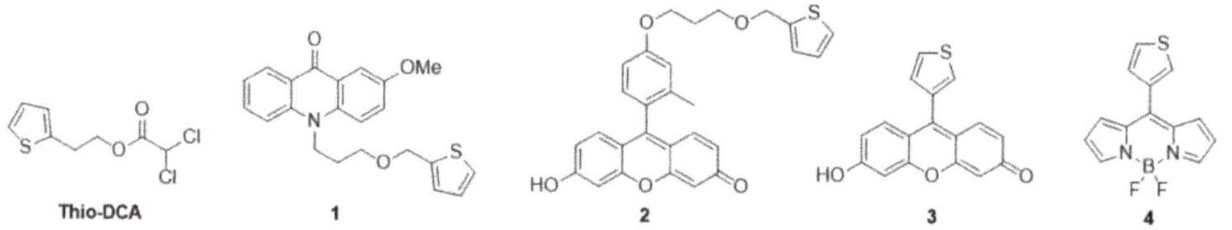

Chart 1. DCA-based drug Thio-DCA and thiophene-containing fluorescent dyes (acridone **1**, xanthene **2–3**, and BODIPY **4**) synthesized in this work.

2. Results
2.1. Synthesis of Thiophene-Modified Fluorescent Markers

In previous work, we showed that simple acridone-based fluorescent probe **1**, containing a thiophene side group (Chart 1), exhibited enhanced mitochondrial accumulation compared to its thiophene-lacking counterpart [40]. Acridone derivatives are known to be very good DNA intercalating agents and therefore usually accumulate in the nucleus [41]. They are also known to have very long fluorescence lifetimes, τ, which make them very suitable for FLIM imaging [46–48]. In fact, probe **1** permits the quantitative determination of microenvironment dipolarity inside mitochondria using the excellent sensing capabilities of the acridone moiety [40].

Encouraged by these results, we determined the performance of the thiophene group as a general mitochondrial carrier for use in medicinal chemistry applications after its incorporation into other fluorescent compounds with different chemical natures, polarities and lipophilic characteristics (Chart 1). Apart from acridone **1**, we synthesized a xanthene derivative with the thiophene group included on a flexible chain (**2**), a xanthene derivative with the thiophene incorporated in the central ring (**3**) and a BODIPY derivative (**4**).

Both xanthene derivatives, 6-hydroxy-9-(2-methyl-4-(3-(thiophen-2-ylmethoxy) propoxy) phenyl)-3H-xanthen-3-one (**2**) and thiophene-modified xanthene **3**, 6-hydroxy-9-(thiophen-3-yl)-3H-xanthen-3-one, were synthesized using a methodology developed by our group (Scheme 2) [49]. Thus, the addition of an organolithium derivative, obtained by bromine-lithium exchange of the corresponding aryl bromide, to the tert-butyldimethylsilyl ester (TBDMS)-protected xanthene moiety afforded compounds **2** and **3** after acid treatment. Compounds **2** and **3** were subsequently isolated as orange solids. Dye **2** is a derivative of 2-methyl-4-methoxy-phenyl xanthene, one of the so-called Tokyo Green dyes [50]. Finally, the *meso*-thiophene BODIPY, **4**, was prepared following a previously published route [51]. Further details regarding the synthetic protocol employed for each compound in Chart 1, as well as spectroscopic characterization (^{1}H- and ^{13}C-NMR spectral data) and mass spectrometry data, are described in the Experimental section and the Supplementary Materials (SM, Schemes S1–S6 and Figures S1–S16).

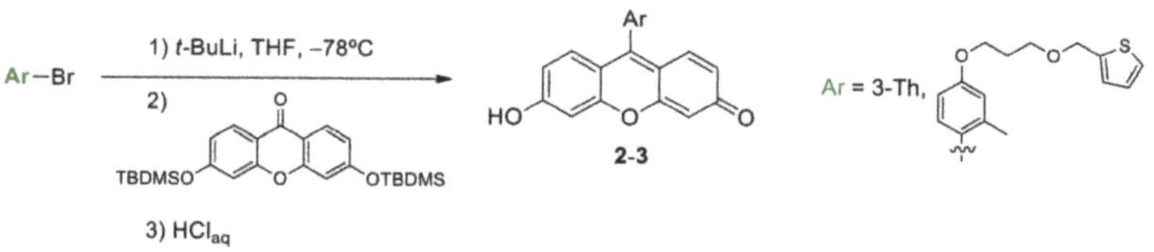

Scheme 2. Synthetic route of compounds **2–3**.

2.2. Thiophene as a General Mitochondrial Delivery Agent

The synthesized thiophene-containing fluorescent markers have different structural and physical features. Whereas acridone **1** and BODIPY **4** are pH-independent and neutral fluorophores, xanthene derivatives **2** and **3** exhibit a prototropic equilibrium between neutral and anionic forms upon deprotonation of the hydroxyl group in the xanthene moiety. Using UV-visible absorption spectroscopy, we confirmed that **1** and **4** exhibited pH-independent spectra (Figure S17 in the SM) and calculated the acid–base equilibrium constant, in terms of pK_a, as 6.28 ± 0.06 and 6.39 ± 0.03 for **2** and **3** (Figure S18), respectively. This mild acidic behavior may already help these dyes localize to the mitochondria [42], but importantly, the presence of the neutral thiophene ring does not alter the acid–base properties or the charge of the dyes. Compound **2** maintained a high emission quantum yield (0.84 ± 0.02) owing to the 2-methyl substituent in the phenyl ring, which keeps it perpendicular to the xanthene plane, decreasing nonradiative deactivation. The perpendicular conformation of an aromatic substituent at the *meso-* position is a well-known requirement for high fluorescence emission efficiency in xanthene [50,52] and BODIPY [53,54] dyes. In contrast, the thiophene ring in xanthene **3** has free rotation, decreasing the fluorescence quantum yield down to 0.14 ± 0.01. In fact, fluorescence lifetime measurements exhibited faster deactivation and hence a lower quantum yield in low viscosity methanol:glycerine mixtures. At 20 °C, the fluorescence lifetime of **3** increased from 1.7 ± 0.1 ns in methanol (viscosity of 0.54 mPa·s) up to 2.54 ± 0.03 ns in a methanol:glycerine mixture of 2.02 mPa·s. This dependence indicates that rotation of the thiophene ring is involved in the deactivation pathway of **3**. Further details on the viscosity dependence of the fluorescence properties of **3** can be found in Figure S19.

Once we ensured that the dyes were photostable enough for imaging applications (Figure S20) and that the presence of the thiophene ring was not detrimental to the fluorescence properties of the dyes, we employed dual-color fluorescence microscopy for the simultaneous imaging of the dyes and mitochondria, which was traced in red using MitoTracker Deep Red (MT). By following the localization of the probe, we could easily detect the transport efficiency of the noncharged carrier to the mitochondria. Figure 1 shows assessment of the effective incorporation of dyes **1** and **2** into the mitochondria with great confidence. Additionally, we used dual-color FLIM microscopy to simultaneously examine the localization of the dyes and their emission kinetics through the fluorescence lifetime values (see the SM and Table S1 for experimental details). Figures S21–S29 in the SM show dual-color FLIM images of dyes **1–4** in live cells, demonstrating clear accumulation in the mitochondria. Nevertheless, a fraction of the dyes was also found in other cellular compartments, confirming that the accumulation is not perfectly specific, and further work may be required to achieve higher selectivity. In fact, the Pearson's correlation coefficient (Table S2) averaged through at least five different images was 0.59 ± 0.10, 0.69 ± 0.07, 0.58 ± 0.12, and 0.67 ± 0.04 for **1**, **2**, **3**, and **4**, respectively. We also obtained the mutual Manders' colocalization coefficients (MCC, Table S2) as a measure of the fraction of coincident pixels in each channel. The MCC values of colocalized dye with MT were 0.46 ± 0.14, 0.64 ± 0.14, 0.58 ± 0.15, and 0.46 ± 0.06 for **1**, **2**, **3**, and **4**, respectively. The MCC values for the MT channel, indicating the fraction of colocalized mitochondrial pixels, were 0.64 ± 0.10, 0.73 ± 0.14, 0.66 ± 0.12, and 0.36 ± 0.12 for **1**, **2**, **3**, and **4**, respectively. These values indicate a good level of colocalization, although accompanied by nonspecificity, as can be visually inspected. Notably, the dye that best localized in the mitochondria was **2**, in which the thiophene group is further apart from the chromophore moiety. In any case, these results indicate that thiophene may be a good carrier for mitochondrial drug delivery.

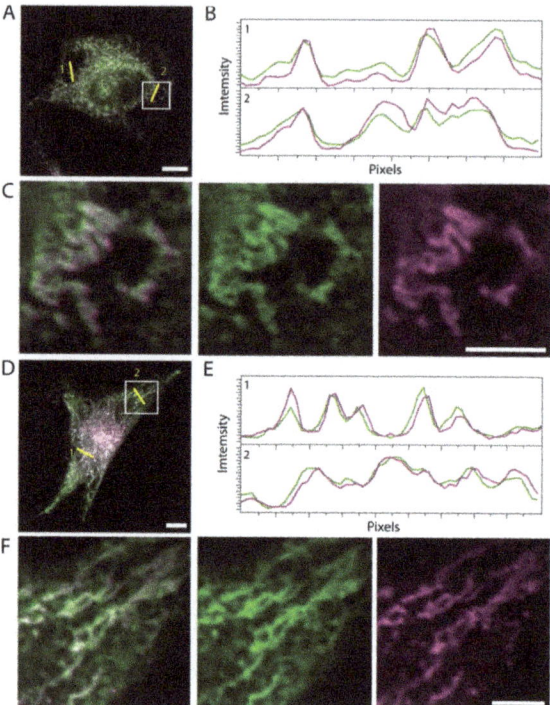

Figure 1. Dual-color confocal microscopy of **1** (**A**–**C**) and **2** (**D**–**F**) in formaldehyde-fixed HeLa cells. (**A**,**D**) Overlaid images of the dye (green) and MT (purple). Scale bars represent 10 μm. (**B**,**E**) Intensity profile traces extracted from the yellow lines in **A**,**D**. (**C**,**F**) Magnified image of the area in the white square, showing the two color channels split. Scale bars represent 5 μm.

Accumulation driven by $\Delta\Psi_m$ is usually related to positively charged lipophilic moieties, such as TPP [13]. Interestingly, dyes **1** and **4** are noncharged and neutral, yet they accumulated in the mitochondria. To evaluate whether $\Delta\Psi_m$ is involved in the accumulation of the dyes in this organelle, we performed colocalization experiments of compound **1** and MT in the presence of BAM-15, a chemical known to disrupt $\Delta\Psi_m$ but not affect the plasma membrane potential and thus prevent drastic consequences on cell viability [55]. After treatment with BAM-15, the mitochondria-tracking dye MT was expelled out of the mitochondria and accumulated in cytoplasmic vacuoles. Interestingly, a similar response was observed with the thiophene-labeled dye **1**, which in part appeared colocalized in the vacuoles with MT but also appeared more homogeneously throughout the cytoplasm (Figure S30). These experiments revealed that $\Delta\Psi_m$ is directly involved in the accumulation of the thiophene-containing dyes in mitochondria. The mitochondrial targeting behavior was similar to that of the MT probe but based on a different carrying mechanism, as MT is a positively charged dye.

2.3. Thio-DCA, a PDHK Inhibitor with Enhanced Effectiveness

Having demonstrated the potential of the thiophene ring to enhance mitochondrial delivery of small organic molecules, we focused our attention on designing an effective mitochondrial chimeric drug, including an active agent and a specific subcellular delivery moiety [56]. The rational design of multifunctional imaging and therapeutic agents using a modular approach is an active field in current theranostics and drug discovery programs [57,58]. As previously described in the introduction, cancer cells rely extensively on the glycolytic pathway to obtain large amounts of metabolic intermediates, which are required as building blocks to sustain their high proliferative rate. In this metabolic reprogramming process, pyruvate is reduced at the end of glycolysis to lactate, and a minor proportion is transported into the mitochondria to be transformed to acetyl-CoA by PDH. This metabolic pathway has been recently targeted in drug screening strategies, with the hypothesis that molecules that could change the preferential metabolism of pyruvate by forcing its entry into mitochondrial metabolism may convey specific toxicity to cancer cells. For this work, we chose DCA as a known PDHK inhibitor capable of reactivating the PDH complex and, presumably, of switching cancer metabolism to foster mitochondria-regulated apoptosis. The main effects of DCA are a decrease in HIF-1α and Bcl-2 in neoplastic cells, followed by an increase in the expression of p-53 upregulated modulator of apoptosis, p-53 and caspases. As a consequence, negative modulation of the transcription of glucose transporter (GLUT) receptors occurs, attenuating the uptake of glucose in tumor cells [59]. Another effect of DCA on tumor cells is the increase in the generation of ROS, allowing the entry of the NADH generated in the Krebs cycle into complex I of the respiratory chain, reactivating PDH and favoring the remodeling of mitochondrial metabolism. This cascade facilitates the opening of the mitochondrial transition pore, which allows the release of proapoptotic mediators, such as cytochrome c and apoptosis-inducing factor, into the cytoplasmic space [60].

Therefore, to enhance the effect of DCA, we synthesized thiophene-modified DCA, Thio-DCA, as depicted in Scheme 3. Further details on the synthesis and characterization can be found in the experimental section and the SM.

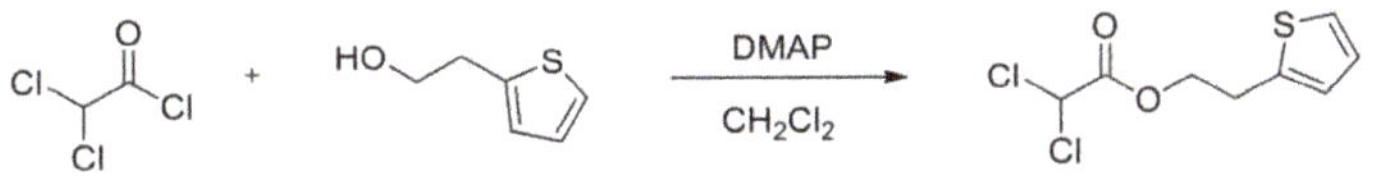

Scheme 3. Synthesis of Thio-DCA.

Regarding the cell lines employed in this work, we focused on breast cancer cells, since there exist different lines conventionally classified according to histological type, tumor grade, lymph node status and immune profile [45]: luminal A (cell line MCF7), luminal B (cell line ZR751), basal (cell line MDA-MB-468), claudin-low (cell line MDA-MB-231), and HER2+ (cell line SKBR3). MDA-MB-468 and MDA-MB-231 are commonly referred to as triple-negative breast cancer lines because of their negative expression of the estrogen receptor (ER), progesterone receptor (PR) and human epidermal growth factor receptor (HER2), presenting high invasiveness and poor prognostic outcome. In contrast, MCF7 and ZR751 are cell lines with a noninvasive low proliferation profile that results in good prognostic clinical outcomes. Finally, SKBR3 is a cell line that is HER2+ but negative for ER and PR. According to its response to treatment, SKBR3 cells show a response to the anti-HER2 therapy trastuzumab and a moderate response to chemotherapy. Therefore, it is relevant to work with all these cell lines due to their different cellular and molecular features and responses to chemotherapies and treatments [45]. Moreover, our recent results showed differences between these cell lines regarding intramitochondrial pH [15], resistance to transaminase inhibition, dependence on NAD+ availability, and sensitivity to alterations in glutamine metabolism [61].

In the first series of experiments, the impact of DCA-induced inhibition of PDHK on cell viability was measured in the aforementioned cell lines. For this purpose, cells were seeded with or without the addition of 10 mM DCA, and after 96 h incubation at 37 °C, cell viability was measured using the well-validated CellTiter Blue assay (see the Experimental section). These experiments permitted us to identify that the MCF7, SKBR3, MDA-MB-231 and MDA-MB-468 cell lines were quite resistant to DCA treatment, displaying cell viability values between 75–90%. Only the ZR751 cell line, with a decrease in cell viability up to

40%, was sensitive to DCA treatment [61]. Given that we wanted to directly compare the enhanced effect of Thio-DCA to the corresponding native DCA we decided not to use the sensitive cell line ZR751 in further experiments and thus only focused on the cell viability of DCA-resistant breast cancer lines upon incubation with Thio-DCA.

Our experiments demonstrated that Thio-DCA presented enhanced, dosage-dependent antitumor activity compared to that presented by DCA for all four studied breast cancer cell lines (Figure 2). The IC_{50} values for Thio-DCA in the four cell lines were 5.9 ± 0.6, 7.8 ± 0.2, 4.0 ± 0.3, and 9.4 ± 0.1 mM for SKBR3, MDA-MB-231, MDA-MB-468, and MCF7, respectively. Thio-DCA at 10 mM exhibited between 4.3- and 9.6-fold increases in antiproliferation activity in the different breast cancer cell lines (Figure 2B) compared to DCA at the same concentration. The lowest value, a 4.3-fold increase, corresponded to MDA-MB-468 cells, mainly because 10 mM DCA caused a mild reduction in cell viability, down to $78 \pm 6\%$ viability. This makes the relative effect of Thio-DCA lower than that of DCA, but Thio-DCA at 10 mM in MDA-MB-468 cells presented the largest reduction in viability, down to $5 \pm 1\%$, among all the tested treatments. For the other three cell lines, 10 mM DCA did not cause any significant reduction in cell viability, confirming the resistance of these cell lines to DCA treatment. Hence, the relative enhancement of the effect of 10 mM Thio-DCA was as large as 8.4–9.6-fold (Figure 2B). Lower concentrations of Thio-DCA still exhibited inhibition. For all cell lines, except MCF7, a Thio-DCA concentration of 5 mM resulted in a significant reduction in cell viability. The largest effect of Thio-DCA was found for the basal line MDA-MB-468. This cell line is characterized by a strong dependence on mitochondrial metabolism [61], and hence, our result is consistent with a larger effect of Thio-DCA due to enhanced mitochondrial delivery of the drug. In contrast, MCF7 cells exhibit glycolysis-dependent metabolism [61], and in turn, the effect of Thio-DCA less notable. The toxic effect of Thio-DCA on MDA-MB-468 cells supports other experimental observations currently in progress by our team that explain the toxicity of DCA treatments in cancer cells, which display a stronger dependency on mitochondrial metabolism. According to our ongoing observations, DCA causes a metabolic collapse of mitochondrial activity due to anaplerotic limitations in response to the DCA-driven activation of the tricarboxylic acid cycle.

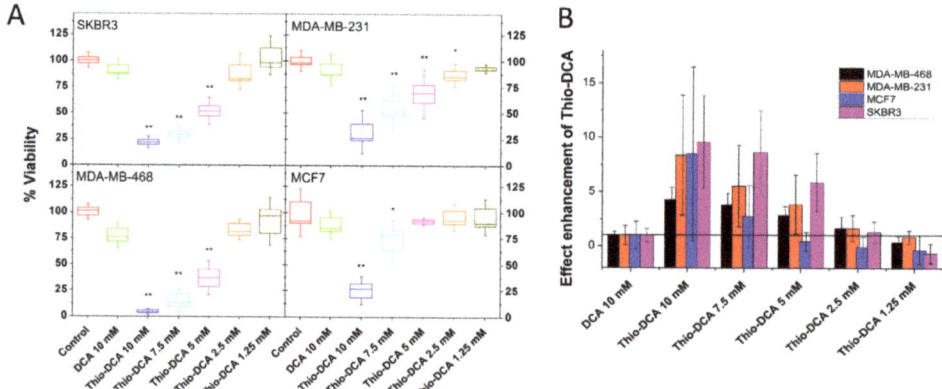

Figure 2. (**A**) Cell viability of SKBR3, MDA-MB-231, MDA-MB-468, and MCF7 breast cancer tumor cells treated with DCA and Thio-DCA at different doses. Squares indicate mean values, box size indicates the standard error of the mean, and whiskers represent the standard deviations. The marked populations were significantly different from the control with 99% (**) or 95% (*) confidence, as indicated by the Holm-Bonferroni and Holm-Sidak tests and the nonparametric Kolmogorov-Smirnov and Mann-Whitney tests. (**B**) Relative enhancement of the reduction in cell viability of Thio-DCA at different doses compared to that of 10 mM DCA.

The thiophene moiety is known to cause cellular toxicity when used at a high dosage due to oxidation by cytochrome P450 [38,39]. This toxicity may, however, be reduced by cellular oxidative stress response by glutathione [38,62]. Hence, we tested the potential toxicity associated with the thiophene moiety using 2-(3-thienyl)ethanol as the model precursor. 2-(3-thienyl)ethanol caused negligible effects on cell viability at concentrations lower than 5 mM. Reaching larger concentrations led to an IC_{50} value of 15 ± 1 mM (Figure S31). Therefore, although the thiophene moiety caused a reduction of cell viability at 10 mM, the effect was not as large as that exhibited by Thio–DCA.

3. Discussion

In seeking new, noncharged organelle-targeting carriers, we found that neutral acridone dyes underwent mitochondrial accumulation when modified with a thiophene ring [40]. Neutral organelle carriers are vastly desired from a synthetic point of view regarding their effect on intraorganelle ionic strength and membrane potentials. Logically, the subsequent step was to test the general applicability of this concept, as we did herein, synthesizing thiophene-containing dyes of different families, charged (xanthenes) and noncharged (acridone and BODIPY), and confirming the enhanced mitochondrial accumulation. We demonstrated the feasibility of the thiophene moiety as a noncharged, nonbasic carrier for targeting mitochondria. All fluorescent derivatives synthesized herein that contained a thiophene group showed good accumulation in mitochondria, although not completely specific in part due to the additional properties that the different fluorescent moieties impart to the molecule as a whole. In previous works, fluorescent dyes containing thiophene groups were reported to be delivered to the mitochondria [63–65], although accumulation in this organelle was justified by hydrophobicity and/or the presence of positive charges in ammonium side groups. For instance, TPP-modified polythiophenes, a construct in which polythiophene is the actual fluorophore, were shown to accumulate in mitochondria [66], although the driving force for mitochondrial delivery was assumed to be the TPP moiety. In contrast, we were able to define the different subcellular localization of dye 1 with respect to thiophene-less acridone [40], demonstrating and confirming herein the enhancement of mitochondrial delivery by the thiophene ring. An underlying active mechanism of mitochondrial accumulation driven by the thiophene ring is supported by the fact that well-known subcellular localization QSAR algorithms [42] cannot predict such organelle targeting for dye 1. A recent algorithm based on machine learning trained with sets of literature data identified key structural motifs for subcellular localization among lysosomes, mitochondria, nucleus and plasma membrane [67]. This algorithm is included in the prediction tool admetSAR 2.0 [68]. The molecules in our work do not hold specific key motifs for mitochondrial localization. In contrast, the thiophene ring was identified by the authors to be a key motif for plasma membrane localization [67]. Interestingly, admetSAR 2.0 successfully predicted that all the molecules in our work would more likely localize in the mitochondria than in lysosomes, nuclei, or the plasma membrane. However, the algorithm also predicted mitochondrial localization for N-(3-hydroxypropyl)-4-methoxyacridone, a compound that localizes in the cell nucleus [40]. Therefore, there is still room for improvement in machine-learning algorithms and QSAR models.

The most promising application, however, was the proof-of-concept of a chimeric drug with enhanced activity, promoted by thiophene-driven mitochondrial accumulation. Thio-DCA exhibited improved toxicity in breast cancer cell lines resistant to the thiophene-lacking counterpart DCA. This larger effect suggests that the inhibitor targets the locations on mitochondrial compartments where metabolic reactions occur. The concept of enhancing the activity of DCA with a mitochondrial carrier was previously reported by Pathak and colleagues, who prepared a chimera of positively charged TPP with three molecules of DCA, so-called Mito-DCA [24]. This molecule exhibited a much more potent effect than DCA alone in tumor cells, even at lower dosages than that reported by us with Thio-DCA. Nevertheless, Mito-DCA contains three DCA moieties per molecule and an overall positive charge that enhances mitochondrial depolarization [24]. In other examples, the anticancer power of haloacetates has been enhanced by incorporating DCA and other derivatives in phospholipid nanoparticles [69]. Increasing the local concentration of the inhibitor through the nanoparticle ensured efficient delivery. Although the doses used for Thio-DCA treatment are still high, they are lower than those employed in recent reports on the use of DCA, usually reaching up to 50 mM [44,70,71], and are similar to DCA concentrations used in sensitive cell lines [72]. The most important observation of our work is, however, that mitochondrial accumulation, promoted by a neutral carrier, enhanced the effect of the drug in several DCA-resistant cell lines. With this proof-of-concept, there is still plenty of room to improve drug efficacy by incorporating it in delivery nanoparticles [69] or supramolecular caging agents [73] and improving drug selectivity by reducing thiophene-associated toxicity by adding substitution radicals to the thiophene ring [38].

It is also informative to consider previous reports on anticancer drug design that involve thiophene cores. These drugs exhibited higher activity than previous inhibitors [74]. Likewise, thiophene-containing natural products, such as the bithiophenes arctinal and arctinol-b, have been shown to have antifungal and antimicrobial activity [75], as well as other cytotoxic effects on tumor cell lines [76]. Thiophene-modified coumarins also exhibit enhanced cytotoxicity towards cancer cell lines, whereas normal fibroblast cells are less affected [77]. In a recent report, Lisboa et al. described a chimeric drug of acridine andmodified thiophene with promising antitumoral activity [78]. We hypothesize that, in some cases, the primary cause of this activity may be inhibitor accumulation in the mitochondria, which is influenced by the thiophene core and enhances the inhibition mechanism by directly targeting where the metabolic reaction occurs.

Our current research lines aim to determine whether different subtypes of breast cancer cells display differential metabolic phenotypes [15,61]. Gaining knowledge about key metabolic features in breast cancer and their functional, molecular and genetic inter-relationships could pave the way for a novel clinical classification, revealing potential therapeutic antimetabolic targets, and diagnostic approaches. The thiophene moiety as a noncharged neutral carrier for targeting mitochondria may represent a considerable advantage to overcome synthetic problems, paving the way to the rational design of new metabolism-targeted anticancer hybrid drugs [78,79]. The full potential of such drugs will be accomplished by incorporating additional substituents to the thiophene ring, aiming for improved selectivity in localization, activity and toxicity.

4. Materials and Methods

4.1. Synthesis Reactions of New Compounds

4.1.1. General Details

All reagents and solvents (CH_2Cl_2, ethyl acetate (EtOAc), hexane, CH_3CN, and methanol (MeOH)) were purchased from standard chemical suppliers and used without further purification. To ensure the dryness of tetrahydrofuran (THF), it was freshly distilled over Na/benzophenone. Anhydrous solvents (dimethylformamide (DMF), CH_2Cl_2 and diethyl ether (Et_2O)) were purchased from standard suppliers. Thin-layer chromatography (TLC) was performed on aluminum-backed plates coated with silica gel 60 (230–240 mesh) with the F_{254} indicator. The spots were visualized with UV light (254 nm and 360 nm) and/or stained with phosphomolybdic acid (10% ethanol solution) and subsequent heating. All chromatographic purifications were performed with silica gel 60 (230–400 mesh). NMR spectra were measured at room temperature. ^1H NMR spectra were recorded at 300, 400, or 500 MHz either in a Varian Direct Drive (Varian Inc., Palo Alto, CA, USA) or Bruker Avance NEO (Bruker BioSpin GmbH, Rheinstetten, Germany). Chemical shifts are reported in ppm using the residual solvent peak as a reference ($CHCl_3$: δ = 7.26 ppm, CH_3OH: δ = 3.31 ppm, and $(CH_3)_2SO$: δ = 2.50 ppm). Data are reported as follows: chemical shift, multiplicity (s: singlet, d: doublet, t: triplet, q: quartet, quint: quintuplet, m: multiplet, dd: doublet of doublets, dt: doublet of triplets, td: triplet of doublets, and bs: broad singlet), coupling constant (*J* in Hz) and integration. ^{13}C NMR spectra were recorded at 75, 101, 126 or 151 MHz using broadband proton decoupling, and chemical shifts are reported in ppm using the residual solvent peaks as a reference (CHCl$_3$: δ = 77.16 ppm, CH$_3$OH: δ = 49.00 ppm, and (CH$_3$)$_2$SO: δ = 39.52 ppm). Carbon multiplicities were assigned by distortionless enhancement by polarization transfer (DEPT) techniques. High-resolution mass spectra (HRMS) were recorded by EI at 70 eV on a Micromass AutoSpec mass spectrometer (Waters Co., Milford, MA, USA) or by ESI on a Waters VG AutoSpec mass spectrometer (Waters Co.). For the synthesis of the compounds described herein, several precursors were required to be prepared, including 2-[3-(4-bromo-3-methyl-phenoxy)propoxymethyl]thiophene (precursor **VII**, Scheme S4 in the SM) and 2,7-di-[*tert*-butyldimethylsilyloxy]-xanthone (precursor **VIII**, Schemes S4 and S5 in the SM). Compounds **1** (Schemes S1–S3) and **4** (Scheme S6) were prepared as previously described, isolated as pure samples and showed NMR spectra identical to reported data [40,51]. Further details on the synthesis and characterization of all the precursors and compounds **1–4**, including ^{1}H NMR and ^{13}C NMR spectra (Figures S1–S16), are compiled in the SM.

4.1.2. Synthesis of 6-hydroxy-9-(2-methyl-4-(3-(thiophen-2-ylmethoxy)propoxy)phenyl)-3H-xanthen-3-one (compound **2**, Scheme S4)

t-BuLi (1.7 M in hexane, 0.96 mL, 1.64 mmol) was added dropwise to a solution of compound **VII** (279 mg, 0.82 mmol) in freshly distilled THF (4 mL) under an Ar atmosphere at −78 °C. After keeping the reaction at that temperature for 20 min, a solution of compound **VIII** (187 mg, 0.41 mmol) in THF (2 mL) was slowly added. Then, the mixture was stirred at −78 °C for 15 min and allowed to reach room temperature. The reaction was monitored by TLC. After consumption of compound **VIII**, 10% HCl (1 mL) was added, promoting a color change from light yellow to orange. Finally, the solvent was removed, and the residue was purified by flash chromatography (SiO$_2$, CH$_2$Cl$_2$/MeOH 9:1) to yield compound **2** (130 mg, 66%) as an orange solid. ^{1}H NMR (400 MHz, MeOD) δ 7.36 (dd, *J* = 5.1, 1.2 Hz, 1H), 7.12 (d, *J* = 8.4 Hz, 1H), 7.08 (d, *J* = 9.7 Hz, 2H), 7.05–7.03 (m, 1H), 7.00 (d, *J* = 2.5 Hz, 1H), 6.9–6.94 (m, 2H), 6.68–6.64 (m, 4H), 4.72 (s, 2H), 4.17 (t, *J* = 6.2 Hz, 2H), 3.72 (t, *J* = 6.1 Hz, 2H), 2.09 (quint, *J* = 6.2 Hz, 2H), 2.02 (s, 3H). ^{13}C NMR (101 MHz, MeOD) δ 179.0 (C), 161.5 (C), 159.7 (C), 156.5 (C), 142.5 (C), 138.9 (C), 132.3 (CH), 131.5 (CH), 127.59 (CH) 127.58 (CH), 126.8 (CH), 126.0 (C), 123.4 (CH), 117.6 (CH), 115.5 (C), 113.3 (CH), 104.5 (CH), 68.3 (CH$_2$), 67.4 (CH$_2$), 66.0 (CH$_2$), 30.7 (CH$_2$), 20.0 (CH$_3$). HRMS (ESI): *m/z* [M+H]$^+$ calculated for C$_{28}$H$_{25}$O$_5$S: 473.1417 found: 473.1416.

4.1.3. Synthesis of 6-hydroxy-9-(thiophen-3-yl)-3H-xanthen-3-one (compound **3**, Scheme S5)

t-BuLi (1.7 M in hexane, 0.66 mL, 1.12 mmol) was added dropwise to a solution of 3-iodothiophene (118 mg, 0.56 mmol) in freshly distilled THF (2 mL) under an Ar atmosphere at −50 °C. After keeping the reaction at that temperature for 20 min, a solution of compound **VIII** (128 mg, 0.28 mmol) in THF (2 mL) was slowly added. Then, the mixture was stirred at −50 °C for 15 min and allowed to reach room temperature. The reaction progress was monitored by TLC. After consumption of compound **VIII**, 10% HCl (1 mL) was added, promoting a color change from light yellow to orange. Finally, the solvent was removed, and the residue was purified by flash chromatography (SiO$_2$, CH$_2$Cl$_2$/MeOH 8:2) to yield compound **3** (48 mg, 59%) as an orange solid. ^{1}H NMR (500 MHz, DMSO-*d*$_6$) δ 7.93–7.87 (m, 2H), 7.32 (dd, *J* = 4.7, 1.4 Hz, 1H), 7.22 (d, *J* = 9.3 Hz, 2H), 6.64 (bs, 4H). ^{13}C NMR (126 MHz, DMSO-*d*$_6$) δ 145.4 (C), 132.2 (C), 130.5 (CH), 129.3 (CH), 128.0 (CH), 127.7 (CH). Several carbons are not observed. HRMS (EI): *m/z* [M]$^+$ calculated for C$_{17}$H$_{10}$O$_3$S: 294.0351 found: 294.0339.

4.1.4. Synthesis of Thio-DCA

4-dimethylaminopyridine (DMAP, 429 mg, 3.51 mmol) was added to a solution of 2-thiopheneethanol (0.26 mL, 2.34 mmol) in CH$_2$Cl$_2$ (5 mL). After 5 min, dichloroacetyl chloride (0.27 mL, 2.81 mmol) was added dropwise. The mixture was stirred at room temperature and monitored by TLC until consumption of starting materials occurred (5–10 min). Celite was then added, and the solvent was removed. The crude material was purified by flash chromatography (SiO$_2$, hexane/EtOAc 9:1) to yield Thio-DCA (512 mg,

91%) as a light yellow liquid. ^{1}H NMR and ^{13}C NMR spectra are shown in the SM. ^{1}H NMR (400 MHz, CDCl$_3$) δ 7.19 (dd, J = 5.1, 1.2 Hz, 1H), 6.96 (dd, J = 5.1, 3.4 Hz, 1H), 6.90 (dd, J = 3.4, 1.2 Hz, 1H), 5.95 (s, 1H), 4.49 (t, J = 6.7 Hz, 2H), 3.25 (t, J = 6.7 Hz, 2H). ^{13}C NMR (75 MHz, CDCl$_3$) δ 164.5 (C), 138.7 (C), 127.2 (CH), 126.1 (CH), 124.5 (CH), 67.6 (CH$_2$), 64.3 (CH), 29.0 (CH$_2$). HRMS (ESI): m/z [M+Na]$^+$ calculated for C$_8$H$_8$O$_2$Cl$_2$SNa: 260.9514 found: 260.9513.

4.2. Instrumentation

Absorption spectra of the different dyes in aqueous solutions were obtained on a Lambda 650 UV–visible spectrophotometer (PerkinElmer, Waltham, MA, USA). The steady-state fluorescence emission and excitation spectra were collected using a Jasco FP-8300 spectrofluorometer (Jasco, Tokyo, Japan). Time-resolved fluorescence decay traces were obtained on a FluoTime 200 SPT spectrofluorometer (PicoQuant GmbH, Berlin, Germany). The concentration of dyes in spectroscopic measurements was between 0.5×10^{-6} and 5×10^{-6} M.

Colocalization studies using dual-color confocal microscopy were performed on a Fluoview FV1000 laser scanning microscope (Olympus, Tokyo, Japan). For imaging compound **2**, compound **3** or MT, the sample was excited with a 405 nm, 488 nm or 635 nm laser line, respectively. Emission from compounds **2** (between 410 and 490 nm) and **3** (between 500 and 580 nm) was collected using a grating, whereas emission from MT was collected with a BA655-755 bandpass filter. Dual-color FLIM experiments were performed on a MicroTime 200 microscope (PicoQuant GmbH, Berlin, Germany) equipped with 440 nm, 470 nm, and 635 nm pulsed diode lasers as excitation sources. Emission from fluorophores **1–4** was separated from that of MT using a 600DCXR dichroic mirror. Different bandpass filters were used for the collection of the fluorescence of **1** (465/30), **2–4** (520/35) and MT (685/70). Further experimental settings for each instrument can be found in the SM and Table S1. The concentration of dyes in the fluorescence imaging experiments was 3×10^{-7} M.

The effect of 2-(3-thienyl)ethanol, DCA or Thio-DCA compounds on cell viability was examined using the CellTiter Blue^{TM} viability assay (Promega Corp. Madison, WI, USA). Cells were plated in quadruplicate in black, cell culture-treated, 96-well, optical, flat-bottom plates at a density of 8×10^4 cells/well. The viability results of different treatments were compared to those of the control (cells in the presence of deuterated DMSO) at both 99% or 95% confidence using the Holm-Bonferroni and Holm-Sidak tests and the nonparametric Kolmogorov-Smirnov and Mann-Whitney tests in Origin 9.0 (OriginLab Corp., Northampton, MA, USA).

Further details about all the experimental methods, procedures and instrumentation can be found in the SM.

4.3. Cell Culture

For the imaging and viability experiments in this work the cell lines 143B (CRL-8303), HeLa (CCL-2), MCF7 (HTB-22), MDA-MB-231 (CRM-HTB-26), and SKBR3 (HTB-30) were acquired from the American Type Culture Collection (ATCC, Manassas, VA, USA), and the lines MDA-MB-468 (ACC 738) and ZR751 (ACC 8701601) were obtained from the Leibniz-Institut DMSZ, German collection of microorganisms and cell cultures GmbH (DMSZ, Braunschweig, Germany). Further details about culture protocols and procedures can be found in the SM.

Supplementary Materials: The following are available online at https://www.mdpi.com/1999-4923/13/2/254/s1: Scheme S1. Synthesis of compounds I and II from 1,3-propanediol.; Scheme S2. Bromination of 2-thiophenemethanol.; Scheme S3. Synthesis of compound 1 from 2-methoxyacridin-9(10H)-one.; Scheme S4. Synthetic route for the preparation of compound 2 starting from 4-bromo-3-methylphenol.; Scheme S5. Nucleophilic addition of 3-iodiothiophene to ketone VIII to obtain xanthene 3.; Scheme S6. Synthesis of BODIPY derivative 4.; Figure S1. 1H-NMR (500 MHz) spectrum of compound II in CDCl3.; Figure S2. 13C-NMR (126 MHz) spectrum of compound II in CDCl3.;

Figure S3. 1H-NMR (500 MHz) spectrum of compound 1 in MeOD.; Figure S4. 13C-NMR (126 MHz) spectrum of compound 1 in MeOD.; Figure S5. 1H-NMR (400 MHz) spectrum of compound V in CDCl3.; Figure S6. 13C-NMR (101 MHz) spectrum of compound V in CDCl3.; Figure S7. 1H-NMR (400 MHz) spectrum of compound VI in CDCl3.; Figure S8. 13C-NMR (101 MHz) spectrum of compound VI in CDCl3.; Figure S9. 1H-NMR (400 MHz) spectrum of compound VII in CDCl3.; Figure S10. 13C-NMR (101 MHz) spectrum of compound VII in CDCl3.; Figure S11. 1H-NMR (400 MHz) spectrum of compound 2 in MeOD.; Figure S12. 13C-NMR (101 MHz) spectrum of compound 2 in CDCl3.; Figure S13. 1H-NMR (500 MHz) spectrum of compound 3 in DMSO-d6.; Figure S14. 13C-NMR (126 MHz) spectrum of compound 3 in DMSO-d6.; Figure S15. 1H-NMR (400 MHz) spectrum of compound Thio-DCA in CDCl3.; Figure S16. 13C-NMR (75 MHz) spectrum of compound Thio-DCA in CDCl3.; Table S1. Dual-color FLIM instrumental settings for colocalization studies of each dye.; Figure S17. Absorption (**A**, **C**) and fluorescence emission (**B**, **D**) spectra of dyes 1 (**A**, **B**) and 4 (**C**, **D**) at different pH values. The excitation wavelength for the emission spectra was 375 nm for compound 1 and 495 nm for compound 4.; Figure S18. Absorption and fluorescence emission dependence with pH of dyes 2 (**A–C**) and 3 (**D–F**) in aqueous solution. **A** and **D**) Absorption spectra at different pH values of dyes 2 (**A**) and 3 (**D**). B and E) Global fittings of the A vs pH data to the general equilibrium equations [15,16] to obtain the ground state pKa values of dyes 2 (**B**) and 3 (**E**). (C and F) Fluorescence emission spectra (λex = 490 nm) of dyes 2 (**C**) and 3 (**F**) in aqueous solution at different pH values.; Figure S19. Average fluorescence lifetime, τ, of dye 3 in methanol:glycerine mixtures of different viscosity at 20, 30 and 40 °C.; Figure S20. Photostability of dyes 1–4 during 2 h of continuous irradiation.; Figure S21. Representative dual-color FLIM images of compound 1 in 143B cells and ρ0206 cells after 20 min of incubation with MT. Panels (**A**) and (**B**) show FLIM images on a pseudo-color scale (between 0 and 17 ns) of the dye's detection channel (left) and the MT detection channel (right). These examples were performed on human osteosarcoma 143B cells (**A**) and ρ0206 cells (**B**). The latter are tumor cells depleted of mitochondrial DNA, thus displaying an extreme metabolic phe-notype due to the absence of respiration [10]. Panels (**C**) and (**D**) show the colocalization images of 1 (green) and MT (red) in 143B cells (**C**) and ρ0206 cells (**D**). Scale bars represent 10 µm. Panels (**E**) and (**F**) show intensity traces in both channels for the depicted lines in images in panels C (for 143B cells) and D (for ρ0206 cells), respectively.; Figure S22. Representative dual-color, super-resolution optical fluctuation imaging (SOFI) of 1 (green channel) and MT (red channel) in formaldehyde-fixed HeLa cells, and intensity plots of the profile lines. Scale bars represent 5 µm.; Figure S23. Mitochondrial localization of compound 1 in 143B cells, after 20 min of incubation with MT, from dual-color FLIM images. Left panels represent the raw intensity images in the 1 channel and the MT channel. Central panels represent the selected region of interest, in cyan for compound 1 and red for MT. Rightmost panels are the overlaid images, with colocalized pixels represented in white color. Scale bars represent 10 µm.; Figure S24. FLIM imaging of compound 1 in 143B cells. The images show the fluorescence lifetime of 1 depicted on a pseudocolor scale between 13 and 16 ns. The leftmost column of images shows colocalized pixels with mitochondria. The central column of images shows non colocalized pixels. The rightmost column of images shows the overall images. Scale bars represent 10 µm. The plots on the right panels represent the pixel distribution of fluorescence lifetime of 1 in each image, localized in mitochondria (black lines) or in other cellular subcompartments (red lines), and the overall lifetime distribution (green lines). Given that the acridone core has a lifetime that depends on the polarity of the microenvironment [18], these data clearly show that the mitochondria matrix is a less polar environment than cellular cytoplasm.; Figure S25. Representative dual-color FLIM images of compound 2 in 143B (**A**, **C**, and **E**) and ρ0206 cells (**B**, **D**, and **F**), after 20 min of incubation with MT. In the FLIM images (**A** and **B**), the dye's detection channel (left) and the MT detection channel (right) are shown separately. The colocalization images (**C** and **D**) of the dye (green) and MT (red) are also shown. Intensity traces in both channels (**E** and **F**) are shown for the depicted lines (marked as 1, 2 and 3) in the colocalization panels. Scale bars represent 10 µm.; Figure S26. Mitochondrial localization of compound 2 in ρ0206 cells, after 20 min of incubation with MT, from dual-color FLIM images. Left panels represent the raw intensity images in the 2 channel and the MT channel. Central panels represent the selected region of interest, in cyan for compound 2 and red for MT. Rightmost panels are the overlaid images, with colocalized pixels represented in white color. Scale bars represent 10 µm.; Figure S27. Mitochondrial localization of compound 3 in MDA-MB-231 cells, after 20 min of incubation with MT, from dual-color FLIM images. Left panels represent the raw intensity images in the 3 channel and the MT channel. Central panels represent the selected region of interest, in cyan for compound 3 and red for MT. Rightmost panels are the overlaid images, with colocalized pixels represented in white color. Scale bars represent 10 μm.; Figure S28. FLIM imaging of compound 3 in MDA-MB-231 cells. The images show the fluorescence lifetime of 3 depicted on a pseudocolor scale between 3 and 6 ns. The leftmost column of images shows colocalized pixels with mitochondria. The central column of images shows non colocalized pixels. The rightmost column of images shows the overall images. Scale bars represent 10 μm. The plots on the right panels represent the pixel distribution of fluorescence lifetime of 3 in each image, localized in mitochondria (black lines) or in other cellular subcompartments (red lines), and the overall lifetime distribution (green lines).; Figure S29. Representative dual-color FLIM images of compound 4 in 143B (**A**, **C**, and **E**) and ρ0206 cells (**B**, **D**, and **F**), after 20 min of incubation with MT. In the FLIM images (**A** and **B**), the dye's detection channel (left) and the MT detection channel (right) are shown separately. The colocali-zation images (**C** and **D**) of the dye (green) and MT (red) are also shown. Intensity traces in both channels (**E** and **F**) are shown for the depicted lines in the colocalization panels. Scale bars represent 10 μm.; Table S2. Pearson's correlation coefficient (PCC) and Manders' colocalization coefficient (MCC) values for the colocalization of dyes 1–4 with the mitochondria tracker MT.[a].; Figure S30. Representative dual-color fluorescence images of compound 1 (green) and the MT tracker (magenta) in 143B cells after 20 min of incubation with BAM15. Scatter plots represent the corre-lation of the intensity values in the green channel vs the red channel. Scale bars represent 10 μm.; Figure S31. Cell viability of SKBR3 breast cancer tumor cells treated with 2-(3-thienyl)ethanol at different doses. Error bars represent standard deviations. Line represents the fit to a dose-response function.

Author Contributions: Conceptualization, M.J.R.-R., M.M., J.M.C. and A.O.; formal analysis, C.R., P.H.-F., V.P.-M., M.C.G.-G., J.M.P., E.G.-F. and A.O.; funding acquisition, M.J.R.-R., J.M.C. and A.O.; investigation, C.R., P.H.-F., V.P.-M., M.C.G.-G., D.M., S.R., E.G.-F. and A.O.; methodology, C.R., D.M., J.M.P., M.J.R.-R., M.M., M.R., S.R., H.De K., J.H., J.M.C. and A.O.; project administration, A.O.; resources, P.H.-F, D.M., S.R., M.R., S.R., H.De K., J.H. and J.M.C.; Supervision, D.M., J.M.P., M.J.R.-R., E.G.-F., M.M., M.R., S.R., H.De K., J.H., J.M.C. and A.O.; visualization, D.M., J.M.P., E.G.-F., S.R. and H.De K.; writing–original draft, C.R. and A.O.; writing–review & editing, C.R., P.H.-F., V.P.-M., M.C.G.-G., D.M., S.R., J.M.P., M.J.R.-R., E.G.-F., M.M., S.R., J.H. and J.M.C. All authors have read and agreed to the published version of the manuscript.

Funding: This research: including APC charges, was funded by the Spanish Agencia Estatal de Investigación (Ministry of Science and Innovation) and the European Regional Development Fund [grant numbers CTQ2014-56370-R, CTQ2014-53598, and CTQ2017-85658-R]; Fundación Ramón Areces; and the initiative Solidaridad Entre Montañas. J.H. acknowledges financial support from the Flemish government through long-term structural funding Methusalem (CASAS2, Meth/15/04).

Data Availability Statement: The data presented in this study are openly available in University of Granada repository, Digibug at http://hdl.handle.net/10481/66449, reference number 10481/66449.

Conflicts of Interest: The authors declare no conflict of interest.

References

1. Scheffler, I.E. Chapter 6: Metabolic Pathways inside Mitochondria. In *Mitochondria*, 2nd ed.; John Wiley & Sons: Hoboken, NJ, USA, 2007.
2. Trotta, A.P.; Chipuk, J.E. Mitochondrial dynamics as regulators of cancer biology. *Cell. Mol. Life Sci.* **2017**, *74*, 1999–2017. [CrossRef]
3. Vyas, S.; Zaganjor, E.; Haigis, M.C. Mitochondria and Cancer. *Cell* **2016**, *166*, 555–566. [CrossRef] [PubMed]
4. Lunt, S.Y.; Heiden, M.G.V. Aerobic Glycolysis: Meeting the Metabolic Requirements of Cell Proliferation. *Ann. Rev. Cell Dev. Biol.* **2011**, *27*, 441–464. [CrossRef] [PubMed]
5. Guerra, F.; Arbini, A.A.; Moro, L. Mitochondria and cancer chemoresistance. *Biochim. Biophys. Acta* **2017**, *1858*, 686–699. [CrossRef] [PubMed]
6. Chen, H.; Chan, D.C. Mitochondrial Dynamics in Regulating the Unique Phenotypes of Cancer and Stem Cells. *Cell Metab.* **2017**, *26*, 39–48. [CrossRef]
7. DeBerardinis, R.J.; Chandel, N.S. Fundamentals of cancer metabolism. *Sci. Adv.* **2016**, *2*, e1600200. [CrossRef]
8. Kalyanaraman, B.; Cheng, G.; Hardy, M.; Ouari, O.; Lopez, M.; Joseph, J.; Zielonka, J.; Dwinell, M.B. A review of the basics of mitochondrial bioenergetics, metabolism, and related signaling pathways in cancer cells: Therapeutic targeting of tumor mitochondria with lipophilic cationic compounds. *Redox Biol.* **2018**, *14*, 316–327. [CrossRef]
9. D'Souza, G.G.M.; Wagle, M.A.; Saxena, V.; Shah, A. Approaches for targeting mitochondria in cancer therapy. *Biochim. Biophys. Acta* **2011**, *1807*, 689–696. [CrossRef]

10. Long, L.; Huang, M.; Wang, N.; Wu, Y.; Wang, K.; Gong, A.; Zhang, Z.; Sessler, J.L. A Mitochondria-Specific Fluorescent Probe for Visualizing Endogenous Hydrogen Cyanide Fluctuations in Neurons. *J. Am. Chem. Soc.* **2018**, *140*, 1870–1875. [CrossRef]
11. Ren, M.; Deng, B.; Zhou, K.; Kong, X.; Wang, J.-Y.; Lin, W. Single Fluorescent Probe for Dual-Imaging Viscosity and H_2O_2 in Mitochondria with Different Fluorescence Signals in Living Cells. *Anal. Chem.* **2017**, *89*, 552–555. [CrossRef]
12. Zhang, X.; Gao, F. Imaging mitochondrial reactive oxygen species with fluorescent probes: Current applications and challenges. *Free Radical Res.* **2015**, *49*, 374–382. [CrossRef]
13. Kumar, N.; Bhalla, V.; Kumar, M. Development and sensing applications of fluorescent motifs within the mitochondrial environment. *Chem. Commun.* **2015**, *51*, 15614–15628. [CrossRef] [PubMed]
14. Xu, W.; Zeng, Z.; Jiang, J.-H.; Chang, Y.-T.; Yuan, L. Discerning the Chemistry in Individual Organelles with Small-Molecule Fluorescent Probes. *Angew. Chem. Int. Ed.* **2016**, *55*, 13658–13699. [CrossRef] [PubMed]
15. Ripoll, C.; Roldan, M.; Contreras-Montoya, R.; Diaz-Mochon, J.J.; Martin, M.; Ruedas-Rama, M.J.; Orte, A. Mitochondrial pH Nanosensors for Metabolic Profiling of Breast Cancer Cell Lines. *Int. J. Mol. Sci.* **2020**, *21*, 3731. [CrossRef] [PubMed]
16. Sánchez, M.I.; Vida, Y.; Pérez-Inestrosa, E.; Mascareñas, J.L.; Vázquez, M.E.; Sugiura, A.; Martínez-Costas, J. MitoBlue as a tool to analyze the mitochondria-lysosome communication. *Sci. Rep.* **2020**, *10*, 3528. [CrossRef]
17. Reshetnikov, V.; Özkan, H.G.; Daum, S.; Janko, C.; Alexiou, C.; Sauer, C.; Heinrich, M.R.; Mokhir, A. N-Alkylaminoferrocene-Based Prodrugs Targeting Mitochondria of Cancer Cells. *Molecules* **2020**, *25*, 2545. [CrossRef]
18. Ong, H.C.; Hu, Z.; Coimbra, J.T.S.; Ramos, M.J.; Kon, O.L.; Xing, B.; Yeow, E.K.L.; Fernandes, P.A.; García, F. Enabling Mitochondrial Uptake of Lipophilic Dications Using Methylated Triphenylphosphonium Moieties. *Inorg. Chem.* **2019**, *58*, 8293–8299. [CrossRef]
19. Jana, B.; Thomas, A.P.; Kim, S.; Lee, I.S.; Choi, H.; Jin, S.; Park, S.A.; Min, S.K.; Kim, C.; Ryu, J.-H. Self-Assembly of Mitochondria-Targeted Photosensitizer to Increase Photostability and Photodynamic Therapeutic Efficacy in Hypoxia. *Chem. A Eur. J.* **2020**, *26*, 10695–10701. [CrossRef] [PubMed]
20. Murphy, M.P. Selective targeting of bioactive compounds to mitochondria. *Trends Biotechnol.* **1997**, *15*, 326–330. [CrossRef]
21. Lei, E.K.; Kelley, S.O. Delivery and Release of Small-Molecule Probes in Mitochondria Using Traceless Linkers. *J. Am. Chem. Soc.* **2017**, *139*, 9455–9458. [CrossRef]
22. Trapella, C.; Voltan, R.; Melloni, E.; Tisato, V.; Celeghini, C.; Bianco, S.; Fantinati, A.; Salvadori, S.; Guerrini, R.; Secchiero, P.; et al. Design, Synthesis, and Biological Characterization of Novel Mitochondria Targeted Dichloroacetate-Loaded Compounds with Antileukemic Activity. *J. Med. Chem.* **2016**, *59*, 147–156. [CrossRef]
23. Ripcke, J.; Zarse, K.; Ristow, M.; Birringer, M. Small-Molecule Targeting of the Mitochondrial Compartment with an Endogenously Cleaved Reversible Tag. *Chembiochem* **2009**, *10*, 1689–1696. [CrossRef]
24. Pathak, R.K.; Marrache, S.; Harn, D.A.; Dhar, S. Mito-DCA: A Mitochondria Targeted Molecular Scaffold for Efficacious Delivery of Metabolic Modulator Dichloroacetate. *ACS Chem. Biol.* **2014**, *9*, 1178–1187. [CrossRef] [PubMed]
25. Zielonka, J.; Joseph, J.; Sikora, A.; Hardy, M.; Ouari, O.; Vasquez-Vivar, J.; Cheng, G.; Lopez, M.; Kalyanaraman, B. Mitochondria-Targeted Triphenylphosphonium-Based Compounds: Syntheses, Mechanisms of Action, and Therapeutic and Diagnostic Applications. *Chem. Rev.* **2017**, *117*, 10043–10120. [CrossRef] [PubMed]
26. Hu, Z.; Sim, Y.; Kon, O.L.; Ng, W.H.; Ribeiro, A.J.M.; Ramos, M.J.; Fernandes, P.A.; Ganguly, R.; Xing, B.; García, F.; et al. Unique Triphenylphosphonium Derivatives for Enhanced Mitochondrial Uptake and Photodynamic Therapy. *Bioconjug. Chem.* **2017**, *28*, 590–599. [CrossRef] [PubMed]
27. Rhee, W.J.; Bao, G. Slow non-specific accumulation of 2′-deoxy and 2′-O-methyl oligonucleotide probes at mitochondria in live cells. *Nucleic Acids Res.* **2010**, *38*, e109. [CrossRef]
28. Perry, S.W.; Norman, J.P.; Barbieri, J.; Brown, E.B.; Gelbard, H.A. Mitochondrial membrane potential probes and the proton gradient: A practical usage guide. *BioTechniques* **2011**, *50*, 98–115. [CrossRef]
29. Jiang, Z.; Liu, H.; He, H.; Yadava, N.; Chambers, J.J.; Thayumanavan, S. Anionic Polymers Promote Mitochondrial Targeting of Delocalized Lipophilic Cations. *Bioconjug. Chem.* **2020**, *31*, 1344–1353. [CrossRef]
30. Gao, P.; Pan, W.; Li, N.; Tang, B. Fluorescent probes for organelle-targeted bioactive species imaging. *Chem. Sci.* **2019**, *10*, 6035–6071. [CrossRef]
31. Buckman, J.F.; Hernández, H.; Kress, G.J.; Votyakova, T.V.; Pal, S.; Reynolds, I.J. MitoTracker labeling in primary neuronal and astrocytic cultures: Influence of mitochondrial membrane potential and oxidants. *J. Neurosci. Meth.* **2001**, *104*, 165–176. [CrossRef]
32. Xu, Z.; Xu, L. Fluorescent probes for the selective detection of chemical species inside mitochondria. *Chem. Commun.* **2016**, *52*, 1094–1119. [CrossRef]
33. Murphy, M.P. How mitochondria produce reactive oxygen species. *Biochem. J.* **2009**, *417*, 1–13. [CrossRef]
34. Abelha, T.F.; Morris, G.; Lima, S.M.; Andrade, L.H.C.; McLean, A.J.; Alexander, C.; Calvo-Castro, J.; McHugh, C.J. Development of a Neutral Diketopyrrolopyrrole Phosphine Oxide for the Selective Bioimaging of Mitochondria at the Nanomolar Level. *Chem. A Eur. J.* **2020**, *26*, 3173–3180. [CrossRef]
35. Limnios, D.; Kokotos, C.G. 2,2,2-Trifluoroacetophenone as an Organocatalyst for the Oxidation of Tertiary Amines and Azines to N-Oxides. *Chem. A Eur. J.* **2014**, *20*, 559–563. [CrossRef]
36. Copéret, C.; Adolfsson, H.; Khuong, T.-A.V.; Yudin, A.K.; Sharpless, K.B. A Simple and Efficient Method for the Preparation of Pyridine N-Oxides. *J. Org. Chem.* **1998**, *63*, 1740–1741. [CrossRef]

37. Pouzet, P.; Erdelmeier, I.; Ginderow, D.; Mornon, J.-P.; Dansette, P.; Mansuy, D. Thiophene S-oxides: Convenient preparation, first complete structural characterization and unexpected dimerization of one of them, 2,5-diphenylthiophene-1-oxide. *J. Chem. Soc. Chem. Commun.* **1995**, 473–474. [CrossRef]
38. Gramec, D.; Mašič, L.P.; Dolenc, M.S. Bioactivation Potential of Thiophene-Containing Drugs. *Chem. Res. Toxicol.* **2014**, *27*, 1344–1358. [CrossRef]
39. Dansette, P.M.; Thang, D.C.; Mansuy, H.E.A.D. Evidence for thiophene-s-oxide as a primary reactive metabolite of thiophene in vivo: Formation of a dihydrothiophene sulfoxide mercapturic acid. *Biochem. Biophys. Res. Comm.* **1992**, *186*, 1624–1630. [CrossRef]
40. Herrero-Foncubierta, P.; González-García, M.D.C.; Resa, S.; Paredes, J.M.; Ripoll, C.; Girón, M.D.; Salto, R.; Cuerva, J.M.; Orte, A.; Miguel, D. Simple and non-charged long-lived fluorescent intracellular organelle trackers. *Dye. Pigment.* **2020**, *183*, 108649. [CrossRef]
41. Thimmaiah, K.; Ugarkar, A.G.; Martis, E.F.; Shaikh, M.S.; Coutinho, E.C.; Yergeri, M.C. Drug–DNA Interaction Studies of Acridone-Based Derivatives. *Nucleosides Nucleotides Nucleic Acids* **2015**, *34*, 309–331. [CrossRef] [PubMed]
42. Horobin, R.W. Predicting Mitochondrial Targeting by Small Molecule Xenobiotics Within Living Cells Using QSAR Models. In *Mitochondrial Medicine: Volume II, Manipulating Mitochondrial Function*; Weissig, V., Edeas, M., Eds.; Springer: New York, NY, USA, 2015; pp. 13–23.
43. Sullivan, L.B.; Gui, D.Y.; Heiden, M.G.V. Altered metabolite levels in cancer: Implications for tumour biology and cancer therapy. *Nat. Rev. Cancer* **2016**, *16*, 680. [CrossRef]
44. Kankotia, S.; Stacpoole, P.W. Dichloroacetate and cancer: New home for an orphan drug? *Biochim. Biophys. Acta Rev. Cancer* **2014**, *1846*, 617–629. [CrossRef]
45. Holliday, D.L.; Speirs, V. Choosing the right cell line for breast cancer research. *Breast Cancer Res.* **2011**, *13*, 215. [CrossRef] [PubMed]
46. Smith, J.A.; West, R.M.; Allen, M. Acridones and quinacridones: Novel fluorophores for fluorescence lifetime studies. *J. Fluoresc.* **2004**, *14*, 151–171. [CrossRef] [PubMed]
47. Gonzalez-Garcia, M.C.; Herrero-Foncubierta, P.; Garcia-Fernandez, E.; Orte, A. Building Accurate Intracellular Polarity Maps through Multiparametric Microscopy. *Methods Protoc.* **2020**, *3*, 78. [CrossRef]
48. Gonzalez-Garcia, M.C.; Herrero-Foncubierta, P.; Castro, S.; Resa, S.; Alvarez-Pez, J.M.; Miguel, D.; Cuerva, J.M.; Garcia-Fernandez, E.; Orte, A. Coupled Excited-State Dynamics in N-Substituted 2-Methoxy-9-Acridones. *Front. Chem.* **2019**, *7*, 129. [CrossRef] [PubMed]
49. Martínez-Peragón, A.; Miguel, D.; Jurado, R.; Justicia, J.; Alvarez-Pez, J.M.; Cuerva, J.M.; Crovetto, L. Synthesis and Photophysics of a New Family of Fluorescent 9-alkyl Substituted Xanthenones. *Chem. A Eur. J.* **2014**, *20*, 447–455. [CrossRef]
50. Urano, Y.; Kamiya, M.; Kanda, K.; Ueno, T.; Hirose, K.; Nagano, T. Evolution of Fluorescein as a Platform for Finely Tunable Fluorescence Probes. *J. Am. Chem. Soc.* **2005**, *127*, 4888–4894. [CrossRef]
51. Choi, S.H.; Kim, K.; Lee, J.; Do, Y.; Churchill, D.G. X-ray diffraction, DFT, and spectroscopic study of N,N'-difluoroboryl-5-(2-thienyl)dipyrrin and fluorescence studies of related dipyrromethanes, dipyrrins and BF2-dipyrrins and DFT conformational study of 5-(2-thienyl)dipyrrin. *J. Chem. Crystallogr.* **2007**, *37*, 315–331. [CrossRef]
52. Paredes, J.M.; Crovetto, L.; Rios, R.; Orte, A.; Alvarez-Pez, J.M.; Talavera, E.M. Tuned lifetime, at the ensemble and single molecule level, of a xanthenic fluorescent dye by means of a buffer-mediated excited-state proton exchange reaction. *Phys. Chem. Chem. Phys.* **2009**, *11*, 5400–5407. [CrossRef]
53. Yu, C.; Jiao, L.; Yin, H.; Zhou, J.; Pang, W.; Wu, Y.; Wang, Z.; Yang, G.; Hao, E. α-/β-Formylated Boron–Dipyrrin (BODIPY) Dyes: Regioselective Syntheses and Photophysical Properties. *Eur. J. Org. Chem.* **2011**, *2011*, 5460–5468. [CrossRef]
54. Jiao, L.; Yu, C.; Wang, J.; Briggs, E.A.; Besley, N.A.; Robinson, D.; Ruedas-Rama, M.J.; Orte, A.; Crovetto, L.; Talavera, E.M.; et al. Unusual spectroscopic and photophysical properties of meso-tert-butylBODIPY in comparison to related alkylated BODIPY dyes. *RSC Adv.* **2015**, *5*, 89375–89388. [CrossRef]
55. Kenwood, B.M.; Weaver, J.L.; Bajwa, A.; Poon, I.K.; Byrne, F.L.; Murrow, B.A.; Calderone, J.A.; Huang, L.; Divakaruni, A.S.; Tomsig, J.L.; et al. Identification of a novel mitochondrial uncoupler that does not depolarize the plasma membrane. *Mol. Metab.* **2014**, *3*, 114–123. [CrossRef] [PubMed]
56. Roman, G.; Popek, T.; Lazar, C.; Kiyota, T.; Kluczyk, A.; Konishi, Y. Drug Evolution Concept in Drug Design: 2. Chimera Method. *Med. Chem.* **2006**, *2*, 175–189. [CrossRef] [PubMed]
57. Borsari, C.; Trader, D.J.; Tait, A.; Costi, M.P. Designing Chimeric Molecules for Drug Discovery by Leveraging Chemical Biology. *J. Med. Chem.* **2020**, *63*, 1908–1928. [CrossRef] [PubMed]
58. Yan, C.; Zhang, Y.; Guo, Z. Recent progress on molecularly near-infrared fluorescent probes for chemotherapy and phototherapy. *Coord. Chem. Rev.* **2021**, *427*, 213556. [CrossRef]
59. Kumar, A.; Kant, S.; Singh, S.M. Novel molecular mechanisms of antitumor action of dichloroacetate against T cell lymphoma: Implication of altered glucose metabolism, pH homeostasis and cell survival regulation. *Chem. Biol. Interact.* **2012**, *199*, 29–37. [CrossRef]
60. Ayyanathan, K.; Kesaraju, S.; Dawson-Scully, K.; Weissbach, H. Combination of Sulindac and Dichloroacetate Kills Cancer Cells via Oxidative Damage. *PLoS ONE* **2012**, *7*, e39949. [CrossRef] [PubMed]
61. Ripoll, C.; Roldan, M.; Ruedas-Rama, M.J.; Martin, M.; Ruedas-Rama, M.J.; Orte, A. Mitochondrial pH Nanosensors for Metabolic profiling of breast cancer cell lines. 2020, in preparation. *Int. J. Mol. Sci.* **2020**, *21*, 3731. [CrossRef]
62. Dreiem, A.; Fonnum, F. Thiophene is Toxic to Cerebellar Granule Cells in Culture After Bioactivation by Rat Liver Enzymes. *Neurotoxicology* **2004**, *25*, 959–966. [CrossRef]
63. Kawazoe, Y.; Shimogawa, H.; Sato, A.; Uesugi, M. A Mitochondrial Surface-Specific Fluorescent Probe Activated by Bioconversion. *Angew. Chem. Int. Ed.* **2011**, *50*, 5478–5481. [CrossRef]

64. Jiang, N.; Fan, J.; Liu, T.; Cao, J.; Qiao, B.; Wang, J.; Gao, P.; Peng, X. A near-infrared dye based on BODIPY for tracking morphology changes in mitochondria. *Chem. Commun.* **2013**, *49*, 10620–10622. [CrossRef]
65. Griesbeck, S.; Zhang, Z.; Gutmann, M.; Lühmann, T.; Edkins, R.M.; Clermont, G.; Lazar, A.N.; Haehnel, M.; Edkins, K.; Eichhorn, A.; et al. Water-Soluble Triarylborane Chromophores for One- and Two-Photon Excited Fluorescence Imaging of Mitochondria in Cells. *Chem. Eur. J.* **2016**, *22*, 14701–14706. [CrossRef]
66. Duca, M.; Dozza, B.; Lucarelli, E.; Santi, S.; Di Giorgio, A.; Barbarella, G. Fluorescent labeling of human mesenchymal stem cells by thiophene fluorophores conjugated to a lipophilic carrier. *Chem. Commun.* **2010**, *46*, 7948–7950. [CrossRef]
67. Yang, H.; Li, X.; Cai, Y.; Wang, Q.; Li, W.; Liu, G.; Tang, Y. In silico prediction of chemical subcellular localization via multi-classification methods. *MedChemComm* **2017**, *8*, 1225–1234. [CrossRef]
68. Yang, H.; Lou, C.; Sun, L.; Li, J.; Cai, Y.; Wang, Z.; Li, W.; Liu, G.; Tang, Y. admetSAR 2.0: Web-service for prediction and optimization of chemical ADMET properties. *Bioinformatics* **2018**, *35*, 1067–1069. [CrossRef] [PubMed]
69. Misra, S.K.; Ye, M.; Ostadhossein, F.; Pan, D. Pro-haloacetate Nanoparticles for Efficient Cancer Therapy via Pyruvate Dehydrogenase Kinase Modulation. *Sci. Rep.* **2016**, *6*, 28196. [CrossRef] [PubMed]
70. de Mey, S.; Dufait, I.; Jiang, H.; Corbet, C.; Wang, H.; Van De Gucht, M.; Kerkhove, L.; Law, K.L.; Vandenplas, H.; Gevaert, T.; et al. Dichloroacetate Radiosensitizes Hypoxic Breast Cancer Cells. *Int. J. Mol. Sci.* **2020**, *21*, 9367. [CrossRef] [PubMed]
71. Tataranni, T.; Agriesti, F.; Pacelli, C.; Ruggieri, V.; Laurenzana, I.; Mazzoccoli, C.; Della Sala, G.; Panebianco, C.; Pazienza, V.; Capitanio, N.; et al. Dichloroacetate Affects Mitochondrial Function and Stemness-Associated Properties in Pancreatic Cancer Cell Lines. *Cells* **2019**, *8*, 478. [CrossRef] [PubMed]
72. Rodrigues, A.S.; Correia, M.; Gomes, A.; Pereira, S.L.; Perestrelo, T.; Sousa, M.I.; Ramalho-Santos, J. Dichloroacetate, the Pyruvate Dehydrogenase Complex and the Modulation of mESC Pluripotency. *PLoS ONE* **2015**, *10*, e0131663. [CrossRef]
73. Fernández-Caro, H.; Lostalé-Seijo, I.; Martínez-Calvo, M.; Mosquera, J.; Mascareñas, J.L.; Montenegro, J. Supramolecular caging for cytosolic delivery of anionic probes. *Chem. Sci.* **2019**, *10*, 8930–8938. [CrossRef] [PubMed]
74. Liu, K.K.C.; Zhu, J.; Smith, G.L.; Yin, M.-J.; Bailey, S.; Chen, J.H.; Hu, Q.; Huang, Q.; Li, C.; Li, Q.J.; et al. Highly Selective and Potent Thiophenes as PI3K Inhibitors with Oral Antitumor Activity. *ACS Med. Chem. Lett.* **2011**, *2*, 809–813. [CrossRef] [PubMed]
75. Hanson, B.A. *Understanding Medicinal Plants. Their Chemistry and Therapeutic Action*; The Haworth Press Inc.: Binghamtom, NY, USA, 2005.
76. Zhang, P.; Liang, D.; Jin, W.; Qu, H.; Cheng, Y.; Li, X.; Ma, Z. Cytotoxic Thiophenes from the Root of *Echinops grijisii* Hance. *Z. Naturforsch.* **2009**, *64c*, 193–196. [CrossRef]
77. Mohareb, R.M.; Megally Abdo, N.Y. Synthesis and Cytotoxic Evaluation of Pyran, Dihydropyridine and Thiophene Derivatives of 3-Acetylcoumarin. *Chem. Pharm. Bull.* **2015**, *63*, 678–687. [CrossRef] [PubMed]
78. Lisboa, T.; Silva, D.; Duarte, S.; Ferreira, R.; Andrade, C.; Lopes, A.L.; Ribeiro, J.; Farias, D.; Moura, R.; Reis, M.; et al. Toxicity and Antitumor Activity of a Thiophene–Acridine Hybrid. *Molecules* **2020**, *25*, 64. [CrossRef]
79. Nepali, K.; Sharma, S.; Sharma, M.; Bedi, P.M.S.; Dhar, K.L. Rational approaches, design strategies, structure activity relationship and mechanistic insights for anticancer hybrids. *Eur. J. Med. Chem.* **2014**, *77*, 422–487. [CrossRef] [PubMed]

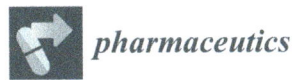

Article

CancerGram: An Effective Classifier for Differentiating Anticancer from Antimicrobial Peptides

Michał Burdukiewicz [1,2], Katarzyna Sidorczuk [3], Dominik Rafacz [2,4], Filip Pietluch [3], Mateusz Bąkała [4], Jadwiga Słowik [4] and Przemysław Gagat [3,*]

1. Faculty of Natural Sciences, Brandenburg University of Technology Cottbus-Senftenberg, 01968 Senftenberg, Germany; michalburdukiewicz@gmail.com
2. Why R? Foundation, 03-214 Warsaw, Poland; dominikrafacz@gmail.com
3. Department of Bioinformatics and Genomics, Faculty of Biotechnology, University of Wrocław, 50-383 Wrocław, Poland; katarzyna.sidorczuk2@uwr.edu.pl (K.S.); filip.pietluch2@uwr.edu.pl (F.P.)
4. Faculty of Mathematics and Information Science, Warsaw University of Technology, 00-662 Warsaw, Poland; matibakala@gmail.com (M.B.); jadwigaslowik5@gmail.com (J.S.)
* Correspondence: przemyslaw.gagat@uwr.edu.pl

Received: 14 October 2020; Accepted: 29 October 2020; Published: 31 October 2020

Abstract: Antimicrobial peptides (AMPs) constitute a diverse group of bioactive molecules that provide multicellular organisms with protection against microorganisms, and microorganisms with weaponry for competition. Some AMPs can target cancer cells; thus, they are called anticancer peptides (ACPs). Due to their small size, positive charge, hydrophobicity and amphipathicity, AMPs and ACPs interact with negatively charged components of biological membranes. AMPs preferentially permeabilize microbial membranes, but ACPs additionally target mitochondrial and plasma membranes of cancer cells. The preference towards mitochondrial membranes is explained by their membrane potential, membrane composition resulting from α-proteobacterial origin and the fact that mitochondrial targeting signals could have evolved from AMPs. Taking into account the therapeutic potential of ACPs and millions of deaths due to cancer annually, it is of vital importance to find new cationic peptides that selectively destroy cancer cells. Therefore, to reduce the costs of experimental research, we have created a robust computational tool, CancerGram, that uses n-grams and random forests for predicting ACPs. Compared to other ACP classifiers, CancerGram is the first three-class model that effectively classifies peptides into: ACPs, AMPs and non-ACPs/non-AMPs, with AU1U amounting to 0.89 and a Kappa statistic of 0.65. CancerGram is available as a web server and R package on GitHub.

Keywords: anticancer peptide (ACP); antimicrobial peptide (AMP); anticancer peptides; antimicrobial peptides; host defense peptides; prediction; random forest

1. Introduction

There are many health care issues that challenge the welfare of humankind; among them, cancer and antimicrobial resistance are of ever-growing concern. According to the World Health Organization, cancer is a leading cause of death globally, responsible for about 9.6 million deaths in 2018 [1], and antimicrobial resistance threatens our ability to treat an increasing number of infectious diseases, with a death toll of tens of thousands of people in Europe and the United States [2,3]. Interestingly, both these challenges could be approached with cationic peptides, antimicrobial peptides (AMPs) and anticancer peptides (ACPs), respectively.

AMPs, also known as host defense peptides, constitute a diverse group of bioactive molecules that provide multicellular organisms with protection against bacteria, fungi, protozoans and viruses [4,5], and microorganisms with weaponry for competition [6,7]. Some AMPs can target cancer cells; this particular group of AMPs is called anticancer peptides (ACPs). AMPs, including ACPs, are short peptides, generally with fewer than 50 amino acids, that are rich in positive and hydrophobic residues, and, consequently, have amphiphilic properties [4,8]. Due to these characteristics, they preferentially interact with negatively charged components of biological membranes, which are typical of the bacterial cell wall and the plasma membrane of cancer but not healthy cells. As a result, AMPs and ACPs lead to membrane micellization and/or permeabilization by forming pores [9–12]. By definition, AMPs target microbial membranes, especially bacterial envelopes, but ACPs, apart from their antimicrobial activity, also exhibit anticancer properties due to slightly different amino acid composition (for details, see [13] and Section 3.1).

One of the promising targets of anticancer therapies are mitochondria, cytoplasmic organelles derived from an ancestor of α-proteobacteria [14–16]. Mitochondria not only provide the energy and building blocks for new cells, but they are also the regulatory centers of redox homeostasis and apoptosis [17]. Interestingly, ACPs can bind to and affect the integrity of the plasma membrane of cancer cells; however, they preferentially disrupt mitochondrial membranes—specifically, they do so at concentrations hundreds of times lower than the concentrations for plasma membrane disruption [18]. The preference is due to the difference in membrane potential that is generated during oxidative phosphorylation at the inner mitochondrial membrane by proton pumps [19]. The membrane potential drives cations and cationic peptides into mitochondria, but because it is steadily increased in cancer cells, it provides even greater killing capacity in the cancerous environment [19–21]. Some preference for targeting mitochondria is also attributed to the fact that mitochondrial membranes still resemble, in terms of composition, the envelope of Gram-negative bacteria, and, therefore, attract AMP-like molecules [22,23]. Moreover, proteins imported into mitochondria carry an N-terminal targeting signal known as the mitochondrial transit peptide, which actually could have evolved from AMPs [24,25]. Since mitochondrial transit peptides show considerable similarity to their presumed progenitors, AMPs might also use the traditional Tom/Tim-dependent pathway to enter mitochondria [26].

Taking into account the therapeutic potential of ACPs, i.e., high target specificity, good efficacy, low toxicity, easy chemical modification and synthesis, it is of vital importance to find new cationic peptides that could target cancer cells [12,27]. Unfortunately, the experimental procedures to identify novel ACPs are time-consuming and expensive. Consequently, there is a demand for efficient and accessible bioinformatics tools that could help indicate potential ACP candidates with high accuracy for further research.

A number of computational approaches have been adopted for ACP prediction; however, there are serious concerns about the quality and quantity of sequences that were used for their development [13]. As a result, these algorithms have problems to discriminate between peptides with similar composition but different activity, i.e., between AMPs and ACPs. Some do not also provide web servers, and, therefore, have limited utility for biologists not well acquainted with bioinformatics ([13] and citations therein).

Our goal was to create a robust three-class model, CancerGram, for differentiating ACPs from AMPs and sequences that are neither ACPs nor AMPs. CancerGram uses n-grams (continuous or discontinuous sequences of n elements) and random forests (a machine learning method) for the classification algorithm. N-grams represent short motifs that are relevant to anticancer, antimicrobial and non-anticancer/non-antimicrobial properties of peptides, and they allow us, in an easily interpretable way, to discriminate between the three classes of molecules. This methodology has already been used with success in our previous projects to develop software for predicting AMPs [28], amyloid proteins [29] and signal peptides [30], and to assess the optimal growth conditions for methanogens [31]. CancerGram addresses the above-mentioned shortcomings of other ACP classifiers using verified data sets from AntiCP 2.0, which is the top-ranking ACP predictor [13]. However, compared to AntiCP 2.0, the decision making process of CancerGram is performed at the same time between three classes of sequences, i.e., ACPs, AMPs and non-ACPs/non-AMPs; therefore, it is convenient from the point of view of the user.

2. Materials and Methods

2.1. Data Sets

The data sets used to develop CancerGram were acquired from Agrawal et al. [13]. The training and validation data sets contained, respectively, 689 and 172 experimentally verified ACPs, 689 and 172 AMPs without anticancer activity and 776 and 194 non-ACP/non-AMP sequences (the negative data set). After the removal of peptides shorter than 5 amino acids, the data sets were used for CancerGram training and validation of its performance. The final numbers of sequences in each class are presented in Table 1. Since we could not repeat the benchmark analyses for AntiCP 2.0 [13], to compare its performance with CancerGram, we downloaded 2952 experimentally verified ACPs from CancerPPD [32], APD3 [33] and DRAMP [34] database and 4118 AMPs from dbAMP database [35]. We removed the most similar sequences using CD-HIT [36], assuming 0.95 and 0.60 identity threshold for ACPs and AMPs, respectively. Next, we removed sequences that were already contained in the training and validation data sets of CancerGram and AntiCP 2.0 [13]. As a result, we obtained an unbiased data set, termed independent, containing 57 ACPs and 769 AMPs (Table 1).

Table 1. Data set sizes used for training and validation of CancerGram.

Data Set	ACP	AMP	Negative
Training	686	689	776
Validation	171	170	194
Independent	57	769	0

2.2. Cross-Validation

We divided the ACP, AMP and non-ACP/non-AMP training data sets into five groups (folds), ensuring approximately the same sequence length distribution in each group for each data set. Next, we performed the fivefold cross-validation on both the mer and peptide layers of the model (for details, see Section 2.4 and Figure 1). The results of the cross-validation are presented in Table 2 and Figure 4.

Table 2. Results of fivefold cross-validation.

Measure	Mer Layer	Peptide Layer
Accuracy	0.64 (+/−0.01)	0.76 (+/−0.021)
AU1U	0.79 (+/−0.006)	0.89 (+/−0.008)
KapS	0.44 (+/−0.015)	0.64 (+/−0.032)

2.3. Extraction of Encoded N-Grams

In order to create the three-class model, we divided each sequence from the training data sets into overlapping subsequences of 5 amino acids (5-mers); the length of 5 amino acids represents the shortest ACPs in our data sets. Consequently, we obtained 11,496 ACP, 15,826 AMP and 18,587 non-ACP/non-AMP 5-mers. From each 5-mer, we extracted n-grams, i.e., sequences of n elements. We analyzed continuous and discontinuous n-grams of size ranging from 1 to 3. In the case of discontinuous n-grams, bigrams (n-grams of size 2) could contain a gap of length from 1 to 3 (e.g., L_N, C__G, K___K), whereas in trigrams (n-grams of size 3), there is only a single gap between the first and the second and/or the second and the third amino acid (e.g., K_L_L, AK_F, L_SA). The gap corresponds to the presence of any amino acid. The n-gram presence was then counted and binarized for each 5-mer. The binarization of n-grams means that if an n-gram is present (at least once) in the 5-mer, it obtains the value of 1, and 0 if it is absent (Figure 1A).

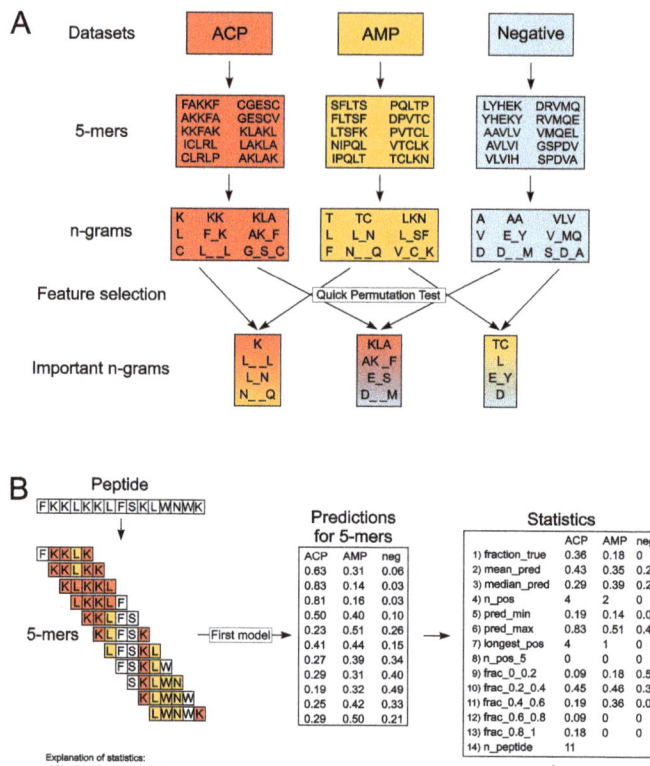

Figure 1. Schematic representation of n-gram extraction (**A**) and decision-making procedure in CancerGram (**B**). The training data sets include ACP (shaded in red), AMP (shaded in yellow) and non-ACP/non-AMP sequences (the negative data set, shaded in blue). Each peptide from the training data sets was divided into subsequences of 5 amino acids (5-mers). For each 5-mer, we extracted continuous and discontinuous n-grams of size ranging from 1 to 3, and exemplary n-grams are presented in boxes shaded in colors respective to the data sets. The informative n-grams for CancerGram training were selected by Quick Permutation Test for all combinations of the data sets, and they are shaded in: (i) red-yellow for the ACP/AMP data set, (ii) red-blue for the ACP/Negative data set, and (iii) yellow-blue for the AMP/Negative data set (**A**). To make a prediction, CancerGram first divides a peptide into 5-mers and then, for each 5-mer, makes a prediction if it is an ACP, AMP or non-ACP/non-AMP (the first model). To scale the prediction from 5-mers to the level of a peptide, numerous statistics are calculated, and on their basis, CancerGram makes the final prediction (the second model) (**B**).

2.4. Model Training with Random Forests

To select the informative n-grams, we performed Quick Permutation Test (QuiPT) [37] on each combination of classes (ACP/AMP data set, ACP/Negative data set and AMP/Negative data set) with p-value threshold 0.0001. We obtained 1883 informative n-grams and used them for CancerGram training. We trained the first random forest model on binarized occurrences of informative n-grams in 5-mers using the ranger R package [38]. The number of trees was set to 2000 and mtry parameter, i.e., the number of variables randomly sampled as candidates at each split, to the default value.

In order to scale the information found in 5-mers to the level of a peptide, we calculated numerous statistics for each peptide and for each class (Figure 1B) according to the methodology used in our previous projects [28]. These statistics were subsequently used to train the second random forest model predicting the class of a given peptide (ACP, AMP or non-ACP/non-AMP). In this case, both the mtry parameter and number of trees (500) were set to the default values. Consequently, the model is composed of stacked random forests [39], where the first one evaluates the probability of each 5-mer derived from a peptide as ACP, AMP or non-ACP/non-AMP, and the second considers statistical results for all mers from the given peptide and decides whether the whole peptide is ACP, AMP or non-ACP/non-AMP (Figure 1B).

3. Results and Discussion

3.1. Composition and Properties of ACPs and AMPs

The amino acid composition that characterizes both ACPs and AMPs (Figures 2 and 3) defines their properties, such as positive charge, hydrophobicity and amphipathicity, and they, in turn, determine their propensity for damaging bacterial and cancer cell membranes [40]. First, the positively charged molecules are driven electrostatically to the negatively charged membranes, and then their hydrophobicity and amphipathicity allows them to penetrate into the membrane and destabilize it in a detergent-like manner (carpet model) and/or by forming pores (barrel-stave or toroidal model) [9–12].

From the three above properties, only the positive charge differentiates the ACP group from AMPs because the upper limit of the positive charge is elevated for ACPs (Figure 2). This is the result of a high frequency of lysine (K), which is a predominant amino acid component of ACPs [13]. Interestingly, arginine (R), which is another basic amino acid, is slightly depleted in ACPs in comparison with AMPs and peptides from the negative data set (Figure 3). The decrease in arginine residues may, however, be beneficial for ACPs as its side chain, compared to lysine's, exhibits higher affinity for zwitterionic (neutral) membranes of healthy cells, and, therefore, is much more toxic [27].

Apart from its positive charge, lysine is also hydrophobic in nature and, as stated above, the hydrophobicity is another important property of both ACPs and AMPs. Peptides with higher hydrophobicity could be able to penetrate deeper into the hydrophobic core of the cell membrane, and, consequently, exhibit stronger propensity to permeabilize it [41]. ACPs are much richer in lysine (K), leucine (L), alanine (A) and phenylalanine (F) compared to AMPs and the peptides from the negative data set (Figure 3) [13]. In addition to its rather weak hydrophobic properties, alanine is also a good helix-forming residue; ACPs are known to form α-helical structures [40]. The last hydrophobic amino acid that deserves attention, tryptophan (W), is generally rare in proteins, but there seems to be more of it in ACPs compared to the other analyzed data sets though it is not statistically significant (Supplementary Tables S1–S3). Tryptophan serves an important role by helping peptides enter cancer cells via the endocytic pathway, thereby traversing the plasma membrane [42,43].

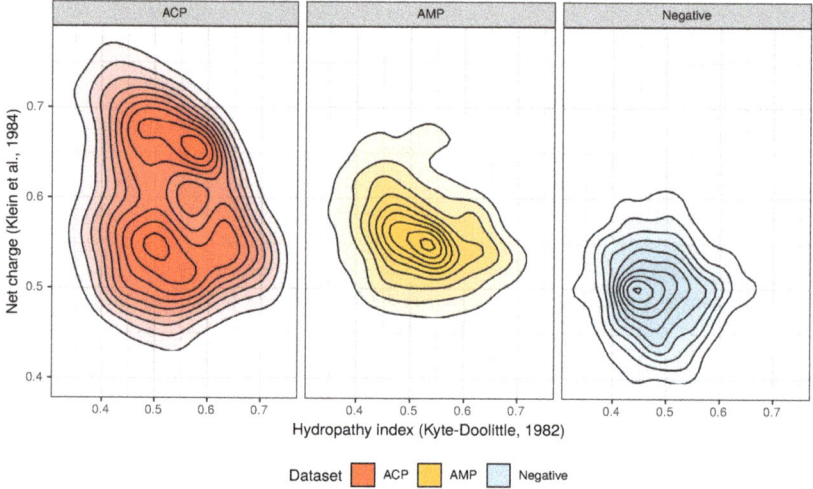

Figure 2. Distribution of the hydropathy index and net charge for anticancer peptides (ACPs), antimicrobial peptides (AMPs) and non-ACP/non-AMP sequences (Negative).

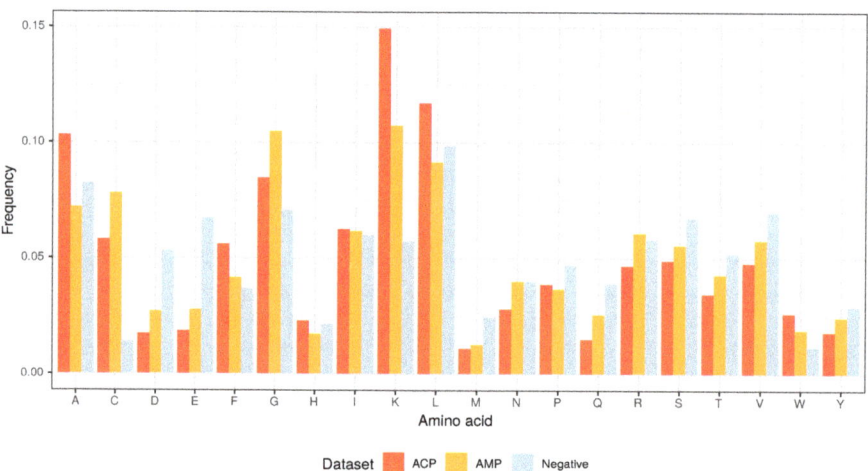

Figure 3. Amino acid composition of ACPs, AMPs and non-ACP/non-AMP sequences (Negative).

The other two amino acids that are abundant in ACPs, but not as much as in AMPs, are glycine (G) and cysteine (C) (Figure 3). The former is known to provide peptides with conformational flexibility and the latter to stabilize and maintain their proper motif and domain structure [43].

Although ACPs and AMPs are generally considered to be similar in terms of properties and the mode of action, the differences in their amino acid composition are significant enough (Supplementary Tables S1–S3) to find informative motifs that characterize them and non-ACPs/non-AMPs, thereby training an effective model for predicting ACPs.

3.2. CancerGram Performance

In order to evaluate the performance of CancerGram, we have chosen three measures: (i) accuracy, (ii) mean AUC (area under the ROC curve) for binary comparisons of each class against each other

(AU1U) and (iii) Kappa statistic (KapS) [44]. Accuracy is the simplest and the most common measure to evaluate the performance of a classifier. In the case of CancerGram, it simply provides the fraction of well-predicted ACPs, AMPs and non-ACPs/non-AMPs. A better measure is AU1U, the approximation of AUC for multi-class models. It informs the user of how much the model is able to distinguish between the three classes of peptides, i.e., ACPs, AMPs and non-ACPs/non-AMPs. A more general interpretation is that AU1U represents the probability that, e.g., a randomly selected ACP will be ranked higher in the ACP class than a random AMP or non-ACP/non-AMP. The values of both accuracy and AU1U range from 0 to 1, where 0.5 means a useless, i.e., a random classifier [45]. The last measure used to evaluate CancerGram is KapS, and it contains the information about how much better the model performs compared to the classifier that simply guesses at random according to the number of elements in each class. KapS evaluates the degree of agreement between CancerGram predictions and the true labels [46]. It takes values in $[-1, 1]$, where 0 means a random classifier and values above 0.80 indicate an excellent one [47]. All measures were calculated using the measures R package [48]. The results of CancerGram validation are presented in Table 3 and the results of the fivefold cross-validation are presented in Table 2 and Figure 4.

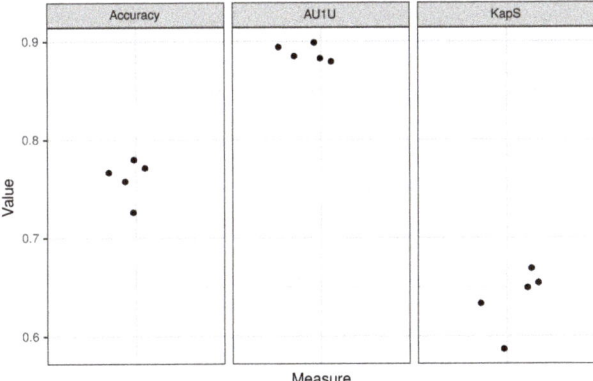

Figure 4. Results of fivefold cross-validation for the peptide layer of the model. Each dot corresponds to a single fold.

CancerGram is a robust model with AU1U amounting to 0.89. The value of KapS 0.65 (0.64 for fivefold cross-validation) informs us that CancerGram is a good model [47]. The least informative measure for the three-class model is the accuracy because, among other things, it does not take into account the distribution of the misclassification among classes, and it is equal to 0.77 (0.76 for fivefold cross-validation). From the point of view of the researcher interested in screening for ACPs, the most important issue is the restrictiveness of the model in terms of false ACP predictions. Accordingly, CancerGram falsely identifies only 1.5% of the non-ACPs/non-AMPs as ACPs (3 out of 194 from the validation data set) and less than 16% AMPs (27 out of 170 from the validation data set).

Table 3. Results of predictions on the validation data sets.

Measure	Value
Accuracy	0.77
AU1U	0.89
KapS	0.65

CancerGram is not only an effective model for ACPs prediction but also the only three-class model available at present. The other ACP classifiers represent binary models, and they have problems with distinguishing between sequences with similar amino acid composition but different activity, i.e., ACPs and AMPs [13]. AntiCP 2.0 has overcome the problem; however, the greatest disadvantage of AntiCP 2.0 is that the biologist may become confused about which model they should use from the ones available on the AntiCP 2.0 web server. The first one is a binary model that differentiates between ACPs and AMPs, and the second between ACPs and non-ACPs [13].

In order to compare the CancerGram and AntiCP 2.0 [13] performance, we decided to test their predictive power towards classification of ACPs and AMPs, which is most challenging for ACP predictors [13]. Interestingly, we could not use the validation data set bacause the final version of AntiCP 2.0 [13] was possibly trained not only on the training but also the validation data set; we were not able to repeat their benchmark analyses. Therefore, we constructed an independent data set containing 57 ACP and 769 AMP sequences. Since CancerGram is a three-class model, we had to binarize its prediction, i.e., the prediction results for AMPs and non-ACPs/non-AMPs were summed and represent the AMP class. CancerGram outperformed AntiCP 2.0 [13] in terms of AUC, accuracy, specificity and the Matthews correlation coefficient (MCC) (Table 4). Sensitivity and specificity indicate the proportion of ACPs and AMPs that were correctly identified as ACPs and AMPs, respectively. Precision reflects the proportion of predicted ACPs that are truly ACPs, and MCC represents a reliable metric for binary classifiers, i.e., a balanced measure of correlation coefficient between predictions and true labels. We also compared the performance of CancerGram with mACPpred [49] because it has recently been published but not included in Agrawal et al. [13] as the benchmark on the validation data set. The mACPpred model, similarly to AntiCP 2.0 [13], is also not as robust as CancerGram and, moreover, compared to AntiCP 2.0 [13] and CancerGram, it tends to predict AMPs as ACPs, i.e., it generates numerous false positive results (low specificity) (Table 5).

Table 4. Comparison of CancerGram and AntiCP 2.0 [13] performance on the independent data set. AntiCP 2.0 predictions were obtained using model 1 of the standalone version with default values of threshold (0.5) and window length (10). CancerGram predictions were binarized. The low values of the Matthews correlation coefficient (MCC), precision and sensitivity are due to the large number of AMPs (769) and low number of ACPs (57) in the independent data set.

Software	MCC	Precision	Sensitivity	Specificity	Accuracy	AUC
CancerGram	0.15	0.17	0.30	0.89	0.85	0.60
AntiCP 2.0	0.07	0.10	0.32	0.79	0.76	0.53

Table 5. Comparison of CancerGram and mACPpred [49] performance on the validation data set, from which sequences used for mACPpred training were removed. The final data set contained 128 ACPs and 170 AMPs. CancerGram predictions were binarized.

Software	MCC	Precision	Sensitivity	Specificity	Accuracy	AUC
CancerGram	0.57	0.78	0.71	0.85	0.79	0.83
mACPpred	0.21	0.48	0.90	0.27	0.54	0.68

3.3. Prediction of Mitochondria-Targeted ACPs with CancerGram

We also wanted to check the predictive power of CancerGram toward ACPs that have been experimentally verified to target mitochondria of cancer cells. By searching the literature, we did find 12 ACPs that were not included in our training data sets (Table 6). The results of the analysis are presented in Table 7. As expected, CancerGram correctly identified most of them, i.e., eight sequences, although it identified GW-H1, lactoferricin B and pleuricidin NRC-03 as AMPs, and A_9K as a non-ACP/non-AMP.

Table 6. Experimentally verified ACPs targeting mitochondria of cancer cells.

Peptide	Sequence	Reference
A_9K	AAAAAAAAAK	[50]
hCAP-18	FRKSKEKIGKEFKRIVQRIKDFLRNLVPRTES	[51,52]
HPRP-A1-TAT	FKKLKKLFSKLWNWKRKKRRQRRR	[53]
KLA	KLAKLAKKLAKLAK	[54–56]
Lactoferricin B	FKCRRWQWRMKKLGAPSITCVRRAF	[57,58]
Magainin 1	GIGKFLHSAGKFGKAFVGEIMKS	[59]
Mastoparan-C	LNLKALLAVAKKIL	[60,61]
NGR Peptide 1	CNGRCGGKLAKLAKKLAKLAK	[56]
GW-H1	GYNYAKKLANLAKKFANALW	[62]
Pleurocidin NRC-03	GRRKRKWLRRIGKGVKIIGGAALDHL	[63]
R7-kla	RRRRRRRKLAKLAKKLAKLAK	[64]
RGD-4C-GG-(KLAKLAK)$_2$	ACDCRGDCFCGGKLAKLAKKLAKLAK	[56]

Table 7. Prediction results for experimentally verified ACPs targeting mitochondria of cancer cells.

Peptide	ACP	AMP	Negative	Decision
A_9K	0.10	0.32	0.58	Negative
GW-H1	0.31	0.64	0.06	AMP
hCAP-18	0.96	0.04	0.00	ACP
HPRP-A1-TAT	0.66	0.33	0.01	ACP
KLA	1.00	0.00	0.00	ACP
Lactoferricin B	0.10	0.90	0.00	AMP
Magainin 1	0.63	0.32	0.05	ACP
Mastoparan-C	0.96	0.04	0.00	ACP
NGR Peptide 1	0.65	0.35	0.00	ACP
Pleurocidin 03	0.00	1.00	0.00	AMP
R7-kla	0.96	0.04	0.00	ACP
RGD-4C-GG-(KLAKLAK)$_2$	0.98	0.02	0.00	ACP

4. Conclusions

Based on data sets from Agrawal et al. [13], we have compared ACPs, AMPs and non-ACP/non-AMP sequences in terms of their amino acid composition. In the case of ACPs, the upper limit of the positive charge was elevated, mostly due to the high content of lysine, which is not only basic but also hydrophobic. The other residues that are overrepresented in ACPs, compared to AMPs and non-ACPs/non-AMPs, are all hydrophobic and include leucine, alanine, phenylalanine and tryptophan [13]. The positive charge, hydrophobicity and amphipathicity are responsible for AMP and ACP selectivity towards microbial membranes and, in the case of ACPs, also for targeting the cancer plasma and mitochondrial membranes. The latter are derived from α-proteobacteria and, due to their bacterial inheritance [22,23] and the potential generated during oxidative phosphorylation [18–20], should be preferred over the plasma membrane.

ACPs and AMPs are generally considered to be similar in terms of properties and the mode of action; however, we did find informative n-grams (amino acid motifs) that well differentiate them from each other and non-ACPs/non-AMPs, thereby allowing us to train an effective random forest model for ACP prediction. CancerGram is the only three-class model available at present and, moreover, it is better at discriminating between anticancer and antimicrobial peptides than other top-ranking predictors, including AntiCP 2.0 [13] and mACPpred [49]. The benchmark results also indicate that our methodology has an advantage over the methodology of Agrawal et al. [13] because, despite training our model on the same data sets, CancerGram outperformed AntiCP 2.0 on the independent data set. CancerGram is easy to use and does not require any other action other than pasting a sequence or sequences into the query box of the web server (see Appendix A). CancerGram does not predict sequences shorter than 5 amino acids, and the user should remember that it was trained on sequences up to 50 amino acids in length, i.e., it was not designed for predicting anticancer proteins.

Since new anticancer agents are desperately needed, CancerGram can be used for ACP screening to identify the best candidates for further experimental procedures. Short cationic peptides represent good antitumor agents because they are small, relatively cheap to produce and easy to modify in order to further increase their anticancer properties and stability or to lower their toxicity to healthy cells [12,27].

Supplementary Materials: The following are available at http://www.mdpi.com/1999-4923/12/11/1045/s1, Table S1: Average amino acid percentages for ACPs and AMPs. The differences in amino acid composition between ACPs and AMPs were statistically evaluated using the Mann–Whitney U test with Benjamini–Hochberg correction. Table S2: Average amino acid percentages for ACPs and the negative data set. The differences in amino acid composition between ACPs and the negative data set were statistically evaluated using the Mann–Whitney U test with Benjamini–Hochberg correction. Table S3: Average amino acid percentages for AMPs and the negative data set. The differences in amino acid composition between AMPs and the negative data set were statistically evaluated using the Mann–Whitney U test with Benjamini–Hochberg correction.

Author Contributions: Author Contributions: Conceptualization, M.B. (Michał Burdukiewicz) and P.G.; formal analysis, M.B. (Michał Burdukiewicz), K.S. and P.G.; funding acquisition, M.B. (Michał Burdukiewicz), K.S., F.P. and P.G.; investigation, M.B. (Michał Burdukiewicz), K.S. and P.G.; methodology, M.B. (Michał Burdukiewicz), K.S., D.R., F.P., M.B. (Mateusz Bąkała), J.S. and P.G.; project administration, M.B. (Michał Burdukiewicz) and P.G.; software, M.B. (Michał Burdukiewicz), K.S., D.R. and F.P.; supervision, M.B. (Michał Burdukiewicz) and P.G.; validation, F.P. and P.G.; visualization, K.S.; writing—original draft preparation, K.S. and P.G.; writing—review and editing, M.B. (Michał Burdukiewicz), K.S., F.P. and P.G. All authors have read and agreed to the published version of the manuscript.

Funding: This work was supported by National Science Centre grant 2017/26/D/NZ8/00444 to PG and MB, National Science Centre grant 2018/31/N/NZ2/01338 to KS and National Science Centre grant 2019/35/N/NZ8/03366 to FP.

Conflicts of Interest: The authors declare no conflict of interest.

Abbreviations

The following abbreviations are used in this manuscript:

AUC	Area under the ROC curve
AU1U	AUC for binary comparisons of each class against each other
ACP	Anticancer peptides
AMP	Antimicrobial peptides
KapS	Kappa statistic
MCC	Matthews correlation coefficient
A	Alanine
R	Arginine
N	Asparagine
D	Aspartic acid
C	Cysteine
E	Glutamic acid
Q	Glutamine
G	Glycine
H	Histidine
I	Isoleucine
L	Leucine
K	Lysine
M	Methionine
F	Phenylalanine
P	Proline
S	Serine

Appendix A. Availability and Implementation

The code necessary to reproduce the analysis presented in this paper is available in the repository: https://github.com/BioGenies/CancerGram-analysis.

The CancerGram prediction web server is available at: http://biongram.biotech.uni.wroc.pl/CancerGram/.

References

1. Cancer. Available online: https://www.who.int/news-room/fact-sheets/detail/cancer (accessed on 13 October 2020).
2. Cassini, A.; Högberg, L.D.; Plachouras, D.; Quattrocchi, A.; Hoxha, A.; Simonsen, G.S.; Colomb-Cotinat, M.; Kretzschmar, M.E.; Devleesschauwer, B.; Cecchini, M.; et al. Attributable deaths and disability-adjusted life-years caused by infections with antibiotic-resistant bacteria in the EU and the European Economic Area in 2015: A population-level modelling analysis. *Lancet Infect. Dis.* **2019**, *19*, 56–66. [CrossRef]
3. CDC. *Antibiotic Resistance Threats in the United States, 2019*; Centres for Disease Control and Prevention, US Department of Health and Human Services: Washington, DC, USA, 2019.
4. Ahmed, A.; Siman-Tov, G.; Hall, G.; Bhalla, N.; Narayanan, A. Human antimicrobial peptides as therapeutics for viral infections. *Viruses* **2019**, *11*, 704. [CrossRef] [PubMed]
5. Mookherjee, N.; Anderson, M.A.; Haagsman, H.P.; Davidson, D.J. Antimicrobial host defence peptides: Functions and clinical potential. *Nat. Rev. Drug Discov.* **2020**, *19*, 311–332. [CrossRef] [PubMed]
6. Raffatellu, M. Learning from bacterial competition in the host to develop antimicrobials. *Nat. Med.* **2018**, *24*, 1097–1103. [CrossRef]
7. Suneja, G.; Nain, S.; Sharma, R. Microbiome: A Source of Novel Bioactive Compounds and Antimicrobial Peptides. In *Microbial Diversity in Ecosystem Sustainability and Biotechnological Applications*; Springer: Berlin, Germany, 2019; pp. 615–630.
8. Felício, M.R.; Silva, O.N.; Gonçalves, S.; Santos, N.C.; Franco, O.L. Peptides with dual antimicrobial and anticancer activities. *Front. Chem.* **2017**, *5*, 5. [CrossRef]
9. Travkova, O.G.; Moehwald, H.; Brezesinski, G. The interaction of antimicrobial peptides with membranes. *Adv. Colloid Interface Sci.* **2017**, *247*, 521–532. [CrossRef]
10. Gaspar, D.; Veiga, A.S.; Castanho, M.A. From antimicrobial to anticancer peptides. A review. *Front. Microbiol.* **2013**, *4*, 294. [CrossRef]
11. Marquette, A.; Bechinger, B. Biophysical investigations elucidating the mechanisms of action of antimicrobial peptides and their synergism. *Biomolecules* **2018**, *8*, 18. [CrossRef]
12. Tornesello, A.L.; Borrelli, A.; Buonaguro, L.; Buonaguro, F.M.; Tornesello, M.L. Antimicrobial peptides as anticancer agents: Functional properties and biological activities. *Molecules* **2020**, *25*, 2850. [CrossRef]
13. Agrawal, P.; Bhagat, D.; Mahalwal, M.; Sharma, N.; Raghava, G.P.S. AntiCP 2.0: An updated model for predicting anticancer peptides. *Brief. Bioinf.* **2020**. [CrossRef]
14. Martin, W.F.; Neukirchen, S.; Zimorski, V.; Gould, S.B.; Sousa, F.L. Energy for two: New archaeal lineages and the origin of mitochondria. *BioEssays* **2016**, *38*, 850–856. [CrossRef] [PubMed]
15. Fan, L.; Wu, D.; Goremykin, V.; Xiao, J.; Xu, Y.; Garg, S.; Zhang, C.; Martin, W.F.; Zhu, R. Phylogenetic analyses with systematic taxon sampling show that mitochondria branch within Alphaproteobacteria. *Nat. Ecol. Evol.* **2020**, *4*, 1213–1219. [CrossRef] [PubMed]
16. Jeena, M.; Kim, S.; Jin, S.; Ryu, J.H. Recent progress in mitochondria-targeted drug and drug-free agents for cancer therapy. *Cancers* **2020**, *12*, 4. [CrossRef]
17. Newmeyer, D.D.; Ferguson-Miller, S. Mitochondria: Releasing power for life and unleashing the machineries of death. *Cell* **2003**, *112*, 481–490. [CrossRef]
18. Szewczyk, A.; Wojtczak, L. Mitochondria as a pharmacological target. *Pharmacol. Rev.* **2002**, *54*, 101–127. [CrossRef]
19. Zorova, L.D.; Popkov, V.A.; Plotnikov, E.Y.; Silachev, D.N.; Pevzner, I.B.; Jankauskas, S.S.; Babenko, V.A.; Zorov, S.D.; Balakireva, A.V.; Juhaszova, M.; et al. Mitochondrial membrane potential. *Anal. Biochem.* **2018**, *552*, 50–59. [CrossRef] [PubMed]

20. Houston, M.A.; Augenlicht, L.H.; Heerdt, B.G. Stable differences in intrinsic mitochondrial membrane potential of tumor cell subpopulations reflect phenotypic heterogeneity. *Int. J. Cell Biol.* **2011**, *2011*. [CrossRef]
21. Constance, J.E.; Lim, C.S. Targeting malignant mitochondria with therapeutic peptides. *Ther. Deliv.* **2012**, *3*, 961–979. [CrossRef]
22. Bansal, S.; Mittal, A. A statistical anomaly indicates symbiotic origins of eukaryotic membranes. *Mol. Biol. Cell* **2015**, *26*, 1238–1248. [CrossRef]
23. Rappocciolo, E.; Stiban, J. Prokaryotic and mitochondrial lipids: A survey of evolutionary origins. In *Bioactive Ceramides in Health and Disease*; Springer: Berlin, Germany, 2019; pp. 5–31.
24. Wollman, F.A. An antimicrobial origin of transit peptides accounts for early endosymbiotic events. *Traffic* **2016**, *17*, 1322–1328. [CrossRef]
25. Garrido, C.O.; Caspari, O.D.; Choquet, Y.; Wollman, F.A.; Lafontaine, I. An antimicrobial origin of targeting peptides to endosymbiotic organelles. *Cells* **2020**, *9*, 1795. [CrossRef]
26. Dudek, J.; Rehling, P.; van der Laan, M. Mitochondrial protein import: Common principles and physiological networks. *Biochim. Et Biophys. Acta (BBA)-Mol. Cell Res.* **2013**, *1833*, 274–285. [CrossRef] [PubMed]
27. Huang, Y.; Feng, Q.; Yan, Q.; Hao, X.; Chen, Y. Alpha-helical cationic anticancer peptides: A promising candidate for novel anticancer drugs. *Mini Rev. Med. Chem.* **2015**, *15*, 73–81. [CrossRef]
28. Burdukiewicz, M.; Sidorczuk, K.; Rafacz, D.; Pietluch, F.; Chilimoniuk, J.; Rödiger, S.; Gagat, P. Proteomic Screening for Prediction and Design of Antimicrobial Peptides with AmpGram. *Int. J. Mol. Sci.* **2020**, *21*, 4310. [CrossRef]
29. Burdukiewicz, M.; Sobczyk, P.; Rödiger, S.; Duda-Madej, A.; Mackiewicz, P.; Kotulska, M. Amyloidogenic motifs revealed by n-gram analysis. *Sci. Rep.* **2017**, *7*, 12961. [CrossRef]
30. Burdukiewicz, M.; Sobczyk, P.; Chilimoniuk, J.; Gagat, P.; Mackiewicz, P. Prediction of signal peptides in proteins from malaria parasites. *Int. J. Mol. Sci.* **2018**, *19*, 3709. [CrossRef]
31. Burdukiewicz, M.; Gagat, P.; Jabłoński, S.; Chilimoniuk, J.; Gaworski, M.; Mackiewicz, P.; Marcin, Ł. PhyMet2: A database and toolkit for phylogenetic and metabolic analyses of methanogens. *Environ. Microbiol. Rep.* **2018**, *10*, 378–382.
32. Tyagi, A.; Tuknait, A.; Anand, P.; Gupta, S.; Sharma, M.; Mathur, D.; Joshi, A.; Singh, S.; Gautam, A.; Raghava, G.P. CancerPPD: A database of anticancer peptides and proteins. *Nucleic Acids Res.* **2014**, *43*, D837–D843. [CrossRef]
33. Wang, G.; Li, X.; Wang, Z. APD3: The antimicrobial peptide database as a tool for research and education. *Nucleic Acids Res.* **2015**, *44*, D1087–D1093. [CrossRef] [PubMed]
34. Kang, X.; Dong, F.; Shi, C.; Liu, S.; Sun, J.; Chen, J.; Li, H.; Xu, H.; Lao, X.; Zheng, H. DRAMP 2.0, an updated data repository of antimicrobial peptides. *Sci. Data* **2019**, *6*, 148. [CrossRef]
35. Jhong, J.H.; Chi, Y.H.; Li, W.C.; Lin, T.H.; Huang, K.Y.; Lee, T.Y. dbAMP: An integrated resource for exploring antimicrobial peptides with functional activities and physicochemical properties on transcriptome and proteome data. *Nucleic Acids Res.* **2018**, *47*, D285–D297. [CrossRef] [PubMed]
36. Fu, L.; Niu, B.; Zhu, Z.; Wu, S.; Li, W. CD-HIT: Accelerated for clustering the next-generation sequencing data. *Bioinformatics* **2012**, *28*, 3150–3152. [CrossRef] [PubMed]
37. Burdukiewicz, M.; Sobczyk, P.; Lauber, C. *Biogram: N-Gram Analysis of Biological Sequences*; GitHub: San Francisco, CA, USA, 2020.
38. Wright, M.N.; Ziegler, A. ranger: A Fast Implementation of Random Forests for High Dimensional Data in C++ and R. *J. Stat. Softw.* **2017**, *77*, 1–17. [CrossRef]
39. Bell, J.; Larson, M.; Kutzler, M.; Bionaz, M.; Löhr, C.V.; Hendrix, D. miRWoods: Enhanced Precursor Detection and Stacked Random Forests for the Sensitive Detection of microRNAs. *PLoS Comput. Biol.* **2019**, *15*, e1007309. [CrossRef]
40. Huang, Y.B.; He, L.Y.; Jiang, H.Y.; Chen, Y.X. Role of helicity on the anticancer mechanism of action of cationic-helical peptides. *Int. J. Mol. Sci.* **2012**, *13*, 6849–6862. [CrossRef] [PubMed]
41. Huang, Y.b.; Wang, X.f.; Wang, H.y.; Liu, Y.; Chen, Y. Studies on mechanism of action of anticancer peptides by modulation of hydrophobicity within a defined structural framework. *Mol. Cancer Ther.* **2011**, *10*, 416–426. [CrossRef]
42. Bhunia, D.; Mondal, P.; Das, G.; Saha, A.; Sengupta, P.; Jana, J.; Mohapatra, S.; Chatterjee, S.; Ghosh, S. Spatial position regulates power of tryptophan: Discovery of a major-groove-specific nuclear-localizing, cell-penetrating tetrapeptide. *J. Am. Chem. Soc.* **2018**, *140*, 1697–1714. [CrossRef]

43. Chiangjong, W.; Chutipongtanate, S.; Hongeng, S. Anticancer peptide: Physicochemical property, functional aspect and trend in clinical application. *Int. J. Oncol.* **2020**, *57*, 678–696. [CrossRef]
44. Ferri, C.; Hernández-Orallo, J.; Modroiu, R. An experimental comparison of performance measures for classification. *Pattern Recognit. Lett.* **2009**, *30*, 27–38. [CrossRef]
45. Hand, D.J.; Till, R.J. A simple generalisation of the area under the ROC curve for multiple class classification problems. *Mach. Learn.* **2001**, *45*, 171–186. [CrossRef]
46. Ben-David, A. About the relationship between ROC curves and Cohen's kappa. *Eng. Appl. Artif. Intell.* **2008**, *21*, 874–882. [CrossRef]
47. Ranganathan, P.; Pramesh, C.; Aggarwal, R. Common pitfalls in statistical analysis: Measures of agreement. *Perspect. Clin. Res.* **2017**, *8*, 187. [CrossRef]
48. Bischl, B.; Lang, M.; Kotthoff, L.; Schiffner, J.; Richter, J.; Studerus, E.; Casalicchio, G.; Jones, Z.M. mlr: Machine Learning in R. *J. Mach. Learn. Res.* **2016**, *17*, 1–5.
49. Boopathi, V.; Subramaniyam, S.; Malik, A.; Lee, G.; Manavalan, B.; Yang, D.C. mACPpred: A support vector machine-based meta-predictor for identification of anticancer peptides. *Int. J. Mol. Sci.* **2019**, *20*, 1964. [CrossRef]
50. Xu, H.; Chen, C.X.; Hu, J.; Zhou, P.; Zeng, P.; Cao, C.H.; Lu, J.R. Dual modes of antitumor action of an amphiphilic peptide A9K. *Biomaterials* **2013**, *34*, 2731–2737. [CrossRef] [PubMed]
51. Farsinejad, S.; Gheisary, Z.; Samani, S.E.; Alizadeh, A.M. Mitochondrial targeted peptides for cancer therapy. *Tumor Biol.* **2015**, *36*, 5715–5725. [CrossRef]
52. Yitzchak, H. Disease Treatment Via Antimicrobial Peptides Or Their Inhibitors. U.S. Patent 8202835 B2, 19 June 2012.
53. Hao, X.; Yan, Q.; Zhao, J.; Wang, W.; Huang, Y.; Chen, Y. TAT modification of alpha-helical anticancer peptides to improve specificity and efficacy. *PLoS ONE* **2015**, *10*, e0138911. [CrossRef]
54. Javadpour, M.M.; Juban, M.M.; Lo, W.C.; Bishop, S.M.; Alberty, J.B.; Cowell, S.M.; Becker, C.L.; McLaughlin, M.L. De novo antimicrobial peptides with low mammalian cell toxicity. *J. Med. Chem.* **1996**, *39*, 3107–3113. [CrossRef]
55. Horton, K.L.; Kelley, S.O. Engineered apoptosis-inducing peptides with enhanced mitochondrial localization and potency. *J. Med. Chem.* **2009**, *52*, 3293–3299. [CrossRef]
56. Ellerby, H.M.; Arap, W.; Ellerby, L.M.; Kain, R.; Andrusiak, R.; Del Rio, G.; Krajewski, S.; Lombardo, C.R.; Rao, R.; Ruoslahti, E.; et al. Anti-cancer activity of targeted pro-apoptotic peptides. *Nat. Med.* **1999**, *5*, 1032–1038. [CrossRef]
57. Bellamy, W.; Takase, M.; Yamauchi, K.; Wakabayashi, H.; Kawase, K.; Tomita, M. Identification of the bactericidal domain of lactoferrin. *Biochim. Et Biophys. Acta (BBA) Protein Struct. Mol. Enzymol.* **1992**, *1121*, 130–136. [CrossRef]
58. Eliassen, L.T.; Berge, G.; Leknessund, A.; Wikman, M.; Lindin, I.; Løkke, C.; Ponthan, F.; Johnsen, J.I.; Sveinbjørnsson, B.; Kogner, P.; et al. The antimicrobial peptide, lactoferricin B, is cytotoxic to neuroblastoma cells in vitro and inhibits xenograft growth in vivo. *Int. J. Cancer* **2006**, *119*, 493–500. [CrossRef]
59. Cruz-Chamorro, L.; Puertollano, M.A.; Puertollano, E.; de Cienfuegos, G.Á.; de Pablo, M.A. In vitro biological activities of magainin alone or in combination with nisin. *Peptides* **2006**, *27*, 1201–1209. [CrossRef] [PubMed]
60. Argiolas, A.; Pisano, J.J. Isolation and characterization of two new peptides, mastoparan C and crabrolin, from the venom of the European hornet, Vespa crabro. *J. Biol. Chem.* **1984**, *259*, 10106–10111. [PubMed]
61. Chen, X.; Zhang, L.; Wu, Y.; Wang, L.; Ma, C.; Xi, X.; Bininda-Emonds, O.R.; Shaw, C.; Chen, T.; Zhou, M. Evaluation of the bioactivity of a mastoparan peptide from wasp venom and of its analogues designed through targeted engineering. *Int. J. Biol. Sci.* **2018**, *14*, 599–607. [CrossRef] [PubMed]
62. Chen, Y.L.S.; Li, J.H.; Yu, C.Y.; Lin, C.J.; Chiu, P.H.; Chen, P.W.; Lin, C.C.; Chen, W.J. Novel cationic antimicrobial peptide GW-H1 induced caspase-dependent apoptosis of hepatocellular carcinoma cell lines. *Peptides* **2012**, *36*, 257–265. [CrossRef]
63. Hilchie, A.; Doucette, C.; DM, P.; Patrzykat, A.; Douglas, S.; Hoskin, D.W. Pleurocidin-family cationic antimicrobial peptides are cytolytic for breast carcinoma cells and prevent growth of tumor xenografts. *Breast Cancer Res.* **2011**, *13*, R102. [CrossRef]

64. Law, B.; Quinti, L.; Choi, Y.; Weissleder, R.; Tung, C.H. A mitochondrial targeted fusion peptide exhibits remarkable cytotoxicity. *Mol. Cancer Ther.* **2006**, *5*, 1944–1949. [CrossRef]

Publisher's Note: MDPI stays neutral with regard to jurisdictional claims in published maps and institutional affiliations.

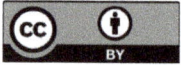

© 2020 by the authors. Licensee MDPI, Basel, Switzerland. This article is an open access article distributed under the terms and conditions of the Creative Commons Attribution (CC BY) license (http://creativecommons.org/licenses/by/4.0/).

MDPI
St. Alban-Anlage 66
4052 Basel
Switzerland
Tel. +41 61 683 77 34
Fax +41 61 302 89 18
www.mdpi.com

Pharmaceutics Editorial Office
E-mail: pharmaceutics@mdpi.com
www.mdpi.com/journal/pharmaceutics

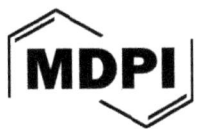

www.ingramcontent.com/pod-product-compliance
Lightning Source LLC
LaVergne TN
LVHW070049120526
838202LV00101B/1899